Advances in Schizophrenia Research
2009

Wagner F. Gattaz · Geraldo Busatto
Editors

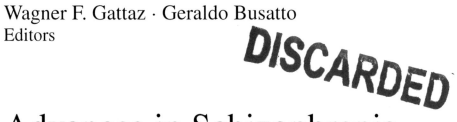

Advances in Schizophrenia
Research
2009

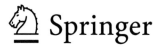 Springer

Editors

Wagner F. Gattaz
Department and Institute of Psychiatry
Faculty of Medicine
University São Paulo
05403-903 São Paulo-SP
Brazil
gattaz@usp.br

Geraldo Busatto
Department and Institute of Psychiatry
Faculty of Medicine
University São Paulo
05403-903 São Paulo-SP
Brazil
geraldo.busatto@hcnet.usp.br

ISBN 978-1-4419-0912-1   e-ISBN 978-1-4419-0913-8
DOI 10.1007/978-1-4419-0913-8
Springer New York Dordrecht Heidelberg London

Library of Congress Control Number: 2009935333

Printed on acid-free paper

Springer is part of Springer Science+Business Media (www.springer.com)

Preface

Schizophrenia remains a mighty challenge to psychiatry, with its causes and underlying brain mechanisms yet to be fully uncovered. Currently available treatments are neither universally effective nor without unwanted effects. These aspects, together with the high prevalence of schizophrenia, its often debilitating nature and associated family/social burden, make this mental disorder one of the most complex public health issues of our times.

The *Advances in Schizophrenia* series intends to become a key reference in this field. Our aim is to provide comprehensive and up-to-date reviews of the wide range of research studies carried out around to world with the purposes of solving the schizophrenia puzzle and providing clues to new forms of treatment and prevention for this disorder.

A special feature of the series is its truly broad scope, virtually encompassing all fields of schizophrenia research: epidemiology and risk factors; psychopathology; diagnostic boundaries; cognition; outcome and prognosis; pathophysiology; genetics; pharmacological and psychological forms of treatment and rehabilitation; community care; and stigma.

The first volume of the series is related to the 6th Symposium on the Search for the Causes of Schizophrenia, held in Sao Paulo, Brazil, in February 2009. We have been organizing the Search-Meetings since 1986. During these 22 years we have managed to keep the main characteristic of this series: the "Search" remains a non-commercial meeting, with a limited number of invited guest speakers and participants. A group of prominent scientists from different centers around the world were invited to provide scholar reviews on the state of the art in each of the above areas, as well as their view on the perspectives for the future. The content table of this book reflects the program of the 6th edition of this meeting and is consistent with our aim to comprehensively cover all relevant areas of research into schizophrenia.

Of the five previous meetings we organized with our friend Heinz Haefner, three took place in Heidelberg and the last two in Brazil. These meetings resulted in five books, edited by Heinz and one of us (WFG) and published by Springer. In this 6th Search, for personal reasons, Heinz could not participate in the preparations of the meeting and in the edition of this book. Nevertheless, we thought that this would be an excellent occasion to dedicate this 6th Search and the first volume of this *Advances in Schizophrenia* series to Heinz Haefner. We feel that Heinz Haefner deserves this homage as one of the most influential psychiatrists of our time, who has given important contributions to both the knowledge about schizophrenia and the care of its sufferers.

In a time of global economic crisis we are indebted to those companies that, in spite of sensitive reductions in their budgets, have given us the financial support for the meeting, which resulted in the production of this book. Therefore, in our name and if we may, in the name of all participants of the 6th Search and authors of this book, we would like to thank, indeed, the unrestricted educational grants provided by Janssen-Cilag, Eli Lilly, and Astra Zeneca.

São Paulo, November 2009   Wagner F. Gattaz
                                                                       Geraldo Busatto

Contents

Contributors

Judith Allardyce Department of Psychiatry and Neuropsychology, South Limburg Mental Health Research and Teaching Network, EURON, Maastricht University, PO Box 616 (DRT 10), 6200 MD Maastricht, The Netherlands, j.allardyce@clinmed.gla.ac.uk

Patrizia A. Baldwin Molecular and Cellular Therapeutics, Royal College of Surgeons in Ireland, Dublin, Ireland; Cavan-Monaghan Mental Health Service, St. Davnet's Hospital, Monaghan, Ireland

David Browne Molecular and Cellular Therapeutics, Royal College of Surgeons in Ireland, Dublin, Ireland; Cavan-Monaghan Mental Health Service, St. Davnet's Hospital, Monaghan, Ireland

Tom Burns University of Oxford, Warneford Hospital, Oxford, OX3 7JX, UK, tom.burns@psych.ucla.edu

Geraldo F. Busatto Department and Institute of Psychiatry, Faculty of Medicine, University of São Paulo, 05403–903, São Paulo, SP, Brazil, geraldo.busatto@hcnet.usp.br

Tyrone D. Cannon Departments of Psychology and Psychiatry and Biobehavioral Sciences, University of California, Los Angeles, California, USA, cannon@psych.ucla.edu

José A.S. Crippa Laboratory of Psychiatric Neuroimaging (LIM21) Department and Institute of Psychiatry, Faculty of Medicine - University of São Paulo, 05403–903, São Paulo - SP - Brazil, jcrippa@fmrp.usp.br

Anthony S. David Section of Cognitive Neuropsychiatry, Institute of Psychiatry, KCL, London SE5 8AF, UK, anthony.david@iop.kcl.ac.uk

Louisa Degenhardt National Drug and Alcohol Research Centre, University of New South Wales, Sydney, New South Wales, Australia, l.degenhardt@unsw.edu.au

Emmanuel Dias-Neto Laboratory of Neuroscience, Department and Institute of Psychiatry, Faculty of Medicine, University of São Paulo, 05403–903, São Paulo, SP, Brazil, emmanuel@usp.br

Peter Falkai Department of Psychiatry and Psychotherapy, University of Goettingen, von Siebold Str. 5, 37075 Goettingen, Germany, pfalkai@gwdg.de

Daniel Freeman Department of Psychology, Institute of Psychiatry, King's College London, Denmark Hill, London, SE5 8AF, UK, d.freeman@iop.kcl.ac.uk

Marta Di Forti Institute of Psychiatry, Box PO63, De Crespigny Park, London, SE5 8AF, UK, m.diforti@iop.kcl.ac.uk

Wolfgang Gaebel Department of Psychiatry and Psychotherapy, Heinrich-Heine-University Düsseldorf, Clinics of the Rhineland Regional Council, Bergische Landstraße 2, D-40629 Düsseldorf, Germany, wolfgang.gaebel@uni-duesseldorf.de

Wagner F. Gattaz Department and Institute of Psychiatry, Faculty of Medicine, University of São Paulo, 05403–903, São Paulo, SP, Brazil, gattaz@usp.br

Ayana Gibbs Section of Cognitive Neuropsychiatry, Institute of Psychiatry, KCL, London SE5, UK, agibbs@uci.edu

Anthony A. Grace Departments of Neuroscience, Psychiatry and Psychology, A210 Langley Hall, University of Pittsburgh, Pittsburgh, PA 15260, USA, graceaa@pitt.edu

Michael F. Green Department of Psychiatry and Biobehavioral Sciences, Semel Institute for Neuroscience and Human Behavior, University of California; Mental Illness Research, Education, and Clinical Center, VISN 22, VA Greater Los Angeles Healthcare System, Los Angeles, USA, mgreen@ucla.edu

Oliver Gruber Department of Psychiatry and Psychotherapy, University of Goettingen, von Siebold Str. 5, 37075 Goettingen, Germany, ogruber@gwdg.de

Robin J. Hennessy Molecular and Cellular Therapeutics, Royal College of Surgeons in Ireland, Dublin, Ireland, rhennessy@rcsi.ie

Oliver Howes Institute of Psychiatry, Box PO63, De Crespigny Park, London, SE5 8AF, UK, o.howes@iop.kcl.ac.uk

James L. Kennedy Neurogenetics Section, Centre for Addiction and Mental Health, University of Toronto, Toronto, ON, Canada, james_kennedy@camh.net

Robert S. Kern Department of Psychiatry and Biobehavioral Sciences, Semel Institute for Neuroscience and Human Behavior, University of California; Mental Illness Research, Education, and Clinical Center, VISN 22, VA Greater Los Angeles Healthcare System, Los Angeles, USA, rkern@ucla.edu

Eoin J. Killackey Orygen Youth Research Centre, University of Melbourne, Melbourne, Victoria, Australia, eoin@unimelb.edu.au

Tara Kingston Molecular and Cellular Therapeutics, Royal College of Surgeons in Ireland, Dublin, Ireland; Cavan-Monaghan Mental Health Service, St. Davnet's Hospital, Monaghan, Ireland, kingstontara@yahoo.co.uk

Anthony Kinsella Molecular and Cellular Therapeutics, Royal College of Surgeons in Ireland, Dublin, Ireland

James B. Kirkbride Department of Psychiatry, University of Cambridge, Cambridge, UK, jbk25@cam.ac.uk

Mark F. Lenzenweger Department of Psychology, State University of New York at Binghamton; Department of Psychiatry and Personality Disorders Institute, Weill College of Medicine at Cornell University, New York, USA, mlenzen@binghamton.edu

Shôn Lewis Professor of Adult Psychiatry and Head, Community-Based Medicine Research School University of Manchester, shon.lewis@manchester.ac.uk

Richard J. Linscott Department of Psychology, University of Otago, Dunedin, New Zealand, linscott@psy.otago.ac.nz

Daniel Martins-de-Souza Laboratory of Neuroscience, Department and Institute of Psychiatry, Faculty of Medicine, University of São Paulo, 05403–903, São Paulo, SP, Brazil, java99@unicamp.br

Paulo R. Menezes Departamento de Medicina Preventiva, Faculdade de Medicina, Universidade de São Paulo, São Paulo, Brazil, pmenezes@usp.br

Andreas Meyer-Lindenberg Central Institute of Mental Health, Zentralinstitut für Seelische Gesundheit, J5, 68159 Mannheim, Germany, a-meyer-lindenberg@zi-mannheim.de

Patrick D. McGorry Orygen Youth Research Centre, University of Melbourne, Melbourne, Victoria, Australia, pmcgorry@unimelb.edu.au

John McGrath Queensland Centre for Mental Health Research, The Park Centre for Mental Health, Wacol, QLD 4076, Australia, john_mcgrath@qcmhr.uq.edu.au

Philip McGuire Section of Neuroimaging, Institute of Psychiatry, OASIS, SLAM NHS Trust, London, p.mcguire@iop.kcl.ac.uk

B. Moghaddam Department of Neuroscience, University of Pittsburgh, Pittsburgh, PA, USA, moghaddam@bns.pitt.edu

Robin M. Murray Institute of Psychiatry, Box PO63, de Crespigny Park, London SE5 8AF, UK, robin.murray@iop.kcl.ac.uk

Barnaby Nelson Orygen Youth Research Centre, University of Melbourne, Melbourne, Victoria, Australia, nelsonb@unimelb.edu.au

Keith H. Nuechterlein Department of Psychiatry and, Biobehavioral, Sciences, Semel Institute for Neuroscience and Human Behavior, University of California, Los Angeles, USA, keithn@ucla.edu

Eadbhard O'Callaghan DETECT Early Psychosis Service, Co. Dublin, Ireland, eadbhard@gmail.com

Elida P.B. Ojopi Laboratory of Neuroscience, Department and Institute of Psychiatry, Faculty of Medicine, University of São paulo, 05403–903, São Paulo, SP, Brazil, elida@usp.br

Olabisi Owoeye Molecular and Cellular Therapeutics, Royal College of Surgeons in Ireland, Dublin, Ireland; Cavan-Monaghan Mental Health Service, St. Davnet's Hospital, Monaghan, Ireland

Eleni Parlapani Department of Psychiatry and Psychotherapy, University of Goettingen, von Siebold Str. 5, 37075 Goettingen, Germany

Maxine X. Patel Section of Cognitive Neuropsychiatry, Institute of Psychiatry, KCL, London SE5 8AF, UK, m.patel@iop.kcl.ac.uk

A.L. Pehrson Department of Neuroscience, University of Pittsburgh, Pittsburgh, PA, USA, pehrson@pitt.edu

Richie Poulton Dunedin Multidisciplinary Health and Development Research Unit, Department of Preventive and Social Medicine, Dunedin School of Medicine, University of Otago, Dunedin, New Zealand, richie.poulton@otago.ac.nz

Babu Rankapalli Clinical Assistant Professor of Psychiatry, University of Florida Medical School, Gainesville, Florida, USA, akbabu_2001@yahoo.com

Mathias Riesbeck Department of Psychiatry and Psychotherapy, Heinrich-Heine-University, Düsseldorf, Germany

Marco A. Romano Silva Laboratorio de Neurociencias, Universidade Federal de Minas Gerais, Belo Horizonte, MG, Brazil, romano-silva@ufmg.br

Wulf Rössler Department of General and Social Psychiatry, Psychiatric University Hospital Zurich, Militärstrasse 8, 8021 Zürich, Switzerland, roessler@dgsp.uzh.ch

Vincent Russell Cavan-Monaghan Mental Health Service, Cavan General Hospital, Cavan, Ireland; Department of Psychiatry, Royal College of Surgeons in Ireland, Dublin, Ireland

Bart P.F. Rutten Department of Psychiatry and Neuropsychology, School of Mental Health and Neuroscience, Maastricht University Medical Centre, EURON, SEARCH, Maastricht, 6200 MD, The Netherlands

Maristela S. Schaufelberger Laboratory of Psychiatric Neuroimaging (LIM21) Department and Institute of Psychiatry, Faculty of Medicine - University of São Paulo, 05403–903, São Paulo - SP - Brazil, maristela_ss@yahoo.com.br

Andrea Schmitt Department of Psychiatry and Psychotherapy, University of Goettingen, von Siebold Str. 5, 37075 Goettingen, Germany, aschmit@gwdg.de

Paul J. Scully Molecular and Cellular Therapeutics, Royal College of Surgeons in Ireland, Dublin, Ireland; Cavan-Monaghan Mental Health Service, St. Davnet's Hospital, Monaghan, Ireland

Renan P. Souza Neurogenetics Section, Centre for Addiction and Mental Health, Toronto, ON, Canada, renandesouza@camh.net

Rajiv Tandon University of Florida Medical School, Gainesville, Florida, USA, tandon@ufl.edu

Jim Van Os Department of Psychiatry and Neuropsychology, School of Mental Health and Neuroscience, Maastricht University Medical Centre, EURON, SEARCH, Maastricht, 6200 MD, The Netherlands; Division of Psychological Medicine, Institute of Psychiatry, London SE5 8AF, UK, j.vanos@sp.unimaas.nl

John L. Waddington Molecular and Cellular Therapeutics, Royal College of Surgeons in Ireland, Dublin, Ireland; Cavan-Monaghan Mental Health Service, St. Davnet's Hospital, Monaghan, Ireland, jwadding@rcsi.ie

Wolfgang Wölwer Department of Psychiatry and Psychotherapy, Heinrich-Heine-University, Düsseldorf, Germany, woelwer@uni-duesseldorf.de

Alison R. Yung Orygen Youth Research Centre, University of Melbourne, Melbourne, Victoria, Australia, ryung@unimelb.edu.au

Marcus V. Zanetti Laboratory of Psychiatric Neuroimaging (LIM21) Department and Institute of Psychiatry, Faculty of Medicine - University of São Paulo, 05403–903, São Paulo - SP - Brazil, marcus_zanetti@yahoo.com.br

Jürgen Zielasek Department of Psychiatry and Psychotherapy, Heinrich-Heine-University, Düsseldorf, Germany, juergen.zielasek@lvr.de

Part I
Epidemiology And Risk Factors

Incidence and Outcome of Schizophrenia Across the Globe

Paulo R. Menezes

Introduction

Ten years ago, during the "IV Search for the Causes of Schizophrenia" meeting, one of the main issues regarding the epidemiology of schizophrenia was the meaning and implications of universality and uniformity in incidence rates for the disease in different places and cultures (Jablensky 1999; Eaton 1999). Most of the evidence upon which the interpretation of data and conclusions were based came from the "Ten Country Study", coordinated by the World Health Organization (WHO) (Sartorius et al. 1986; Jablensky et al. 1992). In that study, also known as the "Determinants of Severe Mental Disorder" study (DOSMeD), incidence rate estimates were obtained for 8 of the 12 participating centres, two of which were from Chandigarh (urban and rural areas), in India. The study also generated relevant data on the outcome of schizophrenia in different cultures. Interpretation of the results from the "Ten Country Study" led to the widespread beliefs that the incidence of schizophrenia is similar across populations and cultures and that its prognosis is more favourable for persons who live in low- and middle-income countries (LAMICs) compared to those living in high-income countries, notions that can be seen in recent publications in the most prestigious scientific medical journals (e.g. Mueser and McGurk 2004).

Epidemiology is the study of the distribution and determinants of health-related states or events in specified populations and the application of this study to control of health problems. Epidemiologists attempt to identify determinants of diseases in populations by examining who is more likely to develop the disease (person), where the disease is commonest (place), and when it is most likely to occur (time), which includes trends over long periods of time. The notion that prevailed in the 1980s and the 1990s, that schizophrenia would occur at similar rates in all populations across the globe, irrespective of individual or group characteristics and life trajectories,

P.R. Menezes (✉)
Departamento de Medicina Preventiva, Faculdade de Medicina, Universidade de São Paulo, São Paulo, Brazil
e-mail: pmenezes@usp.br

W.F. Gattaz, G. Busatto (eds.), *Advances in Schizophrenia Research 2009*,
DOI 10.1007/978-1-4419-0913-8_1, © Springer Science+Business Media, LLC 2010

3

implied that it would be inaccessible for epidemiological investigations, since heterogeneity in incidence between groups and populations is required for epidemiologists to be able to identify potential risk factors. In this respect, schizophrenia would be a very special illness, because it would not only equally affect the rich and the poor, men and women, irrespective of religion or political affiliation, but also be more lenient with those living in less-developed societies regarding its prognosis, notwithstanding the lack of access to mental health care for those suffering from schizophrenia in those societies.

Interest on the epidemiology of schizophrenia and psychoses in general, especially the incidence and outcome of schizophrenia, has been much renewed over recent years. Systematic reviews have shown that there is wide variation in incidence rates of schizophrenia across populations, regions, and groups and that this variation cannot be accounted for on a methodological basis only (McGrath et al. 2004; Cantor-Graae and Selten 2005; March et al. 2008). Such variation is consistent for persons (e.g. migrants) and places (e.g. urban vs. rural areas and between cities and neighbourhoods), but there is controversy regarding trends over time (Kirkbride et al. 2008).

In this chapter, I will present the main results of some recent systematic reviews that examined the incidence of schizophrenia and its variation according to persons and places, new original data that were published after or concomitantly with these reviews, and discuss needs and directions for future research in this area. I will also briefly discuss issues concerning the outcome of schizophrenia, with particular emphasis on the notion of a better prognosis for schizophrenia in LAMICs.

Incidence of Schizophrenia

A turning point in the revival of interest in the epidemiology of schizophrenia was the systematic review conducted by McGrath et al. (2004) on the incidence of the disorder. The main scientific questions were as follows: (1) What is the range of incidence rates? (2) Is there a sex difference in the incidence of schizophrenia? (3) Is there a difference in incidence rates according to urban vs. rural place of residence? (4) What are the central tendency and distribution of incidence rate ratios between native born and migrant groups? The authors searched for studies published between 1965 and 2001 and were able to identify 100 core studies, 23 cohort studies, 24 migrant studies, and 14 studies on other special groups. One hundred and seventy incidence rates were extracted from 55 core studies in 33 countries. The median incidence rate was 15.2/100,000, with central 80% estimates varying from 8 to 43/100,000, a fivefold difference (Fig. 1). The study also showed that men are more likely to develop schizophrenia than women, with a median male:female rate ratio of 1.4. Studies from urban settings yielded higher incidence rates than those from mixed urban–rural settings, and rates among migrants tended to be higher than those for native-born individuals, with a median rate ratio of 4.6. The authors concluded that there is substantial variation in the incidence of schizophrenia and that

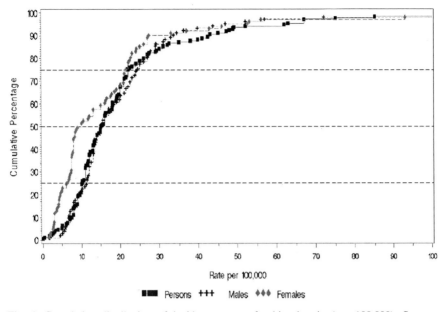

Fig. 1 Cumulative distribution of incidence rates of schizophrenia (per 100,000). Source: McGrath et al. (2004)

the axiom of uniform incidence across populations and cultures cannot be sustained by existing evidence. The data gathered by this systematic review also allowed examining whether the incidence of schizophrenia varied according to economic status of the country (Saha et al. 2006a) and latitude of the centres where the studies were conducted (Saha et al. 2006b). There was no association between economic status of country and incidence of schizophrenia, but rates were significantly higher in centres located at higher latitudes compared to low- and medium-latitude centres. However, the authors stressed that there were only three studies from low-income countries and nine from middle-income countries, and that only two studies were from centres in the Southern Hemisphere, which limits conclusions regarding the questions examined.

Some recent studies present new data on the incidence of schizophrenia across the globe, three of them conducted in LAMICs and three from the Southern Hemisphere (Table 1) (Selten et al. 2005; Kirkbride et al. 2006; Amminger et al. 2006; Menezes et al. 2007; Burns and Esterhuizen 2008; Coid et al. 2008). The Aetiology and Ethnicity in Schizophrenia and Other Psychoses (ÆSOP) study (Kirkbride et al. 2006) aimed at investigating the excess of psychosis incidence in migrant groups in the United Kingdom, using the same methodology in three centres with distinct population profiles (Southeast London, Nottingham, and Bristol). Case ascertainment took place between 1997 and 1999. A surveillance of all psychiatric services where potential cases of first-episode psychosis might have had their first contact was carried out on a regular basis, and direct standardized assessments were made

Table 1 Selected results of recent research that estimated the incidence of psychoses and schizophrenia across the globe

Authors	Study	Centre(s)	Design	Inception period / Age range / Number of cases	Incidence (per 100,000) of psychoses (P) non-affective psychosis (NA) schizophrenia (S)
Amminger et al. (2006)	EPPIC	Australia— northern Melbourne	Reference centre / Medical records + direct assessments	1997–2000 / 15–29 / 1,019	Males P 167 (154–179) / Females P 81 (72–90)
Burns and Esterhuizen (2008)	South Africa	South Africa— Umgungundlovu	Hospital admissions / Medical records	2005 / 15–49 / 160	NA 31.0 (13.4–53.0)
Coid et al. (2008)	ELFEP	UK— East London	All psychiatric services / Direct assessment	1996–1998 / 1998–2000 / 18–64 / 484	P 50.2 (45.5–54.9) / NA 36.8 (32.8–40.7)
Kirkbride et al. (2006)	AESOP	UK— Southeast London, Nottingham, and Bristol	All psychiatric services / Direct assessment	1997–1999 / 16–64 / 568	London P 49.4 (43.6–55.3), NA 37.4 (32.3–42.5) / Nottingham P 23.9 (20.6–27.2), NA 13.1 (10.6–15.5) / Bristol P 20.4 (15.1–25.7), NA 13.2 (8.9–17.4)
Menezes et al. (2007)	SaoPaulo	Brazil— São Paulo	All psychiatric services / Direct assessment	2002–2004 / 18–64 / 367	P 15.8 (14.3–17.6) / NA 10.0 (8.7–11.4)
Selten et al. (2005)	Surinam	Surinam	All psychiatric services / Direct assessment	2002–2003 / 15–54 / 64	S 16.8 (12.3–22.5)

by trained investigators for most participants. A symptom checklist was completed for those who declined to participate, and consensus on diagnoses was given. A total of 568 first-episode cases were included in the study, for a denominator of 1,631,442 person-years at risk. The incidence of all psychoses in Southeast London was 49/100,000 (95% confidence interval (CI): 44–55), much higher than the incidences of 24/100,000 (95% CI: 21–27) observed in Nottingham and 21/100,000 (95% CI: 15–26) in Bristol. Similar differences between the three centres were observed for the incidence of non-affective psychoses. The ÆSOP study showed that the incidence of psychoses and schizophrenia vary not only between countries but also within countries.

The East London First Episode Psychosis (ELFEP) study was designed to answer whether the incidence of psychoses differs across migrant groups and the host population, to examine whether the increased risk associated with migration decreases in subsequent generations born in the United Kingdom and to investigate whether the risk of psychosis among migrants is modified by gender and diagnostic category (Coid et al. 2008). Identification and inclusion of first-episode psychosis cases followed a strategy similar to that used in the ÆSOP study, with regular surveillance of all psychiatric services where someone who lived in the areas defined for the study might seek help for a psychotic episode. Three hundred and sixty-two first-episode cases included in the study received the diagnosis of non-affective psychosis for 828,546 person-years at risk, yielding an age- and sex-standardized incidence of 37/100,000 (95% CI: 33–41), confirming the high incidence of non-affective psychosis in London inner city areas as compared to rates found in other UK centres.

In Australia, the incidence of psychosis was estimated using data from the Early Psychosis Prevention and Intervention Centre (EPPIC), a community-based specialized service for individuals aged 15–29 years who present with a first psychotic episode in north-western Melbourne (Amminger et al. 2006). During the period between 1997 and 2000, 1,019 individuals (687 males) fulfilled criteria for first-episode psychosis, which generated incidence estimates of 167/100,000 for males and 81/100,000 for females. These rates were much higher than those found in previous studies.

Selten et al. (2005) estimated the incidence of schizophrenia in the Surinam. The country, located in the Amazon region in South America, has a population of almost half million people, constituted mostly by African Surinamese (41%), East Indians (37%), and Javanese (15%). Mental health care is provided by the Psychiatric Centre Surinam, and there are six psychiatrists in the country. The authors tried to identify and directly assess all cases of psychosis aged 15–54 years who had had a first contact during a 1-year period, from 2002 to 2003. Sixty-four first contact cases were identified and assessed by the investigators, yielding an incidence of schizophrenia of 16.8/100,000, which is quite close to the median value found in the systematic review by McGrath et al. (2004).

Burns and Esterhuizen (2008) estimated the incidence of psychosis in the District of Umgungundlovu, which is composed of seven municipalities, in the eastern coast of South Africa. One hundred and sixty cases of first-episode non-affective psychoses were identified through the review of medical records of all psychiatric admissions for 2005 in the catchment area. The overall incidence of non-affective psychoses was 31.0/100,000, but there was a fourfold difference of incidence rates between municipalities, ranging from 13.4 to 53.0. However, the estimates for each municipality were not very precise, and this may explain at least in part such wide variation between very close geographic areas. Incidence rates were positively correlated with municipal income inequality ($r = 0.84$; $p = 0.04$).

In Brazil, the incidence of first-episode psychosis was estimated in schizophrenia and other psychoses at unveiling and long-term outcome study (SaoPaulo) (Menezes et al. 2007). The study was conducted in São Paulo, one of the largest cities in the world, situated in the southeast region of the country. The metropolitan area of São Paulo has a population of approximately 18 million inhabitants and is the economic centre of Brazil. The area covered by the study had a population of about 1 million people and was economically very heterogeneous. All psychiatric services, public and private, where those living in the geographical areas defined for the study were scrutinized and potential first-episode cases were identified and contacted. Direct interviews and diagnostic assessment with the SCID took place whenever possible, when the first-episode status was confirmed. In the case of a refusal to be interviewed, the diagnosis was given by consensus using all available information from medical records and key informants. A leakage study was also carried out in order to identify first-episode cases that might have been missed at the time of their first contact with a psychiatric service due to a psychotic episode. Three hundred and sixty-seven first-episode psychosis cases were identified from 2002 to 2005, yielding incidences of 15.8/100,000 (95% CI: 14.3–17.6) for all psychoses and 10.0/100,000 (95% CI: 8.7–11.4) for non-affective psychoses. Such rates were much lower than those previously expected for such a large conurbation in a LAMIC.

Migration and Risk of Schizophrenia

The increased incidence of psychosis and schizophrenia in migrants, as compared with native individuals, has been perhaps one of the most investigated aspects of the epidemiology of schizophrenia over the last 20 years. A systematic review (Cantor-Graae and Selten 2005) of English language publications between 1977 and 2003 identified 18 studies that examined this issue, one being from Australia and all others from Europe. The summary relative risk (RR) from the overall meta-analysis with first- and second-generation migrants (50 estimates) was 2.9 (95% CI: 2.5–3.4), which is much higher than most associations between risk factors and disease for almost all non-communicable diseases in general epidemiology. The analysis comparing incidence of schizophrenia among first-generation migrants with incidence in native populations (40 estimates) yielded a summary RR of 2.7 (95% CI: 2.3–3.2), and the analysis with second-generation migrants (7 estimates) yielded a summary RR of 4.5 (95% CI: 1.5–13.1), suggesting that the risk of schizophrenia is even higher among the children of immigrants. However, there was significant heterogeneity between studies' results, indicating that migrant groups cannot be considered uniformly, as if they all presented the same increased incidence of psychosis. Indeed, significantly greater RRs for migrants from LAMICs and areas where the majority of the population is black were observed. The authors of this systematic review proposed long-term exposure to social defeat or experiences of discrimination as a possible mechanism behind such association.

Recent studies on the incidence of psychosis among immigrants have been published, aimed at testing specific hypotheses related to the association between migration status and increased risk for psychosis, in the United Kingdom, Sweden, and Israel (Fearon et al. 2006; Coid et al. 2008; Kirkbride et al. 2008; Corcoran et al. 2008; Leão et al. 2006; Weiser et al. 2008) (Table 2). The ÆSOP study (Fearon et al. 2006) was designed to estimate the degree of increase in the incidence of schizophrenia in the African-Caribbean population in the United Kingdom, to explore whether such higher risk also applied to other psychoses, and whether the incidence of schizophrenia and other psychoses was also increased among other ethnic minority groups in the United Kingdom. Afro-Caribbeans and Black-Africans showed very high incidence rates for both schizophrenia and mania in men and in women, in all age groups, six to nine times than the incidence of schizophrenia and mania found for the White British population in the three centres that took part in the study (Southeast London, Nottingham, and Bristol). The incidence of schizophrenia and other psychoses was also moderately increased among other ethnic minority groups, but statistical power was limited to detect differences in these smaller ethnic minority groups despite the large size of the population at risk and absolute number of first-episode cases. The authors concluded that the increased incidence of psychosis in these groups may be the consequence of additional risk factors in immigrants, particularly Black-Caribbeans and Black-Africans, or of a higher prevalence of risk factors common to the general population.

Another population-based study conducted in the United Kingdom, the East London First-Episode Psychosis Study (ELFEP), examined whether the increased incidence of schizophrenia and other psychoses was independent of socioeconomic status and extended to the second generation of immigrants, regardless of their ethnic group (Coid et al. 2008; Kirkbride et al. 2008). The ELFEP study confirmed higher incidence of psychosis among all ethnic minority groups, after adjustment for gender, age, and socioeconomic status (SES). After controlling for SES, the RRs for first- and second-generation Afro-Caribbeans and Black-Africans were less pronounced than those found in the ÆSOP study, but the strength of the association was still high.

In Sweden, Leão et al. (2006) investigated whether the increased incidence of schizophrenia and other psychoses observed in some immigrant groups relative to the incidence observed for native Swedish is still present in the next generation and whether having one parent born in Sweden decreases this risk. They used the unique Swedish registers to link databases with individual socio-demographic and socioeconomic characteristics and data from the national hospital discharge. Two million and two hundred persons were followed up either until their first psychiatric admission or till the end of the study. Compared to the incidence of schizophrenia and other psychoses among Swedes, all first- and second-generation migrants

Table 2 Selected results of recent research that estimated rate ratios (95% confidence intervals) for the incidence of psychoses and schizophrenia among migrants compared to the incidence in native populations

Authors	Country	Migration status	Confounding	Exposure groups	Schizophrenia	All psychoses
Fearon et al. (2006)	UK	Ethnic minority groups	Age	Afro-Caribbean	9.1 (6.6–12.6)	6.7 (5.4–8.3)
				Black-African	5.8 (3.9–8.4)	4.1 (3.2–5.3)
				Mixed	2.6 (1.2–6.4)	2.7 (1.8–4.2)
				White others	2.5 (1.6–3.9)	1.6 (1.1–2.2)
Kirkbride et al. (2008)	UK	Ethnic minority groups	Age Gender SES	Afro-Caribbean	3.1 (2.1–4.5)	2.7 (2.0–3.7)
				Black-African	2.6 (1.8–3.8)	2.5 (1.8–3.3)
				White other	1.2 (0.8–2.0)	1.8 (1.3–2.4)
				Bangladeshi	1.1 (0.8–1.7)	1.0 (0.7–1.3)
Leão et al. (2006)	Sweden	First- and second-generation immigrants	Age Income	First-generation Finns	Women 2.5 (2.2–2.9) / Men 1.6 (1.4–1.8)	Women[a] 2.3 (2.0–2.7) / Men[a] 2.3 (2.0–2.8)
				Second-generation Finns	2.3 (1.9–2.9) / 2.3 (1.9–2.7)	2.3 (1.8–2.8) / 2.3 (1.9–2.8)
Weiser et al. (2008)	Israel	First-generation migrant adolescents	Gender SES	Russians	1.6 (1.1–2.2)	
				Ethiopians	3.0 (1.9–4.7)	
Corcoran et al. (2008)	Israel	Second-generation migrants	Paternal and maternal age Maternal education Paternal social class Sex Birth order	Father only	0.9 (0.7–1.2)	
				Mother only	1.0 (0.8–1.3)	
				Both parents	0.9 (0.7–1.1)	

[a]Other psychoses.

showed higher rates. The rate ratios for risk of schizophrenia and other psychoses were more pronounced for immigrants from Finland. First- and second-generation Finns showed more than twice the risk for schizophrenia and other psychoses, even after controlling for age and income, with the exception of first-generation men, who showed a 60% increase in risk. Having one parent born in Sweden did not reduce the risk of psychosis in the second generation of migrants.

Using data from the Israeli Draft Board for over 660,000 adolescents, linked with the National Psychiatric Hospitalization Case Registry, Weiser et al. (2008) also found increased incidence of schizophrenia among adolescent migrants to Israel, which was independent of SES. Adolescents who migrated from Russia had approximately 60% increase in the risk of schizophrenia, whereas those who migrated from Ethiopia were three times as likely as adolescents born in Israel to develop schizophrenia.

Corcoran et al. (2008) investigated whether the incidence of schizophrenia was increased among second-generation immigrants to Israel in a population-based cohort of almost 90,000 offspring born in Jerusalem between 1964 and 1976. Six hundred and thirty-seven first psychiatric admissions with schizophrenia-related diagnoses were identified until the end of 1997, by linkage of the cohort data set with Israel's Psychiatric Registry. The authors found no difference in risk of schizophrenia among second-generation migrants from West Asia, North Africa, or Europe and industrialized countries.

Urbanization and Neighbourhood

Interest in the spatial distribution of schizophrenia and the possible influence of the urban environment date back to the early twentieth century, as seen in the classic ecological work by Faris and Dunham (1939) on the distribution of psychosis in Chicago. The association they described, between poor inner city areas and higher rates of hospital admissions with a diagnosis of schizophrenia, stimulated research on possible risk factors for schizophrenia related to the social environment and the debate on the relationship between socioeconomic position and risk of psychosis. However, interest in this line of investigation decreased sharply in the second half of the last century, until the 1990s, when new, well-conducted epidemiological investigations, mostly cohort studies from European countries, present consistent results for a positive association between urbanicity and incidence of schizophrenia. Krabbendam and Van Os (2005) conducted a meta-analysis of results from 10 such studies, all from developed countries, and found that on average the risk of schizophrenia in urban areas was about twice the risk in rural areas. The increased incidence of schizophrenia in urban areas could not be attributed to confounding or selection bias, such as distance from psychiatric services. The authors argued that mechanisms behind this association are not clear, but possibly involve gene–environment interactions.

March et al. (2008) conducted a systematic review of studies from developed countries, published in English between 1950 and 2007, which investigated the spatial distribution of psychosis. They identified 20 studies examining the incidence of psychosis according to urbanicity and 24 studies comparing the incidence of psychosis between neighbourhoods. All studies on urbanicity and psychosis were carried out in Western Europe, except for one from the United States. Overall, urbanicity was associated with about a twofold increase in the incidence of schizophrenia, as compared to less-urbanized or rural areas, a result similar to that found by Krabbendam and Van Os (2005). The timing of exposure to urbanization was examined in several studies. Increased incidence of psychosis was associated with higher degrees of urbanization at birth in Sweden, the Netherlands, and Denmark. A cumulative association between urban environment and risk of psychosis was described in a study from Denmark (Pedersen and Mortensen 2001). The longer the exposure to urban residence from birth onwards, the higher the risk of developing a psychotic episode. On the other hand, in a study in the Netherlands, those not born in urban areas but who lived in urban centres later in life did not have increased risk for psychosis, whereas those born in urban areas had higher risk, regardless of residence status at the illness onset (Marcelis et al. 1999). In face of these data, March et al. (2008) consider that such increased incidence cannot be simply attributed to social drift and probably represents a true association. The challenge now is to unravel the aetiological mechanisms behind this association.

Of the 24 studies on the association between neighbourhood and incidence of psychosis, 20 were from European countries and 4 from the United States. The great majority of these studies reported heterogeneity of incidence rates at the level of administrative geographic units, such as districts, electoral wards, or other small area units. One of the major methodological difficulties in the investigation of the relationship between neighbourhood and its characteristics with incidence of schizophrenia is the assessment of the timing of exposure. In fact, most studies reviewed by March et al. (2008) only assessed neighbourhood exposure at the time of first contact with psychiatric services, which makes exclusion of drift as an alternative explanation for the observed association more difficult.

In summary, the evidence accumulated so far has consistently shown spatial variation in incidence rates of schizophrenia, according to levels of both urbanization and neighbourhoods. The association between urbanicity and increased risk for psychosis seems to indicate that factors acting early in the life course increase the risk of developing schizophrenia, whereas the association with neighbourhood suggests a role for more proximal risk factors, possibly more related to social processes. March et al. (2008) argue that the confirmation of spatial heterogeneity in the incidence of schizophrenia is relevant from a health services perspective, for it allows more adequate service provision. Another, more central question for the understanding of the aetiological components and mechanisms of schizophrenia is What are the actual exposures producing the observed heterogeneity? They propose that future research might focus on key social pathways, understanding such pathways as chains of social processes that produce specific conditions and exposures in a given place and time. Therefore, place would be a more appropriate concept for epidemiological research on schizophrenia.

Outcome of Schizophrenia

The outcome of schizophrenia across the globe is still an object of debate among the scientific community. Current literature often states that the prognosis is better for persons living in LAMICs compared to those living in rich countries (Mueser and McGurk 2004; Isaac et al. 2007; Menezes et al. 2006). Data supporting this belief come mostly from the series of cross-national studies coordinated by the WHO (WHO 1979; Jablensky et al. 1992; Harrison et al. 2001). In those investigations, the proportion of recovery in the 2-year outcome assessment in centres from LAMICs was significantly higher than that observed in centres from developed countries (WHO 1979; Jablensky et al. 1992). The long-term follow-up of the cohorts that took part in the WHO studies showed that the most important predictor of long-term outcome was the short-term outcome (Harrison et al. 2001). There was heterogeneity of outcome between participating centres, but the investigators did not associate a better prognosis with living in a LAMIC. Instead, they pointed to the need of further research to clarify the role of the cultural context on the course and outcome of schizophrenia. Some recent reviews on the outcome of schizophrenia in different populations came to conflicting conclusions (Menezes et al. 2006; Isaac et al. 2007; Cohen et al. 2008).

Menezes et al. (2006) conducted a systematic review of prospective studies examining outcome in first-episode non-affective psychosis published between 1966 and 2003. Thirty-seven studies, all of them published after 1980 and more than half from 2000 onwards, met the inclusion criteria for the review, summing up 4,100 first-episode cases with a mean follow-up of 3 years. Eighty-five per cent of the studies were conducted in developed countries. Outcome definitions and measures varied considerably, the most common being "good" and "poor" outcomes, but other categories included re-admission, relapse, employment and education, social functioning, and the use of the Global Assessment of Functioning from DSM-III and DSM-IV. Considering all studies that used the "good" and "poor" categories of outcome, the proportion of participants classified as having a "good" outcome was 42%, whereas 27% were classified as having a "poor" outcome. Predictors of good outcome were a combination of pharmacotherapy and psychosocial therapy, lack of epidemiological representativeness of the sample, and study origin from a developing country. Interestingly, studies with samples that were not population based tended to show better outcomes. This may be due to selection bias operating at the level of access to care in special services, such as teaching hospitals or specialized services, where patients who manage to receive care may have higher socioeconomic status, family support, or adherence to treatment, for instance. Despite the finding of better outcome being predicted by a developing country origin of the study, the authors of the review did not discuss why that would be so.

Isaac et al. (2007) reviewed the literature concerning the outcome of schizophrenia in LAMICs, verifying that the belief of a better outcome came from results of three centres in India. The lack of a systematic approach to identify studies from LAMICs may have contributed to the limited number of investigations reviewed by Isaac et al. (2007). Nevertheless, the authors point to the scarcity of empirical data from LAMICs, stressing that lack of resources (funding, technical expertise, manpower) may be a main reason for this situation.

Recently, Cohen et al. (2008) strongly questioned the axiom of better prognosis for schizophrenia in LAMICs, also pointing out that such notion has been based on a very limited amount of evidence coming from the WHO series of investigations on the outcome of schizophrenia in different cultures. They performed a comprehensive literature review of research on schizophrenia outcome from LAMICs and found 23 investigations from 11 countries. These studies showed marked methodological heterogeneity, with retrospective and prospective designs, incident and prevalent samples, follow-up periods ranging from 1 to 20 years, and population- and service-based samples. Outcomes were presented for several domains and assessed in different ways. Notwithstanding these obstacles for comparison of results, the authors managed to examine the evidence for better outcome regarding clinical outcome, patterns of course, disability and social outcomes (marital status and employment), lack of treatment, mortality and suicide, gender differences, and role of families. They observed wide variation in results for clinical outcome, with the proportion of individuals presenting with chronic severe psychotic symptoms at follow-up ranging from 0.0 to 30%, and the proportion showing a chronic pattern of course ranging from <5% to more than 50%. Similar variations were observed for disability and social outcomes. Studies that reported data on mortality, in general, showed rates higher than those from the general population where cases came from, due to both increased suicide rates and natural causes of death. Contrary to beliefs that the outcome of schizophrenia in LAMICs is more benign regardless of adequate treatment or not, the data reviewed provided evidence that those who did not have access to adequate care had worse outcomes than those who received biomedical treatment. Regarding the role of families, the available data show that families give support to their relatives who suffer from schizophrenia, but there is conflict, burden, and breakdown caused by the presence of the ill person in the family environment. The authors concluded that there is wide variability in the outcome of schizophrenia in LAMICs as well as in developed countries, and new epidemiological, clinical, and ethnographic research is needed to address several questions, including

- What is the proportion of prevalent cases of schizophrenia that are receiving psychiatric care?
- What are the effects of biomedical and other treatments on the outcome of schizophrenia across the globe?
- How clinical and social outcomes vary between groups and populations, and which are the factors influencing prognosis?
- What is the impact of caring for a member with schizophrenia on families?
- What are the pathways to care and which socio-cultural factors influence help-seeking decisions?
- What are the circumstances that lead to high mortality among those suffering from schizophrenia?

Perspectives

The systematic synthesis of most available research to date on the incidence of schizophrenia and other psychoses has produced new insight into the epidemiology of schizophrenia across the globe, allowing more adequate interpretation of the wealth of existing data and stimulating new research. However, data on the incidence and outcome of schizophrenia across the globe are still scarce, especially in LAMICs, where most of those who suffer from schizophrenia live. When data are available, they help policy makers to decide on how to improve health-care provision and investigators in generating hypotheses and unveiling mechanisms on the aetiology of schizophrenia. What seems well-established knowledge can be questioned by new good-quality data. The unexpectedly low incidence of psychosis in São Paulo is a good example. It suggests that mechanisms operating in rich countries, which are represented by the consistent association between urbanization and schizophrenia, may not be the same in other populations. Humanity has gained better perspectives for the suffering and burden caused by several non-communicable diseases, such as cancer and cardiovascular diseases, presented by careful and extensive epidemiological investigation. Consistent investment on research into the epidemiology of schizophrenia, particularly in LAMICs, may bring major contributions to our understanding of the aetiology of schizophrenia and other psychoses and improvement to the lives of those who are directly or indirectly affected by these disorders.

Acknowledgment   PRM is partly funded by the CNPq-Brazil.

References

Amminger, G. P., Harris, M. G., Conus, P., Lambert, M., Elkins, K. S., Yuen, H. P., Mcgorry, P. D. Treated incidence of first-episode psychosis in the catchment area of EPPIC between 1997 and 2000. Acta Psychiatrica Scandinavica 114: 337–345, 2006

Burns, J. K., Esterhuizen, T. Poverty, inequality and the treated incidence of first-episode psychosis. An ecological study from South Africa. Social Psychiatry and Psychiatric Epidemiology 43: 331–335, 2008

Cantor-Graae, E., Selten, J. P. Schizophrenia and migration: A meta-analysis and review. American Journal of Psychiatry 162: 12–24, 2005

Cohen, A., Patel, V., Thara, R., Gureje, O. Questioning an axiom: Better prognosis for schizophrenia in the developing world? Schizophrenia Bulletin 34: 229–244, 2008

Coid, J. W., Kirkbride, J. B., Barker, D., Cowden, F., Stamps, R., Yang, M., Jones, P. B. Raised incidence rates of all psychoses among migrant groups: Findings from the east London first episode psychosis study. Archives of General Psychiatry 65: 1250–1258, 2008

Corcoran, C., Perrin, M., Harlap, S., Deutsch, L., Fennig, S., Manor, O., Nahon, D., Kimhy, D., Malaspina, D., Susser, E. Incidence of schizophrenia among second-generation immigrants in the Jerusalem Perinatal Cohort. Schizophrenia Bulletin 2008 [epub ahead of printing]

Eaton, W. W. Evidence for universality and uniformity of schizophrenia around the World: assessment and implications. In: Gattaz, W. F., Häfner, H. (eds.), Search or the Causes of Schizophrenia. Vol. IV Balance of the Century, Springer-Verlag, Berlin, pp. 21–33, 1999

Faris, R., Dunham, H. Mental Disorders in Urban Areas. University of Chicago Press, Chicago, 1939

Fearon, P., Kirkbride, J. B., Morgan, C., Dazzan, P., Morgan, K., Lloyd, T., Hutchinson, G., Tarrant, J., Lun Alan Fung, W., Holloway, J., Mallett, R., Harrison, G., Leff, J., Jones, P. B., Murray, R. M., Muga, F., Mietunen, J., Ashby, M., Hayhurst, H., Craig, T., Mccabe, J., Samele, C., Gwenzi, E., Sharpley, M., Vearnals, S., Hutchinson, G., Burnett, R., Kelly, J., Orr, K., Salvo, J., Greenwood, K., Raune, D., Lambri, M., Jones, S., Auer, S., Rohebak, P., Mcintosh, L., Doody, G., Window, S., Williams, P., Bagalkote, H., Dow, B., Boot, D., Farrant, A., Jones, S., Simpson, J., Moanette, R., Sirip Suranim, P. Z., Ruddell, M., Brewin, J., Medley, I. Incidence of schizophrenia and other psychoses in ethnic minority groups: Results from the MRC AESOP Study. Psychological Medicine 36: 1541–1550, 2006

Harrison, G., Hopper, K., Craig, T., Laska, E., Siegel, C., Wanderling, J., Dube, K. C., Ganev, K., Giel, R., An Der Heiden, W., Holmberg, S. K., Janca, A., Lee, P. W. H., León, C. A., Malhotra, S., Marsella, A. J., Nakane, Y., Sartorius, N., Shen, Y., Skoda, C., Thara, R., Tsirkin, S. J., Varma, V. K., Walsh, D., Wiersma, D. Recovery from psychotic illness: A 15- and 25-year international follow-up study. British Journal of Psychiatry 178: 506–517, 2001

Isaac, M., Chand, P., Murthy, P. Schizophrenia outcome measures in the wider international community. British Journal of Psychiatry 191(Suppl 50): s71–s77, 2007

Jablensky, A. The 100-year epidemiology of schizophrenia. In: Gattaz, W. F., Häfner, H. (eds.), Search for the Causes of Schizophrenia. Vol. IV Balance of the Century, Springer-Verlag, Berlin, pp. 3–19, 1999

Jablensky, A., Sartorius, N., Ernberg, G., Anker, M., Korten, A., Cooper, J. E., Day, R., Bertelsen, A. Schizophrenia: manifestations, incidence and course in different cultures. A World Health Organization ten-country study. Psychological Medicine Monograph Supplement 20: 1–97, 1992

Kirkbride, J. B., Barker, D., Cowden, F., Stamps, R., Yang, M., Jones, P. B., Coid, J. W. Psychoses, ethnicity and socio-economic status. British Journal of Psychiatry 193: 18–24, 2008

Kirkbride, J. B., Croudace, T., Brewin, J., Donoghue, K., Mason, P., Glazebrook, C., Medley, I., Harrison, G., Cooper, J. E., Doody, G. A., Jones, P. B. Is the incidence of psychotic disorder in decline? Epidemiological evidence from two decades of research. International Journal of Epidemiology 38(5): 1255–1264, 2008

Kirkbride, J. B., Fearon, P., Morgan, C., Dazzan, P., Morgan, K., Tarrant, J., Lloyd, T., Holloway, J., Hutchinson, G., Leff, J. P., Mallett, R. M., Harrison, G. L., Murray, R. M., Jones, P. B. Heterogeneity in incidence rates of schizophrenia and other psychotic syndromes: Findings from the 3-center äSOP study. Archives of General Psychiatry 63: 250–258, 2006

Krabbendam, L., Van Os, J. Schizophrenia and urbanicity: A major environmental influence – Conditional on genetic risk. Schizophrenia Bulletin 31: 795–799, 2005

Leão, T. S., Sundquist, J., Frank, G., Johansson, L. M., Johansson, S. E., Sundquist, K. Incidence of schizophrenia or other psychoses in first- and second-generation immigrants: A National Cohort Study. Journal of Nervous and Mental Disease 194: 27–33, 2006

Marcelis, M., Takei, N., Van Os, J. Urbanization and risk for schizophrenia: Does the effect operate before or around the time of illness onset? Psychological Medicine 29: 1197–1203, 1999

March, D., Hatch, S. L., Morgan, C., Kirkbride, J. B., Bresnahan, M., Fearon, P., Susser, E. Psychosis and place. Epidemiologic Reviews 30: 84–100, 2008

Mcgrath, J., Saha, S., Welham, J., El Saadi, O., Maccauley, C., Chant, D. A systematic review of the incidence of schizophrenia: The distribution of rates and the influence of sex, urbanicity, migrant status and methodology. BMC Medicine 2, 2004

Menezes, N. M., Arenovich, T., Zipursky, R. B. A systematic review of longitudinal outcome studies of first-episode psychosis. Psychological Medicine 36: 1349–1362, 2006

Menezes, P. R., Scazufca, M., Busatto, G., Coutinho, L. M. S., Mcguire, P. K., Murray, R. M. Incidence of first-contact psychosis in São Paulo, Brazil. British Journal of Psychiatry 191(Suppl 51): s102–s106, 2007

Mueser, K. T., Mcgurk, S. R. Schizophrenia. Lancet 363: 2063–2072, 2004

Pedersen, C. B., Mortensen, P. B. Evidence of a dose-response relationship between urbanicity during upbringing and schizophrenia risk. Archives of General Psychiatry 58: 1039–1046, 2001

Saha, S., Chant, D. C., Welham, J. L., Mcgrath, J. J. The incidence and prevalence of schizophrenia varies with latitude. Acta Psychiatrica Scandinavica 114: 36–39, 2006a

Saha, S., Welham, J., Chant, D., Mcgrath, J. Incidence of schizophrenia does not vary with economic status of the country: Evidence from a systematic review. Social Psychiatry and Psychiatric Epidemiology 41: 338–340, 2006b

Sartorius, N., Jablensky, A., Korten, A., Ernberg, G., Anker, M., Cooper, J. E., Day, R. Early manifestations and first-contact incidence of schizophrenia in different cultures. A preliminary report on the initial evaluation phase of the WHO Collaborative Study on determinants of outcome of severe mental disorders. Psychological Medicine 16: 909–928, 1986

Selten, J. P., Zeyl, C., Dwarkasing, R., Lumsden, V., Kahn, R. S., Van Harten, P. N. First-contact incidence of schizophrenia in Surinam. British Journal of Psychiatry 186: 74–75, 2005

Weiser, M., Werbeloff, N., Vishna, T., Yoffe, R., Lubin, G., Shmushkevitch, M., Davidson, M. Elaboration on immigration and risk for schizophrenia. Psychological Medicine 38: 1113–1119, 2008

WHO Schizophrenia: An International Follow-Up Study. John Wiley and Sons, Chichester, 1979

Gene–Environment Interactions for Searchers: Collaboration Between Epidemiology and Molecular Genetics

Jim van Os, Bart P.F. Rutten, and Richie Poulton

Introduction

Attempts to discover genes that relate directly to psychotic disorder (i.e., the simple "main effects" approach) have been frustrating and often disappointing, resulting in the expression of methodological concerns (Harrison and Weinberger 2005; Norton et al. 2006) (Collier 2008; Sullivan 2008; O'Donovan et al. 2008; Crow 2008). On the other hand, epidemiological research has unveiled high observed rates of schizophrenia in large cities, immigrant populations, traumatised individuals and cannabis users, at least some of which is thought to be the result of underlying environmental exposures. Exciting findings in other areas of psychiatry have motivated researchers to turn their attention to better understanding the complex ways in which nature interacts with nurture to produce psychosis. This genotype × environmental interaction (hereafter G×E) approach differs from the linear gene–phenotype approach by positing a causal role not for either genes or environment in isolation, but for their synergistic co-participation in the cause of psychosis where the effect of one is conditional on the other (EU-GEI 2008). For example, genes may moderate the psychotogenic effects of dopamine agonist drugs of abuse, or the environment may moderate the level of expression of a gene that is on the causal pathway to psychotic disorder. G×E seems a particularly suitable approach for understanding the development of psychosis because this phenotype is known to be associated with environmentally mediated risks (Cannon and Clarke 2005; Van Os et al. 2005), yet people display considerable heterogeneity in their response to those environmental exposures.

The structure of this article is as follows. First, the principles of genetic epidemiology as relevant for the study of gene–environment interaction will be reviewed briefly. Second, a brief overview will be given on what "the environment" may consist of in studies of G×E and how environmental mechanisms may be

J. van Os (✉)
Department of Psychiatry and Neuropsychology, School of Mental Health and Neuroscience, Maastricht University Medical Centre, EURON, SEARCH, Maastricht, 6200 MD, The Netherlands; Division of Psychological Medicine, Institute of Psychiatry, London SE5 8AF, UK
e-mail: j.vanos@sp.unimaas.nl

W.F. Gattaz, G. Busatto (eds.), *Advances in Schizophrenia Research 2009*,
DOI 10.1007/978-1-4419-0913-8_2, © Springer Science+Business Media, LLC 2010

uncovered using "functional enviromics". Third, the main $G \times E$ findings with regard to psychotic disorders will be reviewed, with a particular focus on epidemiological studies that used indirect measures of genetic risk including twin and adoption studies, family studies and psychometric risk studies. Most of the findings using direct molecular genetic measures of genetic risk will be reviewed elsewhere in this issue. Fourth, considerations will be given to possible underlying mechanisms followed by a discussion of future research and directions.

Ecogenetics

Traditional epidemiology was concerned mainly with environmental risks. Conversely, genetic researchers of complex disorders have mostly focused on molecular genetic approaches, in which the environment and interaction between genes and environment were treated as a power-reducing nuisance term. Awareness has been growing, however, that direct or indirect measures of genetic variation can be considered as a conventional epidemiological risk factor in association studies (Sham 1996) and that epidemiological theory can be readily applied to genetically sensitive data sets (Susser and Susser 1989; Ottman 1990). Thus, epidemiologists and human geneticists have been gradually integrating their respective fields of research into a new discipline called genetic epidemiology (Khoury et al. 1993). Within genetic epidemiology, the term *ecogenetics* refers to the study of specific gene–environment relationships (Motulsky 1977). Within an ecogenetic framework, several types of gene–environment relationships are relevant for the study of complex disorders, representing different biologically plausible mechanisms by which genes and environment can co-influence disease outcome (Khoury et al. 1993; Kendler and Eaves 1986; Ottman 1996; Plomin et al. 1977; Van Os and Marcelis 1998).

Ecogenetics in Psychiatry

Until recently, the conventional wisdom within psychiatry and behavioural genetics was that $G \times E$ was exceedingly rare and difficult to demonstrate. The revival of interest in $G \times E$ derives largely from (1) failures of direct gene–phenotype association studies to uncover genes related to susceptibility for psychiatric disorders and the realisation that their multifactorial aetiology likely includes many complicated interactive effects requiring more advanced approaches (Hamer 2002; Rutter 2006); (2) work demonstrating the operation of $G \times E$ in many other branches of medicine; and (3) recent evidence of $G \times E$ within psychiatry (Moffitt et al. 2005).

The recent $G \times E$ findings in psychiatry suggest that genes are likely to influence disorder mostly indirectly, via their impact upon physiological pathways, and work by increasing (or decreasing) the likelihood of developing a psychiatric disorder, rather than as direct *causes* of disorder per se. Thus, the notion of "a gene for. . ." is misleading and diverts attention from more important issues (Kendler 2005, 2006). Further, some theorists now suggest that (1) additive, non-interactive genetic effects may be less common than previously assumed (cf. Colhoun et al. 2003); (2) studying genes in isolation from known environmental risks may fail to detect important genetic influences; and (3) traditional notions of multiplicative interaction are probably not appropriate for "real-world" interactions (Darroch 1997), particularly given the ubiquity of some environmental exposures (Moffitt et al. 2005; Rutter et al. 2006). Thus, biological synergism (co-participation of causes to some outcome) between environmental exposure and background genetic vulnerability is thought to be common in multifactorial disorders such as psychosis. The classic problem, however, is how co-participation between causes in nature (biological synergism) can be inferred from statistical manipulations with research data (statistical interaction), in particular with regard to the choice of additive (change in risk occurs by adding a quantity) or multiplicative (change in risk occurs by multiplying with a quantity) models. It has been shown that the true degree of biological synergism can be better estimated from—but is not the same as—the additive statistical interaction rather than the much more often used multiplicative interaction (Darroch 1997).

Genetic Moderation of Sensitivity to Environment

According to the concept of genetic moderation of sensitivity to the environment, differences in genetic endowment explain why people respond differently to the same environment (Fig. 1). Most evidence for this type of G×E in psychosis has come indirectly from twin and adoption studies, and a variety of naturalistic designs in which non-specific genetic contributions have been assessed. More recently, researchers have obtained information about how variation in specific measured genes interacts with specific measured environments (Moffitt et al. 2005). Genetic moderation of environmental sensitivity gives rise to *synergism*, or *interaction*, as the biological effects of G and E are dependent on each other in such a way that exposure to neither or either one alone does not result in the outcome in question, whereas exposure to both does. For example, a well-known example of gene–environment interaction is the observation that among Orientals, alcohol sensitivity is strongly regulated by genetic polymorphism of the aldehyde dehydrogenase (*ALDH2*) gene. Similarly, there is strong evidence that some polymorphisms may be involved in psychiatric disorders. For example, the gene encoding the serotonin transporter (5-HTT) contains a regulatory variation (5-HTTLPR), the short ("s")

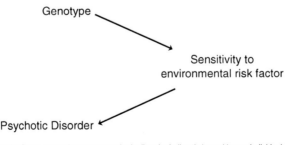

In the figure, genes impact on psychotic disorder indirectly by making an individual more sensitive to the psychotogenic effect of an environmental pathogen.

Fig. 1 Gene × environment interaction: genes controlling environmental sensitivity

allele of which is associated with lower transcriptional efficiency of the promoter as compared to the long ("l") allele. Data from animal and human research indicate that 5-HTTLPR may interact with environmental adversity to cause depression, reflecting underlying developmental mechanisms that affect the structural connectivity, and, as a consequence, functional interactions, within a neural circuit involved in the regulation of emotional reactivity and extinction of fear (Canli and Lesch 2007; Champoux et al. 2002; Wellman et al. 2007; Caspi et al. 2003; Jacobs et al. 2006) (Fig. 2).

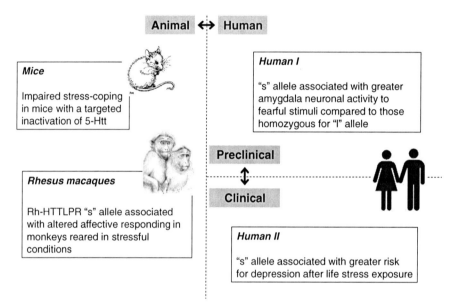

Fig. 2 Promoter activity of the 5-HTT gene is modified by sequence elements within the proximal regulatory region; the short ("s") allele is associated with lower transcriptional efficiency of the promoter as compared to the long ("l") allele: converging evidence of G×E in the depression from animal to human, human to animal, and preclinical to clinical and clinical to preclinical

Although gene–environment synergism is likely prevalent, other models of disease causation, including models that imply that there is no synergism (synergism is zero), may also likely apply, although likely to a lesser degree. For example, an individual may get schizophrenia only if in possession of a certain type of vulnerability conferred by either genetic or environmental factors. An environmental factor could disrupt early brain development in the same manner as a genetic mutation. In this model, synergism is zero and the effect of genes and environment is said to be *additive*.

Environmental Impact on DNA Sequence and Methylation

Apart from genes impacting on sensitivity for environmental risk factors, G×E in psychotic disorder may also take the form of environmental factors impacting either the DNA sequence (causing de novo mutations) or DNA methylation (causing altered gene expression through epimutations). The most suggestive epidemiological evidence for such mechanisms in psychosis comes from studies linking advanced paternal age to the risk of schizophrenia in the offspring (Malaspina et al. 2001; Zammit et al. 2003; Byrne et al. 2003; Sipos et al. 2004). Paternal age varies as a function of the sociocultural environment (Weisfeld and Weisfeld 2002). The observed paternal age effect on schizophrenia may consist of mutagenesis, causing de novo spontaneous mutations, which would then propagate and accumulate in successive generations of sperm-producing cells. Alternatively, the mechanism underlying the paternal age effect may be genomic imprinting (Flint 1992). Genomic imprinting is the phenomenon whereby a small subset of all the genes in the genome is expressed according to their parent of origin. Some imprinted genes are expressed from a maternally inherited chromosome and silenced on the paternal chromosome, whereas other imprinted genes show the opposite expression pattern and are only expressed from a paternally inherited chromosome (Wilkinson et al. 2007). One of the mechanisms for gene silencing is DNA methylation. The inherited methylation pattern is maintained in somatic cells but is erased and re-established late in spermatogenesis for paternally imprinted genes, a process that could become impaired as age advances.

Although research on DNA methylation as an "epigenetic" mechanism underlying G×E in psychiatry is in an early phase, this field appears promising. For example, early maternal behaviour in animals can affect offspring stress sensitivity through altered DNA methylation of key neuronal receptor genes involved in the stress response (Weaver et al. 2004; Meaney and Szyf 2005). Environmentally induced epigenetic mechanisms may explain a range of epidemiological findings including typical age-of-onset incidence curves, monozygotic twin discordance, sex differences, possible risk-increasing effects of prenatal factors associated with in utero folate deficiency (a key component of DNA methylation) (Susser et al. 1996; Zammit et al. 2007; Smits et al. 2004) and possible risk-increasing effects of developmental trauma (Read et al. 2005). A fascinating report from Denmark is suggestive of epigenetic effects involving urban birth and upbringing. Thus, the authors demonstrated that the risk-increasing effect associated with urban birth of the older sibling "carries over" to increase the risk of schizophrenia in the next sibling who was born in a rural area (Pedersen and Mortensen 2006). This evidence is compatible with transmission of a germline epimutation associated with the urban environment. For further details on epigenetics in the context of G×E, refer to the article by Oh et al. (this issue).

Gene–Environment Correlation

In contrast to G×E, gene–environment correlation (hereafter rGE) refers to how differences in an individual's genotype can "drive" differential environmental exposure (Fig. 3). In rGE, exposure to environmental events is not a random phenomenon but rather stems (at least partly) from differences in genetic make-up

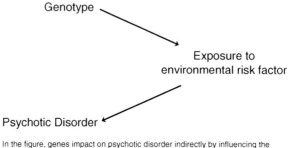

In the figure, genes impact on psychotic disorder indirectly by influencing the probability that an individual becomes exposed to an environmental pathogen.

Fig. 3 Gene × environment correlation: genes controlling environmental exposure

(Plomin et al. 1977). rGEs come in three main forms. *Passive* rGE refers to environmental influences linked to genetic effects external to the person. For example, parents create the early child-rearing environment as well as provide genetic material to their offspring. Passive rGE occurs when parental behaviour, which is partly under genetic control, influences the nature of the early child-rearing environment. Thus, parental genes can exert an influence on the child via the environment, but whose effects are independent of the child itself. In contrast, *Active* rGE (e.g., selection of specific environments or "niche picking") and *Evocative* rGE arise largely as a result of genetic factors nested within the individual (Rutter et al. 2006). Evocative rGE refers to the impact of the child's behaviour on their social environment, in particular the responses they elicit from people around them. One person's preference for sporting activities over another person's penchant for artistic endeavours, thus selecting themselves into different environments, is an example of active rGE, while the different responses elicited from the social environment by gregarious versus shy individuals exemplify evocative rGE. Combining examples of rGE and G×E in one illustrative situation: rGE might manifest as arguments and disagreements preceding marital dissolution, yet G×E may determine who becomes depressed as a result of that relationship breakdown.

Confounding of G × E by rGE

In studies aimed at detecting gene–environment interactions, rGE is noise and must be ruled out. In other words, the "E" in G×E must be shown to be a true environmentally mediated effect rather than a genetic epiphenomenon. For example, does the genetic liability for schizophrenia increase the psychotogenic effect of cannabis or does schizophrenia genetic liability increase the likelihood of *using* cannabis? Experimental paradigms (see below) are able to deal effectively with this problem by randomly assigning participants to the exposed and unexposed conditions. In observational designs, however, confounding by rGE is difficult to rule out but can be tested separately. An interesting example concerns urbanicity and schizophrenia. As discussed below, four independent studies have suggested that the urban environment may contribute to the onset of psychotic disorder in individuals at genetic risk (i.e., evidence for G×E). An alternative explanation, however, is that the genetic liability for schizophrenia increases the likelihood of moving to the big city, i.e., there may be rGE. A priori this is unlikely, given the fact that the effect of urbanicity on schizophrenia is restricted to the window of childhood and adolescence: children do not make the family decision to move to the big city, regardless of whether they are genetically inclined to do so or not. Two twin studies from Australia and the Netherlands on urban mobility support this notion (Whitfield et al. 2005; Willemsen et al. 2005). The Australian study showed more evidence for influence of genetic factors on urban mobility than the Dutch study. However, genetic influence in the Australian study was mostly apparent in older individuals who were well past the age at risk for onset of schizophrenia; environmental factors accounted for most of the variation in younger individuals. The reason for the discrepancy in genetic contribution to urban mobility between the Australian and the Dutch study is likely related to contextual factors. Just as the heritability of alcoholism has been shown to differ as a function of societal availability (severe restriction resulting in alcohol use only by those who are genetically most predisposed), so was the genetic influence on urban mobility shown to vary as a function of base rate of the urban outcome, which was only 10% in Australia versus around 30–50% (very heavy and heavy urbanisation) in the Netherlands. More evidence of genetic influence in Australia therefore may, in part, be the result of the lower base rate of urbanicity. Thus, the conclusion from the Australian and Dutch twin studies is that there are likely only very few human characteristics beyond any genetic influence, including urban mobility. However, in young adulthood, the age range during which psychotic disorder typically declares itself, environmental more than genetic factors may influence exposure to the risk environment that urbanicity represents (van Os 2005), making rGE unlikely.

Another important issue in rGE is that genetic effects on the outcome can be direct or indirect (Fig. 4). For example, genes may have an effect on both the outcome and the environmental exposure, while the environment has no effect on the outcome. In this case, the observed association between the environment and the outcome is genetically confounded (Fig. 4a). On the other hand, genes may have an effect on the environment, but no direct effect on the outcome, as only the environment has a causal effect (Fig. 4b). This is the situation where the environment is on the causal pathway between genes and environment, a situation that can help in providing evidence for a true causal contribution of an environmental factor to disease (Katan 1986) (referred to sometimes as "Mendelian randomisation"; Davey Smith and Ebrahim 2005). For example, evidence in the situation of Fig. 4b of an association between the gene and the outcome can only be explained if there is a true causal relationship between the environmental risk factor and the outcome. Given random assortment of genes from parents to offspring during gamete formation and conception, gene–outcome associations representing gene–causal exposure associations are not generally susceptible to the reverse causation or confounding that may plague conventional observational studies.

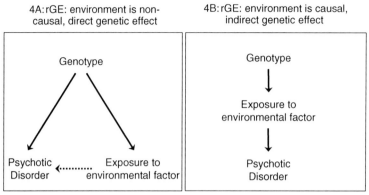

dotted arrow: confounded association

Fig. 4 Gene × environment correlation (rGE): causality of environment

The Environment, Experimental Ecogenetics and Functional Enviromics

The Environment and Psychosis

Here, we refer to the environment broadly as all non-genetic influences that are associated with at least two exposure states. Sometimes, a distinction is made between "biological" and "social" environmental exposures but such a distinction may not be helpful as long as the underlying mechanisms, which are likely overlapping, are not elucidated. There are a number of environmental exposures that are associated with psychotic disorders and symptoms and for which a mechanism of gene–environment interaction has been proposed. These environmental exposures are summarised in Box 1, together with an indication to what degree the evidence for an association with schizophrenia is supported by meta-analytic estimates from systematic reviews. The most solid evidence for an association with schizophrenia and related psychosis outcomes is for paternal age, migration, urbanicity and cannabis use, the latter two particularly in the case of exposure during development.

Environmental Measurement and Experimental Ecogenetics

There are legitimate concerns about how to accurately capture the environmental risk exposure history of participants. This task is particularly challenging when measuring psychosocial risk factors whose negative effects may act cumulatively across long periods of the life course. Equally challenging are the inherent difficulties in precisely measuring "unit exposure" for illicit substances such as cannabis, which can be ingested in different forms, with different THC levels, using different methods. Measuring tobacco intake is comparatively straightforward but even this presents problems with accuracy of recall over long periods.

Box 1 Published Environmental Exposures for Psychosis for which G×E has been Suggested (M+, at least one positive meta-analytic estimate; M+/−, inconclusive meta-analytic estimate; M−, no meta-analytic estimate available)

Environmental variables with likely impact in foetal life:

1. M+: Maternal pregnancy complications, in particular foetal hypoxia and proxies for foetal folate deficiency.
2. M+/−: Prenatal maternal infection, prenatal maternal stress, prenatal maternal folate deficiency.
3. M+: Paternal age.
4. M−: Prenatal exposure to chemical agents (e.g., lead).

Environmental variables with likely impact in early life:

5. M−: Quality of early rearing environment (institutional care, school, parents).
6. M+/−: Childhood trauma (abuse or neglect).

Environmental variables with likely impact in middle childhood/ adolescence:

7. M+: Urban environment during development: a variable indicating the level of population density, or size of a city within a country, of the place where the individual was growing up (between the ages of 5 and 15 years).
8. M+: Cannabis use.
9. M+: Migration.
10. M+/−: Stressful life events.
11. M−: Traumatic brain injury.

Measures of the wider social environment:

12. M−: Neighbourhood measures of social fragmentation, social capital and social deprivation.

Measures of the micro-environment in the flow of daily life:

13. M−: Small daily life stressors, assessed using momentary assessment technology, subtly impacting on affect, salience and reward.

Henquet et al. (2006) have introduced the term "experimental ecogenetics" in human psychosis research to refer to some obvious advantages: (i) randomisation precludes confounding by not only known but, critically, also unknown confounders; (ii) rGE is not an issue if "G" is randomly allocated to "E"; and (iii) it is relatively easy to make the sample size match the required power. In Fig. 5, an example is given of how the association between migration and schizophrenia, and possible genetic moderation thereof, can be examined in the context of an experimental ecogenetic design, by reducing migration to an experimental exposure of "social hostility" and by reducing the psychosis outcome to an experimental outcome of "abnormal salience attribution", and testing the association between exposure and outcome in a genetically sensitive test design.The advent of controlled experiments with virtual reality environments may similarly represent an important asset for the study of environmental exposures (Freeman et al. 2003).

A further issue is that the environment can be conceptualised at many levels that may all be relevant to behavioural phenotypes associated with schizophrenia, varying from minor stressors in the flow of daily life as assessed by momentary assessment technologies (Myin-Germeys et al. 2001) to contextual effects of the wider social environment such as neighbourhood type or ethnic density (Kirkbride et al. 2007; Boydell et al. 2001). Finally, some environmental risks such as "urbanicity" and "ethnicity" are proxies for as-yet unidentified environmental or possibly even partly genetic factors (Pedersen and Mortensen 2006; Selten et al. 2007).

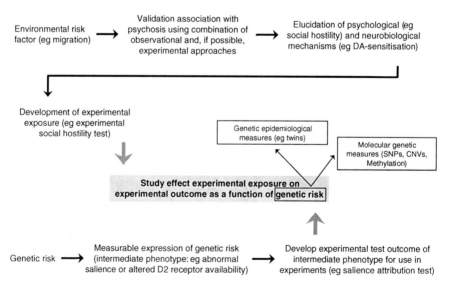

Fig. 5 Development of experimental G × E approaches

Functional Enviromics

Functional enviromics, or the study of the mechanisms underlying environmental impact on the individual to increase the risk for psychopathology, is still in its infancy, with many hypotheses yet to be tested (EU-GEI 2008). These include effects of the environment on (i) developmental programming and adult functional circuits of the brain, (ii) neuroendocrine and neurotransmitter functioning, (iii) patterns of interpersonal interactions that may shape risk for later psychopathology and (iv) affective and cognitive processing (Rutter 2005). Conversely, hypotheses need to be tested about the neural mechanism by which genetic variation may increase susceptibility to environmental stressors. These mechanisms and their underlying pathophysiological pathways need to be clarified in order to develop a priori gene–environment interaction research paradigms (Caspi and Moffitt 2006) (EU-GEI 2008). For example, it has been suggested that there may be synergistic effects of genes and environment in bringing about a "sensitisation" (Featherstone et al. 2007; Tenn et al. 2005) of mesolimbic dopamine neurotransmission (Howes et al. 2004; Collip et al. 2008). This hypothesis is supported by (i) evidence quantifying the impact of stress and dopamine agonist drugs on mesolimbic dopamine release and subsequent sensitisation (Boileau et al. 2006; Arnsten and Goldman Rakic 1998; Covington and Miczek 2001), as well as stress-dopamine agonist cross-sensitisation (Yui et al. 2000; Nikulina et al. 2004; Hamamura and Fibiger 1993); (ii) evidence indicating that genetic risk for schizophrenia is associated with underlying alterations in the dopamine system, including increased dopamine synaptic availability (Hirvonen et al. 2005), increased striatal dopamine synthesis (Huttunen et al. 2008; Meyer-Lindenberg et al. 2002) and increased dopamine reactivity to stress (Brunelin et al. 2008; Myin-Germeys et al. 2005); and (iii) human and animal evidence that effects of environmental risk factors associated with schizophrenia have lasting effects on dopamine neurotransmission including developmental trauma (Hall et al. 1999), defeat stress associated with ethnic minority group (Covington and Miczek 2001; Tidey and Miczek 1996), prenatal hypoxia (Juarez et al. 2003, 2005; Venerosi et al. 2004) and prenatal maternal immune activation (Ozawa et al. 2006) (Meyer et al. 2008).

Thus, although there is evidence to suggest that many other neurotransmitter systems can also be targeted, a case can be made, as an example of functional enviromics, for investigating genetic variation affecting dopamine neurotransmission in interaction with environmental risk factors such as stress and dopamine agonist drugs. Molecular genetic and functional genomic studies focusing on genes associated with dopamine neurotransmission suggest that this gene group may be useful for G×E studies. For example, a recent large study focusing on gene–gene interaction (epistasis) and functional effects suggested that a network of interacting dopaminergic polymorphisms may increase risk for schizophrenia (Talkowski et al. 2008). Evidence for epistasis between genes impacting dopamine signalling can be validated using a neural systems-level intermediate phenotype approach in humans. Recent work of this type, using a prefrontal function fMRI phenotype, similarly suggests epistasis between polymorphisms in genes that control dopamine

signalling (Buckholtz et al. 2007; Meyer-Lindenberg et al. 2006). More specifically, there is evidence that schizophrenia may be characterised by a combination of
prefrontal cortical dysfunction and subcortical dopaminergic disinhibition (Meyer-
Lindenberg et al. 2002). Research has shown that the valine-allele carriers of a functional polymorphism in the catechol-*O*-methyltransferase gene (COMT Val^{158}Met),
an important enzyme regulating prefrontal dopamine turnover, predicted increased
dopamine synthesis in the midbrain, suggesting that this allele may increase the
risk for schizophrenia in interaction with, for example, stress and dopamine agonist
drugs (Meyer-Lindenberg et al. 2005). Several studies suggest that valine-allele carriers may indeed be more sensitive to the psychotogenic effects of drugs of abuse or
stress (Henquet et al. 2006; Caspi et al. 2005; Stefanis et al. 2007).

There are examples of many other avenues that may be explored in functional enviromics. Thus, a recent systematic review suggested that more than 50%
of genes potentially associated with schizophrenia, particularly AKT1, BDNF,
CAPON, CCKAR, CHRNA7, CNR1, COMT, DNTBP1, GAD1, GRM3, IL10,
MLC1, NOTCH4, NRG1, NR4A2/NURR1, PRODH, RELN, RGS4, RTN4/NOGO
and TNF, are subject to regulation by hypoxia and/or are expressed in the vascula-
ture (Schmidt-Kastner et al. 2006). Thus, future studies of genes proposed as candidates for susceptibility to schizophrenia should include their possible regulation
by physiological or pathological hypoxia during development as well as their potential role in gene–environment interactions involving events inducing hypoxia during
early development (Nicodemus et al. 2008).

Epidemiological G×E Studies in Psychosis

Epidemiological Findings

Two robust epidemiological findings suggest that "genes" and "environments" operate interactively to produce schizophrenia. First, there is widespread geographic,
temporal, ethnic and other demographic variation in the incidence of schizophrenia (McGrath et al. 2004; Kirkbride et al. 2006), reinforcing the aetiological role
played by environmental factors. Second, there is marked variability in people's
responses to these environmental risk factors, ranging from obvious vulnerability
to extreme resilience. This well-recognised heterogeneity in response points to the
operation of G×E. A number of studies have examined G×E using indirect measures of genetic risk, such as being a relative, a twin or adopted away offspring
of a person with schizophrenia, or the level of psychometric psychosis proneness
in a person as an expression of distributed genetic risk for psychotic disorder (see
below). The advantage of these studies is that the measure of genetic risk, while
non-specific and therefore not able to capture gene–environment interactions with
very specific mechanisms, is nevertheless (i) well validated and (ii) represents the
complete net genetic load including all gene–gene interactions. While newer studies
using direct molecular genetic measures of genetic risk have the advantage of using

specific measures, they are also prone to false-positive findings, given the enormous amount of molecular genetic variation that can be used for G×E modelling, and the absence of all other factors influencing genetic risk in the model of G×E using a small contribution to genetic variation in the form of an SNP. Therefore, epidemiological studies using indirect measures of genetic risk remain useful and may point the way to G×E studies using direct measures of genetic risk; to date, they remain the most informative. A review of these findings is presented here.

Findings from Twin, Adoption and Family Studies

Twin and adoption studies provide strong but non-specific evidence for the involvement of both genes and environmental factors in the aetiology of schizophrenia (Gottesman and Shields 1976). Both have shown moderate-to-high heritability for schizophrenia but even monozygotic twins show only 50% concordance, underscoring the likelihood of environmental influences and G×E synergism for producing psychotic symptoms and disorder (Van Os and Sham 2003). Findings from several adoption studies are consistent with G×E in the development of psychotic disorders. For example, Carter et al. (2002) compared, in a 25-year longitudinal study, 212 children of schizophrenic mothers with 99 children of normal parents in terms of exposure to environmental risk (i.e., institutional care and family instability). Very few cases of psychosis were identified in those families without a history of schizophrenia but, among those with a family history, strong environmental effects were observed. Consistent with this, Tienari et al. (2004) compared adopted-away offspring ($N = 145$) of mothers with a history of psychotic illness with those without illness ($N = 158$). Measures of the rearing environment in the adoptive home were obtained (measures on scales of "critical/conflictual", "constricted" and "boundary problems") and revealed strong effects for those with a biological predisposition (odds ratio around 10), which were absent in those with low genetic risk (odds ratio around 1).

Findings in support of G×E also come from migration designs, which, for example, have demonstrated a higher risk of psychosis among Caribbean immigrants to the United Kingdom compared to the majority population in the United Kingdom (Cantor-Graae and Selten 2005). Further, family studies of UK-born Afro-Caribbeans have demonstrated a particularly high risk of schizophrenia among the siblings of young, Afro-Caribbean patients (15.9% compared to 1.8% in siblings of white patients), whereas the rates of schizophrenia among the white and Afro-Caribbean parents were similar (8.4 and 8.9%, respectively) (Sugarman and Craufurd 1994).

Studies Using a Psychometric Psychosis Liability Approach

Subtle subclinical expression of psychosis can be measured in the general population (Van Os et al. 2000). There is evidence that this phenotype of "psychometric psychosis proneness" represents in part the distributed genetic risk for psychotic disorder, suggesting it could be used as a proxy to represent the factor "G" in studies of $G \times E$, although to the degree that environmental factors contribute to the psychometric psychosis proneness measure these cannot be excluded as a source of confounding. Thus, Vollema et al. (2002)Vollema and colleagues reported that scores on the positive dimension of a schizotypy questionnaire administered to relatives of patients with psychotic disorders corresponded to their genetic risk of psychosis. Fanous et al. (2001) demonstrated that interview-based positive and negative symptoms in schizophrenia predicted their equivalent subclinical symptom dimensions in non-psychotic relatives, implying an aetiological continuum between the subclinical and the clinical psychosis phenotypes. Kendler and Hewitt (1992) studied twins from the general population and concluded that the variance in most self-reported schizotypy scales, except for perceptual aberration, involved substantial genetic contributions. MacDonald et al. (2001) found in their general population-based twin study only one common schizotypy factor, mainly explained by perceptual aberration, magical ideation, schizotypal cognitions and, to a lesser extent, social anhedonia. The common schizotypy factor was influenced by shared environmental, non-shared environmental and possibly genetic effects. Recently, a general population female twin study by Linney et al. (2003) showed that additive genetic and unique environmental effects influenced self-reported psychotic experiences. The multivariate structural equation model generated two independent latent factors, namely a positive (i.e., cognitive disorganisation, unusual experiences and delusional ideation) and a negative dimension (i.e., cognitive disorganisation and introvertive anhedonia), suggesting different aetiological mechanisms for the various scales of the subclinical psychosis phenotype. In a recent, general population study using both self-reported and interview-based measures of positive and negative dimensions of psychotic experiences in 257 subjects belonging to 82 families, significant family-specific variations for both positive and negative subclinical psychosis dimensions were demonstrated, with between-family proportions of total variance between 10 and 40%. Thus, both the positive and the negative dimensions of subclinical psychosis show familial clustering in samples unselected for psychiatric disease (Hanssen et al. 2006). Operationalising the genetic effect "G" along these lines, Henquet et al. (2005) showed that a psychometric measure of psychosis proneness interacted with cannabis use to predict the likelihood of developing psychotic symptoms. In this study, rGE was unlikely to have been a confounder since no association between baseline psychosis proneness and subsequent use of cannabis was observed. Nonetheless, confounding cannot be ruled out entirely because the proxy genetic measure of psychometric psychosis proneness will also be influenced by environmental factors. As a complement to the observational designs described above, Verdoux et al. (2003) used a quasi-experimental "experience sampling" method, and obtained similar findings showing that psychosis liability moderated the effect of cannabis in terms of "switching on" psychotic symptoms in the flow of daily life. For more details on possible gene × cannabis interactions, we refer to the article by Henquet et al. (this issue). Other studies using psychometric psychosis liability as a proxy measure for genetic risk were able to demonstrate $G \times E$

with childhood urbanicity (Spauwen et al. 2006a) (see below for more details) and childhood trauma (Spauwen et al. 2006b).

Summary of Epidemiological G×E Studies to Date

In Table 1, the different epidemiological G×E studies are summarised. For each study, the proxy genetic factor, the proxy environmental factor and the main findings as well as main limitations are summarised. Environmental exposures used in G×E studies include migration, urbanicity, obstetric complications, cannabis, stress, developmental trauma and others. In most studies, the effect of genes and environment alone was rather small, and the bulk of their effect mediated through gene–environment interactions.

Epidemiological Replications of Gene–Urbanicity Interaction

The finding that the rate of psychotic disorder is higher in children and adolescents growing up in an urban environment is well replicated (Krabbendam and van Os 2005) and unlikely to be confounded entirely by rGE due to selective drift to urban areas in those at genetic risk for psychosis (Van Os 2004; Pedersen and Mortensen 2001), although rGE may operate to some degree (Pedersen and Mortensen 2006; Selten et al. 2007) as it will in the case of many environmental risks (van Os et al. 2005). "Urbanicity" is a proxy for an as-yet unidentified environmental factor(s) prevalent in urban areas and, if causal, may contribute to up to 20–30% of the incidence of psychotic disorder in some countries (Van Os 2004). For this reason, urbanicity is an interesting factor to study in the context of G×E. Four studies in the Netherlands, Germany, Israel and Denmark have attempted to examine gene–urbanicity interactions using epidemiological designs and indirect measures of genetic risk (Spauwen et al. 2006; Van Os et al. 2003, 2004; Weiser et al. 2007). All studies found evidence for gene–urbanicity interaction and are summarised in Table 2. Clearly, the possibility of interaction between an environmental exposure in urban areas and genetic risk is in need of further study, focusing on (i) the precise nature of the urban exposure, for example, growing up in an area lacking in trust and cohesion, (ii) the psychological and neurobiological mechanism of the environmental exposure in order to develop rational hypotheses about gene–environment interaction, (iii) the nature of the genetic variation involved, and ultimately (iv) the mechanism of the gene–environment interactions.

Future Prospects

To date, the study of gene–environment interactions has largely been epidemiological, where genotype, risk exposure and disorder are studied as they occur in the population (Khoury et al. 2004). A key contribution of a robust G×E comes from

Table 1 First-generation studies of proxy gene–environment interaction in psychotic disorder

Proxy genetic variable	Proxy environmental variable	Findings	Remarks
Positive family history (FH)	Ethnic group	Familial morbid risk for psychotic disorder higher in siblings of African-Caribbean probands than in those of white probands (Sugarman and Craufurd 1994; Hutchinson et al. 1996)	➤ May be informative; however, preferably environmental exposure status and clinical status are measured in both cases *and* all first-degree relatives and analyses are adjusted for age, sex and number of relatives ➤ Level of misclassification may be high because many unaffected relatives may carry the high-risk genotype ➤ *Absence* of an association between positive family history and environmental exposure does *not* rule out gene–environment interaction, and *presence* of an association does not rule out *lack* of gene–environment interaction (Marcelis et al. 1998) ➤ Evidence can be considered stronger if replicated (e.g., urbanicity findings) ➤ Testing for interaction on additive scale likely more informative (Darroch 1997)
	Urban birth	No association between urban birth and a positive family history for psychotic disorder (Mortensen et al. 1999); however, interaction was tested on multiplicative rather than additive scale (see below)	
	Obstetric complications	Mostly inconclusive findings with regard to family history (Nimgaonkar et al. 1988; Kunugi et al. 1996; O'Callaghan et al. 1992)	
	Birth in winter/spring	Positive, negative and inconclusive associations with family history (Baron and Gruen 1988; Shur 1982; Pulver et al. 1992; Dassa et al. 1996)	
	Stressful life events	Positive association with family history (Van Os et al. 1994)	
	Urbanicity	Evidence for synergism between urban environment (proxy environmental risk) and family history (proxy genetic risk) when tested on additive scale (Van Os et al. 2003)	

Table 1 (continued)

Proxy genetic variable	Proxy environmental variable	Findings	Remarks
Having an identical twin with psychotic disorder	Being discordant for psychotic disorder	Children of both affected and non-affected twin in discordant pair have higher rate of psychotic disorder (Kringlen and Cramer 1989; Fischer 1971; Gottesman and Bertelsen 1989)	⋏ Suggests environmental factor is necessary for the expression of high-risk genotype in affected twin or inhibition of protective genotype in unaffected twin
Biological parent with psychotic disorder	Growing up in dysfunctional adoptive family environment	Risk of psychotic disorder spectrum disorder or psychotic disorder-associated thought disorder higher in high-risk adoptees who had been brought up in dysfunctional adoptive family environment (Tienari et al. 2004, 1994; Wahlberg et al. 1997, 2004).	⋏ Risk of psychotic disorder spectrum disorder 3% in the absence of environmental risk and 62% in the presence of environmental risk. This difference seems extremely high ⋏ Children destined to develop psychotic disorder may have contributed to dysfunctional family environment rather than the other way round
	Institutional care, family instability	Very few cases of psychosis were identified in those families without a history of psychotic disorder but, among those with a family history, strong environmental effects were observed (Carter et al. 2002)	⋏ Case–control comparison difficult as many other factors may be involved

Table 1 (continued)

Proxy genetic variable	Proxy environmental variable	Findings	Remarks
	Having positive relationships with father and mother	High-risk children with positive parental relationships had lower risk for developing psychotic disorder (Carter et al. 1999)	➤ May suggest a negative G×E
Having neither, one or two parents with psychotic disorder	Obstetric complications	The greater the proxy genetic risk, the greater the effect of obstetric complications, in particular foetal hypoxia, on ventricular enlargement (the psychotic disorder endophenotype) (Cannon et al. 1993, 2002)	➤ Genetic risk may increase the risk of obstetric complication (rGE). ➤ Genetic risk may increase the risk of heavy alcohol consumption or head injury resulting in greater OC effect sizes
Having a parent with psychotic disorder and additionally having an electrodermal abnormality as a child	Paternal absence	Higher rate of paternal absence in children who subsequently developed psychotic disorder (Walker 1981)	➤ Status of electrodermal abnormality as a marker of genetic risk for psychotic disorder unclear
Having an MZ twin with psychotic disorder	Sharing the same chorion with the co-twin	Concordance rate was higher for MZ twins whose marker suggested they were monochorionic than those whose marker indicated they were dichorionic (Davis and Phelps 1995)	➤ These results are compatible with an environmental factor in the prenatal environment facilitating expression of genetic risk for psychotic disorder

Table 1 (continued)

Proxy genetic variable	Proxy environmental variable	Findings	Remarks
Having expression of genetically influenced psychometric psychosis liability	Early trauma	Evidence that trauma and psychometric psychosis liability synergistically increase the risk for psychosis persistence over time (Spauwen et al. 2006)	⋏ Difficult to disentangle rGE from G×E ⋏ Psychometric psychosis liability very indirect measure of genetic risk
	Cannabis use	Evidence that cannabis and psychometric psychosis liability synergistically increase the risk for psychosis persistence over time (Henquet et al. 2005; see also Verdoux et al. 2003)	
	Growing up in urban environment	Evidence that urbanicity and psychometric psychosis liability synergistically increase the risk for psychosis persistence over time (Spauwen et al. 2006)	

Table 1 (continued)

Proxy genetic variable	Proxy environmental variable	Findings	Remarks
Being a member of a schizophrenia pedigree	Traumatic brain injury	Within the schizophrenia pedigrees but not bipolar pedigrees, traumatic brain injury was associated with a greater risk of schizophrenia, consistent with synergistic effects between genetic vulnerability for schizophrenia and traumatic brain injury	➢ Similar comments as for positive family history
None	Having an older father	Having an older father is associated with an increased risk of schizophrenia in the offspring (Malaspina et al. 2001; Zammit et al. 2003; Byrne et al. 2003; Sipos et al. 2004)	➢ The underlying mechanism of this association may represent a special case of gene–environment interaction whereby the environment impacts on DNA sequence (de novo mutation) or DNA methylation (affecting gene expression). Thus, age of the father is a variable that is partly under control from the sociocultural environment, and older age may have an effect on DNA methylation in sex cells (the inherited methylation pattern in humans is maintained in somatic cells but is erased and re-established late in spermatogenesis for paternally imprinted genes, a process that could become impaired as age advances). Alternatively, advanced paternal age may lead to an increased rate of de novo mutations in gametes

Table 2 Studies of gene–urbanicity interactions

Study	Country	Measure genetic risk	Measure urbanicity	Psychosis outcome	Rate unexposed[a]	Rate E[b]	Rate G[c]	Rate GE[d]
Van Os et al. (2003)	The Netherlands	Family history psychosis	Population density – dichotomous	Psychotic disorder	0.85%	1.59%	3.01%	9.72%
Van Os et al. (2004)	Denmark	Family history psychotic disorder	Five categories from capital city to rural area – five levels	Psychotic disorder	Summary increase in incidence associated with urbanicity in individuals WITHOUT family history: 0.054%		Summary increase in incidence associated with urbanicity in individuals WITH family history: 0.22%	
Spauwen et al. (2006)	Germany	Psychometric psychosis liability	City of Munich versus surrounding villages – dichotomous	Psychotic symptoms	14.2%	12.1%	14.9%	29%
Weiser et al. (2007)	Israel	Cognitive impairment endophenotype	Population density – five levels	Psychotic disorder	Summary increase in incidence associated with urbanicity in cognitively non-vulnerable group: 0.011%		Summary increase in incidence associated with urbanicity in cognitively vulnerable group: 0.10%	

[a]Those exposed to neither urbanicity nor genetic risk.
[b]Those exposed to urbanicity only.
[c]Those exposed to genetic risk only.
[d]Those exposed to both urbanicity and genetic risk.

knowing that three apparently unconnected factors (gene, environmental risk factor and disorder) are in fact causally linked (Moffitt et al. 2005). However, there are a number of methodological concerns that continue to challenge genetic-epidemiological research, mainly because observational methods struggle to achieve the degree of control that is possible using experimental designs (EU-GEI 2008; Caspi and Moffitt 2006). Concerns are listed below.

The Ideal Sample Size for G×E Research

Clearly the optimal sample size required to detect G×E will vary according to the design used. For example, case–control studies will generally require very large sample sizes simply because the genetic effects are expected to be small. However, even with prospective cohort studies, large sample sizes may be required when the environmental risk factor(s) and/or disorder of interest occur at low frequencies. However, large sample sizes are not always necessary, or desirable given the costs of amassing large samples. Indeed, sample size requirements can be substantially reduced with high-quality measurement of environmental risk factors, especially when measures are repeated over time (Wong et al. 2003); in particular, the use of momentary assessment technologies with many repeated measures holds promise for the detection of subtle gene–environment interactions (Myin-Germeys et al. 2001; Wichers et al. 2007a, b). Other methods to reduce sample size, based on selection of extreme exposure groups, may also apply (Boks et al. 2007).

Biostatistics

It is likely that mass genome-wide molecular genetic approaches, "enriched" with a few measures of "environmental" exposures, will create invalid and confusing findings, largely because of the extent of multiple testing and the opportunities for post hoc analyses afforded by such studies. It is of paramount importance to consider the study of G×E as a separate discipline, requiring a highly specialised and multidisciplinary approach taking both environment and genes seriously. A hypothesis-driven strategy focusing on final common pathways in which biological synergism between genetic and environmental mechanisms takes place, fed by information from functional enviromics and functional genomics pointing to promising neural systems and processes, may constitute the most productive approach. In combination, this will enable a translational approach for systematically studying the effect of environmental manipulations on neural systems linked to genetic risk for schizophrenia. However, even a hypothesis-driven approach is likely to face major challenges in the area of biostatistics. Even allowing for, as discussed earlier, the major problem of how to bridge the gap between statistical interaction (statistical manipulations of data) and biological synergism (biological processes in nature), which currently cannot be estimated directly (Van Os and Sham 2003), solutions to, for example, modelling multiple ambiguous haplotype × environment interactions need to be developed (Lake et al. 2003). Fortunately, software allowing for modelling complicated interactions is currently being incorporated in several statistical programs (Li and Stephens 2003; Lange et al. 2004).

Which Endophenotypes to Study?

In order to elucidate converging pathways that are the site of biological synergism between genes and environments, a wide range of approaches employing intermediate (or endo-) phenotypes may be used. For example, one may focus on the domain of neural systems-level intermediate phenotypes (Meyer-Lindenberg et al. 2006; Murray et al. 2008; Barkus et al. 2007), cognition (Filbey et al. 2008; Toulopoulou et al. 2007; Barnett et al. 2007a, b; Bombin et al. 2008), neuroanatomy (van Haren et al. 2008; Boos et al. 2007; Marcelis et al. 2003), salience attribution (Jensen et al. 2008; Kapur 2003), treatment response (Arranz and de Leon 2007), measures of course and outcome (Verdoux et al. 1996), subclinical psychosis expression (Stefanis et al. 2004; Schurhoff et al. 2003, 2007), neurotic symptoms (Zinkstok et al. 2008) and dynamic cerebral phenotypes in early-onset groups (Arango et al. 2008). The appeal of studying endophenotypes is obvious in that, compared to clinical diagnoses which are often characterised by substantial heterogeneity, endophenotypes appear to be cleaner, simpler constituents of psychopathology and (maybe falsely) promise improved chances of detecting true gene effects. Nonetheless, questions remain about which endophenotypes, for which disorder, are most worthy of study in a G×E framework. One argument against the use of endophenotypes is their apparently lower heritability estimates than the clinical phenotype (Greenwood et al. 2007). Although at first glance this may seem a valid argument, lower heritability estimates are only to be expected if endophenotypes reflect the "pure" contribution of genes and the clinical phenotype additionally represents the contribution of gene–environment interactions. The reason for this is that heritability estimates are derived from genetic epidemiological studies that estimate simple genetic and simple environmental contributions to schizophrenia liability. Unfortunately, these studies do not model the contribution of gene–environment interactions (G×E), because researchers tend to not include direct measures of the environment in such studies, thus precluding the quantification of gene–environment interactions. Therefore, the heritability of schizophrenia may be 80%, but simulations show that gene–environment interactions may make up the bulk of this proportion (Van Os and Sham 2003). Thus, endophenotypes may be more suitable measures of "pure" genetic risk, as heritability estimates of the clinical disorder may be inflated by gene–environment interactions. Further research on this issue is needed.

Multiple Tests

As mentioned earlier, there are legitimate concerns about low prior probability testing for associations between a large number of polymorphisms (for example, via

SNP chips) and specific disorders in the absence of some guiding theory that will allow researchers to sort true from false-positive associations. Guarding against "fishing trips" is important if we are to advance our understanding of how G×E operates in the development of schizophrenia.

Conclusion

Not only is there meta-analytic support for environmental effects on schizophrenia risk, evidence is now accumulating that environmental exposures are impacting on the risk for psychotic disorder in co-participation with genetic factors and that effects of genes and environment in isolation are likely small or non-existent.

Embracing a G×E approach has implications for gene discovery. That is, selecting and/or stratifying samples based on documented environmental risk exposure may help not only in the quest to identify new susceptibility genes for psychotic disorders but also in unravelling the pathway(s) to the onset of first-episode psychosis. For molecular genetic research, this means that the strategy of "brute force" (Collier 2008), used to compensate for loss of power due to underlying G×E by inclusion of huge samples of many thousands of patients and hundreds of thousands of markers along the genome, may be complemented by imaginative approaches based on environmental stratification. Genetic odds ratio of 1.1 in non-stratified samples may be considerably higher in exposed samples. In addition, distal tiny genetic contributions by themselves explain little if more proximal interactions with environmental component causes, explaining the underlying pathophysiology.

It is obvious that more funding needs to be directed to G×E research – after nearly 1,500 inconclusive molecular genetic investigations in schizophrenia complementary approaches no longer need to be excluded. The European Network of Schizophrenia Networks for the Study of Gene–Environment Interactions (EU-GEI) (EU-GEI 2008) has suggested that part of the funding may be necessary to bring together the multitude of disciplines, currently working in isolation of each other, which is necessary for the study of gene–environment interactions.

Future research needs to better integrate epidemiological and experimental paradigms focusing on functional enviromics and functional genomics (Caspi and Moffitt 2006; EU-GEI 2008). This is desirable because neither traditional genetic epidemiology nor epidemiologic studies on isolated environmental factors can tell us much about the biological mechanisms involved in a G×E. These approaches are complementary, with each informing the other, and ideally should be used in unison for best effect. Many (but by no means all) of the challenges confronting genetic epidemiology listed above can be addressed using experimental designs with their advantages of greater experimental control and precision. However, these benefits have to be balanced against the loss of ecological validity that can sometimes result.

Epidemiologists should be encouraged to incorporate more physiological (i.e., mechanistic) measures in their studies and to move beyond two-way interactions to models involving multiple genes and environments, as well as gene–gene and environment–environment interactions.

Acknowledgment Parts of this chapter appeared as: van Os, J., Poulton, R. (2008). Environmental vulnerability and genetic-environmental interactions. In: *The Recognition and Management of Early Psychosis: A Preventive Approach*, 2nd edition (eds. H. Jackson and P. McGorry). Cambridge University Press: Cambridge; van Os J, Rutten BP, Poulton R. Gene-environment interactions in schizophrenia: review of epidemiological findings and future directions. Schizophrenia Bulletin 34:1066–1082, 2009.

References

Arango C, Moreno C, Martinez S, Parellada M, Desco M, Moreno D, Fraguas D, Gogtay N, James A, Rapoport J. (2008). Longitudinal brain changes in early-onset psychosis. Schizophr Bull 34:341–53.

Arnsten AF, Goldman Rakic PS. (1998). Noise stress impairs prefrontal cortical cognitive function in monkeys: evidence for a hyperdopaminergic mechanism. Arch Gen Psychiatry 55: 362–8.

Arranz MJ, de Leon J. (2007). Pharmacogenetics and pharmacogenomics of schizophrenia: a review of last decade of research. Mol Psychiatry 12:707–47.

Barkus E, Stirling J, Hopkins R, McKie S, Lewis S. (2007). Cognitive and neural processes in non-clinical auditory hallucinations. Br J Psychiatry Suppl 51:s76–s81.

Barnett JH, Heron J, Ring SM, Golding J, Goldman D, Xu K, Jones PB. (2007b). Gender-specific effects of the catechol-*O*-methyltransferase Val108/158Met polymorphism on cognitive function in children. Am J Psychiatry 164:142–9.

Barnett JH, Jones PB, Robbins TW, Muller U. (2007a). Effects of the catechol-*O*-methyltransferase Val158Met polymorphism on executive function: a meta-analysis of the Wisconsin Card Sort Test in schizophrenia and healthy controls. Mol Psychiatry 12:502–9.

Baron M, Gruen R. (1988). Risk factors in schizophrenia. Season of birth and family history [see comments]. Br J Psychiatry 152:460–5.

Boileau I, Dagher A, Leyton M, Gunn RN, Baker GB, Diksic M, Benkelfat C. (2006). Modeling sensitization to stimulants in humans: an [11C]raclopride/positron emission tomography study in healthy men. Arch Gen Psychiatry 63:1386–95.

Boks MP, Schipper M, Schubart CD, Sommer IE, Kahn RS, Ophoff RA. (2007). Investigating gene environment interaction in complex diseases: increasing power by selective sampling for environmental exposure. Int J Epidemiol 36:1363–9.

Bombin I, Arango C, Mayoral M, Castro-Fornieles J, Gonzalez-Pinto A, Gonzalez-Gomez C, Moreno D, Parellada M, Baeza I, Graell M, Otero S, Saiz PA, Patino-Garcia A. (2008). DRD3, but not COMT or DRD2, genotype affects executive functions in healthy and first-episode psychosis adolescents. Am J Med Genet B Neuropsychiatr Genet 147:873–9.

Boos HB, Aleman A, Cahn W, Pol HH, Kahn RS. (2007). Brain volumes in relatives of patients with schizophrenia: a meta-analysis. Arch Gen Psychiatry 64:297–304.

Boydell J, van Os J, McKenzie K, Allardyce J, Goel R, McCreadie RG, Murray RM. (2001). Incidence of schizophrenia in ethnic minorities in London: ecological study into interactions with environment. BMJ 323:1336–8.

Brunelin J, d'Amato T, van Os J, Cochet A, Suaud-Chagny MF, Saoud M. (2008). Effects of acute metabolic stress on the dopaminergic and pituitary–adrenal axis activity in patients with schizophrenia, their unaffected siblings and controls. Schizophr Res 100:206–211.

Buckholtz JW, Sust S, Tan HY, Mattay VS, Straub RE, Meyer-Lindenberg A, Weinberger DR, Callicott JH. (2007). fMRI evidence for functional epistasis between COMT and RGS4. Mol Psychiatry 12:893–5, 885.

Byrne M, Agerbo E, Ewald H, Eaton WW, Mortensen PB. (2003). Parental age and risk of schizophrenia: a case–control study. Arch Gen Psychiatry 60:673–8.

Canli T, Lesch KP. (2007). Long story short: the serotonin transporter in emotion regulation and social cognition. Nat Neurosci 10:1103–9.

Cannon M, Clarke MC. (2005). Risk for schizophrenia – broadening the concepts, pushing back the boundaries. Schizophr Res 79:5–13.

Cannon TD, Mednick SA, Parnas J, Schulsinger F, Praestholm J, Vestergaard A. (1993). Developmental brain abnormalities in the offspring of schizophrenic mothers. I. Contributions of genetic and perinatal factors [see comments]. Arch Gen Psychiatry 50:551–64.

Cannon TD, van Erp TG, Rosso IM, Huttunen M, Lonnqvist J, Pirkola T, Salonen O, Valanne L, Poutanen VP, Standertskjold-Nordenstam CG. (2002). Fetal hypoxia and structural brain abnormalities in schizophrenic patients, their siblings, and controls. Arch Gen Psychiatry 59: 35–41.

Cantor-Graae E, Selten JP. (2005). Schizophrenia and migration: a meta-analysis and review. Am J Psychiatry 162:12–24.

Carter JW, Parnas J, Cannon TD, Schulsinger F, Mednick SA. (1999). MMPI variables predictive of schizophrenia in the Copenhagen High-Risk Project: a 25-year follow-up. Acta Psychiatr Scand 99:432–40.

Carter JW, Schulsinger F, Parnas J, Cannon T, Mednick SA. (2002). A multivariate prediction model of schizophrenia. Schizophr Bull 28:649–82.

Caspi A, Moffitt TE, Cannon M, McClay J, Murray R, Harrington H, Taylor A, Arseneault L, Williams B, Braithwaite A, Poulton R, Craig IW. (2005). Moderation of the effect of adolescent-onset cannabis use on adult psychosis by a functional polymorphism in the catechol-O-methyltransferase gene: longitudinal evidence of a gene × environment interaction. Biol Psychiatry 57:1117–27.

Caspi A, Moffitt TE. (2006). Gene–environment interactions in psychiatry: joining forces with neuroscience. Nat Rev Neurosci 7:583–90.

Caspi A, Sugden K, Moffitt TE, Taylor A, Craig IW, Harrington H, McClay J, Mill J, Martin J, Braithwaite A, Poulton R. (2003). Influence of life stress on depression: moderation by a polymorphism in the 5-HTT gene. Science 301:386–9.

Champoux M, Bennett A, Shannon C, Higley JD, Lesch KP, Suomi SJ. (2002). Serotonin transporter gene polymorphism, differential early rearing, and behavior in rhesus monkey neonates. Mol Psychiatry 7:1058–63.

Colhoun HM, McKeigue PM, Davey Smith G. (2003). Problems of reporting genetic associations with complex outcomes. Lancet 361:865–72.

Collier DA. (2008). Schizophrenia: the polygene princess and the pea. Psychol Med 1–5.

Collip D, Myin-Germeys I, Van Os J. (2008). Does the concept of "sensitization" provide a plausible mechanism for the putative link between the environment and schizophrenia? Schizophr Bull 34:220–5.

Covington HE, 3rd, Miczek KA. (2001). Repeated social-defeat stress, cocaine or morphine. Effects on behavioral sensitization and intravenous cocaine self-administration "binges". Psychopharmacology (Berl) 158:388–98.

Crow TJ. (2008). The emperors of the schizophrenia polygene have no clothes. Psychol Med 1–5.

Darroch J. (1997). Biologic synergism and parallelism [see comments]. Am J Epidemiol 145: 661–8.

Dassa D, Sham PC, Van Os J, Abel K, Jones P, Murray RM. (1996). Relationship of birth season to clinical features, family history, and obstetric complication in schizophrenia. Psychiatry Res 64:11–7.

Davey Smith G, Ebrahim S. (2005). What can mendelian randomisation tell us about modifiable behavioural and environmental exposures? BMJ 330:1076–9.

Davis JO, Phelps JA. (1995). Twins with schizophrenia: genes or germs? Schizophr Bull 21:13–8.

EU-GEI. (2008). European Network of Schizophrenia Networks for the Study of Gene Environment Interactions. Schizophrenia aetiology: do gene–environment interactions hold the key? Schizophr Res 102:21–6.

Fanous A, Gardner C, Walsh D, Kendler KS. (2001). Relationship between positive and negative symptoms of schizophrenia and schizotypal symptoms in nonpsychotic relatives. Arch Gen Psychiatry 58:669–673.

Featherstone RE, Kapur S, Fletcher PJ. (2007). The amphetamine-induced sensitized state as a model of schizophrenia. Prog Neuropsychopharmacol Biol Psychiatry 31:1556–71.

Filbey FM, Toulopoulou T, Morris RG, McDonald C, Bramon E, Walshe M, Murray RM. (2008). Selective attention deficits reflect increased genetic vulnerability to schizophrenia. Schizophr Res 101:169–75.

Fischer M. (1971). Psychoses in the offspring of schizophrenic monozygotic twins and their normal co-twins. Br J Psychiatry 118:43–52.

Flint J. (1992). Implications of genomic imprinting for psychiatric genetics. Psychol Med 22:5–10.

Freeman D, Slater M, Bebbington PE, Garety PA, Kuipers E, Fowler D, Met A, Read CM, Jordan J, Vinayagamoorthy V. (2003). Can virtual reality be used to investigate persecutory ideation? J Nerv Ment Dis 191:509–14.

Gottesman, II, Bertelsen A. (1989). Confirming unexpressed genotypes for schizophrenia. Risks in the offspring of Fischer's Danish identical and fraternal discordant twins [see comments]. Arch Gen Psychiatry 46:867–72.

Gottesman, II, Shields J. (1976). A critical review of recent adoption, twin, and family studies of schizophrenia: behavioral genetics perspectives. Schizophr Bull 2:360–401.

Greenwood TA, Braff DL, Light GA, Cadenhead KS, Calkins ME, Dobie DJ, Freedman R, Green MF, Gur RE, Gur RC, Mintz J, Nuechterlein KH, Olincy A, Radant AD, Seidman LJ, Siever LJ, Silverman JM, Stone WS, Swerdlow NR, Tsuang DW, Tsuang MT, Turetsky BI, Schork NJ. (2007). Initial heritability analyses of endophenotypic measures for schizophrenia: the consortium on the genetics of schizophrenia. Arch Gen Psychiatry 64:1242–50.

Hall FS, Wilkinson LS, Humby T, Robbins TW. (1999). Maternal deprivation of neonatal rats produces enduring changes in dopamine function. Synapse 32:37–43.

Hamamura T, Fibiger HC. (1993). Enhanced stress-induced dopamine release in the prefrontal cortex of amphetamine-sensitized rats. Eur J Pharmacol 237:65–71.

Hamer D. (2002). Genetics. Rethinking behavior genetics. Science 298:71–2.

Hanssen M, Krabbendam L, Vollema M, Delespaul P, Van Os J. (2006). Evidence for instrument and family-specific variation of subclinical psychosis dimensions in the general population. J Abnorm Psychol 115:5–14.

Harrison PJ, Weinberger DR. (2005). Schizophrenia genes, gene expression, and neuropathology: on the matter of their convergence. Mol Psychiatry 10:40–68; image 5.

Henquet C, Krabbendam L, Spauwen J, Kaplan C, Lieb R, Wittchen HU, van Os J. (2005). Prospective cohort study of cannabis use, predisposition for psychosis, and psychotic symptoms in young people. BMJ 330:11.

Henquet C, Rosa A, Krabbendam L, Papiol S, Fananas L, Drukker M, Ramaekers JG, van Os J. (2006). An experimental study of catechol-o-methyltransferase Val158Met moderation of delta-9-tetrahydrocannabinol-induced effects on psychosis and cognition. Neuropsychopharmacology 31:2748–57.

Hirvonen J, van Erp TG, Huttunen J, Aalto S, Nagren K, Huttunen M, Lonnqvist J, Kaprio J, Hietala J, Cannon TD. (2005). Increased caudate dopamine D2 receptor availability as a genetic marker for schizophrenia. Arch Gen Psychiatry 62:371–8.

Howes OD, McDonald C, Cannon M, Arseneault L, Boydell J, Murray RM. (2004). Pathways to schizophrenia: the impact of environmental factors. Int J Neuropsychopharmacol 7(Suppl 1):S7–S13.

Hutchinson G, Takei N, Fahy TA, Bhugra D, Gilvarry C, Moran P, Mallett R, Sham P, Leff J, Murray RM. (1996). Morbid risk of schizophrenia in first-degree relatives of white and African-Caribbean patients with psychosis. Br J Psychiatry 169:776–80.

Huttunen J, Heinimaa M, Svirskis T, Nyman M, Kajander J, Forsback S, Solin O, Ilonen T, Korkeila J, Ristkari T, McGlashan T, Salokangas RK, Hietala J. (2008). Striatal dopamine synthesis in first-degree relatives of patients with schizophrenia. Biol Psychiatry 63:114–7.

Jacobs N, Kenis G, Peeters F, Derom C, Vlietinck R, van Os J. (2006). Stress-related negative affectivity and genetically altered serotonin transporter function: evidence of synergism in shaping risk of depression. Arch Gen Psychiatry 63:989–96.

Jensen J, Willeit M, Zipursky RB, Savina I, Smith AJ, Menon M, Crawley AP, Kapur S. (2008). The formation of abnormal associations in schizophrenia: neural and behavioral evidence. Neuropsychopharmacology 33:473–9.

Juarez I, De La Cruz F, Zamudio S, Flores G. (2005). Cesarean plus anoxia at birth induces hyperresponsiveness to locomotor activity by dopamine D2 agonist. Synapse 58: 236–42.

Juarez I, Silva-Gomez AB, Peralta F, Flores G. (2003). Anoxia at birth induced hyperresponsiveness to amphetamine and stress in postpubertal rats. Brain Res 992:281–7.

Kapur S. (2003). Psychosis as a state of aberrant salience: a framework linking biology, phenomenology, and pharmacology in schizophrenia. Am J Psychiatry 160:13–23.

Katan MB. (1986). Apolipoprotein E isoforms, serum cholesterol, and cancer. Lancet 1:507–8.

Kendler KS, Eaves LJ. (1986). Models for the joint effect of genotype and environment on liability to psychiatric illness. Am J Psychiatry 143:279–89.

Kendler KS, Hewitt J. (1992). The structure of self-report schizotypy in twins. J Personal Disord 6:1–17.

Kendler KS. (2005). "A gene for…": the nature of gene action in psychiatric disorders. Am J Psychiatry 162:1243–52.

Kendler KS. (2006). Reflections on the relationship between psychiatric genetics and psychiatric nosology. Am J Psychiatry 163:1138–46.

Khoury MJ, Beaty TH, Cohen BH. (1993). Genetic Epidemiology. Oxford: Oxford University Press.

Khoury MJ, Millikan R, Little J, Gwinn M. (2004). The emergence of epidemiology in the genomics age. Int J Epidemiol 33:936–44.

Kirkbride JB, Fearon P, Morgan C, Dazzan P, Morgan K, Tarrant J, Lloyd T, Holloway J, Hutchinson G, Leff JP, Mallett RM, Harrison GL, Murray RM, Jones PB. (2006). Heterogeneity in incidence rates of schizophrenia and other psychotic syndromes: findings from the 3-center AeSOP study. Arch Gen Psychiatry 63:250–8.

Kirkbride JB, Morgan C, Fearon P, Dazzan P, Murray RM, Jones PB. (2007). Neighbourhood-level effects on psychoses: re-examining the role of context. Psychol Med 37:1413–25.

Krabbendam L, van Os J. (2005). Schizophrenia and urbanicity: a major environmental influence – conditional on genetic risk. Schizophr Bull 31:795–9.

Kringlen E, Cramer G. (1989). Offspring of monozygotic twins discordant for schizophrenia. Arch Gen Psychiatry 46:873–7.

Kunugi H, Nanko S, Takei N, Saito K, Murray RM, Hirose T. (1996). Perinatal complications and schizophrenia. Data from the Maternal and Child Health Handbook in Japan. J Nerv Ment Dis 184:542–6.

Lake SL, Lyon H, Tantisira K, Silverman EK, Weiss ST, Laird NM, Schaid DJ. (2003). Estimation and tests of haplotype–environment interaction when linkage phase is ambiguous. Hum Hered 55:56–65.

Lange C, DeMeo D, Silverman EK, Weiss ST, Laird NM. (2004). PBAT: tools for family-based association studies. Am J Hum Genet 74:367–9.

Li N, Stephens M. (2003). Modeling linkage disequilibrium and identifying recombination hotspots using single-nucleotide polymorphism data. Genetics 165:2213–33.

Linney YM, Murray RM, Peters ER, MacDonald AM, Rijsdijk F, Sham PC. (2003). A quantitative genetic analysis of schizotypal personality traits. Psychol Med 33:803–16.

MacDonald AW, Pogue-Geile MF, Debski TT, Manuck S. (2001). Genetic and environmental influences on schizotypy: a community-based twin study. Schizophr Bull 27:47–58.

Malaspina D, Harlap S, Fennig S, Heiman D, Nahon D, Feldman D, Susser ES. (2001). Advancing paternal age and the risk of schizophrenia. Arch Gen Psychiatry 58: 361–7.

Marcelis M, Suckling J, Woodruff P, Hofman P, Bullmore E, van Os J. (2003). Searching for a structural endophenotype in psychosis using computational morphometry. Psychiatry Res 122:153–67.

Marcelis M, Van Os J, Sham P, Jones P, Gilvarry C, Cannon M, McKenzie K, Murray R. (1998). Obstetric complications and familial morbid risk of psychiatric disorders. Am J Med Genet 81:29–36.

McGrath J, Saha S, Welham J, El Saadi O, MacCauley C, Chant D. (2004). A systematic review of the incidence of schizophrenia: the distribution of rates and the influence of sex, urbanicity, migrant status and methodology. BMC Med 2:13.

Meaney MJ, Szyf M. (2005). Environmental programming of stress responses through DNA methylation: life at the interface between a dynamic environment and a fixed genome. Dialogues Clin Neurosci 7:103–23.

Meyer U, Nyffeler M, Schwendener S, Knuesel I, Yee BK, Feldon J. (2008). Relative prenatal and postnatal maternal contributions to schizophrenia-related neurochemical dysfunction after in utero immune challenge. Neuropsychopharmacology 33:441–56.

Meyer-Lindenberg A, Kohn PD, Kolachana B, Kippenhan S, McInerney-Leo A, Nussbaum R, Weinberger DR, Berman KF. (2005). Midbrain dopamine and prefrontal function in humans: interaction and modulation by COMT genotype. Nat Neurosci 8:594–6.

Meyer-Lindenberg A, Miletich RS, Kohn PD, Esposito G, Carson RE, Quarantelli M, Weinberger DR, Berman KF. (2002). Reduced prefrontal activity predicts exaggerated striatal dopaminergic function in schizophrenia. Nat Neurosci 5:267–71.

Meyer-Lindenberg A, Nichols T, Callicott JH, Ding J, Kolachana B, Buckholtz J, Mattay VS, Egan M, Weinberger DR. (2006). Impact of complex genetic variation in COMT on human brain function. Mol Psychiatry 11:867–77, 797.

Moffitt TE, Caspi A, Rutter M. (2005). Strategy for investigating interactions between measured genes and measured environments. Arch Gen Psychiatry 62:473–81.

Mortensen PB, Pedersen CB, Westergaard T, Wohlfahrt J, Ewald H, Mors O, Andersen PK, Melbye M. (1999). Effects of family history and place and season of birth on the risk of schizophrenia [see comments]. N Engl J Med 340:603–8.

Motulsky AG. (1977). Ecogenetics: genetic variation in susceptibility to environmental agents. In: Armendares S, Lisker R. (eds.), Human Genetics. Amsterdam, Excerpta Medica, pp. 375–85.

Murray GK, Corlett PR, Clark L, Pessiglione M, Blackwell AD, Honey G, Jones PB, Bullmore ET, Robbins TW, Fletcher PC. (2008). How dopamine dysregulation leads to psychotic symptoms? Abnormal mesolimbic and mesostriatal prediction error signalling in psychosis. Mol Psychiatry 13:239.

Myin-Germeys I, Marcelis M, Krabbendam L, Delespaul P, van Os J. (2005). Subtle fluctuations in psychotic phenomena as functional states of abnormal dopamine reactivity in individuals at risk. Biol Psychiatry 58:105–10.

Myin-Germeys I, Van Os J, Schwartz JE, Stone AA, Delespaul PA. (2001). Emotional reactivity to daily life stress in psychosis. Arch Gen Psychiatry 58:1137–44.

Nicodemus KK, Marenco S, Batten AJ, Vakkalanka R, Egan MF, Straub RE, Weinberger DR. (2008). Serious obstetric complications interact with hypoxia-regulated/vascular-expression genes to influence schizophrenia risk. Mol Psychiatry 13:873–7.

Nikulina EM, Covington HE, 3rd, Ganschow L, Hammer RP, Jr, Miczek KA. (2004). Long-term behavioral and neuronal cross-sensitization to amphetamine induced by repeated brief social defeat stress: Fos in the ventral tegmental area and amygdala. Neuroscience 123:857–65.

Nimgaonkar VL, Wessely S, Murray RM. (1988). Prevalence of familiality, obstetric complications, and structural brain damage in schizophrenic patients. Br J Psychiatry 153:191–7.

Norton N, Williams HJ, Owen MJ. (2006). An update on the genetics of schizophrenia. Curr Opin Psychiatry 19:158–64.

O'Callaghan E, Gibson T, Colohan HA, Buckley P, Walshe DG, Larkin C, Waddington JL. (1992). Risk of schizophrenia in adults born after obstetric complications and their association with early onset of illness: a controlled study [see comments]. BMJ 305:1256–9.

O'Donovan MC, Craddock N, Owen MJ. (2008). Schizophrenia: complex genetics, not fairy tales. Psychol Med 1–3.

Ottman R. (1990). An epidemiologic approach to gene–environment interaction. Genet Epidemiol 7:177–85.

Ottman R. (1996). Gene–environment interaction: definitions and study designs. Prev Med 25: 764–70.

Ozawa K, Hashimoto K, Kishimoto T, Shimizu E, Ishikura H, Iyo M. (2006). Immune activation during pregnancy in mice leads to dopaminergic hyperfunction and cognitive impairment in the offspring: a neurodevelopmental animal model of schizophrenia. Biol Psychiatry 59:546–54.

Pedersen CB, Mortensen PB. (2001). Evidence of a dose–response relationship between urbanicity during upbringing and schizophrenia risk. Arch Gen Psychiatry 58:1039–46.

Pedersen CB, Mortensen PB. (2006). Are the cause(s) responsible for urban–rural differences in schizophrenia risk rooted in families or in individuals? Am J Epidemiol 163:971–8.

Plomin R, DeFries JC, Loehlin JC. (1977). Genotype–environment interaction and correlation in the analysis of human behavior. Psychol Bull 84:309–22.

Pulver AE, Liang KY, Brown CH, Wolyniec P, McGrath J, Adler L, Tam D, Carpenter WT, Childs B. (1992). Risk factors in schizophrenia. Season of birth, gender, and familial risk [see comments]. Br J Psychiatry 160:65–71.

Read J, van Os J, Morrison AP, Ross CA. (2005). Childhood trauma, psychosis and schizophrenia: a literature review with theoretical and clinical implications. Acta Psychiatr Scand 112:330–50.

Rutter M, Moffitt TE, Caspi A. (2006). Gene–environment interplay and psychopathology: multiple varieties but real effects. J Child Psychol Psychiatry 47:226–61.

Rutter M. (2005). How the environment affects mental health. Br J Psychiatry 186:4–6.

Rutter M. (2006). Genes and Behaviour: Nature-Nurture Interplay Explained. Malden, MA, USA: Blackwell Publishing.

Schmidt-Kastner R, van Os J, Steinbusch HWMS, Schmitz C. (2006). Gene regulation by hypoxia and the neurodevelopmental origin of schizophrenia. Schizophr Res 84:253–71.

Schurhoff F, Szoke A, Chevalier F, Roy I, Meary A, Bellivier F, Giros B, Leboyer M. (2007). Schizotypal dimensions: an intermediate phenotype associated with the COMT high activity allele. Am J Med Genet B Neuropsychiatr Genet 144:64–8.

Schurhoff F, Szoke A, Meary A, Bellivier F, Rouillon F, Pauls D, Leboyer M. (2003). Familial aggregation of delusional proneness in schizophrenia and bipolar pedigrees. Am J Psychiatry 160:1313–9.

Selten JP, Cantor-Graae E, Kahn RS. (2007). Migration and schizophrenia. Curr Opin Psychiatry 20:111–5.

Sham P. (1996). Genetic epidemiology. Br Med Bull 52:408–33.

Shur E. (1982). Season of birth in high and low genetic risk schizophrenics. Br J Psychiatry 140:410–5.

Sipos A, Rasmussen F, Harrison G, Tynelius P, Lewis G, Leon DA, Gunnell D. (2004). Paternal age and schizophrenia: a population based cohort study. BMJ 329:1070.

Smits L, Pedersen C, Mortensen P, Van Os J. (2004). Association between short birth intervals and schizophrenia in the offspring. Schizophr Res 70:49–56.

Spauwen J, Krabbendam L, Lieb R, Wittchen HU, Van Os J. (2006a). Evidence that the outcome of developmental expression of psychosis is worse for adolescents growing up in an urban environment. Psychol Med 407–15.

Spauwen J, Krabbendam L, Lieb R, Wittchen HU, van Os J. (2006b). Impact of psychological trauma on the development of psychotic symptoms: relationship with psychosis proneness. Br J Psychiatry 188:527–33.

Stefanis NC, Henquet C, Avramopoulos D, Smyrnis N, Evdokimidis I, Myin-Germeys I, Stefanis CN, Van Os J. (2007). COMT Val158Met moderation of stress-induced psychosis. Psychol Med 37:1651–6.

Stefanis NC, Van Os J, Avramopoulos D, Smyrnis N, Evdokimidis I, Hantoumi I, Stefanis CN. (2004). Variation in catechol-o-methyltransferase val158 met genotype associated with schizotypy but not cognition: a population study in 543 young men. Biol Psychiatry 56: 510–5.

Sugarman PA, Craufurd D. (1994). Schizophrenia in the Afro-Caribbean community. Br J Psychiatry 164:474–80.

Sullivan PF. (2008). The dice are rolling for schizophrenia genetics. Psychol Med 1–4.

Susser E, Neugebauer R, Hoek HW, Brown AS, Lin S, Labovitz D, Gorman JM. (1996). Schizophrenia after prenatal famine. Further evidence [see comments]. Arch Gen Psychiatry 53:25–31.

Susser E, Susser M. (1989). Familial aggregation studies. A note on their epidemiologic properties. Am J Epidemiol 129:23–30.

Talkowski ME, Kirov G, Bamne M, Georgieva L, Torres G, Mansour H, Chowdari KV, Milanova V, Wood J, McClain L, Prasad K, Shirts B, Zhang J, O'Donovan MC, Owen MJ, Devlin B, Nimgaonkar VL. (2008). A network of dopaminergic gene variations implicated as risk factors for schizophrenia. Hum Mol Genet 17:747–58.

Tenn CC, Fletcher PJ, Kapur S. (2005). A putative animal model of the "prodromal" state of schizophrenia. Biol Psychiatry 57:586–93.

Tidey JW, Miczek KA. (1996). Social defeat stress selectively alters medocorticolimbic release: an in vivo microdialysis study. Brain Research 721:140–9.

Tienari P, Wynne LC, Moring J, Lahti I, Naarala M, Sorri A, Wahlberg KE, Saarento O, Seitamaa M, Kaleva M, et al. (1994). The Finnish adoptive family study of schizophrenia. Implications for family research [see comments]. Br J Psychiatry Suppl:20–6.

Tienari P, Wynne LC, Sorri A, Lahti I, Laksy K, Moring J, Naarala M, Nieminen P, Wahlberg KE. (2004). Genotype–environment interaction in schizophrenia-spectrum disorder. Long-term follow-up study of Finnish adoptees. Br J Psychiatry 184:216–22.

Toulopoulou T, Picchioni M, Rijsdijk F, Hua-Hall M, Ettinger U, Sham P, Murray R. (2007). Substantial genetic overlap between neurocognition and schizophrenia: genetic modeling in twin samples. Arch Gen Psychiatry 64:1348–55.

van Haren NE, Bakker SC, Kahn RS. (2008). Genes and structural brain imaging in schizophrenia. Curr Opin Psychiatry 21:161–7.

Van Os J, Fahy TA, Bebbington P, Jones P, Wilkins S, Sham P, Russell A, Gilvarry K, Lewis S, Toone B, et al. (1994). The influence of life events on the subsequent course of psychotic illness. A prospective follow-up of the Camberwell Collaborative Psychosis Study. Psychol Med 24:503–13.

Van Os J, Hanssen M, Bak M, Bijl RV, Vollebergh W. (2003). Do urbanicity and familial liability coparticipate in causing psychosis? Am J Psychiatry 160:477–82.

Van Os J, Hanssen M, Bijl R-V, Ravelli A. (2000). Straus (1969) revisited: a psychosis continuum in the general population? Schizophr Res 45:11–20.

van Os J, Henquet C, Stefanis N. (2005). Cannabis-related psychosis and the gene–environment interaction: comments on Ferdinand et al. 2005. Addiction 100:874–5.

Van Os J, Krabbendam L, Myin-Germeys I, Delespaul P. (2005). The schizophrenia envirome. Curr Opin Psychiatry 18:141–5.

Van Os J, Marcelis M. (1998). The ecogenetics of schizophrenia: a review. Schizophr Res 32: 127–35.

van Os J, Pedersen CB, Mortensen PB. (2004). Confirmation of synergy between urbanicity and familial liability in the causation of psychosis. Am J Psychiatry 161: 2312–4.

Van Os J, Sham P. (2003). Gene–environment interactions. In: Murray RM, Jones PB, Susser E, Van Os J, Cannon M. (eds.), The Epidemiology of Schizophrenia. Cambridge, Cambridge University Press, pp. 235–54.

Van Os J. (2004). Does the urban environment cause psychosis? Br J Psychiatry 184:287–8.

van Os J. (2005). Commentary on residential location papers by Whitfield et al. (2005) and Willemsen et al. (2005). Twin Res Hum Genet 8:318–9.

Venerosi A, Valanzano A, Cirulli F, Alleva E, Calamandrei G. (2004). Acute global anoxia during C-section birth affects dopamine-mediated behavioural responses and reactivity to stress. Behav Brain Res 154:155–64.

Verdoux H, Gindre C, Sorbara F, Tournier M, Swendsen JD. (2003). Effects of cannabis and psychosis vulnerability in daily life: an experience sampling test study. Psychol Med 33:23–32.

Verdoux H, Van Os J, Sham P, Jones P, Gilvarry K, Murray R. (1996). Does familiality predispose to both emergence and persistence of psychosis? A follow-up study. Br J Psychiatry 168:620–6.

Vollema MG, Sitskoorn MM, Appels MC, Kahn RS. (2002). Does the Schizotypal Personality Questionnaire reflect the biological-genetic vulnerability to schizophrenia? Schizophr Res 54:39–45.

Wahlberg KE, Wynne LC, Hakko H, Laksy K, Moring J, Miettunen J, Tienari P. (2004). Interaction of genetic risk and adoptive parent communication deviance: longitudinal prediction of adoptee psychiatric disorders. Psychol Med 34:1531–41.

Wahlberg KE, Wynne LC, Oja H, Keskitalo P, Pykalainen L, Lahti I, Moring J, Naarala M, Sorri A, Seitamaa M, Laksy K, Kolassa J, Tienari P. (1997). Gene–environment interaction in vulnerability to schizophrenia: findings from the Finnish Adoptive Family Study of Schizophrenia. Am J Psychiatry 154:355–62.

Walker E. (1981). Attentional and neuromotor functions of schizophrenics, schizoaffectives, and patients with other affective disorders. Arch Gen Psychiatry 38:1355–8.

Weaver IC, Cervoni N, Champagne FA, D'Alessio AC, Sharma S, Seckl JR, Dymov S, Szyf M, Meaney MJ. (2004). Epigenetic programming by maternal behavior. Nat Neurosci 7:847–54.

Weiser M, van Os J, Reichenberg A, Rabinowitz J, Nahon D, Kravitz E, Lubin G, Shmushkevitz M, Knobler HY, Noy S, Davidson M. (2007). Social and cognitive functioning, urbanicity and risk for schizophrenia. Br J Psychiatry 191:320–4.

Weisfeld GE, Weisfeld CC. (2002). Marriage: an evolutionary perspective. Neuro Endocrinol Lett 23(Suppl 4):47–54.

Wellman CL, Izquierdo A, Garrett JE, Martin KP, Carroll J, Millstein R, Lesch KP, Murphy DL, Holmes A. (2007). Impaired stress-coping and fear extinction and abnormal corticolimbic morphology in serotonin transporter knock-out mice. J Neurosci 27:684–91.

Whitfield JB, Zhu G, Heath AC, Martin NG. (2005). Choice of residential location: chance, family influences, or genes? Twin Res Hum Genet 8:22–6.

Wichers M, Myin-Germeys I, Jacobs N, Peeters F, Kenis G, Derom C, Vlietinck R, Delespaul P, Van Os J. (2007a). Genetic risk of depression and stress-induced negative affect in daily life. Br J Psychiatry 191:218–23.

Wichers MC, Myin-Germeys I, Jacobs N, Peeters F, Kenis G, Derom C, Vlietinck R, Delespaul P, van Os J. (2007b). Evidence that moment-to-moment variation in positive emotions buffer genetic risk for depression: a momentary assessment twin study. Acta Psychiatr Scand 115:451–7.

Wilkinson LS, Davies W, Isles AR. (2007). Genomic imprinting effects on brain development and function. Nat Rev Neurosci 8:832–43.

Willemsen G, Posthuma D, Boomsma DI. (2005). Environmental factors determine where the Dutch live: results from the Netherlands twin register. Twin Res Hum Genet 8:312–7.

Wong MY, Day NE, Luan JA, Chan KP, Wareham NJ. (2003). The detection of gene–environment interaction for continuous traits: should we deal with measurement error by bigger studies or better measurement? Int J Epidemiol 32:51–7.

Yui K, Goto K, Ikemoto S, Ishiguro T. (2000). Stress induced spontaneous recurrence of methamphetamine psychosis: the relation between stressful experiences and sensitivity to stress. Drug Alcohol Depend 58:67–75.

Zammit S, Allebeck P, Dalman C, Lundberg I, Hemmingson T, Owen MJ, Lewis G. (2003). Paternal age and risk for schizophrenia. Br J Psychiatry 183:405–8.

Zammit S, Lewis S, Gunnell D, Smith GD. (2007). Schizophrenia and neural tube defects: comparisons from an epidemiological perspective. Schizophr Bull 33:853–8.

Zinkstok J, van Nimwegen L, van Amelsvoort T, de Haan L, Yusuf MA, Baas F, Linszen D. (2008). Catechol-O-methyltransferase gene and obsessive-compulsive symptoms in patients with recent-onset schizophrenia: preliminary results. Psychiatry Res 157:1–8.

The Natural History of the Course and Outcome of Schizophrenia

Judith Allardyce and Jim van Os

Background

Understanding a disease's pathological trajectory, by describing its progression and course, from the *time an individual is exposed to causal factors* until recovery or death, is just as important as aetiological understandings, when considering strategies to deal with disease prevention and control (Bhopal 2002; Wynne 1988). The natural history describes the uninterrupted trajectory in an individual of the biological and symptom development of a disorder from the moment it is initiated by exposure to its risk factors. However, there is very little information regarding the natural history of schizophrenia. Why is this? First, throughout history psychotic symptoms (with associated disability), i.e. the manifest cases, have resulted in institutional care or other medical, religious or cultural interventions, which influence the longitudinal progression, and certainly from the 1950s the vast majority of individuals diagnosed with schizophrenia have received antipsychotic medication; therefore, our contemporary studies examining course are unlikely to reflect the true natural history. Second, studies of natural history ideally require a disease-free population to be closely followed up either until the population is no longer at risk of the disease or until death. However, to date, most studies for pragmatic reasons have depended on cohorts in contact with clinical services; such samples are likely to be the people with the most severe symptoms or with significant associated disability, i.e. a need for care. There is mounting evidence, however, that these manifest cases are only a proportion of the people within the total population who have psychotic symptoms (Wiles et al. 2006; Olfson et al. 2002; Verdoux et al. 1998; van Os et al. 2000). Using the metaphor of the iceberg (Last 1963), these symptoms represent the tip of the iceberg, visible and measurable; however, in most diseases like the iceberg the majority of cases lurk unseen, unmeasured and forgotten by clinicians. Epidemiological studies which set out to examine the course and outcome of disease and forget this

J. Allardyce (✉)
Department of Psychiatry and Neuropsychology, South Limburg Mental Health Research and Teaching Network, EURON, Maastricht University, PO Box 616 (DRT 10), 6200 MD Maastricht, The Netherlands
e-mail: j.allardyce@clinmed.gla.ac.uk

W.F. Gattaz, G. Busatto (eds.), *Advances in Schizophrenia Research 2009*,
DOI 10.1007/978-1-4419-0913-8_3, © Springer Science+Business Media, LLC 2010

ubiquitous iceberg phenomenon by merely examining the clinically manifest cases are weak and potentially misleading (Last 2004). The unidentified subclinical cases may be missed cases or they may represent variants of the same pathological process or spectrum of disease. The goal of epidemiological studies of the course of disease is therefore to define the nature and causes of these subclinical and clinical spectrum variants by quantifying disease progression within aggregated populations and also at the individual level in order to develop models to reliably predict outcome. Such studies of the causes and consequences of psychotic processes should ideally be representative of the spectrum of psychosis; studies based on selected prodromal/or cases fulfilling diagnostic criteria for disorder are from the tip of the iceberg and may well give an erroneous view, especially when their findings are used in the evaluation of screening or early intervention strategies. Third, causal agents rarely act in isolation to increase risk, rather their effects are cumulative and act across a wide range of developmental periods perhaps even over decades. The long latency between exposure of causal factors and the eventual development of schizophrenia (the incubation period) means that studies designed to examine the nature and causes of the variation in course require population cohorts to be followed up and closely observed over decades or that cases have to retrospectively recall psychopathology and exposures, which is inherently fraught with bias, especially over such long incubation periods. Fourth, there is no reason to assume that the risk factors for the emergence of schizophrenia and those influencing its persistence are congruent (the discrete effect model); therefore, to fully describe the course of schizophrenia and its determinants from initial exposure of causal agents requires studies to span across the incubation period, onset and persistence of symptoms. Due to the above issues we do not have well-defined descriptions of the natural history of schizophrenia, and so have to try and piece together its progression inferred from a group of recent population studies examining subclinical psychotic-like experiences, such as brief low-grade psychotic experiences (in late childhood early adolescence) which demonstrably predict later onset of psychotic disorder and the (mostly older) studies examining the course of symptoms and disability, after diagnosis of disorder is made.

Nature of the Symptom Trajectory Prior to Diagnosis of Disorder

The Dunedin Multidisciplinary Health and Development study is a longitudinal follow-up of a representative birth cohort of 1,037 children born in Dunedin, New Zealand, during the year 1972–1973, which has not only sequentially assessed childhood developmental indices but also serially collected self-reported psychopathology (ages 11, 13, 15, 18 and 21 years) with further psychiatric interviews having been carried out at ages 11 and 26 years. The investigators examined whether self-reported delusional beliefs and hallucinatory experiences at age 11 years would predict schizophreniform psychiatric disorder at age 26 years (Poulton et al. 2000). By age 11 years, nearly 15% of the total cohort reported some psychotic experience. Children were grouped according to the strength/frequency of their psychotic experiences (at age 11 years): the majority of children had no psychotic symptoms (control group ($n = 654$)), an intermediate group had weak symptoms ($n = 95$) and a small proportion had symptoms described as strong ($n = 12$). At age 26 years, 2% of the controls had a diagnosis of schizophreniform disorder, compared with 9.5% in the weak-symptom group and 25% in the strong-symptom group. Early psychotic experiences specifically increased the risk for schizophreniform disorder moderately in the weak-symptom group (odds ratio 5.1, 95% confidence interval 1.7–18.3) and strongly in the strong-symptom group (odds ratio 16.4, 95% confidence interval 3.9–67.8), compared to controls. While 25% of the strong-symptom group had developed schizophreniform disorder, a further 70% (although not fulfilling the full diagnostic criteria for schizophreniform disorder) still reported some psychotic symptoms (*persistence of pre-clinical psychotic experiences*) at the age of 26 years and 90% had occupational and social difficulties. The strong-symptom group also manifest impairments in motor, language and cognitive ability, suggesting that pervasive and persistent psychotic experiences may be indicators of an underlying ongoing psychotic process, reflecting increased genetic liability. The weak-symptom group, on the other hand, did not have such prominent developmental abnormalities, although they had significant receptive language impairment, suggesting a weaker genetic liability. Replication of this transition from subclinical psychotic experiences to full-blown psychotic disorder over time comes from a longitudinal general population study in The Netherlands (The Netherlands Mental Health Survey and Incidence Study; NEMESIS) (Hanssen et al. 2005). In order to identify new cases of subclinical psychotic experiences, the investigators followed up the cohort for 1 year. Individuals who reported subclinical psychotic experiences at the 1-year assessment, but not at baseline, were considered *incident cases*. Next, a second-wave follow-up (over 2 years) allowed the risk of transition of subclinical to clinical psychotic disorder (both affective and non-affective psychosis) in the *incident case* group compared with the future risk of psychosis risk in the group of individuals with no clinical or subclinical psychotic experiences (controls). The *incident cases* were at significantly higher risk of developing psychotic disorders compared to the controls (odds ratio 65.1, 95% confidence interval 19.4–218.1) and the positive predictive value over 2 years was 8%. There was a dose–response relationship in the association between the number of subclinical psychotic experiences and the transition to clinical psychosis going from a risk of around 30 in individuals who had only one subclinical psychotic experience (odds ratio 27.3, 95% confidence interval 5.2–143.6) to a much higher risk in individuals who had multiple subclinical experiences (odds ratio 211.2, 95% confidence interval 51.6–864.1). In both the Dunedin Cohort and the Nemesis study, transition from subclinical to clinical psychotic disorder was higher in individuals characterised by persistent subclinical psychotic experiences. In the Nemesis study, transition was also partly dependent on the emotional context of the subclinical psychotic experience. Subclinical psychotic experiences (represented by the portion of the iceberg below the water line) have been found to be relatively common, in general population surveys, with a prevalence of around 15%. However, most are brief, self-limiting developmental phenomena. The reasons as to why approximately 15% of children have subclinical psychotic experiences during development and the others do not are not fully established, but they may in part reflect the shared genetic liability for psychosis continuously distributed in the general population but understanding why some people with such symptoms go on to develop psychotic disorder and others do not is important for our understanding of the natural history of psychotic disorders.

A Dynamic Model of Psychosis Evolution: Proneness-Persistence-Impairment Hypothesis

In two large independent general population samples, NEMESIS and EDPD (the early developmental health and incidence survey), investigators examined the hypothesis that these relatively common, subclinical developmental psychotic experiences could become abnormally persistent when synergistically combined with known risk factors for onset of psychotic disorders (the study used cannabis, urban upbringing and developmental trauma) (Cougnard et al. 2007). Over a follow-up period of 3 years, the studies found the rates of subclinical psychotic experiences, which *persisted* to be relatively low, to be 26% (NEMESIS) and 31% (EDSP); however, rates of persistence increased progressively with higher baseline doses of exposure to known risk factors. This suggests that environmental determinants of psychotic disorders may in part operate by driving up the rates of subclinical psychotic experiences, which become persistent in individuals with a genetic liability for psychosis. A dynamic model of psychosis evolution or proneness-persistence-impairment model may best conceptualise this trajectory from developmental expression of psychosis liability (transitory subclinical psychotic symptoms) to more intrusive persistent subclinical psychotic symptoms to significant impairment and dysfunction and the eventual onset of psychotic disorder. Such a model provides a framework for further investigation of the ontogenesis of psychotic disorders. Although the psychosis-proneness-persistence-impairment model of psychosis offers a possible insight into the underlying mechanism for development of psychosis, its estimated positive predictive power of around 40% for persistent subclinical symptoms ability to estimate onset of future psychotic disorders is still too low to be useful as a general population screening test (Van Os et al. 2008).

Studies of the Course and Outcome of Psychosis: Evidence from Clinical Samples of Patients Diagnosed with Schizophrenia

The pervading clinical and societal view of schizophrenia is of a debilitating progressive disorder of poor outcome, a legacy from Kraepelin's studies of the course of psychoses in patients admitted to a large custodial institution in Germany, during the late nineteenth century. He combined a number of clinical syndromes into a single disease entity (dementia praecox) due to his clinical observation that they seemed to share a poor outcome (estimated permanent cure: range 2.6–16%). However, the asylum provided long-term residential care for people with the most severe, complex and debilitating conditions (that is, a biased sample, skewed towards the worst outcomes), which is unlikely to fully reflect the complete range of outcomes for schizophrenia, a fact recognised by Kraepelin himself (Kraepelin 1971). While most clinicians no longer work in long-term custodial settings, clinical caseloads remain principally of patients requiring sustained contact with clinical service, rather than a truly representative sample of everyone ever diagnosed with schizophrenia so perpetuating the clinical illusion of schizophrenia as an *invariably*chronic and deteriorating disorder (Harding et al. 1987d).

Methodological Difficulties in Defining the Course and Outcome of Schizophrenia After Diagnosis

During the last century, many studies have attempted to examine the outcome of schizophrenia; yet despite this best effort, the data on longitudinal course remain weak principally due to the innate methodological difficulties associated with follow-up studies, which are especially sensitive to confounding and bias (Van Os 2008):

1. *Variation in the populations from which patients are selected*: Many studies have relied on in-patients samples only. However, approximately 20% of schizophrenic patients are never admitted to hospital and they may differ from those admitted in important variables associated with outcome (Driessen et al. 1998)
2. *Variation in diagnostic criteria*: Lack of concordance between different classification systems may result in different samples being identified. When 'broad' concepts of schizophrenia are employed, the results are more favourable than studies using 'narrow' definitions (Harrison and Mason 1993). Follow-up studies for patients who have been diagnosed using ICD-9/10 on average yield prognostically more favourable results than those using the narrower more restrictive criteria found in DSM III and later (Westermeyer and Harrow 1984; Hegarty et al. 1994). Furthermore, if the diagnostic criteria for schizophrenia are repeatedly modified over time (e.g. with revisions of DSM or ICD), it may lead to subtle variation in the course and outcome, which makes the systematic combination of the results difficult.
3. *Variation in the length of illness before entry into the follow-up study*: If this varies then subjects with an admixture of follow-up epochs and levels of symptom persistence are being examined.
4. *Variation in length of follow-up*: In general the longer time of follow-up, the less representative a single cross-sectional measure of course will be, but here validity is highly dependent on the quality of the sources of information of any retrospective assessment. A number of instruments with reported good reliability have now been developed to record course retrospectively, e.g. the

semi-operationalised instrument of the WHO Life Chart (WHO 1992; Sartorius et al. 1996).

5. *Variability of completeness of follow-up*: In any follow-up study, a proportion of cases will be lost to follow-up due to death, migration, refusal or are untraceable for other reasons. Many of the studies have high rates of attrition (greater than 20%) and were carried out at a time when the researcher was unable to take account for this attrition (using imputation methods or other latent variable methods) during the analyses; however, loss to follow-up may be related to particular patterns of course and outcome, which will bias towards a particular outcome. It is possible that patients with better outcome are less likely to be followed up.

6. *Variation in the concepts and methods used to assess course and outcome*: There is no single measure of course and outcome of schizophrenia, and widely different concepts are used in different studies. Qualitative summary terms, such as 'recovery' 'improvement' or 'deterioration', are likely to obfuscate intra-individual variability over time; furthermore, such terms are used inconsistently. Outcome is a multidimensional construct (at least three domains should be considered: symptom severity, functional impairment and disability in social and occupational roles). However, these domains are related and few studies have used data reduction techniques to deal with the problems of multiple analyses. Furthermore in some individuals, their outcome status will vary considerably as a function of the actual outcome measure or domain used. That is, a person may continue to work in spite of moderate chronic psychotic symptoms or may have low rating of positive psychotic symptoms but significant social disability due to grumbling negative symptoms or residual anxiety (Strauss and Carpenter 1974). This is demonstrated in Table 1 (van Os 2008). Lastly, few studies have been able to examine serial follow-up measures and have to depend on a single outcome measure which is less representative of longitudinal course especially when follow-up is long and therefore many studies have not explored the dynamic adaptive variability of course and when they have there is no consistency in course descriptors used. Some authors suggest that the variation in course could be described accurately in three or four types (Shepherd et al. 1989) to as many as 70 or so descriptors (Huber et al. 1980).

7. *Variation in the characteristics of the general population*: For example, social outcomes (e.g. unemployment) will be influenced by the general unemployment rates in the area.

8. *Variation in statistical techniques and adjustment of confounding*: Statistical methods, which deal with multiple comparisons made at different time points, were not available or not available at the time of publication of the many studies. And many investigators have not had sufficient resources to collect adequate data on potential confounding variables when assessing potential predictor (or prognostic indicators).

9. *Variation in long-term management of schizophrenia*: Finally, treatment varies across time and place, which may differentially modify the natural history of the disorder.

Table 1

Study	N	Event rate	Upper limit	Lower limit	definition of poor outcome
Muller, 1951 (Germany)	200	0.41	0.34	0.48	insidious chronic course, continual need for full time care
Bland, 1978 (Alberta)	43	0.16	0.05	0.27	severe chronic social and /or intellectual deficit
Stephens, 1978 (Baltimore)	349	0.30	0.25	0.35	"unimproved" evidence of chronic sustained psychotic symptoms
Ciompi, 1980 (Switzerland)	289	0.18	0.14	0.22	severe chronic phase
Salokangas, 1983 (Finland)	161	0.24	0.18	0.31	continous psychotic symptoms
Rabiner, 1986 (New York)	36	0.44	0.28	0.61	relapsed or in-episode evidence of psychotic symptoms
Sartorius, 1986 (Multinational)	1352	0.40	0.37	0.42	unremitting psychotic symptoms
Shephard, 1989 (UK)	107	0.43	0.34	0.52	remained impaired throughout follow up
SSRG, 1989 (Scotland)	49	0.39	0.25	0.52	psychotic symptoms present at follow up
Marneros, 1992 (Germany)	355	0.17	0.13	0.21	psychotic symptoms present at follow up
Thara, 1994 (India)	76	0.07	0.01	0.12	continous psychotic symptoms
an der Heiden, 1995 (Germany)	56	0.59	0.46	0.72	moderate to severe symptoms ar follow up and
Mason, 1996 (UK)	58	0.34	0.22	0.47	continous symptoms in the 2 years prior to folllow up
Weiselgren, 1996 (Sweden)	101	0.14	0.07	0.21	"poor outcome" evidence of ongoing persistant psychotic symptoms
Ganev, 1998 (Bulgaria)	55	0.45	0.32	0.59	chronic continous psychotic sxymptoms
Wiersma, 1998 (Netherlands)	82	0.11	0.04	0.18	chronic continous psychotic sxymptoms
Vanquez-Barques, 1999 (Spain)	76	0.09	0.03	0.16	chronic continous psychotic sxymptoms
Sterling, 2003 (UK)	49	0.06	-0.01	0.13	GAF score =1 at follow up

0.0   0.5   1.0

Study	N	Event rate	Upper limit	Lower limit	definition of good outcome
Muller, 1951 (Germany)	200	0.33	0.26	0.40	recovered or substantially improved at time of discharge
Bland, 1978 (Alberta)	43	0.21	0.09	0.33	symptomatic recovery with no social or intellectual deficit
Stephens, 1978 (Baltimore)	349	0.24	0.20	0.29	"recovered" included patients with symptoms but no social impairment
Ciompi, 1980 (Switzerland)	289	0.27	0.22	0.32	remitted completely or had only mild residual symptoms
Salokangas, 1983 (Finland)	161	0.55	0.47	0.62	complete recovery or occasional mild psychotic symptoms
Rabiner, 1986 (New York)	36	0.56	0.39	0.72	symptomatic remission for at least 3 months prior to assessment
Sartorius, 1986 (Multinational)	1352	0.39	0.36	0.42	one episode with no or minimal symptoms at follow up
Shephard, 1989 (UK)	107	0.22	0.15	0.30	had no relapse during follow up
SSRG, 1989 (Scotland)	49	0.37	0.23	0.50	asymptomatic and functioning adequately
Marneros, 1992 (Germany)	355	0.07	0.04	0.10	full remission
Thara, 1994 (India)	76	0.17	0.09	0.26	complete recovery without relapse during follow up period
an der Heiden, 1995 (Germany)	56	0.25	0.14	0.36	full recovery over follow up period
Mason, 1996 (United Kingdom)	58	0.52	0.39	0.65	full remission
Weiselgren, 1996 (Sweden)	101	0.30	0.21	0.39	dichotomised variable "good outcome" versus "poor outcome"
Ganev, 1998 (Bulgaria)	55	0.38	0.25	0.51	complete remission
Wiersma, 1998 (Netherlands)	82	0.27	0.17	0.36	complete remission
Vanquez-Barques, 1999 (Spain)	76	0.32	0.21	0.42	symptomatic recovery may have residual symptoms
Sterling, 2003 (UK)	49	0.47	0.33	0.61	categorical measure GAF score =4

0.0   0.5   1.0

Evidence from Recent Meta-analytical Studies of Outcome of Schizophrenia

Systematic review of prospectively designed studies examining the outcome of first-episode schizophrenia (and other psychosis) published during the period 1966–2003 found good outcome in 42%, intermediate outcome in 35% and poor outcome in 27% of the samples with a diagnosis of schizophrenia. However, these pooled estimates should be interpreted with caution as they have combined studies which used different definitions of schizophrenia, have different sample biases, compare outcome categories which may be incomparable, e.g. good outcome in one study is equivalent to intermediate outcome in another, and the outcome typologies are broad and do not fully reflect the enormous heterogeneity of trajectories; furthermore, the degree of completeness of the follow-up varied considerably across the studies. This frequency distribution is comparable with the findings from an earlier meta-analysis, which is hampered by similar threats to comparability (Hegarty 1994; Menezes et al. 2006; Bromet et al. 2005).

In order to augment the findings of these studies, we review important follow-up studies which have been published in the last decade, which were all epidemiologically defined representative samples of first admission or first contact schizophrenia (spectrum) disorder operationally defined using modern classification system (ICD, DSM or RDC) of long-term follow-up (greater than 10 years). Most of these studies were excluded from a recently published systematic review of outcome due to its strict definition of prospective (Menezes et al. 2006). Here we review such studies where although the assessment of course may often have been retrospective and rather limited, the cross-sectional clinical outcome measures were gathered prospectively and included a face-to-face interview with the patient and where possible informant information from family or psychiatric services was sought. Eight separate cohorts were identified (Tables 2–4), which had useful information on long-term outcome (Eaton et al. 1998; Wiersma et al. 1998; Mason et al. 1995, 1996, 1997; Ganev 1998; Hans-Jürgen Möller 2000; Jäger 2004; Harrow et al. 2000; Herbener and Harrow 2001; Racenstein et al. 2002;

Table 2

Cohort studied	Follow-up time (years)	Mean age of presentation (years)	Standard deviation
Groningen (NL)	15	23	–
Nottingham (UK)	13	29	7.01
Sofia (Bulgaria)	16	27.2	8.08
Munich (Germany)	15	30.10	11.8
Chicago (USA)	20	22.9	3.91
Manchester (UK)	10	26.3	10
Madras (India)	20	24.5	6.5
Singapore	20	23.30	2.43

Table 3

Cohort	Statistics for each study					Event rate and 95% CI
	Event rate	Lower limit	Upper limit	Z-Value	p-Value	
Groningen (The Netherlands)	0.512	0.405	0.618	0.221	0.825	
Nottingham (United Kingdom)	0.672	0.551	0.773	2.751	0.006	
Sofia (Bulgaria)	0.350	0.241	0.478	-2.287	0.022	
Munich (Germany)	0.632	0.518	0.732	2.267	0.023	
Chicago (United States of America)	0.643	0.525	0.746	2.356	0.018	
Manchester (United Kingdom)	0.563	0.470	0.651	1.319	0.187	
Madras (India)	0.500	0.398	0.602	0.000	1.000	

-1.00   -0.50   0.00   0.50   1.00

Meta Analysis

Table 4

Study name	Statistics for each study					Event rate and 95% CI
	Event rate	Lower limit	Upper limit	Z-Value	p-Value	
Groningen (The Netherlands)	0.768	0.665	0.847	4.580	0.000	
Nottingham (United Kingdom)	0.848	0.764	0.907	6.146	0.000	
Sofia (Bulgaria)	0.917	0.815	0.965	5.134	0.000	
Munich (Germany)	0.921	0.880	0.949	10.284	0.000	
Chicago (United States of America)	0.808	0.755	0.851	9.120	0.000	
Manchester (United Kingdom)	0.438	0.349	0.530	-1.319	0.187	
Madras (India)	0.844	0.754	0.906	5.817	0.000	
Singapore	0.721	0.676	0.763	8.552	0.000	

-1.00   -0.50   0.00   0.50   1.00

Meta Analysis

Herbener et al. 2005; Stirling et al. 2003; Kua 2003; Thara et al. 1994). There is still significant methodological and clinical heterogeneity between these long-term studies, e.g. the use of first admission, first contact and recent contact with services used in different studies, i.e. lead time bias (differential stage of disorder at entry to follow-up study). While all studies have used reliable tools for the assessment of outcome such as the WHO Life Chart or a Global assessment of functioning (symptom) score, these are only recognised as valid for the period around the time of the outcome assessment (maximum of 2 years). Therefore, we have only weak information regarding the intervening years and tells us little about the pathological trajectory or the dynamic interplay between the patient, disorder and environment. All these caveats notwithstanding, there is relative heterogeneity of some important methodological considerations. With regard to the age of onset of the samples being compared (Table 2), sex distribution (Table 3), and the loss to follow-up (attrition rates) (Table 4). The statistical combination of these studies concurs with other meta-analyses finding, 41% of the samples being in remission at the time of outcome assessment (Table 5).

Taken together, the evidence from recently published systematic reviews generally supports the following conclusions. (1) The course of schizophrenia is highly variable both *within* patient and *between* patients, even after taking account of methodological heterogeneity across studies. There is a broad range of possible course patterns ranging from complete recovery to continuous unremitting psychopathology, cognitive performance and social functioning. Between such extremes, a substantial number of patients present with multiple episodes of psychosis interspersed with partial remission. However, our current rudimentary typologies of good/bad outcome, remitted and unremitted, do not allow us to tease out the within-class heterogeneity. (2) Less than half of patients diagnosed with schizophrenia show substantial clinical improvement after follow-up time averaging 6 years. While these estimates are more optimistic than the earlier reports based on observations in institutional settings, they importantly emphasise the fact that schizophrenia

Table 5

Cohort name	Statistics for each study					Event rate and 95% CI
	Event rate	Lower limit	Upper limit	Z-Value	p-Value	
Groningen (The Netherlands)	0.268	0.184	0.374	-4.025	0.000	
Nottingham (United Kingdom)	0.418	0.306	0.538	-1.338	0.181	
Sofia (Bulgaria)	0.350	0.241	0.478	-2.287	0.022	
Munich (Germany)	0.355	0.256	0.468	-2.487	0.013	
Chicago (United States of America)	0.429	0.318	0.546	-1.191	0.234	
Manchester (United Kingdom)	0.469	0.335	0.608	-0.428	0.668	
Madras (India)	0.474	0.365	0.585	-0.459	0.647	
Singapore	0.463	0.414	0.512	-1.495	0.135	
	0.407	0.356	0.460	-3.390	0.001	

-1.00   -0.50   0.00   0.50   1.00

Meta Analysis

is more often associated with persistent chronic disability that profoundly affects a person's development and quality of life. (3) Examining the trends in course and outcome over the last century revealed substantial gains in favourable outcome from the 1920s until the 1970s, after which the gradient seemed to reverse (slightly). This biphasic trend may reflect developments in treatment, changes in diagnostic criteria across the decades as well as possible sampling bias. It has been suggested that this secular trend observed represents a benign metamorphosis in the course and outcome of schizophrenia (Harrison and Mason 1993; Zubin et al. 1983); moreover, the virtual disappearance of the most lethal form of catatonia was evident even before the introduction of antipsychotics. The reasons for this are unclear but may reflect changes in health-care provision and the development of psychological, social and rehabilitation approaches to treatment. Unfortunately, the current cannon of outcome studies (as published) does not lend itself to easily disentangling direct disease effects from environmental factors, which may influence the persistence of the disorder. (4) There may be some fluctuation in course, with the greatest variability being in the first 5–10 years, after which the course tends to plateau out. However, cross-sectional outcome measures of psychopathology are not found to be dependent on study duration, suggesting no clear pattern of deterioration (McGlashan 1988). (5) On average, patients with a diagnosis of schizophrenia have the poorest outcome, with schizo-affective patients occupying an intermediate position between schizophrenia and affective psychosis; however, diagnostic categories of psychosis poorly predict outcome. (6) Course and outcome estimates vary depending on the diagnostic classification used. Patients diagnosed using broadly defined schizophrenia have generally better outcomes compared to the narrowly defined (post-DSM III) schizophrenia. (7) The vast majority of the outcome studies to date come from Western Europe and the United States; there is little information from the developing economy states. (8) There is no reliable set of predictors for course and outcome yet identified. Furthermore, the predictive value of putative prognostic indicators is generally poor and likely to depend on the duration of illness (stage) and the projection time. Significant methodological differences in definition of predictor variables, adjustments for other known risk factors, differential attrition rates (loss to follow-up) and variation in outcome measurement reduce the comparability of studies on the prediction of prognosis and make exploratory subgroup analyses difficult despite a large number of published studies. Best estimates to date suggest that all known prognostic factors or psychopathology explain only a small amount of the total variance in outcome (estimates at around 30%, depending on the outcome domain under study), which translates into low predictive power.

Future Directions

To understand the natural history of psychosis, it will not be enough to simply continue to repeat the studies using clinical samples (first episode) or high-risk samples of people with 'at-risk mental states' or prodromal syndromes, to fully understand the dynamic nature of the pathological trajectory and its mutability with environmental factors will eventually require to study a more population-based approach of the whole spectrum of psychotic experiences. Furthermore, the statistical combination of outcome studies for schizophrenia more or less concurs, with around 40% of people having good outcome. The current typologies obfuscate marked *within* outcome category heterogeneity, and tell us very little about the course and its dynamic interplay with psychological and environmental factors. Our current literature base has employed classical epidemiological approaches with analyses being based on linear deterministic models of diagnoses or subsets of diagnoses resulting in biologically immutable (or partially mutable through treatment) outcomes. However, even from some of these outcome studies published over 20 years ago (Harding et al. 1987a, b, c), there is evidence suggesting marked variability within the individual, suggesting that it is not the disease which is immutable but rather the persons' liability, and the outcome is actual fact of the consequence of the interplay of the biological, social and psychological factors (Fig. 1) (Harding et al. 1987d). The current typologies may be clinically helpful; we have to try and tease out which constructs are the best discriminators of important functional outcomes, and if we wish to understand the causal determinants of persistence, we may have to employ different statistical methods which take into consideration the continuous fluid and dynamic nature of the construct, perhaps using growth mixture modelling or other latent variable techniques. We will have to better elucidate the relationship between the different clinical and functional domains of outcome as current measures. A recent study examining this issue using mixture modelling techniques for data reduction purposes, on outcome at 5 years, yielded three ordered classes, which varied by the level of outcome severity, from best, with little residual disability of clinical symptomology, to worst, with severe and chronic symptoms and social disability. There were however clear monotonic changes in the level of symptomology and disability across the classes, while the methodology employed in this study, latent class analysis (LCA), can make no firm assumptions about the underlying latent

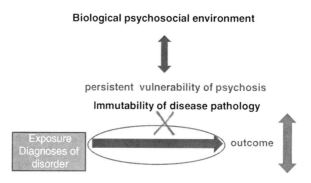

Fig. 1 Biological psychosocial environment

structure of outcome. The ordered classes suggest a dimensional outcome gradient (Fig. 2) (Allardyce 2009). Further research examining outcome using fine-grained assessment of outcomes, and latent variable modelling employed to better understand the relationships between the outcome measures, as they emerge would be informative.

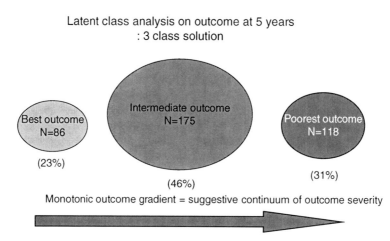

Fig. 2 Latent class analysis on outcome at 5 years: three class solution

References

Allardyce Jv, J. Outcome of psychosis at 5-year follow-up. Submitted 2009.

Bhopal R. Natural History, Spectrum, Iceberg, Population Patterns and Screening. Concepts of Epidemiology. Oxford: Oxford University Press; 2002, 132–62.

Bromet EJ, Naz B, Fochtmann LJ, Carlson GA, Tanenberg-Karant M. Long-term diagnostic stability and outcome in recent first-episode cohort studies of schizophrenia. Schizophrenia Bulletin 2005 July 1; 31(3):639–49.

Cougnard A, Marcelis M, Myin-Germeys I, De Graaf R, Vollebergh W, Krabbendam L, et al. Does normal developmental expression of psychosis combine with environmental risk to cause persistence of psychosis? A psychosis proneness-persistence model. Psychological Medicine 2007 Apr; 37(4):513–27.

Driessen G, Gunther N, Bak M, van Sambeek M, van Os J. Characteristics of early- and late-diagnosed schizophrenia: implications for first-episode studies. Schizophrenia Research 1998 Sep 7; 33(1–2):27–34.

Eaton WW, Thara R, Federman E, Tien A. Remission and relapse in schizophrenia: the Madras Longitudinal Study. Journal of Nervous & Mental Disease 1998 Jun; 186(6):357–63.

Ganev K, Onchev G, Ivanov P. A 16-year follow-up study of schizophrenia and related disorders in Sofia, Bulgaria. Acta Psychiatrica Scandinavica 1998; 98(3):200–7.

Möller HJ, Bottlender R, Wegner U, Wittmann J, Strauss A. Long-term course of schizophrenic, affective and schizoaffective psychosis: focus on negative symptoms and their impact on global indicators of outcome. Acta Psychiatrica Scandinavica 2000; 102(s407):54–7.

Hanssen M, Bak M, Bijl R, Vollebergh W, van Os J. The incidence and outcome of subclinical psychotic experiences in the general population. British Journal of Clinical Psychology 2005 Jun; 44(Pt 2):181–91.

Harding CM, Brooks GW, Ashikaga T, Strauss JS, Breier A. The Vermont longitudinal study of persons with severe mental illness, II: long-term outcome of subjects who retrospectively met DSM-III criteria for schizophrenia. American Journal of Psychiatry 1987a Jun; 144(6): 727–35.

Harding CM, Brooks GW, Ashikaga T, Strauss JS, Breier A. The Vermont longitudinal study of persons with severe mental illness, I: Methodology, study sample, and overall status 32 years later. American Journal of Psychiatry 1987b Jun; 144(6):718–26.

Harding CM, Strauss JS, Hafez H, Lieberman PB. Work and mental illness. I. Toward an integration of the rehabilitation process. Journal of Nervous & Mental Disease 1987c Jun; 175(6):317–26.

Harding CM, Zubin J, Strauss JS. Chronicity in schizophrenia: fact, partial fact, or artifact? Hospital & Community Psychiatry 1987d May; 38(5):477–86.

Harrison G, Mason P. Schizophrenia – falling incidence and better outcome? The British Journal of Psychiatry 1993 Oct 1; 163(4):535–41.

Harrow M, Grossman LS, Herbener ES, Davies EW. Ten-year outcome: patients with schizoaffective disorders, schizophrenia, affective disorders and mood-incongruent psychotic symptoms. The British Journal of Psychiatry 2000 Nov 1; 177(5):421–6.

Hegarty JD, Baldessarini RJ, Tohen M, Waternaux C, Oepen G. One hundred years of schizophrenia: a meta-analysis of the outcome literature [see comment]. American Journal of Psychiatry 1994 Oct; 151(10):1409–16.

Herbener ES, Harrow M, Hill SK. Change in the relationship between anhedonia and functional deficits over a 20-year period in individuals with schizophrenia. Schizophrenia Research 2005; 75(1):97–105.

Herbener ES, Harrow M. Longitudinal assessment of negative symptoms in schizophrenia/schizoaffective patients, other psychotic patients, and depressed patients. Schizophrenia Bulletin 2001 Jan 1; 27(3):527–37.

Huber G, Gross G, Schuttler R, Linz M. Longitudinal studies of schizophrenic patients. Schizophrenia Bulletin 1980; 6(4):592–605.

Jäger M, Bottlender R, Strauses A, Möller HJ. Fifteen-year follow-up of ICD-10 schizoaffective disorders compared with schizophrenia and affective disorders. Acta Psychiatrica Scandinavica 2004; 109(1):30–7.

Kraepelin E. Dementia Praecox and Paraphrenia, 1919 (translated by Barkley RM). New York: Robert E. Kreiger; 1971.

Kua J, Wong KE, Kua EH, Tsoi WF. A 20-year follow-up study on schizophrenia in Singapore. Acta Psychiatrica Scandinavica 2003; 108(2):118–25.

Last J. The challenge of epidemiology: issues and selected readings. In: Buck C (ed) The Challenge of Epidemiology: Issues and Selected Readings Pan American Health Organization, PAHO, 2004, 917–22.

Last J. The iceberg "completing the clinical picture" in general practice. The Lancet 1963; ii:28–31.

Mason P, Harrison G, Croudace T, Glazebrook C, Medley I. The predictive validity of a diagnosis of schizophrenia. A report from the International Study of Schizophrenia (ISoS) coordinated by the World Health Organization and the Department of Psychiatry, University of Nottingham. The British Journal of Psychiatry 1997 April 1; 170(4):321–7.

Mason P, Harrison G, Glazebrook C, Medley I, Croudace T. The course of schizophrenia over 13 years. A report from the International Study on Schizophrenia (ISoS) coordinated by the World Health Organization. The British Journal of Psychiatry 1996 November 1; 169(5):580–6.

Mason P, Harrison G, Glazebrook C, Medley I, Dalkin T, Croudace T. Characteristics of outcome in schizophrenia at 13 years. The British Journal of Psychiatry 1995 Nov 1; 167(5):596–603.

McGlashan TH. A selective review of recent North American long-term followup studies of schizophrenia. Schizophrenia Bulletin 1988; 14(4):515–42.

Menezes NM, Arenovich T, Zipursky RB. A systematic review of longitudinal outcome studies of first-episode psychosis. Psychological Medicine 2006 Oct; 36(10):1349–62.

Olfson M, Lewis-Fernandez R, Weissman MM, Feder A, Gameroff MJ, Pilowsky D, et al. Psychotic Symptoms in an Urban General Medicine Practice. American Journal of Psychiatry 2002 Aug 1; 159(8):1412–9.

Poulton R, Caspi A, Moffitt TE, Cannon M, Murray R, Harrington H. Children's self-reported psychotic symptoms and adult schizophreniform disorder:A 15-year longitudinal study. Archives of General Psychiatry 2000 Nov 1; 57(11):1053–8.

Racenstein JM, Harrow M, Reed R, Martin E, Herbener E, Penn DL. The relationship between positive symptoms and instrumental work functioning in schizophrenia: A 10 year follow-up study. Schizophrenia Research 2002; 56(1–2):95–103.

Sartorius N, Gulbinat W, Harrison G, Laska E, Siegel C. Long-term follow-up of schizophrenia in 16 countries. A description of the International Study of Schizophrenia conducted by the World Health Organization. Social Psychiatry & Psychiatric Epidemiology 1996 Sep; 31(5):249–58.

Shepherd M, Watt D, Falloon I, Smeeton N. The natural history of schizophrenia: a five-year follow-up study of outcome and prediction in a representative sample of schizophrenics. Psychological Medicine – Monograph Supplement 1989; 15:1–46.

Stirling J, White C, Lewis S, Hopkins R, Tantam D, Huddy A, et al. Neurocognitive function and outcome in first-episode schizophrenia: a 10-year follow-up of an epidemiological cohort. Schizophrenia Research 2003; 65(2–3):75–86.

Strauss JS, Carpenter WT, Jr. The prediction of outcome in schizophrenia. II. Relationships between predictor and outcome variables: a report from the WHO international pilot study of schizophrenia. Archives of General Psychiatry 1974 Jul; 31(1):37–42.

Thara R, Henrietta M, Joseph A, Rajkumar S, Eaton WW. Ten-year course of schizophrenia – the Madras longitudinal study. Acta Psychiatrica Scandinavica 1994 Nov; 90(5):329–36.

Van Os J. The clinical epidemiology of schizophrenia. In: B. Kaplan, V. Sadock and P. Ruiz (eds) Kaplan & Sadock's Comprehensive Textbook of Psychiatry, 9th edition. London: Lippincott Williams & Wilkins; 2008.

Van Os J, Hanssen M, Bijl RV, Ravelli A. Strauss (1969) revisited: a psychosis continuum in the general population? Schizophrenia Research 2000; 45(1–2):11–20.

Verdoux H, Maurice-Tison S, Gay B, Van Os J, Salamon R, Bourgeois ML. A survey of delusional ideation in primary-care patients. Psychological Medicine 1998; 28(01):127–34.

Westermeyer JF, Harrow M. Prognosis and outcome using broad (DSM-II) and narrow (DSM-III) concepts of schizophrenia. Schizophrenia Bulletin 1984; 10(4):624–37.

WHO. Who Coordinated Multi-Centred Study on the Course and Outcome of Schizophrenia. Geneva: WHO; 1992.

Wiersma D, Nienhuis FJ, Slooff CJ, Giel R. Natural course of schizophrenic disorders: A 15-Year Followup of a Dutch Incidence Cohort. Schizophrenia Bulletin 1998 January 1; 24(1):75–85.

Wiles NJ, Zammit S, Bebbington P, Singleton N, Meltzer H, Lewis G. Self-reported psychotic symptoms in the general population: Results from the longitudinal study of the British National Psychiatric Morbidity Survey. The British Journal of Psychiatry 2006 June 1; 188(6):519–26.

Wynne LC. The Natural Histories of Schizophrenic Processes. Schizophrenia Bulletin 1988; 14(4):653–9.

Zubin J, Magaziner J, Steinhauer SR. The metamorphosis of schizophrenia: from chronicity to vulnerability. Psychological Medicine 1983 Aug; 13(3):551–71.

Impact of Contextual Environmental Mechanisms on the Incidence of Schizophrenia and Other Psychoses

James B. Kirkbride

Introduction

We do not know, in most cases, how far social failure and success are due to heredity, and how far to environment. But environment is the easier of the two to improve.

JBS Haldane, 1892–1964

Substitute "schizophrenia and other psychoses" for "social failure and success" and the relevancy of JBS Haldane's quote to the search for the causes of psychotic disorders becomes immediately apparent. If we accept Tim Crow's powerful assertion that psychosis is the price *Homo sapiens* pay for language (Crow 2000) then there shall be no requirement to bastardise the quote at all.

This hypothesis builds upon the work of previous scientists to have considered why schizophrenia persists in the population despite its apparent genetic disadvantage. From an evolutionary perspective, Kuttner et al. (1967) postulated that schizophrenia was an inherently human disorder, inextricably bound to our development of functions to realise complex social relations, intelligence and, as Crow supports, language. In his influential work, Professor Crow (2000) suggests that a process of lateralisation in the brain at some shared point in our ancestry, leading to the asymmetry of function but not form, allowed humans to evolve this unique capacity that marks us out from other species. Put simply, when abnormalities in this lateralisation process occur, the result is psychosis, a misinterpretation of thoughts and messages received and processed by the brain, leading to the common positive symptoms of psychosis: delusions and hallucinations.

This superficially intuitive theory – that psychosis is a uniquely human phenomenon – assumes that the phenomenology and epidemiology of the disorder is globally ubiquitous. If the disorder were to occur equally worldwide, this would

J.B. Kirkbride (✉)
Department of Psychiatry, University of Cambridge, Cambridge, UK
e-mail: jbk25@cam.ac.uk

W.F. Gattaz, G. Busatto (eds.), *Advances in Schizophrenia Research 2009*,
DOI 10.1007/978-1-4419-0913-8_4, © Springer Science+Business Media, LLC 2010

support a common genetic mutation in the brain of less evolved *Homo* species
– perhaps even of a single gene [*sic*] (Crow 1995) – which led to both the extra
functionality of language and higher order cognitive processing, and the devastating
effects of psychosis. Geographical homogeneity in incidence would suggest that this
genetic change occurred at a common point in our ancestry, prior to the speciation
event that would allow *Homo sapiens* to leave Africa and populate every continent
on Earth. The genetic advantages conferred by our capacity for language would be
so great that it would not only lead to the extinction of all other *Homo* species, but
that psychosis, the unfortunate by-product of our evolutionary advantage, would be
the price humans paid for language. Crow (2000) argues that the inextricable connection of psychosis to language resolves the central paradox of schizophrenia: that
it is maintained in the population, despite considerable disadvantage to those who
bear it, because it confers such massive evolutionary advantages to the remainder of
the population.

Two recent developments in our understanding of schizophrenia and other psychoses do not support the exact mechanisms of Crow's hypothesis (though these
developments do not exclude the possibility that his general theory remains correct). First, the great hope that schizophrenia would be a disorder resulting from
mutation of a single gene has not been borne out by the research (Owen et al. 2005).
Rather, several genes, presumably of small effect, are likely to interact with each
other (and, most likely, the environment) to provide a polygenetic basis for the origins of psychotic disorder. Sadly, there have been few consistent replications for
candidate schizophrenia genes from linkage or association studies, but there is hope
that future genome-wide association studies (GWASs) may elucidate risk genes for
psychoses (Collier 2008). Further epigenetic processes – changes to the expression
of genes rather than the sequence itself – may provide another layer of complexity,
which psychiatric researchers are only beginning to get a handle on. While the focus
of the remainder of this chapter is on the environment and psychosis, it is important
to acknowledge that genes, epigenetic processes and the environment are likely to be
inexplicably linked. For a full review of the latest genetic findings in schizophrenia
research see Part III.

The second development in our understanding of psychosis to challenge the
mechanism of Crow's *speciation* hypothesis is that one of its central tenets –
that the incidence of psychosis is equal worldwide – can no longer be supported.
This view was largely based on the erroneous interpretation of the World Health
Organization's (WHO) Ten Country study in which the authors reported nearly
a threefold difference in incidence between centres with the highest and lowest rates (Jablensky et al. 1992). Because this variation only reached statistical
significance for broadly defined schizophrenia, the results were misinterpreted
by some as providing evidence for homogeneity in the incidence of narrowly
defined schizophrenia. It is now apparent that this conclusion was premature. The
inconclusive results of the WHO study could better be attributed to an absence
of evidence rather than the evidence of absence. Several epidemiological studies – of increasing methodological rigour – have now shown considerable variation in the incidence of psychotic disorders (McGrath et al. 2004; March et al.

2008), not only along the classic demographic dimensions of age and sex but by ethnicity, immigration, social class and, importantly, place. The view that schizophrenia and other psychotic disorders are egalitarian, indiscriminately affecting people with an equal probability wherever they live in the world, can no longer be sustained.

This variation has major implications for schizophrenia research, not only because it counters a widely held misconception in psychiatry but because it implicates that the environment is aetiologically relevant to the onset of psychosis, either through direct main effects or through more complex contextual mechanisms interacting with individual-level risk, including genetic susceptibility and possible epigenetic processes. In this chapter, I will highlight the exact contextual mechanisms for schizophrenia that have thus far been identified. Since, as Haldane notes, the environment is (presently) more eminently modifiable than our genetic code, it seems logical that putative prevention strategies for schizophrenia will necessarily require us to elucidate those environments – or the contextual mechanisms through which different environments impinge upon different individuals – which increase the probability (risk) of developing psychosis.

In the following chapter, I will briefly delineate the scope of this chapter and define what is meant by a "contextual environmental mechanism". I will outline the evidence supporting variation in the incidence of schizophrenia by major socioenvironmental factors including ethnicity and place, before reviewing the main candidate socioenvironmental risk factors that have been proposed to explain higher incidence rates of psychoses in immigrant groups and certain geographical locales. As we shall see, some of these environmental factors are likely to be highly contextual, with evidence emerging that individual risk is embedded within socioenvironmental experience. I will then consider the compelling public health prerogative that argues for the identification and removal of people from "risky" environments in order to successfully prevent psychosis. I conclude by attempting to place the evidence for contextual mechanisms in psychosis into a broader theory of psychosis onset. In doing so, I hope to demonstrate that far from disproving Crow's (1995) hypothesis, the presence of heterogeneity in the incidence of schizophrenia can still be consistent with his theory, although in the light of new genetic and environmental evidence, with some modification.

Epidemiological and Clinical Scope of the Chapter

Both incidence (new cases) and prevalence (new and existing cases) can offer important epidemiological clues as the aetiological basis of disease. However, for schizophrenia, and psychiatric disorders more generally, prevalence rates are less aetiologically useful because they are a function not only of the number of new cases but of the death rate for people with psychosis, and course and duration of illness, all of which are confounded by treatment. This is not to say that prevalence is unimportant. Understanding the prevalence of psychosis – particularly the lifetime prevalence – gives us an understanding of the expected burden of psychosis in different populations. Such information is therefore pivotal for planning effective mental health-care services. The lifetime prevalence of schizophrenia is typically estimated at around 1% (Regier et al. 1988; Kessler et al. 1994), although a recent meta-analysis has found variation along some dimensions including socioeconomic and migrant status (Saha et al. 2005). Such variation may be attributable to the incidence of disorder, or care and treatment thereafter, and illustrates the difficulty in separating out possible causal mechanisms from effects of service provision and treatment.

Incidence rates potentially offer more clues about the aetiological basis of schizophrenia because they should be less influenced by issues inherent to prevalence rates. Most studies interested in putative variation in schizophrenia and its possible contextual environmental correlates have used incident cases of disorder over prevalent cases because the possible effects of treatment and survival on estimates can be minimised. Studies that include incident cases typically refer to cases of psychoses in their first episode of disorder. Since schizophrenia and other psychoses may present a recurring, chronic episodic pattern, it is important to ensure that cases have not previously presented to services. Incident cases can be included in several epidemiological study designs including cross-sectional, case–control and cohort studies. Each design has a number of different strengths and weaknesses and each lends progressive degrees of support for causal associations between the putative exposure variable and outcome (it is beyond the scope of this chapter to provide an introduction to psychiatric epidemiology, but for an excellent primer on the subject see Susser et al., 2006b). In this chapter, I therefore limit the scope to studies based on incident cases of schizophrenia, wherever possible.

Although this chapter is written for the *6th Search for the Causes of Schizophrenia*, it is almost impossible to provide a complete introduction to the contextual mechanisms that influence the risk – or incidence – of disorder, without drawing upon evidence for complementary and/or contrasting associations between putative environmental factors and other psychotic disorders. In advance of the release of DSM-V, there has been considerable debate about the value of a categorical classification of psychotic disorders over a dimensional approach (Allardyce et al. 2007), which instead draws together common symptoms such as positive or negative symptoms, mania or substance abuse. This thinking is in line with the idea that a dimensional approach is more sensitive to an underlying continuum of psychosis liability in the population (van Os 2003). It is difficult to discuss contextual mechanisms for schizophrenia without drawing upon evidence from other relevant psychotic disorders or even from population-based samples of psychosis-like experiences. Therefore, while schizophrenia is the foremost focus of this chapter, I will also, where relevant, draw upon findings that provide support for, or against, contextual mechanisms in relation to other psychotic disorders, such as bipolar disorder and the depressive psychoses. Here, I also include literature on both narrowly defined schizophrenia (such as DSM-IV 295.xx or ICD-10 F20) and the broader definition, which extends to other non-affective psychoses including schizophreniform disorder and schizoaffective disorder (i.e., DSM-IV 295.xx, 297.xx 298.8, 298.9, or ICD-10 F20-29).

Defining Contextual Mechanisms and Variables

Just what do we mean by "contextual" variables and mechanisms? For the purposes of this chapter, a contextual *mechanism* is defined as the process through which an environmental exposure may act differentially upon an individual's risk of developing schizophrenia, depending on their individual-level characteristics. A good example is that of the relationship between the increased risk of schizophrenia for people of ethnic minority status and the level of ethnic density in the neighbourhood in which they live (Boydell et al. 2001). For some ethnic minority individuals, risk appears to increase when they live in neighbourhoods where ethnic minority groups make up a smaller proportion of the overall neighbourhood total (see below). Such a cross-level interaction between individual ethnicity and neighbourhood-level ethnic density potentially moves us closer to the aetiological genesis of elevated rates of psychoses in ethnic minority groups, generating important hypotheses about putative causal mechanisms. The importance of contextual environmental mechanisms in the aetiology of schizophrenia is only likely to increase over the forthcoming decades as we attempt to elucidate why so many people are exposed to ubiquitous factors such as urbanicity or black and minority ethnic status, yet so few people go on to develop psychosis. In this volume, Jim van Os discussed how such contextual mechanisms – interactions between genes, epigenetics and the environment – involving genetic interplay may be important. In this chapter, I consider how the wider social environment may act differentially upon individuals to dictate individual risk of psychoses.

To confuse the issue, environmental-level variables, also termed neighbourhood-level variables or societal-level variables, have often also been called contextual *variables* in order to distinguish them from individual-level attributes. Throughout this chapter, however, a "contextual" *mechanism* will refer to the more specific process whereby the effect of an individual-level attribute on psychosis risk is conditional upon an environmental-level variable. Because our understanding of how contextual mechanisms may affect the risk of psychoses is at an embryonic stage, both those environmental-level characteristics that increase the risk of schizophrenia for all groups and those that have been shown to operate via contextual mechanisms will be included in this review. It may be that we have yet to elucidate the exact contextual mechanisms for environmental factors that appear to ubiquitously raise rates, or they may genuinely increase risk for all individuals. Regardless, it is worthy to include such factors here. It is also important to note that we should be as equally aware of environmental factors that *lower* the incidence of schizophrenia (protective factors) as we are about those factors that *raise* rates (risk factors). To limit the scope of this chapter, I have restricted the discussion to environmental factors in the social sphere; for viral hypotheses of schizophrenia, see Brown et al. (2004, 2005) or Cannon et al. (2003).

Variation in the Incidence of Schizophrenia and Other Psychoses

Estimates of the Incidence of Schizophrenia

It is more difficult to answer the question *"what is the incidence of schizophrenia?"* than might have previously been assumed from earlier texts (Tsuang et al. 1995), given recent advances in our understanding of heterogeneity in incidence rates along various sociodemographic and contextual dimensions. Nevertheless, the incidence of schizophrenia and other psychotic disorders is known to be rare. A recent systematic review of the schizophrenia literature (1965–2001) identified 100 "core" incidence studies (McGrath et al. 2004) with a median observed incidence rate of 15.2 per 100,000 person-years (10th–90th percentile: 7.7, 43.0). The distribution of these rates suggested considerable asymmetric variation between studies; 80% of studies reported rates of less than 30 per 100,000 person-years (see Fig. 1). Reasons for this apparent variation may include methodological artefact (Bresnahan et al. 2000), possible changes in incidence over time (see below), sex differences, or ethnic or geographical variation, including urban/rural differences in the incidence of psychosis.

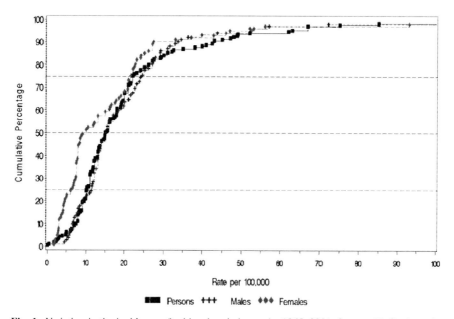

Fig. 1 Variation in the incidence of schizophrenia by study, 1965–2001. Source: McGrath et al. (2004). Truncated on x-axis at 100 per 100,000 person-years. Each box denotes a separate study

Individual-Level Variation in Incidence

We are fortunate that the most fundamental aspects of the epidemiology of schizophrenia and other psychoses – namely incidence rates by age and sex – have been clearly established and almost universally accepted. Due, in part, to the pioneering work of Heinz Hafner (1993), we know that schizophrenia has a distinctive, highly replicable, age and sex distribution, characterised by a young peak age at onset, typically occurring in the mid-twenties for men and a few years later – during the late twenties and early thirties – for women (Hafner et al. 1993; Kirkbride et al. 2006) (see Fig. 2). The incidence of schizophrenia is approximately 40% higher in men than in women (McGrath et al. 2004); however, this varies by age, with women experiencing a secondary peak in incidence around menopause (Fig. 2). Other non-affective psychotic disorders share a similar distribution of rates by age and sex as apparent for schizophrenia. For the affective psychoses, which include bipolar disorder and the depressive psychoses, the age profile remains similar to that in Fig. 2, but there appears to be no difference in incidence rates between men and women (Kirkbride et al. 2006).

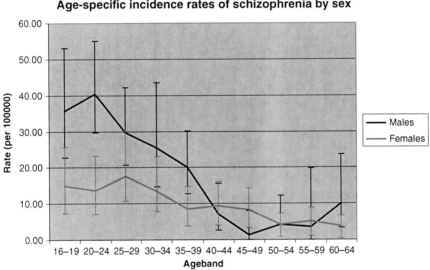

Fig. 2 Typical distribution of the incidence of schizophrenia by age and sex. Source: Kirkbride et al. (2006)

A more controversial axis upon which variation in the incidence of psychotic disorders has been observed is ethnicity/immigration (Singh and Burns 2006). One of the first studies to consider psychotic illness among immigrants was conducted in the United States by Ødegaard, who investigated the rates of hospitalised admissions to psychiatric wards in the 1920s (Ødegaard, 1932). He found that hospitalised admission rates were twice as high for Norwegian immigrants than for the remainder of the American-born population or for Norwegians who had not migrated. To explain the finding, Ødegaard (1932) posited that people who were predisposed to psychotic illness were more likely to emigrate than their healthy peers. More recent research has established that this explanation is extremely unlikely (Selten et al. 2002). Not only does migration require a high degree of cognitive processing, often in excess of that available to someone in the prodromal stage of psychosis, but a recent study of Surinamese immigration to the Netherlands directly tested Ødegaard's selection hypothesis, finding no evidence to support it (Selten et al. 2002). Selten and colleagues (1997) had previously shown that Surinamese immigrants to the Netherlands were at significantly increased risk of schizophrenia compared to the native white Dutch. If Ødegaard's (1932) hypothesis were true, they supposed that rates would no longer remain significantly raised if they imagined that the entire population of Surinam had migrated, but that the additional migrants (those who had, in fact, remained in Surinam) contributed to no further cases of disorder. When they added these additional "migrants" to the denominator, the incidence rate of schizophrenia in this hypothetical Surinamese population in the Netherlands remained raised, thus demonstrating that selection bias was unlikely to explain raised rates in these immigrants.

Elevated rates observed in immigrant groups and their offspring have persisted in spite of improved methodological designs including the following: larger sample sizes; a movement from hospitalised admission-based records to population-based samples; standardised diagnoses, often made blind to the ethnicity of the subject; control for several potential confounding factors including age, sex and socioeconomic status (Kirkbride et al. 2008b); and more accurate estimates of denominator populations. Studies from the United Kingdom (Harrison et al. 1988; King et al. 1994; van Os et al. 1996; Fearon et al. 2006), the Netherlands (Selten et al. 1997; Veling et al. 2006), Sweden (Zolkowska et al. 2001; Cantor-Graae et al. 2005) and Denmark (Cantor-Graae et al. 2003) have all observed raised rates in first-generation immigrants. In the United Kingdom and the Netherlands, rates appear to be most greatly elevated for black Caribbean and African immigrants, who are around 5–10 times more likely to experience a psychotic disorder than the native white population of the host country. That rates in the Caribbean are not elevated to the same extent as the rates for black Caribbean immigrants excludes the possibility that raised rates among immigrants could be attributable to higher rates in the country of origin (Hickling and Rodgers-Johnson 1995; Bhugra et al. 1996; Mahy et al. 1999).

Other immigrant groups also appear to experience elevated rates of psychotic disorder, including Moroccan immigrants in the Netherlands (Veling et al. 2006), immigrants from the Middle East to Sweden (Zolkowska et al. 2001) and non-native white immigrants in Denmark (Cantor-Graae et al. 2003) and the United Kingdom (Fearon et al. 2006; Kirkbride et al. 2008b). Rates appear to be more modestly raised in these groups, typically around twice those of the native white group in the host population. There has been much debate about whether people who migrated to the United Kingdom from the Indian subcontinent are also at increased risk of psychosis. These groups migrated at a similar time as black Caribbean and African immigrants to the United Kingdom (in the three decades following World War II), but some studies have shown that rates do not appear to be as highly elevated, potentially implicating differing experiences of potential contextual environmental factors, such as discrimination, as relevant to schizophrenia risk. Some studies have not found evidence of an increased risk in Asian immigrants compared with their white British counterparts (King et al. 1994), while others have reported modest increases (around 1.6 times the rate in the white British group) (Bhugra et al. 1997). These inconsistent findings may have arisen because of the small sample sizes of Asian groups in some studies, which often did not permit separate analysis of Indian, Pakistani and Bangladeshi groups, which are highly heterogeneous in terms of culture, religion and migratory experiences (Bhopal et al. 1991).

The largest study of schizophrenia in Asian immigrants to date was conducted in a highly heterogeneous population in East London (Kirkbride et al. 2008b). The East London First Episode Psychoses (ELFEP) study was able to estimate robust incidence rates of schizophrenia separately for Indian, Pakistani and Bangladeshi groups. It found that rates in the latter two ethnic groups, although not Indians, were significantly raised compared with the white British group, having adjusted for age and sex differences (Kirkbride et al. 2008b). However, this provided only half the picture. When stratified by sex, it became apparent that Pakistani and Bangladeshi women were at between four and five times the risk of schizophrenia compared with white British women, but that rates for their male counterparts were not elevated in relation to incidence rates for white British men. This suggested that the socioenvironmental factors (see below), which may increase the risk of psychosis for migrants, may be operating differentially by sex in some Asian groups, offering potential clues as to the aetiological role of contextual factors.

From the last two decades of the twentieth century onwards, the offspring of immigrants who had migrated to Europe from the Caribbean, Africa and Asia during the decades following World War II began to enter the critical age period where psychosis risk was greatest. Subsequent studies in these populations have revealed that incidence rates for the so-called "second-generation" offspring are at least the same, if not slightly increased (McGovern and Cope 1987; Harrison et al. 1988; Sugarman and Craufurd 1994; Coid et al. 2008). This suggests that factors allied to migratory processes alone are not sufficient to explain the raised rates in immigrants and their offspring, and that other factors – allied to post-migratory experiences – may be aetiologically important in the onset of psychoses. Contemporary research has begun to investigate whether the increased individual risk faced by immigrants and people of black and minority ethnic (BME) status is conditional upon contextual mechanisms, such as ethnic density (see below).

Ever since Faris and Dunham (1939) observed higher rates of schizophrenia in the poorer areas of Chicago, researchers have investigated whether individual-level socioeconomic status was associated with psychosis (Hollingshead and Redlich 1958; Goldberg and Morrison 1963; Dohrenwend and Dohrenwend 1969). Several studies (Hollingshead and Redlich 1958; Dohrenwend and Dohrenwend 1969), but not all (Goldberg and Morrison 1963), have observed an inverse association between socioeconomic status and schizophrenia, but it is unclear whether this association is a consequence of downward drift (Goldberg and Morrison 1963; Jones et al. 1993). The best evidence with regard to the potential causal influence of socioeconomic status on psychoses comes from studies that have measured socioeconomic status of the parent at birth, rather than the current or highest socioeconomic status of the subject with schizophrenia, thus minimising the potential effect of downward social drift. There is some evidence that parental socioeconomic status is associated with an increased risk of schizophrenia (Werner et al. 2007), but the effect appears to be restricted to the very poorest socioeconomic groups and is typically small (Byrne et al. 2004). Further, these associations have not been observed using prospectively collected longitudinal birth cohorts, which suggest socioeconomic status at birth is similar between those who do and do not go on to develop psychoses in adulthood (Jones et al. 1994, 1998). Social class may only therefore be a weak risk indicator, or marker, for other correlated socioenvironmental and sociodemographic factors related to urbanicity or ethnicity (Bresnahan and Susser 2003).

Temporal Variation in Incidence Rates of Schizophrenia and Other Psychoses

Understanding the past, current and likely future incidence of psychotic disorders is essential for effective health-care planning. It is also important for potential hypothesis generation: Tim Crow (1995) argues that the maintenance of schizophrenia in the population at a constant rate, despite the manifest evolutionary disadvantage faced by the sufferer, supports its inherent link with the evolution of language. However, assessing whether the incidence of schizophrenia has changed over time is riddled with methodological difficulties. Several studies during the 1980s and the 1990s reported a decline in the incidence of schizophrenia (Eagles et al. 1988; Der et al. 1990; Geddes et al. 1993; Munk-Jorgensen and Mortensen 1993; Osby et al. 2001). It has been suggested that the re-organisation of mental health care in the developed world during this time, with a movement towards outpatient rather than in-patient care, may have explained this apparent decline (Harrison et al. 1991), but this has not been equivocally demonstrated (Eagles 1991; Munk-Jorgensen and Mortensen 1993). More recently, it has been suggested that changes in diagnostic fashion may account for this decline (Osby et al. 2001), and Allardyce et al. (2000) have found some evidence to support this assertion using data from Scotland (Eagles et al. 1988; Geddes et al. 1993). Temporal changes in factors close to birth have been investigated (Suvisaari et al. 1999), such as declining obstetric complications or improving maternal nutrition, but the evidence base is contradictory (see Bresnahan et al. (2005) for a review).

In the United Kingdom, at least, the current evidence does not support (Brewin et al. 1997; Allardyce et al. 2000; Kirkbride et al. 2008d), and possibly counters (Castle et al. 1991; Boydell et al. 2003), a decline in the incidence of broadly defined schizophrenia. Increases in the incidence of psychotic disorders in inner London between 1965 and 1997 (Boydell et al. 2003) may have been largely attributable to the increased proportion of BME and immigrant groups in the area over this period (van Os et al. 1996; Boydell et al. 2001), illustrating the need to measure and understand changes in the prevalence of putative environmental factors over time as well.

Geographical Variation in Incidence Rates of Schizophrenia and Other Psychoses

Before considering the contextual mechanisms that underpin variation in the incidence of schizophrenia, it is important to demonstrate that such variation exists. Homogeneity in rates, after all, would not permit us to elucidate the potential aetiological components that contribute to the risk of psychosis. In this volume, Paulo Menezes showed that the incidence of schizophrenia varies between different populations across the globe, in contrast to the prevailing dogma (McGrath 2006).

Variation in the incidence of schizophrenia on a smaller, neighbourhood scale has been demonstrated since Faris and Dunham (1939) first showed that higher administrative rates of schizophrenia were found in inner-city census tracts of Chicago, more than 70 years ago. They found that these tracts had higher rates of poverty, greater proportions of immigrants and higher levels of social isolation. There is now considerable evidence that the rate of schizophrenia rises with increasing urbanicity and varies geographically (March et al. 2008). For a long time, it was argued that higher rates of schizophrenia in urban areas were a result of reverse causation; it was not so much that living in the city was in some way toxic, but that people who would go on to develop schizophrenia were more likely to drift into poorer, inner-city areas because of difficulties securing access to employment and affordable housing during the prodromal phase of disorder. Such social drift was a double-edged sword, since those who remained mentally well were more likely to be able to move up and out from the inner-city areas. It is highly possible that both social drift and social causation simultaneously contribute to the higher rates of psychotic disorders in urban areas, perhaps in a cyclical fashion, which propels vulnerable individuals into environments that ever increase the risk of developing schizophrenia.

A series of studies in the late 1990s and early twenty-first century have demonstrated that social drift cannot explain all the increased rates of schizophrenia associated with urbanicity. In a landmark study, Lewis et al. (1992) analysed data from a cohort of nearly 50,000 male conscripts to the Swedish army, for whom they linked residency during upbringing to any later hospitalised first admission of schizophrenia. They found that the incidence of schizophrenia for those conscripts who had been brought up in cities was 65% higher than for those conscripts brought up in rural areas. Notably, this association persisted after adjustment for several potential confounds, including cannabis use, parental divorce and a family history of psychiatric disorder. Support for a genuinely causal association between urbanicity and risk of schizophrenia grew following the publication of a second study by Mortensen et al. (1999), who demonstrated, through a prospectively collected cohort of 1.75 million people in Denmark, that this association was evident from birth. Further, the longer the people had resided in urban areas – and the more urban their environment – the greater the risk of schizophrenia later in life.

Recent studies have estimated that a significant proportion of the variation in incidence rates – now placed at around 8% – can be attributed to characteristics associated with neighbourhood level or environmental characteristics (van Os et al. 2000; Kirkbride et al. 2007b). Even in highly urbanised areas variation in the incidence of schizophrenia – not accounted for by individual-level confounders – remains evident (Kirkbride et al. 2007a). An interesting contrast here is the apparent absence of evidence for variation in the incidence of the affective psychoses by place. Thus, a national study in Denmark (Pedersen and Mortensen 2006), a city-wide study in Chicago (Faris and Dunham 1939), a rural study in Ireland (Scully et al. 2004) and urban studies in Southeast London (Kirkbride et al. 2007a) and Mannheim (Maylaih et al. 1989) have all failed to observe any significant neighbourhood-level variation in incidence of the affective psychoses. Although in some individual studies a lack of statistical power may have explained the absence of any observed variance, this is unlikely to explain the consistent direction of these results, including a cohort study of over 2 million people by Pedersen and Mortensen (2006). Thus, it appears that the effect of the environment on psychotic disorder may be limited to schizophrenia, having implications for the genesis of psychosis. Further, a tantalising finding from van Os' group (Kaymaz et al. 2006) suggested that for people with bipolar disorder, risk *did* increase with urbanicity, but only in those with comorbid psychotic symptoms, providing more evidence that the association with urbanicity is specific to the "psychotic" component of disorder. The absence of any variation in the incidence of unipolar depression at the neighbourhood level would also attest to this hypothesis (Weich et al. 2003).

The Role of Contextual Mechanisms on the Incidence of Schizophrenia

Although there is now good evidence that the incidence of schizophrenia varies geographically, the exact mechanisms that link exposure to ubiquitous environmental factors, such as urbanicity and immigration, to an increased risk of developing psychotic disorder remain to be elucidated. In response, researchers have pursued two related lines of enquiry in an attempt to discover how exposure to certain environmental characteristics may contribute to the onset of schizophrenia. First, research has tested whether putative environmental factors increase (or decrease) the risk of schizophrenia equally for all individuals or whether certain environments are more risky for individuals with certain characteristics, i.e. are there interactions that make individual risk of schizophrenia contextual upon exposure to putative environmental factors? Thus, researchers have become interested in testing cross-level interactions between individuals and neighbourhood-level environmental characteristics. We shall refer to these as "context-specific" exposure variables. Second, as well as considering how contextual mechanisms may affect the incidence (or risk) of schizophrenia, researchers have also attempted to drill down beneath "classic" exposures such as ethnic minority status, immigrant status and urban living – which can only be proxy measures for other underlying socioenvironmental risk factors – in order to elucidate more specific risk factors for schizophrenia and other psychotic disorders. Moving from broad risk indicators for schizophrenia, i.e. urbanicity, to specific risk factors, i.e. social disadvantage (Morgan et al. 2008), will only help to improve our understanding of the aetiological role of the social environment in psychosis onset. We shall refer to these as "context-refining" exposure variables.

Both streams of epidemiological research are important since it may turn out that different aspects of the environment operate differently upon the risk of schizophrenia, with some aspects increasing the risk for certain individuals contextually while others increase risk similarly for all exposed individuals. We shall consider both of these in turn.

Context-Specific Environmental Exposure Variables and the Incidence of Schizophrenia

One of the first contextual mechanisms to be considered in relation to the incidence of schizophrenia was the relationship between individual ethnicity and neighbourhood-level ethnic density. Tapping into the idea that social isolation may be a risk factor for schizophrenia, researchers posited whether the incidence of schizophrenia was greater for people from ethnic minority groups when they lived in neighbourhoods where ethnic minorities made up a smaller proportion of the overall neighbourhood total population. Several recent studies (Boydell et al. 2001; Kirkbride et al. 2008a; Veling et al. 2008) have found evidence to support the ethnic density effect, suggesting that being socially isolated may increase one's risk of schizophrenia. It is interesting to note that this is far from a new finding; one of Faris and Dunham's (1939) lesser-known findings was that they found evidence of a contextual effect of ethnic density.

van Os et al. (2000) pursued the idea that social isolation may be important in the onset and risk of schizophrenia by considering whether the incidence of schizophrenia for single people also varied contextually, depending on the proportion of other single people in the community. They found that the risk of schizophrenia in Maastricht was approximately doubled for single people living in neighbourhoods where the overall proportion of single people in the neighbourhood was below the city average, compared with single people living in neighbourhoods with above-average proportions of single people. The authors suggested this finding was compatible with the theory that social isolation was relevant to an increased risk of schizophrenia. For single people in neighbourhoods with fewer people living alone, their opportunity for social interaction may have decreased, resulting in greater social isolation and associated risk of psychosis. In neighbourhoods with greater opportunities for social interaction with other single people, the incidence of schizophrenia was lower.

Whether reverse causation explains these findings should be considered. On the one hand, the results were obtained from cross-sectional studies, making it difficult to determine whether exposure (single marital status) occurred before or after the onset of schizophrenia. Since people with schizophrenia are more likely to be living alone, it follows that the association between single marital status and schizophrenia is attributable to reverse causation. On the other hand, while van Os et al.'s (2000) work showed that the incidence of schizophrenia was higher for single people than for married persons (attributable to reverse causation), this was contextual upon the proportion of people living alone in the neighbourhood. It is more difficult to attribute this person–environment interaction to reverse causality, because it operates in the opposite direction to that which would be expected if reverse causation was in operation. If people with schizophrenia were more likely to drift into more socially fragmented and isolated neighbourhoods, one would expect to see a *higher* incidence of schizophrenia for single people living in neighbourhoods with *higher* proportions of people living alone – such neighbourhoods are typically more fragmented, deprived and transient. Instead, in van Os et al.'s (2000) study, we see the opposite: the incidence of schizophrenia is *higher* for single people living in neighbourhoods with *lower* proportions of people living alone. This does not readily fit with the possibility of reverse causation: neighbourhoods with fewer single people are usually more residentially stable, affluent and socially cohesive. It does not follow that people with schizophrenia would selectively drift into such areas.

Research interest in whether the social environment mediated the risk of schizophrenia has led researchers to consider the contextual influence of a range of neighbourhood-level socioenvironmental variables that may act as markers for social isolation.

With respect to ethnicity, Kirkbride et al. (2007b) have extended findings on ethnic density by considering a related concept of ethnic fragmentation: the extent to which a given ethnic group lives in a spatially cohesive residential pattern. We found that as ethnic fragmentation increased, the overall incidence of schizophrenia in those neighbourhoods increased. This remained significant after adjustment for individual-level age and sex, and neighbourhood-level socioeconomic deprivation and ethnic density. It will be important to test whether this ecological finding is truly contextual; is the incidence of schizophrenia for black and minority ethnic groups conditional upon the level of ethnic fragmentation in their neighbourhood, as observed for ethnic density?

Veling et al. (2007) have also considered possible mediating, contextual influences on the risk of schizophrenia for black and minority ethnic groups. Their research focused on whether racial discrimination in the community influenced risk of schizophrenia. Using first-episode data from the Netherlands, they demonstrated that the incidence of schizophrenia was significantly elevated for various black and minority ethnic groups (compared with the native white Dutch). The magnitude of this excess risk increased in proportion to the level of discrimination each ethnic group perceived itself as receiving (measured from a separate, population-based cross-sectional survey in the Netherlands). Thus, Moroccans, who were perceived as experiencing greatest discrimination, also had the highest incidence of schizophrenia. This important finding suggests that discrimination may be a negative environmental exposure that increases the risk of psychotic disorder. The findings above all support this possible mechanism, by suggesting that environmental factors (ethnic density, ethnic cohesion and social support and cohesion), which may buffer individuals from the experience of discrimination or other stressful events associated with urban living or minority status, result in lower rates of schizophrenia in those communities.

It is salient to note that these contextual findings are also supported by studies of individual-level risk factors. For example, in the Aetiology and Ethnicity in Schizophrenia and Other Psychoses (ÆSOP) study, Morgan et al. (2008) studied a series of first-episode cases, and controls, and looked for differences in their levels of social disadvantage, measured across six domains: education, housing, employment, relationships, social networks and living arrangements. The authors found that the odds ratio for schizophrenia increased in a dose–response manner with increasing social disadvantage. Interestingly, this association was observed for the white British and black Caribbean groups separately, but the prevalence of social disadvantage events was considerably greater in both black Caribbean cases and controls than their white British counterparts. This suggests that the impact of social disadvantage is context specific, here having a greater impact in the black Caribbean population. This supports a related finding by the same group showing that disadvantage during childhood – indexed by aberrant separation from one or both parents – increases later risk of psychotic disorder for white British, black Caribbean and black African groups to the same extent, but that the impact (prevalence) of these separation events was considerably greater for black cases and controls (Morgan et al. 2007).

The increased incidence of schizophrenia associated with smoking cannabis may also be contextually dependent (see also John McGrath in Part V). Smoking cannabis appears to increase one's risk of experiencing psychosis (Henquet et al. 2005). Early concerns that the relationship may have been attributable to self-medication of psychotic patients – reverse causation – appear to have been tempered, as prospectively collected longitudinal data, and subsequent meta-analyses, have found that the risk of psychosis is increased by around 41% in those who have ever smoked cannabis (Moore et al. 2007). Interestingly, this relationship appears to operate in a dose–response manner, such that the risk of psychosis increases with more frequent use (Moore et al. 2007) and earlier age at onset (Arseneault et al. 2002), although whether this is due to greater cumulative exposure to cannabis (van Os et al. 2002; Zammit et al. 2002) or exposure at critical periods of brain development – such as adolescence – still requires to be elucidated fully. Pursuing this line of enquiry, some researchers have posited whether exposure to cannabis – an environmental risk factor – was contextually dependent on individual genetic susceptibility (see also John McGrath in Part V). One prospective birth cohort study (Caspi et al. 2005) has observed that the risk of psychotic symptoms and schizophreniform disorder due to cannabis use was modified in the presence of the valine allele at the val[158]met polymorphism of the catechol-O-methyltransferase (COMT) gene, important in regulating dopaminergic activity known to be relevant to the development of positive psychotic symptoms. Researchers found that individuals with the val/val polymorphism were at over 10 times increased risk of schizophreniform disorder if they smoked cannabis during adolescence, but this risk decreased non-significantly to 2.5 times in the val/met group and was close to unity in the met/met group. However, there is considerable debate in the research community as to whether this finding is due to chance (Moore et al. 2007). First, it has yet to be extended to schizophrenia. Second, it has not been replicated in observational research, although there has been a partial replication in an experimental setting (Henquet et al. 2006). Third, this finding was observed in only a subset of the Dunedin sample (people with adolescent-onset cannabis use), and while, as Moore et al. (2007; p. 325) note, "[a]rguments for why earlier use of cannabis might have more harmful effects are intuitively compelling. . .no robust evidence supports this view". Fourth, the interaction observed in the Dunedin cohort was based on statistical rather than on biological synergism (Darroch 1997), and may therefore not reflect a genuine contextual relationship between gene and environment (Jim van Os in Part I). Finally, it is unclear whether the val[158]met polymorphism for COMT is directly associated with an increased risk of psychosis (Allen et al. 2008), leading researchers to question whether it is even a susceptibility gene for schizophrenia (Williams et al. 2007) (although it is important to note that the absence of a direct effect does not preclude the possibility of interactive – contextual – effects).

Context-Refining Environmental Exposure Variables and the Incidence of Schizophrenia

In addition to the socioenvironmental variables mentioned above, which increase the incidence of schizophrenia in a contextually dependent manner, a host of other socioenvironmental variables have been associated with the incidence of schizophrenia in the population as a whole. Whether contextual mechanisms for these environmental factors exist, or whether they elevate rates ubiquitously amongst the "exposed", remains to be elucidated, and will only be borne out by further studies capable of realising the complexity of unearthing possible interactions between genetic, epigenetic, individual and environmental factors in the incidence of schizophrenia. Such environmental factors not only provide signposts for possible contextual mechanisms, but have allowed us to refine our hypotheses as to how seemingly ubiquitous exposure to "urbanicity" or "immigration" may increase the risk of schizophrenia.

Assuming that the association between urbanicity and schizophrenia is causal (Mortensen et al. 1999), urbanicity can only be considered an indicator for other correlated environmental variables that impinge directly on individual risk of schizophrenia. Researchers have been particularly interested in those aspects of the neighbourhood environment that may generate and foster social isolation, since these fit in with possible theories of how social disadvantage may lead to psychosis (Selten and Cantor-Graae 2005). As well as the aforementioned contextual effects, researchers have observed a direct association between the level of social fragmentation or cohesion at the neighbourhood level and the incidence of schizophrenia in that neighbourhood. Important research by Hafner et al. (1969) in Mannheim, Germany, during the 1960s replicated Faris and Dunham's (1939) earlier finding that the incidence of schizophrenia was concentrated in inner-city areas. Similar work by Giggs in Nottingham revealed that the highest rates of schizophrenia were found in inner-city areas characterised by low social cohesion, high residential mobility and other characteristics indexing low social and economic deprivation (Giggs 1973, 1986; Giggs and Cooper 1987). Similar findings have been reported in Bristol (Hare 1956). Remarkably, these findings appear to be stable over long periods of time (Weyerer and Häfner 1989; Loffler and Hafner 1999). More recently, Silver et al. (2002) investigated whether specific structural characteristics of the neighbourhood were associated with the risk of schizophrenia in the Epidemiological Catchment Area (ECA) survey in the United States. They found that for every standard deviation increase in neighbourhood residential mobility – higher population turnover – there was a significant increase in the odds of schizophrenia (OR: 1.27; 95% CI: 1.02, 1.59), after adjustment for age, sex, ethnicity, socioeconomic status and neighbourhood-level socioeconomic deprivation. The authors suggested that their finding supported the hypothesis that in areas with higher levels of social disorganisation – indexed by high residential mobility – it was more difficult for people to form strong social ties that may have otherwise protected them from stressful experiences, which, for some individuals, could lead to the onset of psychotic symptoms.

This hypothesis is supported by other recent epidemiological findings that have investigated the association between social disorganisation and schizophrenia. In Scotland, Allardyce et al. (2005) created a social fragmentation index based on census variables for every postcode sector (population ~5,000). After adjustment for deprivation and urban/rural status, they found that first admission rates were significantly higher in areas characterised by greater social fragmentation. Further evidence that the incidence of schizophrenia is associated with neighbourhood-level social cohesion comes from the ÆSOP study in Southeast London (Kirkbride et al. 2007b, 2008a). We initially used a proxy for social cohesion – voter turnout at local elections – to investigate this link. We found that the incidence of schizophrenia was highest in the neighbourhoods with lowest voter turnout, after adjustment for other important individual- and neighbourhood-level characteristics. Pursuing this theme, we attempted to measure neighbourhood-level social cohesion more accurately through a cross-sectional survey based on methods proposed by social capital theorists (Sampson et al. 1997; McCulloch 2001). From the results of this survey, neighbourhoods were divided into areas with low, medium and high levels of social cohesion. As hypothesised, Kirkbride et al. (2008a) found that the incidence of schizophrenia was significantly higher in neighbourhoods with the lowest level of social cohesion. However, unexpectedly, neighbourhoods with the *highest* level of social capital also had significantly higher rates of schizophrenia compared with wards with medium levels of social cohesion. These relationships persisted despite adjustment for possible confounding by age, sex, ethnicity and socioeconomic deprivation. The authors suggested that while a number of methodological possibilities could not be excluded, their result was consistent with the hypothesis that social cohesion may operate contextually (Drukker et al. 2006). Thus, an individual's risk of schizophrenia was influenced not only by the level of social cohesion or support in the neighbourhood but by their ability to access it. They posited that the risk of schizophrenia might be even greater for individuals living in areas of high social cohesion, but who were unable to access it, than for individuals living in areas with lower social cohesion. Such an explanation is analogous to, and supported by, findings with regard to the ethnic density hypothesis.

This example illustrates the importance of testing potential interactions between neighbourhood-level variables and individual-level characteristics. It is unlikely that all environmental characteristics affect all individuals to the same degree or even in the same way. It will be important for future epidemiological studies to design methodologies that are sensitive to contextual mechanisms that shape individual risk of schizophrenia. It will also be important to study those factors in the environment which are putatively protective against the onset of psychosis. Social cohesion provides one possible example here. For example, the elevated incidence of schizophrenia in Pakistani and Bangladeshi women, but not men, is consistent with the hypothesis that a lack of social support confers an increased risk of disorder. Incidence rates remained elevated after adjustment for socioeconomic status (Kirkbride et al. 2008b) and appeared to be higher for first (non-UK born) rather than second-generation (UK born) women from the Indian subcontinent (Coid et al. 2008). These findings potentially suggest that the protective risk factors afforded to their male counterparts – less discrimination than experienced by black Caribbean and African immigrants and their offspring, and strong social cohesion within Asian communities – lower the risk of schizophrenia. Conversely, for some Asian women – who may have less access to protective factors in the community and who often occupy a more marginal social status in some Asian communities – the risk of psychosis may be greater. This effect may be amplified for first generation migrant women, given additional cultural and language barriers in assimilating in the host community. Such hypotheses on contextually specific social isolation, while intuitively attractive, have yet to be explicitly tested in observational studies in psychiatric epidemiology, and addressing the role of contextual risk and protective factors will be an important advance in our search for the causes of schizophrenia and other psychotic disorders.

In the closing two sections of this chapter, I consider the implications that the identification of contextual mechanisms for psychoses will potentially have for public health and the aetiology of schizophrenia. First I consider the public health impact and imperative for identifying specific contextual socioenvironmental variables that increase the risk of schizophrenia. Second, I conclude by considering the possible biological pathways through which seemingly distal socioenvironmental factors may impinge upon individual characteristics, in some cases via contextual mechanisms, to increase the risk of developing psychotic symptoms and clinical disorder.

The Impact of Socioenvironmental Factors for Schizophrenia and Other Psychoses

If we could identify and remove the contextual exposures that increase the incidence of schizophrenia and other psychoses associated with urban living and ethnic minority status, we could prevent a substantial proportion of new, incident cases of disorder, both globally and nationally.

Recent research from the pooled estimates of two large, epidemiological studies of first episode psychoses in England (ÆSOP and ELFEP) has suggested that if the risk factors – including contextual factors – which increase the risk of psychotic disorders in black and minority ethnic populations could be successfully identified and removed, we could prevent 21.6% of all cases of psychosis. Within specific populations, such as black Caribbean and black African groups, we could prevent a staggering 81.0 and 74.4% of incident cases, respectively (Kirkbride et al. 2008c). The potential public health benefits are no less substantial for those factors allied to urbanicity. Mortensen et al. (1999) placed the population attributable risk fraction for urbanicity in relation to the incidence of schizophrenia at 35%, a figure comparable with that recently observed in the United Kingdom (Kirkbride et al. 2008c). Our data suggest that the synergistic prevention of factors allied to both urbanicity and black and ethnic minority status could lead to an overall reduction in the incidence of non-affective psychoses of 61.7% in England's urban populations (Kirkbride et al. 2008c).

Such *theoretical* public health gains are undoubtedly impressive. They present the *raison d'etre* for psychiatric research to identify the suite of aetiologically contextual factors that underpin associations between ethnic minority status, immigration, urbanicity and an increased risk of psychoses, and implement appropriate interventions against them. Such public health gains would improve the lives of millions of people, both for those who would have gone on to develop psychosis and for those on whom the burden of care would fall. These gains would also present substantial economic savings, in terms of both the direct costs saved to mental health services and indirect costs associated with keeping people in the labour market. Whether such population attributable risk fractions are *tangible*, however, is a more important question. It will be vital that psychiatric epidemiology moves beyond associations between urbanicity and psychosis to identifying the specific contextual mechanisms involved in the aetiology of disorder. It is evident from the above body of work that researchers are beginning to test, and discover, contextual mechanisms associated with the incidence of schizophrenia, but it will be imperative for future studies to tease out the specific interactions between genetic susceptibility, epigenetics (Jim van Os in Part I), other individual-level characteristics and the environment, if we are to develop effective community-based strategies for the prevention of schizophrenia and other psychotic disorders. From a public health perspective, it is salient to remember that schizophrenia is a rare outcome and the increased risk associated with some contextual factors, such as cannabis consumption, while significant, is small. Since the prevalence of exposure to such contextual factors is often high, population-based interventions, for example, to reduce cannabis consumption are likely to have only limited impact in preventing psychoses in the community until we are able to more narrowly identify which individuals, via which contextual mechanisms, are at the greatest increased risk of schizophrenia.

Placing Contextual Mechanisms in Context: From Envirome to Epigenetics

If contextual mechanisms are aetiologically important in the onset of schizophrenia and other psychotic disorders, and the available evidence presented above appears to support this, then for some individuals exposure to socioenvironmental factors must impinge upon normal biological processes in the brain, to manifest the onset of psychotic symptoms. Understanding how environmental exposures are coded and processed by our brains under normal and abnormal conditions will provide great clues about the aetiology of psychoses and allow us to delineate precisely which environments are likely to be risky for different individuals. This will allow us to develop more effective public health interventions aimed at specific environmental triggers. Linking the envirome with the genome will be fundamental to understanding how – and when – contextual, environmental factors increase the risk of psychoses. Several allied disciplines – not least epidemiology, genetics, neuropsychiatry, neuropsychology and neurobiology – will need to be included in such collaborative efforts if we are to begin to understand how seemingly distal environmental effects impinge on biological mechanisms to contribute to the eventual onset of psychoses.

In Fig. 3 I provide a conceptual diagram illustrating how exposures at multiple levels – genetic, epigenetic, individual and environmental – may interact over the life course to govern the risk of schizophrenia. Thus, the *multiple lenses* model suggests that a series of lenses – risk and protective factors – will shape our risk of psychoses (x-axis). Our exposure to these factors changes over time (z-axis), as we move through different environments and as our individual responses and characteristics respond and evolve to these environments (y-axis). Over the life course, our exposure to these environmental lenses is in constant interaction with our genetic susceptibility (fixed at birth) and epigenetic processes (also modifiable over the life course) to determine our risk of psychosis. Psychiatric epidemiology has been influential in establishing that individual-level risk is, in part at least, contextual upon our exposure to environmental factors (ethnic density, cannabis use). Our discipline has also refined the lenses that may be both protective and detrimental to our risk of psychosis. We are beginning to move from fairly broad lenses – urbanicity, social class, ethnicity, immigration and family history of psychosis – to progressively narrower, more specific lenses, such as social cohesion, social support, discrimination, cannabis use and specific genes. The future challenge for psychiatric epidemiology and allied disciplines will be to (i) continue to refine these lenses to elucidate more specific risk and protective factors for psychoses, (ii) understand how these factors interact with each other and with genetic susceptibility to provide contextual

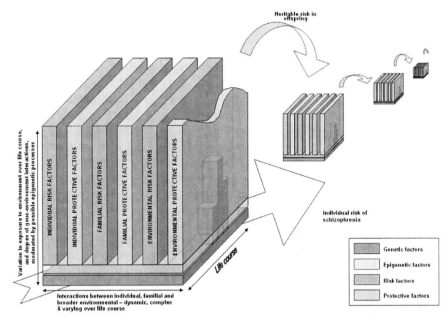

Fig. 3 Multiple lenses model of the aetiology of psychotic disorders

pathways for psychosis and (iii) determine those stages of the life course where exposure to such factors is most critical in terms of increasing the risk for (or protecting people against) psychosis.

This conceptual model is consistent with a *stress-vulnerability* model for psychosis (Nuechterlein and Dawson 1984), which offers one plausible biological explanation for how exposure to a series of contextual risk and protective factors may lead to the onset of psychotic symptoms for certain, presumably genetically susceptible individuals. This model suggests that underlying vulnerability to psychoses is sensitised through a series of negative life events and socioenvironmental stressors (Myin-Germeys et al. 2005; Morgan et al. 2007). There is accumulating evidence that dopaminergic dysregulation presents a candidate biological mechanism through which chronic exposure to social stress may lead to the onset of psychoses (Di Forti et al. 2007). It has been shown –both in animal studies (Robinson et al. 1988) and in patients with schizophrenia (Laruelle et al. 1996) – that when challenged with amphetamine, excessive amounts of striatal dopamine are released. Striatal dopamine is an important neurotransmitter in the misolimbic system critical for processing stimuli as either rewarding or dangerous. Under normal processing, dopamine allows the individual to determine the salience of such stimuli and choose an appropriate response to them (Schultz 2002). It has been proposed that disruption to this dopaminergic pathway through an excess release of dopamine – or hyperdopamingeric dysregulation – leads to aberrant salience of otherwise neutral stimuli, resulting in positive psychotic symptoms more commonly referred to as delusions and hallucinations (Kapur 2003). In Kapur's (2003) heuristic model, he suggests that delusions are "a cognitive effort by the patient to make sense of these aberrantly salient experiences, whereas hallucinations reflect a direct experience of the aberrant salience of internal representations...of percepts and memories". What Kapur (2003) argues is that in the schizophrenic brain aberrant salience persists in the absence of stimuli, leading to a chronic, enduring course of disorder rather than a single acute episode. In turn, antipsychotics work by blocking dopamine from attaching to D_2 receptors in the brain, allowing a reprieve from the positive symptoms associated with schizophrenia.

Repeated exposure to social stressors may also sensitise the mesolimbic dopaminergic system in a similar way to amphetamines and other psychostimulants (Lucas et al. 2004). The process of sensitisation suggests that repeated exposure to such stressors produces an incremental stress response, here assumed to be dopaminergic, until eventually a critical threshold is surpassed, beyond which clinically relevant psychotic experiences begin to manifest themselves. Animal paradigms have demonstrated that repeated exposure to social stressors results in elevated dopaminergic activity (Tidey and Miczek 1996; Lucas et al. 2004) and behavioural sensitisation (Covington and Miczek 2001). Social defeat (Selten and Cantor-Graae 2005) – chronic exposure to a series of negative life events resulting in marginalisation – has been proposed as a parallel model for the onset of psychotic symptoms in humans.

The dopamine hypothesis of schizophrenia thus provides a plausible biological mechanism capable of unifying the plethora of associations reported between various socioenvironmental lenses at multiple levels and the risk of psychoses. Exposure across the life course to a series of lenses, which may be both protective and deleterious, shapes our sensitisation to dopamine, and both determine and govern our vulnerability to stress. For some individuals, without sufficient buffering from the detrimental effects of urban living or minority status – substance abuse (Moore et al. 2007) discrimination (Veling et al. 2007), poverty (Croudace et al. 2000), social isolation (Allardyce et al. 2005) – by protective factors such as social cohesion and support (Kirkbride et al. 2008a), the result of chronic exposure to social stressors would be the onset of psychotic symptoms via dopaminergic dysregulation. It is envisaged that this mechanism would be underpinned by polymorphic variation to susceptibility genes relevant to dopaminergic regulation, including neuregulin (NRG1), dysbindin (DTNBP1), D-amino acid oxidase activator (DAOA) and the aforementioned COMT gene (Di Forti et al. 2007).This contextual hypothesis would help us understand how ubiquitous exposure to environmental stimuli, such as urbanicity or immigrant status, leads to the onset of psychoses in only a few individuals. It also accords with the current literature, which suggests that many genes of small effect may contribute to the onset of psychotic symptoms and that, indeed, there may be many pathways to psychotic disorder, unified via dopaminergic dysregulation, rather that any single aetiological factor (Seeman et al. 2005).

The epidemiological data supporting an association between socioenvironmental factors and the risk of schizophrenia, as presented in this chapter, are consistent with this possibility. Recent studies have shown that markers of social stress, indexed by disadvantage such as discrimination (Veling et al. 2007), immigrant status

(Cantor-Graae and Selten 2005; Kirkbride et al. 2008b), social disadvantage (Morgan et al. 2008), childhood trauma (Bebbington et al. 2004), separation from parents during childhood (Morgan et al. 2007) or socioeconomic deprivation (Croudace et al. 2000) are all associated with an increased risk of schizophrenia. Similarly, in neighbourhoods indexed with greater levels of social isolation (Allardyce et al. 2005), the incidence of schizophrenia has been observed to be higher. Thus, single marital status (van Os et al. 2000), ethnic fragmentation (Kirkbride et al. 2007b) and high levels of residential turnover (Silver et al. 2002), which all index a lack of potential buffers against social stressors, have been shown to be associated with higher rates of psychoses. This risk appears to be contextually dependent: exacerbated for individuals who experience them when they are in the minority (van Os et al. 2000; Boydell et al. 2001; Kirkbride et al. 2008a; Veling et al. 2008).

Concluding Remarks: Future Directions

It is now clear that there is marked variation in the incidence of schizophrenia and other psychoses along several important socioenvironmental dimensions, not least by immigration, ethnicity and place. In the search for the causes of schizophrenia, we now know that certain social and environmental characteristics are likely to increase the risk of disorder. Moreover, a growing body of literature suggests that contextual mechanisms may be important to aetiology: certain environments appear to be more risky for certain individuals. Other environmental factors, such as social cohesion, have been discovered, which appear to be associated with the incidence of schizophrenia but for which no clear contextual effect has yet emerged. It may be that such factors operate independently to increase risk, or it may be that we are still to elucidate the specific contextual mechanisms through which these factors operate. One thing seems clear though: contextual mechanisms are likely to be critical in explaining how seemingly ubiquitous exposure to certain factors (immigration, urbanicity, cannabis use) result in an absolutely low incidence of schizophrenia and other psychoses in the population at risk. Incorporating genetic information into epidemiological studies of contextual processes is only likely to yield greater insights into our understanding of the aetiology of psychotic disorders (Caspi et al. 2005), and adopting prospectively collected, longitudinal data will help to elucidate the critical timing of exposure to socioenvironmental factors over the life course. It is likely that even contextual mechanisms are themselves contextually embedded in time as well as in space.

What implications does this have for Crow's (2000) hypothesis that schizophrenia originated after humans evolved the capacity for language prior to leaving Africa? The answer, I believe, is very little. That the incidence of schizophrenia is not equal worldwide does not have drastic implications for psychiatric genetics. It does not render Crow's hypothesis, or a polygenetic basis of psychosis, or an epigenetic origin for psychosis redundant (Crow 2008). In fact, given that allele frequency often varies widely between populations it seems entirely plausible that a heritable disease could show differing incidences among different populations, especially if the genetic basis for this disease involved multiple genes, incomplete penetrance and/or interaction with environmental factors. Man [sic] could have left Africa with a similar genetic liability for psychosis, and as isolated groups developed differing cultural systems in response to differing environmental terrains, so our propensity to develop psychosis might be influenced by intermediary layers of social networks and support. As much is tentatively proposed to explain the apparent associations between social isolation and schizophrenia today (Allardyce and Boydell 2006). Thus, variation in incidence across the world supports a genetic basis for psychosis, intrinsically linked to our experience and interpretation of environmental exposures. Whether the exact mechanisms prove to be polygenetic or epigenetic, or both, it is likely that differential experiences of environmental cues will determine whether our predisposing genetic susceptibility results in the onset of psychoses.

Future studies will have to overcome several hurdles if we are to successfully advance our aetiological understanding of psychoses, not least the synthesis of traditionally disparate disciplines including genetics, neuroscience and epidemiology. Thus far, separate disciplines have yielded largely inconsistent results in the search for underlying biological pathways for psychoses. The dopamine hypothesis is no exception (Keshavan et al. 2008). Similarly, it has been difficult to elucidate specific genetic and social markers for psychoses, which underpin the three largest risk indicators for psychoses: a family history (Kendler and Diehl 1993), urbanicity (McGrath et al. 2004) and minority status (Cantor-Graae and Selten 2005). But given our relatively crude treatment of genetics (in psychiatric epidemiology) or of the environment (in genetics and neuroscience), or of our failure to elucidate the relevant timing of exposure more generally, it is perhaps not surprising that the literature is littered with such inconsistencies. By beginning to tackle the complexity that lies ahead of us, such as investigating contextual mechanisms, we should begin to observe large and consistent effect sizes for psychosis as we refine risk into a set of ever more specific lenses operating at particular periods of the life course. It is up to us to design methodologies that are sensitive to these complexities. Susser et al. (2006a) have promoted eco-epidemiology as a paradigm through which such grandiose aspirations may be realised, calling for prospective, longitudinal, multifactorial, multilevel studies to represent the gold standard in this respect. The precise aetiological roles of genes and environments – and the contextual mechanisms that link them – will need to be elucidated more fully before we are able to develop effective public mental health strategies against the onset of schizophrenia and other psychoses, but environment is likely to remain the easier of the two to improve. In so doing, we may move closer to realising the large *theoretical* population attributable risks on offer to us.

References

Allardyce, J., Boydell, J. (2006). Environment and Schizophrenia: Review: The Wider Social Environment and Schizophrenia. *Schizophr Bull* **32**(4), 592–598.

Allardyce, J., Gilmour, H., Atkinson, J. et al. (2005). Social fragmentation, deprivation and urbanicity: relation to first-admission rates for psychoses. *Br J Psychiatry* **187**(5), 401–406.

Allardyce, J., McCreadie, R., Morrison, G. et al. (2007). Do symptom dimensions or categorical diagnoses best discriminate between known risk factors for psychosis? *Soc Psychiatry Psychiatr Epidemiol* **42**(6), 429–437.

Allardyce, J., Morrison, G., Van Os, J. et al. (2000). Schizophrenia is not disappearing in southwest Scotland. *Br J Psychiatry* **177**, 38–41.

Allen, N. C., Bagade, S., McQueen, M. B. et al. (2008). Systematic meta-analyses and field synopsis of genetic association studies in schizophrenia: the SzGene database. *Nat Genet* **40**(7), 827–834.

Arseneault, L., Cannon, M., Poulton, R. et al. (2002). Cannabis use in adolescence and risk for adult psychosis: longitudinal prospective study. *Br Med J* **325**(7374), 1212–1213.

Bebbington, P. E., Bhugra, D., Brugha, T. et al. (2004). Psychosis, victimisation and childhood disadvantage: Evidence from the second British National Survey of Psychiatric Morbidity. *Br J Psychiatry* **185**(3), 220–226.

Bhopal, R. S., Phillimore, P., Kohli, H. S. (1991). Inappropriate use of the term 'Asian': an obstacle to ethnicity and health research. *J Public Health Med* **13**(4), 244–246.

Bhugra, D., Hilwig, M., Hossein, B. et al. (1996). First-contact incidence rates of schizophrenia in Trinidad and one-year follow-up. *Br J Psychiatry* **169**(5), 587–592.

Bhugra, D., Leff, J., Mallett, R. et al. (1997). Incidence and outcome of schizophrenia in Whites, African-Caribbeans and Asians in London. *Psychol Med* **27**(4), 791–798.

Boydell, J., Van Os, J., Lambri, M. et al. (2003). Incidence of schizophrenia in south-east London between 1965 and 1997. *Br J Psychiatry* **182**, 45–49.

Boydell, J., van Os, J., McKenzie, K. et al. (2001). Incidence of schizophrenia in ethnic minorities in London: ecological study into interactions with environment. *Br Med J* **323**(7325), 1336–1338.

Bresnahan, M., Susser, E. (2003). Investigating socioenvironmental influences in schizophrenia: conceptual and design issues. In: R. M. Murray, P. B. Jones, E. Susser, J. van Os, M. Cannon (eds.), *The Epidemiology of Schizophrenia*. Cambridge University Press: Cambridge.

Bresnahan, M., Schaefer, C. A., Brown, A. S., Susser, E. S. (2005). Prenatal determinants of schizophrenia: what we have learned thus far? *Epidemiol Psichiatr Soc* **14**(4), 194–197.

Bresnahan, M. A., Brown, A. S., Schaefer, C. A. et al. (2000). Incidence and cumulative risk of treated schizophrenia in the prenatal determinants of schizophrenia study. *Schizophr Bull* **26**(2), 297–308.

van Os, M. Cannon (eds.), *The Epidemiology of Schizophrenia*. Cambridge University Press: Cambridge.

Brewin, J., Cantwell, R., Dalkin, T. et al. (1997). Incidence of schizophrenia in Nottingham – a comparison of two cohorts, 1978–80 and 1992–94. *Br J Psychiatry* **171**, 140–144.

Brown, A. S., Begg, M. D., Gravenstein, S. et al. (2004). Serologic evidence of prenatal influenza in the etiology of schizophrenia. *Arch Gen Psychiatry* **61**(8), 774–780.

Brown, A. S., Schaefer, C. A., Quesenberry, C. P., Jr. et al. (2005). Maternal Exposure to Toxoplasmosis and Risk of Schizophrenia in Adult Offspring. *Am J Psychiatry* **162**(4), 767–773.

Byrne, M., Agerbo, E., Eaton, W. W. et al. (2004). Parental socio-economic status and risk of first admission with schizophrenia – a Danish national register based study. *Soc Psychiatry Psychiatr Epidemiol* **39**(2), 87–96.

Cannon, M., Kendell, R., Susser, E. et al. (2003). Prenatal and perinatal risk factors for schizophrenia. In: R. M. Murray, P. B. Jones, E. Susser, J. van Os, M. Cannon (eds.), *The Epidemiology of Schizophrenia*. Cambridge University Press: Cambridge.

Cantor-Graae, E., Pedersen, C. B., McNeil, T. F. et al. (2003). Migration as a risk factor for schizophrenia: a Danish population-based cohort study. *Br J Psychiatry* **182**, 117–122.

Cantor-Graae, E., Selten, J.-P. (2005). Schizophrenia and migration: a meta-analysis and review. *Am J Psychiatry* **162**(1), 12–24.

Cantor-Graae, E., Zolkowska, K., McNeil, T. F. (2005). Increased risk of psychotic disorder among immigrants in Malmo: a 3-year first-contact study. *Psychol Med* **35**(8), 1155–1163.

Caspi, A., Moffitt, T. E., Cannon, M. et al. (2005). Moderation of the effect of adolescent-onset cannabis use on adult psychosis by a functional polymorphism in the catechol-O-methyltransferase gene: longitudinal evidence of a gene × environment interaction. *Biol Psychiatry* **57**(10), 1117–1127.

Castle, D., Wessely, S., Der, G. et al. (1991). The incidence of operationally defined schizophrenia in Camberwell, 1965–84. *Br J Psychiatry* **159**, 790–794.

Coid, J. W., Kirkbride, J. B., Barker, D. et al. (2008). Raised incidence rates of all psychoses among migrant groups: findings from the East London first episode psychosis study. *Arch Gen Psych* **65**(11), 1250–1258.

Collier, D. A. (2008). Schizophrenia: the polygene princess and the pea. *Psychol Med* **38**(12), 1687–1691.

Covington, H. E., 3rd, Miczek, K. A. (2001). Repeated social-defeat stress, cocaine or morphine. Effects on behavioral sensitization and intravenous cocaine self-administration "binges". *Psychopharmacology (Berl)* **158**(4), 388–398.

Croudace, T. J., Kayne, R., Jones, P. B. et al. (2000). Non-linear relationship between an index of social deprivation, psychiatric admission prevalence and the incidence of psychosis. *Psychol Med* **30**(1), 177–185.

Crow, T. J. (1995). A continuum of psychosis, one human gene, and not much else – the case for homogeneity. *Schizophr Res* **17**(2), 135–145.

Crow, T. J. (2000). Schizophrenia as the price that Homo sapiens pays for language: a resolution of the central paradox in the origin of the species. *Brain Res Rev* **31**(2–3), 118–129.

Crow, T. J. (2008). The emperors of the schizophrenia polygene have no clothes. *Psychol Med* **38**(12), 1681–1685.

Darroch, J. (1997). Biologic synergism and parallelism. *Am J Epidemiol* **145**(7), 661–668.

Der, G., Gupta, S., Murray, R. M. (1990). Is schizophrenia disappearing? *Lancet* **335**(8688), 513–516.

Di Forti, M., Lappin, J. M., Murray, R. M. (2007). Risk factors for schizophrenia – all roads lead to dopamine. *Eur Neuropsychopharmacol* **17**(Suppl 2), S101–S107.

Dohrenwend, B. P., Dohrenwend, B. S. (1969). *Social Status and Psychological Disorder: A Causal Inquiry*. John Wiley & Sons: New York.

Drukker, M., Krabbendam, L., Driessen, G. et al. (2006). Social disadvantage and schizophrenia: a combined neighbourhood and individual-level analysis. *Soc Psychiatry Psychiatr Epidemiol* **41**(8), 595–604.

Eagles, J. M. (1991). The relationship between schizophrenia and immigration: are there alternatives to psychosoical hypotheses? *Br J Psychiatry* **159**: 783–789.

Eagles, J. M., Hunter, D., McCance, C. (1988). Decline in the diagnosis of schizophrenia among 1st contacts with psychiatric-services in Northeast Scotland, 1969–1984. *Br J Psychiatry* **152**, 793–798.

Faris, R. E. L., Dunham, H. W. (1939). *Mental Disorders in Urban Areas*. University of Chicago Press: Chicago.

Fearon, P., Kirkbride, J. B., Morgan, C. et al. (2006). Incidence of schizophrenia and other psychoses in ethnic minority groups: results from the MRC AESOP Study. *Psychol Med* **36**(11), 1541–1550.

Geddes, J. R., Black, R. J., Whalley, L. J. et al. (1993). Persistence of the decline in the diagnosis of schizophrenia among first admissions to Scottish hospitals from 1969 to 1988. *Br J Psychiatry* **163**, 620–626.

Giggs, J. A. (1973). Distribution of schizophrenics in Nottingham. *T I Brit Geogr* **59**, 5–76.

Giggs, J. A. (1986). Mental disorders and ecological structure in Nottingham. *Soc Sci Med* **23**, 945–961.

Giggs, J. A., Cooper, J. E. (1987). Ecological structure and the distribution of schizophrenia and affective psychoses in Nottingham. *Br J Psychiatry* **151**, 627–633.

Goldberg, E. M., Morrison, S. L. (1963). Schizophrenia and social class. *Br J Psychiatry* **109**(463), 785–802.

Hafner, H., Maurer, K., Loffler, W. et al. (1993). The influence of age and sex on the onset and early course of schizophrenia. *Br J Psychiatry* **162**, 80–86.

Hafner, H., Reimann, H., Immich, H. et al. (1969). Inzidenz seelischer Erkrankungen in Mannheim 1965. *Soc Psychiatr* **4**, 127–135.

Hare, E. H. (1956). Mental illness and social condition in Bristol. *J Ment Sci* **102**, 349–357.

Harrison, G., Cooper, J. E., Gancarczyk, R. (1991). Changes in the administrative incidence of schizophrenia. *Br J Psychiatry* **159**, 811–816.

Harrison, G., Owens, D., Holton, A. et al. (1988). A prospective study of severe mental disorder in Afro-Caribbean patients. *Psychol Med* **18**(3), 643–657.

Henquet, C., Murray, R., Linszen, D. et al. (2005). The environment and schizophrenia: the role of cannabis use. *Schizophr Bull* **31**(3), 608–612.

Henquet, C., Rosa, A., Krabbendam, L. et al. (2006). An Experimental Study of Catechol-*O*-Methyltransferase Val(158)Met Moderation of Delta-9-Tetrahydrocannabinol-Induced Effects on Psychosis and Cognition. *Neuropsychopharmacology* **31**(12), 2748–2757.

Hickling, F. W., Rodgers-Johnson, P. (1995). The incidence of first contact schizophrenia in Jamaica. *Br J Psychiatry* **167**(2), 193–196.

Hollingshead, A. B., Redlich, F. C. (1958). *Social Class and Mental Illness*. Wiley: New York.

Jablensky, A., Sartorius, N., Ernberg, G. et al. (1992). Schizophrenia: manifestations, incidence and course in different cultures. A World Health Organization ten-country study. *Psychol Med Monogr Suppl* **20**, 1–97.

Jones, P., Rodgers, B., Murray, R. et al. (1994). Child development risk factors for adult schizophrenia in the British 1946 birth cohort. *Lancet* **344**(8934), 1398–1402.

Jones, P. B., Bebbington, P., Foerster, A. et al. (1993). Premorbid social underachievement in schizophrenia. Results from the Camberwell Collaborative Psychosis Study. *Br J Psychiatry* **162**, 65–71.

Jones, P. B., Rantakallio, P., Hartikainen, A. L. et al. (1998). Schizophrenia as a long-term outcome of pregnancy, delivery, and perinatal complications: a 28-year follow-up of the 1966 north Finland general population birth cohort. *Am J Psychiatry* **155**(3), 355–364.

Kapur, S. (2003). Psychosis as a state of aberrant salience: A framework linking biology, phenomenology, and pharmacology in schizophrenia. *Am J Psychiatry* **160**(1), 13–23.

Kaymaz, N., Krabbendam, L., de Graaf, R. et al. (2006). Evidence that the urban environment specifically impacts on the psychotic but not the affective dimension of bipolar disorder. *Soc Psychiatry Psychiatr Epidemiol* **41**(9), 679–685.

Kendler, K. S., Diehl, S. R. (1993). The genetics of schizophrenia: a current, genetic-epidemiologic perspective. *Schizophr Bull* **19**(2), 261–285.

Keshavan, M. S., Tandon, R., Boutros, N. N. et al. (2008). Schizophrenia, "just the facts": What we know in 2008: Part 3: Neurobiology. *Schizophr Res* **106**(2–3), 89–107.

Kessler, R. C., McGonagle, K. A., Zhao, S. et al. (1994). Lifetime and 12-month prevalence of DSM-III-R psychiatric disorders in the United States. Results from the National Comorbidity Survey. *Arch Gen Psychiatry* **51**(1), 8–19.

King, M., Coker, E., Leavey, G. et al. (1994). Incidence of psychotic illness in London: comparison of ethnic groups. *Br Med J* **309**(6962), 1115–1119.

Kirkbride, J., Boydell, J., Ploubidis, G. et al. (2008a). Testing the association between the incidence of schizophrenia and social capital in an urban area. *Psychol Med* **38**(8), 1083–1094.

Kirkbride, J. B., Coid, J. W., Barker, D. et al. (2008b). Psychoses, ethnicity and socio-economic status. *Br J Psychiatry* **193**(1), 18–24.

Kirkbride, J. B., Coid, J. W., Fearon, P. et al. (2008c). Ethnicity, migration and urbanicity: estimating the public mental health impact of major risk indicators for psychoses. In review.

Kirkbride, J. B., Croudace, T., Brewin, J. et al. (2008d). Is the incidence of psychotic disorder in decline? Epidemiological evidence from two decades of research. *Int J Epidemiol* Aug 25 **38**(5), 1255–1264.

Kirkbride, J. B., Fearon, P., Morgan, C. et al. (2006). Heterogeneity in incidence rates of schizophrenia and other psychotic syndromes: findings from the 3-center ÆSOP study. *Arch Gen Psychiatry* **63**(3), 250–258.

Kirkbride, J. B., Fearon, P., Morgan, C. et al. (2007a). Neighbourhood variation in the incidence of psychotic disorders in Southeast London. *Soc Psychiatry Psychiatr Epidemiol* **42**(6), 438–445.

Kirkbride, J. B., Morgan, C., Fearon, P. et al. (2007b). Neighbourhood-level effects on psychoses: re-examining the role of context. *Psychol Med* **37**(10), 1413–1425.

Kuttner, R. E., Lorincz, A. B., Swan, D. A. (1967). The schizophrenia gene and social evolution. *Psychol Rep* **20**(2), 407–412.

Laruelle, M., Abi-Dargham, A., van Dyck, C. H. et al. (1996). Single photon emission computerized tomography imaging of amphetamine-induced dopamine release in drug-free schizophrenic subjects. *Proc Natl Acad Sci USA* **93**(17), 9235–9240.

Lewis, G., David, A., Andreasson, S. et al. (1992). Schizophrenia and city life. *Lancet* **340**(8812), 137–140.

Loffler, W., Hafner, H. (1999). Ecological patterns of first admitted schizophrenics to two German cities over 25 years. *Soc Sci Med* **49**, 93–108.

Lucas, L. R., Celen, Z., Tamashiro, K. L. K. et al. (2004). Repeated exposure to social stress has long-term effects on indirect markers of dopaminergic activity in brain regions associated with motivated behavior. *Neuroscience* **124**(2), 449–457.

Mahy, G. E., Mallett, R., Leff, J. et al. (1999). First-contact incidence rate of schizophrenia on Barbados. *Br J Psychiatry* **175**, 28–33.

March, D., Hatch, S. L., Morgan, C. et al. (2008). Psychosis and Place. *Epidemiol Rev*, mxn006.

Maylaih, E., Weyerer, S., Hafner, H. (1989). Spatial concentration of the incidence of treated psychiatric disorders in Mannheim. *Acta Psychiatr Scand* **80**(6), 650–656.

McCulloch, A. (2001). Social environments and health: cross sectional national survey. *Br Med J* **323**(7306), 208–209.

McGovern, D., Cope, R. V. (1987). First psychiatric admission rates of first and second generation Afro Caribbeans. *Soc Psychiatr* **22**(3), 139–149.

McGrath, J., Saha, S., Welham, J. et al. (2004). A systematic review of the incidence of schizophrenia: the distribution of rates and the influence of sex, urbanicity, migrant status and methodology. *BMC Medicine* **2**, 13–22.

McGrath, J. J. (2006). Variations in the incidence of schizophrenia: Data versus dogma. *Schizophr Bull* **32**(1), 195–197.

Moore, T. H. M., Zammit, S., Lingford-Hughes, A. et al. (2007). Cannabis use and risk of psychotic or affective mental health outcomes: a systematic review. *The Lancet* **370**(9584), 319–328.

Morgan, C., Kirkbride, J., Hutchinson, G. et al. (2008). Cumulative social disadvantage, ethnicity and first-episode psychosis: a case–control study. *Psychol Med* **38**, 1701–1715.

Morgan, C., Kirkbride, J. B., Leff, J. et al. (2007). Parental separation, loss and psychosis in different ethnic groups: a case–control study. *Psychol Med* **37**(4), 495–503.

Mortensen, P. B., Pedersen, C. B., Westergaard, T. et al. (1999). Effects of family history and place and season of birth on the risk of schizophrenia. *N Engl J Med* **340**(8), 603–608.

Munk-Jorgensen, P., Mortensen, P. B. (1993). Is schizophrenia really on the decrease? *Eur Arch Psychiatry Clin Neurosci* **242**(4), 244–247.

Myin-Germeys, I., Delespaul, P., van Os, J. (2005). Behavioural sensitization to daily life stress in psychosis. *Psychol Med* **35**(5), 733–741.

Nuechterlein, K. H., Dawson, M. E. (1984). A heuristic vulnerability/stress model of schizophrenic episodes. *Schizophr Bull* **10**(2), 300–312.

Degaard, Ø. (1932). Emigration and insanity. *Acta Psychiatr Neurol* (Suppl. 4), 1–206.

Osby, U., Hammar, N., Brandt, L. et al. (2001). Time trends in first admissions for schizophrenia and paranoid psychosis in Stockholm County, Sweden. *Schizophr Res* **47**(2–3), 247–254.

Owen, M. J., Craddock, N., O'Donovan, M. C. (2005). Schizophrenia: genes at last? *Trends Genet* **21**(9), 518–525.

Pedersen, C. B., Mortensen, P. B. (2006). Urbanicity during upbringing and bipolar affective disorders in Denmark. *Bipolar Disorders* **8**(3), 242–247.

Regier, D. A., Boyd, J. H., Burke, J. D., Jr. et al. (1988). One-month prevalence of mental disorders in the United States. Based on five Epidemiologic Catchment Area sites. *Arch Gen Psychiatry* **45**(11), 977–986.

Robinson, T. E., Jurson, P. A., Bennett, J. A. et al. (1988). Persistent sensitization of dopamine neurotransmission in ventral striatum (nucleus accumbens) produced by prior experience with (+)-amphetamine: a microdialysis study in freely moving rats. *Brain Res* **462**(2), 211–222.

Saha, S., Chant, D., Welham, J. et al. (2005). A Systematic Review of the Prevalence of Schizophrenia. *PLoS Med* **2**(5), e141.

Sampson, R. J., Raudenbush, S. W., Earls, F. (1997). Neighborhoods and violent crime: a multilevel study of collective efficacy. *Science* **277**(5328), 918–924.

Schultz, W. (2002). Getting formal with dopamine and reward. *Neuron* **36**(2), 241–263.

Scully, P. J., Owens, J. M., Kinsella, A. et al. (2004). Schizophrenia, schizoaffective and bipolar disorder within an epidemiologically complete, homogeneous population in rural Ireland: small area variation in rate. *Schizophr Res* **67**(2–3), 143–155.

Seeman, P., Weinshenker, D., Quirion, R. et al. (2005). Dopamine supersensitivity correlates with D2High states, implying many paths to psychosis. *Proc Natl Acad Sci USA* **102**(9), 3513–3518.

Selten, J. P., Cantor-Graae, E. (2005). Social defeat: risk factor for schizophrenia? *Br J Psychiatry* **187**(2), 101–102.

Selten, J.-P., Cantor-Graae, E., Slaets, J. et al. (2002). Odegaard's selection hypothesis revisited: schizophrenia in Surinamese immigrants to the Netherlands. *Am J Psychiatry* **159**(4), 669–671.

Selten, J. P., Slaets, J. P., Kahn, R. S. (1997). Schizophrenia in Surinamese and Dutch Antillean immigrants to The Netherlands: evidence of an increased incidence. *Psychol Med* **27**(4), 807–811.

Silver, E., Mulvey, E. P., Swanson, J. W. (2002). Neighborhood structural characteristics and mental disorder: Faris and Dunham revisited. *Soc Sci Med* **55**(8), 1457–1470.

Singh, S. P., Burns, T. (2006). Race and mental health: there is more to race than racism. *Br Med J* **333**(7569), 648–651.

Sugarman, P. A., Craufurd, D. (1994). Schizophrenia in the Afro-Caribbean community. *Br J Psychiatry* **164**(4), 474–480.

Susser, E., Schwartz, S., Morabia, A. (2006a). Eco-epidemiology. In: E. Susser, S. Schwartz, A. Morabia, E. J. Bromet (eds.), *Psychiatric Epidemiology*. Oxford University Press: Oxford.

Susser, E., Schwartz, S., Morabia, A. et al. (2006b). *Psychiatric Epidemiology*. Oxford University Press: Oxford.

Suvisaari, J. M., Haukka, J. K., Tanskanen, A. J. et al. (1999). Decline in the incidence of schizophrenia in Finnish cohorts born from 1954 to 1965. *Arch Gen Psychiatry* **56**(8), 733–740.

Tidey, J. W., Miczek, K. A. (1996). Social defeat stress selectively alters mesocorticolimbic dopamine release: an in vivo microdialysis study. *Brain Res* **721**(1–2), 140–149.

Tsuang, M. T., Tohen, M., Zahner, G. E. P. (1995). *Textbook in Psychiatric Epidemiology*. John Wiley & Sons: New York.

van Os, J. (2003). Is there a continuum of psychotic experiences in the general population? *Epidemiol Psichiatr Soc* **12**(4), 242–252.

van Os, J., Bak, M., Hanssen, M. et al. (2002). Cannabis use and psychosis: a longitudinal population-based study. *Am J Epidemiol* **156**(4), 319–327.

van Os, J., Castle, D. J., Takei, N. et al. (1996). Psychotic illness in ethnic minorities: clarification from the 1991 census. *Psychol Med* **26**(1), 203–208.

van Os, J., Driessen, G., Gunther, N. et al. (2000). Neighbourhood variation in incidence of schizophrenia. Evidence for person–environment interaction. *Br J Psychiatry* **176**, 243–248.

Veling, W., Selten, J.-P., Susser, E. et al. (2007). Discrimination and the incidence of psychotic disorders among ethnic minorities in The Netherlands. *Int J Epidemiol* **36**(4), 761–768.

Veling, W., Selten, J. P., Veen, N. et al. (2006). Incidence of schizophrenia among ethnic minorities in the Netherlands: a four-year first-contact study. *Schizophr Res* **86**(1–3), 189–193.

Veling, W., Susser, E., van Os, J. et al. (2008). Ethnic density of neighborhoods and incidence of psychotic disorders among immigrants. *Am J Psychiatry* **165**(1), 66–73.

Weich, S., Holt, G., Twigg, L. et al. (2003). Geographic variation in the prevalence of common mental disorders in Britain: a multilevel investigation. *Am J Epidemiol* **157**(8), 730–737.

Werner, S., Malaspina, D., Rabinowitz, J. (2007). Socioeconomic status at birth is associated with risk of schizophrenia: population-based multilevel study. *Schizophr Bull* **33**(6), 1373–1378.

Weyerer, S., Häfner, H. (1989). The stability of the ecological distribution of the incidence of treated mental disorders in the city of Mannheim. *Soc Psychiatry Psychiatr Epidemiol* **24**(2), 57–62.

Williams, H. J., Owen, M. J., O'Donovan, M. C. (2007). Is COMT a susceptibility gene for schizophrenia? *Schizophr Bull* **33**(3), 635–641.

Zammit, S., Allebeck, P., Andreasson, S. et al. (2002). Self reported cannabis use as a risk factor for schizophrenia in Swedish conscripts of 1969: historical cohort study. *Br Med J* **325**(7374), 1199.

Zolkowska, K., Cantor-Graae, E., McNeil, T. F. (2001). Increased rates of psychosis among immigrants to Sweden: is migration a risk factor for psychosis? *Psychol Med* **31**(4), 669–678.

Part II
Pathophysiology

Disinhibition of Prefrontal Cortex Neurons in Schizophrenia

B. Moghaddam and A.L. Pehrson

Introduction

A large body of evidence has implicated abnormal functioning of the prefrontal cortex (PFC) in the pathophysiology of schizophrenia (Robbins 1996; Andreasen et al. 1997; Winterer and Wvneinberger 2004; Lewis and Moghaddam 2006). These abnormalities are found at molecular and functional levels and are thought to be the basis of cognitive deficits in individuals with schizophrenia. However, little is known about the physiological mechanisms that contribute to this malfunction. Here we review some of the literature that points to PFC abnormalities in schizophrenia and recent theories that unify the multimodal functional and postmortem findings in schizophrenia.

Previous mechanistic investigations of the pathophysiology of schizophrenia have primarily focused on dopaminergic and cholinergic systems in different subregions of the PFC (Geraud et al. 1987; Goldman-Rakic 1987; Daniel et al. 1989, 1991; Lewis et al. 1992; McGaughy et al. 1996; Robbins 1998). This has been justified by the fact that well-known antipsychotic drugs are thought to exert their therapeutic actions by blocking the dopamine D_2 receptors. Furthermore, manipulation of dopamine receptors in the PFC profoundly affects cognitive functions such as working memory that are dependent on the functional integrity of the PFC (Goldman-Rakic 1987) and disrupted in schizophrenia (Keefe 2001). More recent work has shifted the attention to glutamate and GABA-containing neurons. The glutamatergic afferents to the PFC originate primarily in regions that have been implicated in the etiology and pathophysiology of schizophrenia such as the thalamus, amygdala, and the hippocampus (Jeste and Lohr 1989; Conrad et al. 1991; Harrison et al. 1991; Andreasen et al. 1994, 1999). Dysfunctional glutamate neurotransmission, in particular NMDA receptor-mediated neurotransmission, has been linked to schizophrenia (Kim et al. 1980; Javitt and Zukin 1991; Olney and Farber 1995) primarily because noncompetitive NMDA receptor antagonists such

B. Moghaddam (✉)
Department of Neuroscience, University of Pittsburgh, Pittsburgh, PA, USA
e-mail: moghaddam@bns.pitt.edu

W.F. Gattaz, G. Busatto (eds.), *Advances in Schizophrenia Research 2009*,
DOI 10.1007/978-1-4419-0913-8_5, © Springer Science+Business Media, LLC 2010

as phencyclidine (PCP) and ketamine are psychotomimetic and produce, in healthy individuals, behaviors that resemble the cognitive deficits (Krystal et al. 1994; Malhotra et al. 1996; Adler et al. 1998) and some of the negative and positive symptoms of schizophrenia (Luby et al. 1959; Javitt and Zukin 1991; Krystal et al. 1994). GABA neurons are the most prevalent interneurons in the PFC and are thought to tightly control the activity of PFC afferents (Aradi et al. 2002). Recent studies link schizophrenia to increased $GABA_A$ expression on pyramidal neurons (Benes et al. 1996), reduced expression of the GABA reuptake transporter GAT1 (Woo et al. 1998; Pierri et al. 1999), and reductions in the GABA-synthesizing enzyme GAD_{67} (Akbarian et al. 1995; Volk et al. 2000), suggesting that GABA-mediated inhibitory neurotransmission in the cortex may be disrupted.

Dopamine Dysfunction in Schizophrenia

Altered dopamine neurotransmission has been a suspected cause in some features of schizophrenia for some time and has led to the influential dopamine hypothesis of schizophrenia (Carlsson 1977). This is based largely on observations that dopamine agonists such as amphetamine induce symptoms of psychosis (Randrup and Munkvad 1965), while dopaminergic D_2 receptor antagonists attenuate these symptoms. Indeed, there is a strong correlation between the clinical potency of many antipsychotics and their affinity for the D_2 receptor (Seeman and Lee 1975; Creese et al. 1976) and striatal D_2 receptor occupancy between 60 and 70% predicts clinical response to first-generation antipsychotics such as haloperidol (Kapur et al. 2000; Farde et al. 1988). Further support for altered dopamine neurotransmission in schizophrenia comes from observations that patients with this disease have significantly greater increases in dopamine release than controls under baseline conditions (Abi-Dargham et al. 2000) and in response to acute amphetamine challenge (Breier et al. 1997; Laruelle et al. 1996; Abi-Dargham et al. 1998). Furthermore, a recent meta-analysis reports a small but significant increase in striatal D_2 receptors in patients with schizophrenia (Weinberger and Laruelle 2001). A plausible interpretation of data such as these is that schizophrenia is related to hyperactive dopamine neurotransmission, particularly in the striatum.

But there is also evidence that calls the relationship between hyperactive striatal dopamine and psychotic symptoms into question. For example, although schizophrenia appears to be related to increased basal dopamine release and D_2 receptor density in the striatum, the magnitude of these changes has not been correlated with the severity of the positive symptom cluster (Abi-Dargham et al. 2000; Weinberger and Laruelle 2001). Furthermore, the idea that an overactive dopamine system elicits symptoms of schizophrenia is not supported by the fact that dopamine D_1 antagonists have not been found to have antipsychotic efficacy. Blocking D_1 receptors is generally more effective than D_2 receptors in ameliorating behavioral effects of hyperdopaminergic states in laboratory animals (Arnsten et al. 1994; Cuomo et al. 1986; Kuczenski and Segal 1999). Therefore, symptoms resulting from a hyperactive dopamine system should be more effectively reversed by a D_1 antagonist than a D_2 antagonist, which is not the case in schizophrenia. It should be emphasized that postmortem and genetic studies have generally failed to show a sustained hyperactive dopamine system in schizophrenia, further supporting the idea that D_2 antagonist treatment is not working through reducing postsynaptic dopamine function.

Why do D_2 receptor antagonists have antipsychotic efficacy if there is no underlying dopamine hyperfunction in schizophrenia? One plausible mechanism may be as follows: while both D_1 and D_2 receptors are abundant in all dopamine-innervated regions, their ultrastructural localization is quite distinct. In particular, although D_1 receptors are primarily, if not exclusively, localized postsynaptically, D_2 receptors are localized extensively on presynaptic sites both on dopamine terminals and on non-dopamine terminals, including excitatory glutamatergic axons (Wang and Pickel 2002). The D_2 receptors on dopamine terminals act as autoreceptors and tightly regulate the release of vesicular dopamine (Wolf et al. 1987). The D_2 heteroreceptors on glutamate terminals are thought to mediate an inhibitory influence on glutamate release (Calabresi et al. 1992; Cepeda et al. 2001). Thus, blockade of dopamine D_2 receptors increases the release of dopamine and glutamate, suggesting two possible mechanisms for the therapeutic efficacy of antipsychotic drugs: an increase in glutamate neurotransmission and activation of dopamine neurotransmission at D_1 receptors. This is consistent with the ideas that there exists a D_1 receptor deficiency in schizophrenia (Goldman-Rakic et al. 2004) and that NMDA receptors, as discussed below, may be hypofunctional in schizophrenia.

Glutamate Neurotransmission and Schizophrenia

Exposure to a single low dose of an NMDA receptor antagonist such as phencyclidine (PCP) or ketamine produces schizophrenia-like symptoms in healthy individuals and profoundly exacerbates preexisting symptoms in patients with schizophrenia (Javitt and Zukin 1991; Krystal et al. 1994; Lahti et al. 1995). The symptoms produced by these agents resemble positive and cognitive symptoms of schizophrenia, as well as disruptions in smooth-pursuit eye movements and prepulse inhibition of startle. These effects of NMDA receptor antagonists strongly suggest that glutamate neurotransmission at the NMDA receptor is compromised in schizophrenia (Moghaddam 2003).

In addition to the pharmacological evidence, other lines of work have implicated a role for glutamate neurotransmission in the etiology and pathophysiology of schizophrenia. For example, the majority of the genes that have recently been associated with an increased risk for schizophrenia can influence the function of modulatory sites on the NMDA receptor or intracellular-receptor interacting proteins that link glutamate receptors to signal transduction pathways (Harrison and Owen 2003; Moghaddam 2003). Postmortem studies show changes in glutamate receptor binding, transcription, and subunit protein expression in the prefrontal cortex, thalamus, and the hippocampus of subjects with schizophrenia (Clinton and Meador-Woodruff 2004). Examples include decreases in NR1 subunits of the NMDA receptor in the hippocampus and frontal cortical areas, high expression of excitatory amino acid transporters (EAATs) in the thalamus, and changes in the NMDA receptor-affiliated intracellular proteins such as PSD95 and SAP102 in the prefrontal cortex and thalamus. Another example includes amino acids N-acethylaspartate (NAA) and N-acethylaspartylglutamate (NAAG). Levels of NAA and the activity of the enzyme that cleaves NAA to NAAG and glutamate are altered in the CSF and postmortem tissue from individuals with schizophrenia (Tsai et al. 1995). NAAG is an endogenous ligand for the mGlu3 subtype of glutamate receptor, the gene for which has been implicated in increased propensity to develop schizophrenia. Furthermore, reduced NAA levels are thought to reflect decreased glutamate availability.

Recent imaging studies using a novel SPECT tracer for the NMDA receptor [123I]CNS-1261 (Pilowsky et al. 2005) have reported reduced NMDA receptor binding in the hippocampus of medication-free patients. While this study remains to be replicated in a larger group of patients, it represents the first direct demonstration of NMDA receptor deficiency in schizophrenia. Glutamate neurons regulate the function of other neurons that have been strongly implicated in the pathophysiology of schizophrenia. These include GABA interneuons whose morphology has been altered in schizophrenia (see below) and dopamine neurons, which are the target of antipsychotic drugs.

GABA Neurotransmission and Schizophrenia

Cortical GABAergic neurons are a diverse group of cells, consisting of several subsets that can be distinguished on the basis of morphological, electrophysiological, and biochemical characteristics (for review, please see Benes and Berretta 2001). One set of cortical GABAergic cells that appear to be particularly important in the pathophysiology of schizophrenia includes basket and chandelier neurons. Both of these cell populations have fast-spiking firing patterns, express the calcium-binding protein parvalbumin, and can be differentiated on the basis of their axonal projections. Basket cells are typically multipolar, having several primary dendrite branches, and project a large spread of axons that synapse primarily on pyramidal neuron cell bodies. These axo-somatic projections allow for a strong inhibitory effect on pyramidal cell-firing patterns. Chandelier neurons project axo-axonal terminals (termed cartridges) that synapse exclusively on the initial segment of pyramidal neuron axons. Moreover, these cartridges, which can be identified based on the expression of the GABA reuptake transporter GAT1, are positioned to veto the propagation of action potentials, and therefore also play an important inhibitory role in modulating pyramidal neuron output (Benes and Lange 2001).

There is now a growing line of evidence suggesting altered GABAergic neurotransmission in schizophrenia. Postmortem studies have reported reductions in the density of non-pyramidal cells in the PFC and anterior cingulate cortex (ACC) in patients with schizophrenia (Benes et al. 1991; Benes and Berretta 2001), as well as reductions in the number of parvalbumin-expressing cells in the PFC (Beasley and Reynolds 1997). Furthermore, patients with schizophrenia have significant increases in $GABA_A$ expression on pyramidal neurons in the PFC (Benes et al. 1996) and ACC (Benes et al. 1992), as well as a reduction in the number of cartridges expressing GAT1 (Woo et al. 1998; Pierri et al. 1999).

The most consistently altered marker of GABA function in schizophrenia is reduced expression of GAD_{67}, which has been observed in at least two subtypes of GABA neurons in PFC subregions, including the DLPFC (Akbarian et al. 1995; Lewis et al. 2005). GAD_{67} accounts for the majority of GABA synthesis in the PFC. The reduced GAD_{67} function in subtypes of GABA neurons in schizophrenia, together with disruptions in $GABA_A$ and GAT1 expression (Benes et al. 1996; Woo et al. 1998; Pierri et al. 1999), strongly supports the idea that GABA availability is reduced in cortical synapses. It should, however, be mentioned that GABA synthesis, which is regulated via a process called the GABA shunt (Fig. 1), is quite complex in that reduced activity of GAD may also be reflective of a compensatory effect in response to sustained increases in GABA release. Increased levels of GABA have been shown to downregulate GAD activity in cultures and in specific regions of intact brain including the PFC (Rimvall et al. 1993; Sheikh and Martin 1998). Although postmortem studies in schizophrenia are not generally supportive of activated GABA function, the possible role of this mechanism should not be discounted.

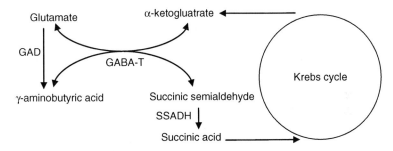

Fig. 1 The GABA shunt is a closed-loop process with the dual purpose of *producing and conserving* the supply of GABA. The first step in the GABA shunt is the transamination of a-ketoglutarate (a-KG) by GABA transaminase (**GABA-T**) into glutamate. **Glutamic acid decarboxylase (GAD)** catalyzes the decarboxylation of glutamate to form GABA. GABA is metabolized by the enzyme **GABA-T**. To conserve the supply of GABA, this transamination occurs when a-KG molecule is present to accept the amino group removed from GABA, forming glutamate. Therefore, a molecule of GABA can be metabolized only if a molecule of precursor is formed

Disinhibition Hypothesis

Given the dominance of the dopamine hypothesis of schizophrenia, earlier attempts to consolidate theories that involved NMDA receptor or GABA deficiency involved a mechanistic cause and effect connection with dopamine hyperactivity. For example, earlier studies examining dopamine turnover or measuring the uptake of labeled dopamine showed that NMDA receptor antagonists increase the release of striatal dopamine (Bowyer et al. 1984; Hiramatsu et al. 1989). This finding contributed to initial versions of an integrated dopamine–glutamate theory, suggesting that NMDA receptor hypofunction may represent a model that mimicked the presumed dopamine hyperfunction state in schizophrenia (Javitt and Zukin 1991; Carlsson et al. 1993). This interpretation, however, could not account for the fact that NMDA receptor antagonists induce a far wider range of schizophrenia-like symptoms than the dopaminergic models and that many of their behavioral effects are independent of dopamine neurotransmission (Krystal et al. 1999). Thus, the theory was modified to include separate roles for cortical versus subcortical glutamate–dopamine interactions, in order to explain the induction of negative and cognitive symptoms in addition to positive symptoms (Weinberger 1987; Davis et al. 1991; Heinz et al. 2003). However, subsequent work using microdialysis or imaging methodologies showed that behaviorally relevant doses of NMDA antagonists do not increase striatal dopamine release in rodents, primate, or humans (Verma and Moghaddam 1996; Adams et al. 2002; Aalto et al. 2002), and dopamine antagonists such as haloperidol do not attenuate PCP-induced psychosis in humans (Aniline and Pitts 1982). Furthermore, behavioral studies have demonstrated that the aberrant behavioral effects of the NMDA receptor antagonists do not require dopamine (Carlsson and Carlsson 1990; Adams and Moghaddam 1998; Chartoff et al. 2005) and are not attenuated by dopamine antagonists (Bakshi et al. 1994; Corbett et al. 1995). These data, and the abundance of postmortem and genetic findings supporting a role for the glutamate system in the pathophysiology of schizophrenia, have led to the proposal that the primary abnormalities in schizophrenia may involve the synaptic signaling machinery in cortical regions and that a dopaminergic abnormality may be a consequence of cortical dysregulation of dopamine neurons. Interestingly, contrary to years of assertion that the PFC stimulates dopamine neuronal activity, stimulation of PFC neurons at physiological frequencies actually decreases dopamine release in the ventral striatum (Jackson et al. 2001). This suggests that the PFC exerts an inhibitory influence over subcortical dopamine presumably through the indirect activation of GABA neurons. Thus, reduced glutamatergic function in the PFC may remove this inhibitory influence and lead to an abnormally overactive subcortical dopamine system in schizophrenia. Recent electrophysiological studies recording from PFC cortical neurons in behaving rodents, in fact, show that a state of NMDA deficiency can lead to reduced burst activity of cortical neurons (Jackson et al. 2004).

Given the lack of direct evidence for a dopaminergic abnormality in schizophrenia, an alternative hypothesis has been that antipsychotic drugs, which are D_2 receptor antagonists, work by modifying the function of cortical (glutamatergic) neurons. A substantial body of evidence demonstrates that dopamine modulates cortical and subcortical glutamatergic transmission (for review, see Seamans and Yang 2004). Notably, electrophysiological studies have revealed a delicate modulatory effect for dopamine on the electrical conductance of cortical excitatory neurons that is neither excitatory nor inhibitory but rather a gating effect that depends on the activity state of target neurons (Lavin and Grace 2001; Durstewitz 2006). Furthermore, D_2 receptors may regulate the temporal organization of electrical activity in the PFC. D_2 receptors also inhibit the release of glutamate (Koga and Momiyama 2000), suggesting that the blockade of D_2 receptors by antipsychotic drugs can overcome a putative state of glutamate deficiency. In support of this mechanism, electrophysiological studies have shown that antipsychotic agents, particularly clozapine, exert positive modulatory effects on the NMDA receptor function in PFC and may attenuate the blockade of these receptors by NMDA receptor antagonists (Gemperle et al. 2003).

A related hypothesis has been that dopamine, GABA, and glutamate interactions may occur through modulating intricate postsynaptic intracellular mechanisms that mediate cross-talks between these transmitter systems in the prefrontal cortex. An example of this is depicted in Fig. 2. Regions other than the PFC that have been

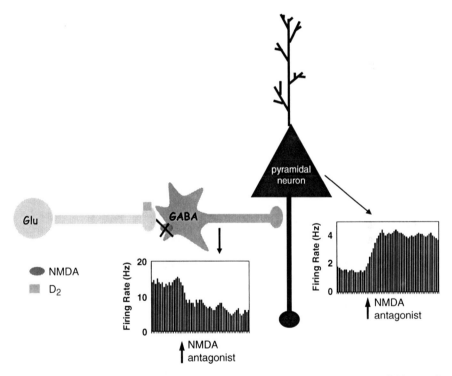

Fig. 2 A simplified circuit representing the basic interplay between glutamate, GABA, and dopamine neurotransmission in the cortex. Under normal conditions, glutamatergic afferents from cortical regions such as the thalamus and hippocampus drive the activity of GABAergic interneurons in the PFC, which serve to maintain inhibitory control of pyramidal neuron activity. Under conditions of NMDA hypofunction, GABAergic activity is reduced and tonic inhibitory control of pyramidal neuron activity is lost. Antagonism of dopamineric D_2 receptors on glutamatergic terminals may increase glutamate release, restoring normal GABAergic inhibitory tone on pyramidal neuron activity

implicated in the pathophysiology of schizophrenia include regions such as the thalamus and hippocampus that provide substantial glutamate projections to PFC subregions. Reduced or dysregulated glutamatergic afferent activity from the thalamus or hippocampus could produce an NMDA hypofunction state in the PFC. A consequence of this may be reduced activity of GABA neurons, in particular parvalbumin-containing interneurons that are strongly driven by these inputs under normal conditions. This condition supports the postmortem findings of reduced GAD activity in the PFC. Inhibition of these neurons then results in dysregulation of PFC afferents leading to increased "noise" level (Jackson et al. 2004) and reduced ability to properly encode task-relevant events. One mechanism to ameliorate this is D_2 inhibition (Homayoun and Moghaddam 2008) because activation of D_2 (and not D_1) receptors has been shown to reduce GABA-mediated inhibition of pyramidal neurons (Seamans and Yang 2004). The ideal pharmacological approach, however, would be to correct the dysregulated glutamate drive or its subsequent effects on inhibitory interneurons.

Thankfully, in the last few years these novel hypotheses are being tested by concrete data from animal and human laboratory studies. A new effort to test novel compounds that have are driven by logical design has begun (Patil et al. 2007; Lewis et al. 2008). After five decades of persevering on the first generation of antipsychotic drugs and the so-called "new generation" that have proved to not to have better efficacy than their antique counterparts (Geddes et al. 2000; Lieberman 2007), there is optimism that a truly new generation of antipsychotics that are more effective in treating schizophrenia is on the horizon.

References

Aalto, S., Hirvonen, J., Kajander, J., Scheinin, H., Nagren, K., Vilkman, H., Gustafsson, L., Syvalahti, E. & Hietala, J. (2002) Ketamine does not decrease striatal dopamine D2 receptor binding in man. Psychopharmacology (Berl) 164:401–406

Abi-Dargham, A., Gil, R., Krystal, J., Baldwin, R. M., Seibyl, J. P., Bowers, M., van Dyck, C. H., Charney, D. S., Innis, R. B. & Laruelle, M. (1998) Increased striatal dopamine transmission in schizophrenia: Confirmation in a second cohort. American Journal of Psychiatry 155: 761–767

Abi-Dargham, A., Rodenhiser, J., Printz, D., Zea-Ponce, Y., Gil, R., Kegeles, L., Weiss, R., Cooper, T., Mann, J., Van Heertum, R., Gorman, J. & Laruelle, M. (2000) Increased baseline occupancy of D2 receptors by dopamine in schizophrenia. Proceedings of the National Academy of Sciences of USA 97:8104–8109

Adams, B. & Moghaddam, B. (1998) Corticolimbic dopamine neurotransmission is temporally dissociated from the cognitive and locomotor effects of phencyclidine. Journal of Neuroscience 18:5545–5554

Adams, B. W., Bradberry, C. W. & Moghaddam, B. (2002) NMDA antagonist effects on striatal dopamine release: microdialysis studies in awake monkeys. Synapse 43:12–18

Adler, C. M., Goldberg, T. E., Malhotra, A. K., Pickar, D. & Breier, A. (1998) Effects of ketamine on thought disorder, working memory, and semantic memory in healthy volunteers. Biological Psychiatry 43:811–816

Akbarian, S., Kim, J. J., Potkin, S. G., Hagman, J. O., Tafazzoli, A., Bunney, W. E., Jr. & Jones, E. G. (1995) Gene expression for glutamic acid decarboxylase is reduced without loss of neurons in prefrontal cortex of schizophrenics [see comments]. Archives of General Psychiatry 52:258–266

Andreasen, N. C., Arndt, S., Swayze, V., II, Cizadlo, T., Flaum, M., O'Leary, D., Erhardt, J. C. & Yuh, W. T. (1994) Thalamic abnormalities in schizophrenia visualized through magnetic resonance image averaging. Science 266:294–298

Andreasen, N. C., Nopoulos, P., O'Leary, D. S., Miller, D. D., Wassink, T. & Flaum, M. (1999) Defining the phenotype of schizophrenia: cognitive dysmetria and its neural mechanisms. Biological Psychiatry 46:908–920

Andreasen, N. C., O'Leary, D. S., Flaum, M., Nopoulos, P., Watkins, G. L., Boles Ponto, L. L. & Hichwa, R. D. (1997) Hypofrontality in schizophrenia: distributed dysfunctional circuits in neuroleptic-naive patients. Lancet 349:1730–1734

Aniline, O. & Pitts, F. N., Jr. (1982) Phencyclidine (PCP): A review and perspectives. Critical Reviews in Toxicology 10:145–177

Aradi, I., Santhakumar, V., Chen, K. & Soltesz, I. (2002) Postsynaptic effects of GABAergic synaptic diversity: regulation of neuronal excitability by changes in IPSC variance. Neuropharmacology 43:511–522

Arnsten, A. F., Cai, J. X., Murphy, B. L. & Goldman-Rakic, P. S. (1994) Dopamine D1 receptor mechanisms in the cognitive performance of young adult and aged monkeys. Psychopharmacology 116:143–151

Bakshi, V. P., Swerdlow, N. R. & Geyer, M. A. (1994) Clozapine antagonizes phencyclidine-induced deficits in sensorimotor gating of the startle response. Journal of Pharmacology & Experimental Therapeutics 271:787–794

Beasley, C. L. & Reynolds, G. P. (1997) Parvalbumin-immunoreactive neurons are reduced in the prefrontal cortex of schizophrenics. Schizophr Res 24:349–355

Benes, F. & Berretta, S. (2001) GABAergic interneurons: implications for understanding schizophrenia and bipolar disorder. Neuropsychopharmacology 25:1–27

Benes, F. M. & Lange, N. (2001) Two-dimensional versus three-dimensional cell counting: a practical perspective. Trends Neuroscience 24:11–17

Benes, F. M., McSparren, J., Bird, E. D., SanGiovanni, J. P. & Vincent, S. L. (1991) Deficits in small interneurons in prefrontal and cingulate cortices of schizophrenic and schizoaffective patients. Archives of General Psychiatry 48:996–1001

Benes, F. M., Vincent, S. L., Alsterberg, G., Bird, E. D. & SanGiovanni, J. P. (1992) Increased GABAA receptor binding in superficial layers of cingulate cortex in schizophrenics. Journal of Neuroscience 12:924–929

Benes, F. M., Vincent, S. L., Marie, A. & Khan, Y. (1996) Up-regulation of GABAA receptor binding on neurons of the prefrontal cortex in schizophrenic subjects. Neuroscience 75: 1021–1031

Bowyer, J. F., Spuhler, K. P. & Weiner, N. (1984) Effects of phencyclidine, amphetamine and related compounds on dopamine release from and uptake into striatal synaptosomes. Journal of Pharmacology & Experimental Therapeutics 229:671–680

Breier, A., Su, T. P., Saunders, R., Carson, R. E., Kolachana, B. S., de Bartolomeis, A., Weinberger, D. R., Weisenfeld, N., Malhotra, A. K., Eckelman, W. C. & Pickar, D. (1997) Schizophrenia is associated with elevated amphetamine-induced synaptic dopamine concentrations: evidence from a novel positron emission tomography method. Proceedings of the National Academy of Sciences USA 94:2569–2574

Calabresi, P., De Murtas, M., Mercuri, N. B. & Bernardi, G. (1992) Chronic neuroleptic treatment: D2 dopamine receptor supersensitivity and striatal glutamatergic transmission. Annals of Neurology 31:366–373

Carlsson, A. (1977) Does dopamine play a role in schizophrenia? Psychological Medicine 7: 583–597

Carlsson, A., Svensson, A. & Carlsson, M. L. (1993) Future strategies in the discovery of new antipsychotic agents: focus on dopamine–glutamate interactions. In: Brunello, N., Mendlewicz, J. & Racagni, G. (eds.) New Generation of Antipsychotic Drugs: Novel Mechanisms of Action, Karger, Basel, pp. 118–129

Carlsson, M. & Carlsson, A. (1990) Interactions between glutamatergic and monoaminergic systems within the basal ganglia – implications for schizophrenia and Parkinson's disease. Trends in Neurosciences 13:272–276

Cepeda, C., Hurst, R. S., Altemus, K. L., Flores-Hernandez, J., Calvert, C. R., Jokel, E. S., Grandy, D. K., Low, M. J., Rubinstein, M., Ariano, M. A. & Levine, M. S. (2001) Facilitated glutamatergic transmission in the striatum of D2 dopamine receptor-deficient mice. Journal of Neurophysiology 85:659–670

Chartoff, E. H., Heusner, C. L. & Palmiter, R. D. (2005) Dopamine is not required for the hyperlocomotor response to NMDA receptor antagonists. Neuropsychopharmacology 30:1324–1333

Clinton, S. & Meador-Woodruff, J. (2004) Abnormalities of the NMDA receptor and associated intracellular molecules in the thalamus in schizophrenia and bipolar disorder. Neuropsychopharmacology 29:1353–1362

Conrad, A., Abebe, T., Ron, A., Forsythe, S. & Scheibel, B. (1991) Hippocampal pyramidal cell disarray in schizophrenia as a bilateral phenomenon. Archives of General Psychiatry 48: 413–417

Corbett, R., Camacho, F., Woods, A. T., Kerman, L. L., Fishkin, R. J., Brooks, K. & Dunn, R. W. (1995) Antipsychotic agents antagonize non-competitive N-methyl-D-aspartate antagonist-induced behaviors. Psychopharmacology (Berl) 120:67–74

Creese, I., Burt, D. & Snyder, S. (1976) Dopamine receptor binding predicts clinical and pharmacological potencies of antischizophrenic drugs. Science 192:481–483

Cuomo, V., Cagiano, R., Colonna, M., Renna, G. & Racagni, G. (1986) Influence of SCH 23390, a DA1-receptor antagonist, on the behavioural responsiveness to small and large doses of apomorphine in rats. Neuropharmacology 25:1297–1300

Daniel, D., Berman, K. & Weinberger, D. (1989) The effect of apomorphine on regional cerebral bloodflow in schizophrenia. Journal of Neuropsychiatry & Clinical Neuroscience 1: 377–384

Daniel, D. G., Weinberger, D. R., Jones, D. W., Zigun, J. R., Cippola, R., Handel, S., Bigelow, L. B., Goldberg, T. E., Berman, K. F. & Kleinman, J. E. (1991) The effect of amphetamine on regional cerebral blood flow during cognitive activation in schizophrenia. Journal of Neuroscience 11:1907–1917

Davis, K. L., Kahn, R. S., Ko, G. & Davidson, M. (1991) Dopamine in schizophrenia: a review and reconceptualization. American Journal of Psychiatry 148:1474–1486

Durstewitz, D. (2006) A few important points about dopamine's role in neural network dynamics. Pharmacopsychiatry 39(Suppl 1):S72–S75

Farde, L., Wiesel, F. A., Halldin, C. & Sedvall, G. (1988) Central D2-dopamine receptor occupancy in schizophrenic patients treated with antipsychotic drugs. Archives of General Psychiatry 45:71–76

Geddes, J., Freemantle, N., Harrison, P. & Bebbington, P. (2000) Atypical antipsychotics in the treatment of schizophrenia: systematic overview and meta-regression analysis. BMJ 321: 1371–1376

Gemperle, A. Y., Enz, A., Pozza, M. F., Luthi, A. & Olpe, H. R. (2003) Effects of clozapine, haloperidol and iloperidone on neurotransmission and synaptic plasticity in prefrontal cortex and their accumulation in brain tissue: an in vitro study. Neuroscience 117:681–695

Geraud, G., Arne-Bes, M., Guell, A. & Bes, A. (1987) Reversibility of hemodynamic hypofrontality in schizophrenia. Journal of Cerebral Blood Flow & Metabolism 7:9–12

Goldman-Rakic, P. S. (1987) Circuitry of primate prefrontal cortex and regulation of behavior by representational memory. In: Plum, F. & Mountcastle, V. (eds.) Handbook of Physiology :The Nervous System, American Physiological Society, Bethesda, MD, pp. 373–417

Goldman-Rakic, P. S., Castner, S. A., Svensson, T. H., Siever, L. J. & Williams, G. V. (2004) Targeting the dopamine D1 receptor in schizophrenia: insights for cognitive dysfunction. Psychopharmacology (Berl) 174:3–16

Harrison, P. J., McLaughlin, D. & Kerwin, R. W. (1991) Decreased hippocampal expression of a glutamate receptor gene in schizophrenia. Lancet 337:450–452

Harrison, P. J. & Owen, M. J. (2003) Genes for schizophrenia? Recent findings and their patho-physiological implications.[comment]. Lancet 361:417–419

Heinz, A., Romero, B., Gallinat, J., Juckel, G. & Weinberger, D. R. (2003) Molecular brain imaging and the neurobiology and genetics of schizophrenia. Pharmacopsychiatry 36(Suppl 3): S152–S157

Hiramatsu, M., Cho, A. K. & Nabeshima, T. (1989) Comparison of the behavioral and biochemical effects of the NMDA receptor antagonists, MK-801 and phencyclidine. European Journal of Pharmacology 166:359–366

Homayoun, H. & Moghaddam, B. (2008) Orbitofrontal Cortex Neurons as a Common Cellular Target for Different Classes of Antipsychotic Drugs. Society for Neuroscience Abstract, Washington DC

Jackson, M., Homayoun, H. & Moghaddam, B. (2004) NMDA receptor hypofunction produces concomitant firing rate potentiation and burst activity reduction in the prefrontal cortex. Proceedings of the National Academy of Sciences of USA 101:6391–6396

Jackson, M. E., Frost, A. & Moghaddam, B. (2001) Stimulation of prefrontal cortex at physiologically relevant frequencies inhibits dopamine release in the nucleus accumbens. Journal of Neurochemistry 78:920–923

Javitt, D. C. & Zukin, S. R. (1991) Recent advances in the phencyclidine model of schizophrenia. American Journal of Psychiatry 148:1301–1308

Jeste, D. & Lohr, J. (1989) Hippocampal pathological findings in schizophrenia. A morphometric study. Archives of General Psychiatry 46:1019–1024

Kapur, S., Zipursky, R., Jones, C., Remington, G. & Houle, S. (2000) Relationship between dopamine D(2) occupancy, clinical response, and side effects: a double-blind PET study of first-episode schizophrenia. American Journal of Psychiatry 157:514–520

Keefe, R. (2001) Neurocognition. In: Breier, A., Tran, P. V., Herrea, J. M., Tollefson, G. D. & Bymaster, F. P. (eds.) Current Issues in the Psychopharmacology of Schizophrenia, Lippincott Williams & Wilkins, Philadelphia, pp. 209–223

Kim, J., Kornhuber, H., Schmid-Burgk, W. & Holzmuller, B. (1980) Low cerebrospinal fluid glutamate in schizophrenic patients and a new hypothesis on schizophrenia. Neuroscience Letters 20:379–382

Koga, E. & Momiyama, T. (2000) Presynaptic dopamine D2-like receptors inhibit excitatory transmission onto rat ventral tegmental dopaminergic neurons. Journal of Physiology 523(Pt 1): 163–173

Krystal, J. H., D'Souza, D. C., Karper, L. P., Bennett, A., Abi-Dargham, A., Abi-Saab, D., Cassello, K., Bowers M. B., Jr., Vegso, S., Heninger, G. R. & Charney, D. S. (1999) Interactive effects of subanesthetic ketamine and haloperidol in healthy humans. Psychopharmacology 145: 193–204

Krystal, J. H., Karper, L. P., Seibyl, J. P., Freeman, G. K., Delaney, R., Bremner, J. D., Heninger, G. R., Bowers, M., Jr. & Charney, D. S. (1994) Subanesthetic effects of the noncompetitive NMDA antagonist, ketamine, in humans: psychotomimetic, perceptual, cognitive, and neuroendocrine responses. Archives of General Psychiatry 51:199–214

Kuczenski, R. & Segal, D. S. (1999) Sensitization of amphetamine-induced stereotyped behaviors during the acute response. Journal of Pharmacology and Experimental Therapeutics 288: 699–709

Lahti, A. C., Koffel, B., LaPorte, D. & Tamminga, C. A. (1995) Subanesthetic doses of ketamine stimulate psychosis in schizophrenia. Neuropsychopharmacology 13:9–19

Laruelle, M., Abi-Dargham, A., van Dyck, C., Gil, R., D'Souza, C., Erdos, J., McCance, E., Rosenblatt, W., Fingado, C., Zoghbi, S., Baldwin, R., Seibyl, J., Krystal, J., Charney, D. & Innis, R. (1996) SPECT imaging of amphetamine-induced dopamine release in drug-free schizophrenic subjects. Proceedings of the National Academy of Sciences USA 93:9235–9340

Lavin, A. & Grace, A. (2001) Stimulation of D1-type dopamine receptors enhances excitability in prefrontal cortical pyramidal neurons in a state-dependent manner. Neuroscience 104: 335–346

Lewis, D. A., Cho, R. Y., Carter, C. S., Eklund, K., Forster, S., Kelly, M. A. & Montrose, D. (2008) Subunit-selective modulation of GABA type A receptor neurotransmission and cognition in schizophrenia. American Journal of Psychiatry 165:1585–1593

Lewis, D. A., Hashimoto, T. & Volk, D. W. (2005) Cortical inhibitory neurons and schizophrenia. Nature Reviews Neuroscience 6:312–324

Lewis, D. A., Hayes, T. L., Lund, J. S. & Oeth, K. M. (1992) Dopamine and neural circuitry of primate prefrontal cortex: implications for schizophrenia research. Neuropsychopharmacology 6:127–134

Lewis, D. A. & Moghaddam, B. (2006) Cognitive dysfunction in schizophrenia: convergence of gamma-aminobutyric acid and glutamate alterations. Archives of Neurology 63: 1372–1376

Lieberman, J. A. (2007) Effectiveness of antipsychotic drugs in patients with chronic schizophrenia: efficacy, safety and cost outcomes of CATIE and other trials. Journal of Clinical Psychiatry 68:e04

Luby, E., Cohen, B., Rosenbaum, G., Gottlieb, J. & Kelley, R. (1959) Study of a new schizophrenomimetic drug-sernyl. American Medical Association Archives of Neurology and Psychiatry 81:363–369

Malhotra, A. K., Pinals, D. A., Weingartner, H., Sirocco, K., Missar, C. D., Pickar, D. & Breier, A. (1996) NMDA receptor function and human coginition: the effects of ketamine in healthy volunteers. Neuropsychopharmacology 14:301–307

McGaughy, J., Kaiser, T. & Sarter, M. (1996) Behavioral vigilance following infusions of 192 IgG-saporin into the basal forebrain: selectively of the following behavioral impairment and relation to cortical AChE-positive fiber density. Behavioral Neuroscience 110:247–265

Moghaddam, B. (2003) Bringing order to the glutamate chaos in schizophrenia. Neuron 40: 881–884

Olney, J. & Farber, N. (1995) Glutamate receptor dysfunction and schizophrenia. Archives of General Psychiatry 52:998–1007

Patil, S. T., Zhang, L., Martenyi, F., Lowe, S. L., Jackson, K. A., Andreev, B. V., Avedisova, A. S., Bardenstein, L. M., Gurovich, I. Y., Morozova, M. A., Mosolov, S. N., Neznanov, N. G., Reznik, A. M., Smulevich, A. B., Tochilov, V. A., Johnson, B. G., Monn, J. A. & Schoepp, D. D. (2007) Activation of mGlu2/3 receptors as a new approach to treat schizophrenia: a randomized Phase 2 clinical trial. Nature Medicine 13:1102–1107

Pierri, J. N., Chaudry, A. S., Woo, T. U. & Lewis, D. A. (1999) Alterations in chandelier neuron axon terminals in the prefrontal cortex of schizophrenic subjects. American Journal of Psychiatry 156:1709–1719

Pilowsky, L. S., Bressan, R. A., Stone, J. M., Erlandsson, K., Mulligan, R. S., Krystal, J. H. & Ell, P. J. (2006) First in vivo evidence of an NMDA receptor deficit in medication-free schizophrenic patients. Molecular Psychiatry 11(2):118–119

Randrup, A. & Munkvad, I. (1965) Special antagonism of amphetamine-induced abnormal behaviour. Inhibition of stereotyped activity with increase of some normal activities. Psychopharmacologia 7:416–422

Rimvall, K., Sheikh, S. N. & Martin, D. L. (1993) Effects of increased gamma-aminobutyric acid levels on GAD67 protein and mRNA levels in rat cerebral cortex. Journal of Neurochemistry 60:714–20

Robbins, T. (1996) Dissociating executive functions of the prefrontal cortex. Philosophical Transactions of the Royal Society of London-Series B: Biological Sciences 351:1463–1470

Robbins, T. W. (1998) Arousal and attention: psychopharmacological and neuropsychological studies in experimental animals. In: Parasuraman, R. (eds.) The Attentive Brain, MIT Press, Cambridge, MA, pp. 189–220

Seamans, J. K. & Yang, C. R. (2004) The principal features and mechanisms of dopamine modulation in the prefrontal cortex. Progress in Neurobiology 74:1–58

Seeman, P. & Lee, T. (1975) Antipsychotic drugs: direct correlation between clinical potency and presynaptic action on dopamine neurons. Science 188:1217–1219

Sheikh, S. N. & Martin, D. L. (1998) Elevation of brain GABA levels with vigabatrin (gamma-vinylGABA) differentially affects GAD65 and GAD67 expression in various regions of rat brain. Journal of Neuroscience Research 52:736–741

Tsai, G., Passani, L. A., Slusher, B. S., Carter, R., Baer, L., Kleinman, J. E. & Coyle, J. T. (1995) Abnormal excitatory neurotransmitter metabolism in schizophrenic brains. Archives of General Psychiatry 52:829–836

Verma, A. & Moghaddam, B. (1996) NMDA receptor antagonists impair prefrontal cortex function as assessed via spatial delayed alternation performance in rats: modulation by dopamine. Journal of Neuroscience 16:373–379

Volk, D. W., Austin, M. C., Pierri, J. N., Sampson, A. R. & Lewis, D. A. (2000) Decreased glutamic acid decarboxylase67 messenger RNA expression in a subset of prefrontal cortical gamma-aminobutyric acid neurons in subjects with schizophrenia. Archives of General Psychiatry 57:237–245

Wang, H. & Pickel, V. M. (2002) Dopamine D2 receptors are present in prefrontal cortical afferents and their targets in patches of the rat caudate-putamen nucleus. Journal of Comparative Neurology 442:392–404

Weinberger, D. R. (1987) Implications of normal brain development for the pathogenesis of schizophrenia. Archives of General Psychiatry 44:660–669

Weinberger, D. R. & Laruelle, M. (2001) Neurochemical and neuropharmacological imaging in schizophrenia. In: Davis, K. L., Charney D., Coyle J. T. & Nemeroff C. (eds.) Neuropsychopharmacology – The Fifth Generation of Progress, Lippincott Williams & Wilkins, Philadelphia, pp. 833–855

Winterer, G. & Weinberger, D. (2004) Genes, dopamine and cortical signal-to-noise ratio in schizophrenia. Trends in Neurosciences 27:683–690

Wolf, M., Deutch, A. & Roth, R.H. (1987) The neuropharmacology of dopamine. In: F.A. Henn, F.A. & DeLisi, L.E. (eds.) Handbook of Schizophrenia Vol. 2 Neurochemistry and Neuropharmacology, Elsevier Science Publishers, Amsterdam, pp. 101–147

Woo, T. U., Whitehead, R. E., Melchitzky, D. S. & Lewis, D. A. (1998) A subclass of prefrontal gamma-aminobutyric acid axon terminals are selectively altered in schizophrenia. Proceedings of the National Academy of Sciences of USA 95:5341–5346

Brain Anatomical Abnormalities in Schizophrenia: Neurodevelopmental Origins and Patterns of Progression over Time

Geraldo F. Busatto, Marcus V. Zanetti, Maristela S. Schaufelberger, and José A.S. Crippa

Introduction

In his first delineation of the concept of *dementia praecox* at the end of the nineteenth century, Emil Kraepelin proposed the existence of progressive degenerative neuronal changes underlying the symptoms of this disorder, soon later renamed as schizophrenia by Eugen Bleuler (see review by DeLisi, 2008). On the basis of Kraepelin's writings, a number of authors have, over several decades, formulated theories proposing that schizophrenia should be seen as a neurodegenerative disorder.

However, by the 1980s, neuropathological investigations had produced little evidence to support the view of schizophrenia as a neurodegenerative condition. In contrast, clinical and epidemiological findings began to provide evidence in favor of the alternative notion that schizophrenia should be seen as a neurodevelopmental disorder (see Falkai et al., this volume). Initial formulations of neurodevelopmental models for schizophrenia proposed that pathological processes would take place during pre- or peri-natal phases of brain development in schizophrenia subjects, remaining relatively static until the outbreak of psychotic symptoms in adolescence–early adulthood, when later brain maturational processes would normally take place (Weinberger, 1987; Murray & Lewis, 1987).

Since then, a wealth of studies using novel neuropathological techniques and in vivo neuroimaging methods have provided greater insights into the origins of brain pathological changes in schizophrenia as well as into the possible patterns of progression of such changes over time.

In this chapter, we provide a concise review of such evidence, with a strong emphasis on in vivo structural magnetic resonance imaging (MRI) studies, and discuss how these findings have been taken as supportive of neurodevelopmental versus neurodegenerative hypotheses of schizophrenia.

G.F. Busatto (✉)
Department and Institute of Psychiatry, University of São Paulo Medical School,
São Paulo, Brazil
e-mail: geraldo.busatto@hcnet.usp.br

W.F. Gattaz, G. Busatto (eds.), *Advances in Schizophrenia Research 2009*,
DOI 10.1007/978-1-4419-0913-8_6, © Springer Science+Business Media, LLC 2010

A Succinct Review of Postmortem Neuropathological Studies of Schizophrenia

In the first half of the twentieth century, psychiatry research was linked to post-mortem neuropathology, supported by the *Kraepelinian* belief of an underlying degenerative neuropathological basis for *dementia praecox*, and also under the influence of the neurohistological investigations of Alois Alzheimer (Bogerts, 1999). Postmortem studies on brain tissue from schizophrenia subjects at that time identified cortical atrophy and cellular abnormalities in the cortex, thalamus, and basal ganglia, but they did not reveal pathological findings similar to those present in classic neurodegenerative illnesses (Bogerts, 1999). It was not until the 1980s that, following the advances in methodological techniques, postmortem neuropathological studies in schizophrenia began to afford more reliable findings. These studies have searched for neurodegeneration markers as those observed in senile dementias, then evolved to the study of cortical cytoarchitecture, and later to the investigation of synapses. Such modern neuropathological studies on schizophrenia have been authoritatively reviewed by several authors (Harrison, 1999, 2004; Bogerts, 1999; Arnold and Rioux, 2001; Kasai, 2002; Harrison and Weinberger, 2005; Glantz et al., 2006). A brief synthesis of their findings is provided in the following paragraphs.

Macroscopic neuropathological investigations have demonstrated that schizophrenia is associated with volumetric reductions in the whole brain, temporal lobe, and thalamus, as well as with enlargement of the ventricular system and basal ganglia. Other findings have included a higher frequency of cavum septum pellucidum (CSP) and an absence of the normal cortical brain asymmetry. However, findings of macroscopic brain volume reductions per se in postmortem studies, although of great value in demonstrating the presence of brain abnormalities in schizophrenia, did not contribute significantly to the understanding of the time onset of such anomalies, as these volume differences might have occurred at early or late stages of illness.

Reactive proliferation and hypertrophy of astrocytes are considered hallmarks of inflammatory or neurodegenerative processes. However, histopathological investigations have demonstrated that these gliotic processes are consistently absent in schizophrenia (Harrison, 2004). Such absence of gliosis strongly suggests that neurodegenerative injuries do not occur in schizophrenia and this has become one of the main pillars of the neurodevelopmental hypothesis for schizophrenia (see Falkai et al., this volume). Also, there is a lack of Alzheimer's disease pathology in post-mortem brain tissue from subjects with schizophrenia. This was initially exemplified by the studies of Arnold et al. (1998), who failed to find either neurodegenerative lesions or neural injury in the ventromedial temporal lobe and frontal cortex in postmortem assessments of elderly patients with schizophrenia, or correlations between behavioral/cognitive deficits and age-related degenerative findings. However, it should be noted that the absence of gliosis per se is not a definite measure to determine the nature of the pathological mechanisms underlying the symptoms of schizophrenia.

Neuropathological studies investigating cytoarchitectural patterns in the brains of schizophrenia subjects have provided important insights regarding cell density, number, size, shape, orientation, localization, and clustering in association with this disorder. The most consistent results have been a reduction in size and increase in density of pyramidal neurons in the hippocampus and dorsolateral prefrontal cortex of schizophrenia subjects and reduced number of neurons in the thalamic mediodorsal nucleus. One other remarkable feature is the presence of aberrant clustered neurons in the entorhinal cortex, hippocampus, cingulate cortex, and in the deep white matter subjacent to the temporal and frontal neocortices. These abnormalities strongly suggest the presence of a brain anomaly that affects neuronal migration, survival, and connectivity. However, these initial postmortem findings have not always been replicated in subsequent studies that used more refined methodologies. What seems to best characterize the hippocampal pathology in schizophrenia is, rather than abnormalities in cell number, changes in morphological cellular parameters in terms of size, organization, and shape (see Falkai et al., this volume).

Glial cells have also been the focus of recent postmortem studies of schizophrenia and they have been found to be reduced in number and function in prefrontal, motor, and anterior cingulate cortices. A reduction in the number and function of oligodendrocytes and ultrastructural alterations of myelin sheets have been described in schizophrenia.

Indirect investigations of synapses have been made possible by evaluating the expression of synaptic proteins, providing information on synaptic density, size, vesicles, or structural abnormalities in the synaptic region. Consistent findings in schizophrenia have been a reduction in presynaptic proteins, such as synaptophysin, synapsin, and complexin II in brain areas such as the hippocampus and parahipocampal gyrus, mainly affecting glutamatergic terminals. Presynaptic protein reductions have also been described in the dorsolateral prefrontal cortex and the thalamus. Dendrites and dendritic spines, evaluated with postsynaptic markers, also seem to be altered in schizophrenia, as shown by a decreased expression of spinophilin, dysbindin, and, with less consistency, the microtubule-associated protein 2 (MAP2). Recently, neurotrophic signaling of brain-derived neurotrophic factor (BDNF) has also been found to be altered in the hippocampus and prefrontal cortex in schizophrenia.

The synaptic and neuron size reduction detected in postmortem investigations of schizophrenia, together with the increased neuronal density, is suggestive of a reduction in the neuropil, which consists of the sum of dendrites, axons, and synapses. Therefore, the reductions in volume and cortical thickness observed in postmortem brain tissue of schizophrenia subjects are likely to be consequential to reduced neuropil elements and cell size but not to neuronal loss.

Postmortem studies suggest that the hippocampus may exhibit different forms of synaptic pathology throughout life, with changes in inhibitory neurons and synapses in the early phase of schizophrenia, and progressive abnormalities, possibly related to glutamatergic excitatoxicity, appearing later over the course of the illness (see Falkai et al., this volume).

In synthesis, postmortem studies demonstrate that neurodegenerative pathology is not the basis of the structural brain abnormalities that are seen in association with schizophrenia, given the absence of gliosis and the lack of Alzheimer's disease pathology in schizophrenia. Rather, postmortem studies have supported the hypothesis of early brain developmental abnormalities in schizophrenia. According to Harrison (2004), the neuropathology of schizophrenia should be considered to be of neurodevelopmental nature involving quantitative, but not qualitative, differences in cytoarchitectural parameters. The presence of cortical neuropil/neuron size reduction and glial cell abnormalities is compatible with deviations in the normal brain processes of wiring, synaptic pruning, and myelinization (Keshavan et al., 1994; Lewis, 1997; Keshavan, 1999), or apoptosis leading to synaptic elimination without cell death (Glantz et al. 2006). Abnormalities on each of these mechanisms would be compatible with the time frame of schizophrenia onset and course (Lencz et al., 2001).

Although postmortem studies have provided invaluable clues for the time onset of the brain changes in schizophrenia, they do not allow, per se, full explanations for the nature and timing of the different pathological processes underlying the disorder. Advances in neuroimaging techniques have allowed the investigation of in vivo brain abnormalities associated with the disorder, with the advantage of assessing subjects not only at the onset of psychosis but also longitudinally with repeated measures over time. This research area is covered in the following sections of this chapter.

In Vivo Structural Neuroimaging Studies: Detection of Volumetric Brain Abnormalities in First-Episode Schizophrenia

To date, the in vivo neuroimaging approach that provided the greatest deal of data informing the pathogenesis of schizophrenia has been the use of structural MRI to compare patients in the early stages of the disorder versus control groups of healthy individuals matched for demographic variables. Studies comparing groups of first-episode psychosis subjects against healthy control samples have provided unequivocal evidence that brain volume abnormalities are detectable at the time of first presentation of schizophrenia symptoms. By minimizing the confounding influence of illness chronicity and long-term exposure to pharmacological treatment, these MRI investigations have provided indications that the brain structural abnormalities associated with schizophrenia antecede the emergence of psychotic symptoms. This has been taken as supportive of neurodevelopmental theories of the disorder (Woods, 1998; Van Haren et al., 2008a).

Morphometric MRI studies of first-episode schizophrenia patients have consistently shown significant global brain volume reductions, mostly in gray matter tissue, as well as enlargement of the ventricular system (Vita et al., 2006; Steen et al., 2006). In order to investigate the presence of regional volume abnormalities across separate cortical and subcortical brain structures, MRI studies of schizophrenia have quantified regional brain volumes using regions of interest (ROIs) placed on selected brain portions. These studies have variably demonstrated volume deficits mainly in the prefrontal and temporal neocortical regions, medial temporal structures (including the hippocampus and parahippocampal gyrus), basal ganglia, thalamus, and anterior cingulate gyrus (Wright et al., 2000; Shenton et al., 2001). Recent meta-analyses of ROI-based MRI studies of schizophrenia have highlighted the findings of whole brain and hippocampal volume reductions, as well as of lateral and third ventricular enlargement (Vita et al., 2006; Steen et al., 2006).

In recent years, there have been several further methodological advances in the field of morphometric MRI. For instance, voxel-based methods have been incorporated to allow the detection of brain volume changes across the entire cerebral volume in an automated fashion. These techniques include the voxel-based morphometry (VBM) approach (which allows voxelwise gray and white matter volume analyses) (Good et al., 2001) and the deformation-based morphometry (DBM) methodology (which enables automated quantifications of differences in brain shape) (Yoon et al., 2006). MRI studies using these techniques have not only confirmed previous findings obtained using the ROI-based approach but also enabled the demonstration of gray matter deficits associated with first-episode schizophrenia in other regions not readily assessable with ROI-based methods, such as the insula (Honea et al., 2005; Schaufelberger et al., 2007). Moreover, it has recently become possible to subject such voxel-based data to powerful computational approaches that allow meta-analyses of the tridimensional coordinates of the foci of gray matter differences between groups from the different studies reported in the literature (Ellison-Wright et al., 2008). Such meta-analytic approach has allowed comparisons of the patterns of brain deficits associated with first-episode psychosis with those of chronic schizophrenia, and such comparisons have indicated that progressive brain abnormalities over the illness course may occur specifically in cortical regions (Ellison-Wright et al., 2008).

One other development in the recent MRI literature of first-episode psychosis has been the incorporation of population-based methods, whereby large numbers of incident cases of psychosis can be recruited from circumscribed geographical regions, spanning the full spectrum of schizophrenia-related disorders. Moreover, such epidemiological approaches allow the inclusion of large numbers of nonpsychotic control individuals from exactly the same geographical areas. In the first study of this kind (the Ætiology and Ethnicity in Schizophrenia and Other Psychoses (AESOP) study), MRI measurements were obtained in 73 first-episode psychosis patients (44 of whom were diagnosed with schizophrenia) and 58 healthy controls from the neighborhood. Subtle findings of decreased hippocampal gray matter as well as enlarged lateral and third ventricle volumes were detected in the schizophrenia group (Morgan et al., 2007).

Also using a population-based approach, we have recently completed a morphometric MRI study of first-episode psychosis in Sao Paulo, Brazil (Schaufelberger et al., 2007). We evaluated a large sample of first-episode psychosis patients ($n=122$, 62 of whom with schizophrenia or schizophreniform disorder) compared to 94 next-door neighbors with no history of psychosis. Using VBM methods, we found gray matter reductions in schizophrenia subjects in the prefrontal, superior temporal, and insular cortices, as well as in the hippocampus, in high consistency with the findings of previous studies using similar image acquisition and analysis methods (Job et al., 2002; Honea et al., 2005). These findings have provided confirmation that brain abnormalities are evident in the early stages of psychosis not only in severely ill subjects (which have predominated in the samples recruited in most previous MRI studies of first-episode schizophrenia) but also in community representative samples of sufferers from milder schizophrenia-related disorders.

One other distinctive feature of our study is that it was the first large MRI investigation of first-episode psychosis outside high-income countries. We found significant reductions in gray matter in Brazilian first-episode psychosis subjects in those same brain regions where gray matter decrements have been detected in patient samples studied in high-income nations, thus indicating that first-episode schizophrenia has a similar neuroanatomic substrate in different environments. This suggests that the supposed better outcome of psychosis in developing countries compared with developed countries (Hopper and Wanderling, 2000) is not related to differences in the brain mechanisms underlying the symptoms of the disorder.

Association Between Focal Brain Developmental Abnormalities and the Diagnosis of Schizophrenia

One additional strategy used in structural MRI investigations of neurodevelopmental versus neurodegenerative models for schizophrenia is regarding the search for focal gross changes that could indicate abnormalities that occurred during early stages of neurodevelopment. If one detects an excess of such findings in schizophrenia samples relative to controls, this provides support to the notion that disturbances in brain development are of critical relevance to the disorder (Murray and Fearon, 1999).

Several case reports described the presence of gross brain abnormalities of neurodevelopmental origin, such as agenesis of the corpus callosum, in patients presenting with schizophrenia symptoms, as documented by computed tomography (CT) or structural MRI scans (Kuhnley et al., 1981; Reveley and Reveley, 1983; Lewis et al., 1988). In addition, there have been many MRI investigations comparing the incidence of medial and midline brain structural anomalies, such as the persistence of CSP and absence of the adhesio interthalamica (AI), between groups of schizophrenia patients and healthy controls. Persistence of CSP and absence of AI both indicate abnormalities in early brain development (Rakic and Yakovlev, 1968). Excessive abnormalities of CSP and AI in patients with schizophrenia could represent early markers of other developmental defects involving some of the midline brain structures that have consistently been linked to schizophrenia, such as the thalamus, hippocampus, and corpus callosum (Nopoulos et al., 1998). This would be in line with neurodevelopmental hypotheses of schizophrenia (Weinberger, 1987; Murray and Lewis, 1987).

A higher prevalence of CSP in groups of patients with schizophrenia in comparison to healthy controls has been observed in a number of structural MRI studies carried out with patient samples in chronic (Rajarethinam et al., 2001; Galarza et al., 2004) or first-episode (DeLisi et al., 1993) stages of the illness. As most MRI studies in this field presented positive results until recently, this type of abnormality became established as one of the most robust neuroimaging findings associated with schizophrenia (Shenton et al., 2001). However, this has come into disrepute more recently, with the publication of several consecutive studies that failed to find significant differences in the prevalence of CSP between schizophrenia patients and controls (de Souza Crippa et al., 2006; Flashman et al., 2007; Takahashi et al., 2007; Rajarethinam et al., 2008).

Recent high-resolution MRI studies, using more quantitative approaches and relatively objective assessment methods, have improved the accuracy of estimates of the prevalence and length of CSP in schizophrenia. In particular, the thin-slice length methodology of counting the number of slices in which a CSP appears in coronal brain views is now considered the state-of-the-art method to assess the presence and severity of this brain abnormality in MRI studies. A CSP with anterior-to-posterior length spanning six or more millimeters has been defined as large (Nopoulos et al., 1997, 1998; Hagino et al., 2001) based on previous postmortem findings (Shunk, 1963), and this landmark is now established as the most sensitive and reliable index to classify CSP findings. Using this method, several MRI studies have reported an increased prevalence of large CSP in schizophrenia (Kasai et al., 2004; Dickey et al., 2007). However, the prevalence of CSP of any size has not been found to differ between patients with schizophrenia and healthy controls in many of these recent reports (Kwon et al., 1998; de Souza Crippa et al., 2006). Based on such pattern of results, it has been speculated that the clinical significance of a CSP in schizophrenia may depend more on its magnitude than simply on its presence or absence (Flashman et al., 2007; Takahashi et al., 2007; Rajarethinam et al., 2008).

Although not always replicated, findings of large CSP in schizophrenia have been associated with family history of psychosis (Uematsu and Kaiya, 1989), duration of the illness (Brisch et al., 1989), poor outcome (Fukuzako and Kodama, 1998), more severe negative symptoms and thinking disturbances (Kasai et al., 2004; Flashman et al., 2007), higher suicide rates (Filipović et al., 2005), and greater cognitive deficits (Nopoulos et al., 2000; Flashman et al., 2007). In addition, schizophrenia patients with large CSP also present more pronounced brain asymmetry and reduced volumes of the left temporal lobe (Nopoulos et al., 1996), bilateral hippocampus (Kwon et al., 1998), bilateral amygdala, and left parahippocampal gyrus (Kasai et al., 2004; Takahashi et al., 2007). Taken together, these findings suggest that schizophrenia subjects with a large CSP may display distinct patterns of disturbed brain morphology and, possibly, more psychopathological impairment.

The AI (or massa intermedia) is a midline structure connecting the medial surfaces of the thalamus on each side across the third ventricle. It usually fuses between the 13th and 14th weeks of gestation (Rosales et al., 1968), but varies in size among individuals. The AI is missing in about 20% of human brains (Carpenter and Sutin, 1983) and seems to be more commonly absent in males than in females (Malobabic et al., 1987; Allen and Gorski, 1991). Absent AI has been reported to be more common among patients with schizophrenia than in healthy subjects (Snyder et al., 1998; Nopoulos et al., 2001; Takahashi et al., 2008), although this finding has not always been replicated (Ettinger et al., 2007). It has been demonstrated that schizophrenia patients without AI also display increased third ventricle volume (Snyder et al., 1998; Meisenzahl et al., 2002; Takahashi et al., 2008), as well as smaller parahippocampal and amygdalar volumes (Takahashi et al., 2008). Furthermore, schizophrenia patients without AI have been found to present with more severe negative symptoms than patients with AI (Takahashi et al., 2008; Meisenzahl et al., 2000, 2002), although such findings have not been replicated by other authors (de Souza Crippa et al., 2006). Two studies evaluated the presence of large CSP and absent AI in the same sample, showing absolutely no (de Souza Crippa et al., 2006) or little (Takahashi et al., 2008) overlap between those two findings.

In conclusion, the issue as to whether there is an excess of brain focal abnormalities indicative of neurodevelopmental anomalies in schizophrenia is not yet resolved. The overall incidence rates of enlarged CSP and absent AI in schizophrenia in the MRI studies reviewed herein show that these are relatively uncommon findings in schizophrenia (de Souza Crippa et al., 2006). Therefore, these midline structural abnormalities should at most be regarded as early neurodevelopmental risk factors that could be associated with a future manifestation of schizophrenia in a subgroup of patients rather than as causative determinants of the disorder.

Progression of Morphologic Brain Changes After the Onset of Psychosis

One powerful way to directly investigate the patterns of progression of brain structural abnormalities associated with schizophrenia is to conduct longitudinal MRI studies, in which morphometric brain measurements are obtained repeatedly over the course of the illness in subjects with first-episode psychosis, in comparison to asymptomatic volunteers also assessed with repeated MRI measurements.

In the first study of this kind, DeLisi et al. (1997) recruited an initial sample of 87 schizophrenia patients at the time of their first psychotic episode and 52 healthy controls and noted a significant increase in lateral ventricle volumes in patients compared to controls. After 5 years, 50 schizophrenia individuals and 20 controls had been reevaluated approximately on an annual basis, and the analysis of such longitudinal data revealed greater left ventricle enlargement in patients relative to controls over time, as well as reduced volumes of the overall left and right cerebral hemispheres, right cerebellum, and isthmus of the corpus callosum. No between-group differences were detected with regard to the volumes of the caudate nucleus, temporal lobe, or hippocampus. After 10 years of follow-up, schizophrenia patients ($n =$ 26) still exhibited ventricular enlargement relative to controls (DeLisi et al., 2004), with no significant differences being observed in temporal lobe measures (DeLisi and Hoff, 2005). However, an unexpected direct correlation between greater ventricle volumes over time and better (rather than worse) outcome was reported (DeLisi et al., 2004).

Since then, several other follow-up MRI studies of schizophrenia have been carried out, with intervals between scans varying from 1 to 5 years. Table 1 summarizes the findings of longitudinal MRI studies conducted to date in samples of adult subjects with first-episode schizophrenia. These studies have provided compelling evidence that brain abnormalities associated with schizophrenia may increase in severity over time, by demonstrating the presence of progressive reductions in total brain (Wood et al., 2001; Cahn et al., 2002) and global gray matter volumes (Cahn et al., 2002), as well as increases in total cerebrospinal fluid spaces (Ho et al., 2003; Bachmann et al., 2004; Nakamura et al., 2007) and lateral ventricle volumes (Lieberman et al., 2001; Cahn et al., 2002, Nakamura et al., 2007; van Haren et al., 2008b). With regard to regional brain changes, longitudinal MRI studies of schizophrenia have detected significantly progressive volume decreases over time in the following: total frontal (Gur et al., 1998; Bachmann et al., 2004, Ho et al., 2003; Nakamura et al., 2007) and temporal lobes (Bachmann et al., 2004; Nakamura et al., 2007); the cingulate gyrus (Koo et al., 2008); the left superior frontal cortex (van Haren et al., 2007); the Heschl gyrus, left planum temporale, and superior temporal gyrus (Kasai et al., 2003a, b; Théberge et al., 2007; van Haren et al., 2007); and the hippocampus (Wang et al., 2008), caudate nucleus (Théberge et al., 2007; van Haren et al., 2007; Wang et al., 2008), and thalamus (van Haren et al., 2007; Wang et al., 2008).

In a notable proportion of the above studies, there have been indications of a direct association between favorable outcome of schizophrenia and lesser brain volume deficits at follow-up (Lieberman et al., 2001; Cahn et al., 2002; Ho et al., 2003; Nakamura et al., 2007; Van Haren et al., 2008b; Hulshoff Pol and Kahn, 2008).

The literature above provides strong support to the notion of schizophrenia as a progressive brain disorder, as argued in several recent authoritative reviews on this topic (Pantelis et al., 2005; van Haren et al., 2008a; DeLisi, 2008; Hulshofff Poll and Kahn, 2008). Several possible mechanisms have been proposed as underlying the progression of brain volume deficits as detected in such longitudinal MRI studies of schizophrenia. These have included persistent abnormal neurotransmission (dopaminergic, glutamatergic, GABA-ergic), neuropil abnormalities (dendrites/synapse density) (Selemon and Goldman-Rakic, 1999), and stress-related hypothalamo-pituitary-adrenal functional hyperactivity (Keshavan et al., 1998; Pantelis et al., 2005), which could lead to reductions in dendritic spines (Chen et al. 2008). It is interesting to note that these explanations do not imply degenerative processes, which is consistent with the arguments raised in the recent neuropathological literature of schizophrenia reviewed in the first part of this chapter.

One additional and particularly interesting hypothesis to explain the schizophrenia-related patterns of progressive brain changes implicates the occurrence of abnormal processes of brain maturation during adult age in association with the disorder. van Haren et al. (2008b), in a 5-year follow-up study of 96

Table 1 Longitudinal MRI studies of adult-onset first-episode schizophrenia

Study	Sample (mean follow-up interval)	Image acquisition and/or analysis methods* (brain regions evaluated)	Main results (changes over time)
DeLisi et al. (1997)	50 FESZ 20 HC (4–5 years)	ROI (hemispheres, TL, STG, cerebellum, AHC, CC, VVLL)	Patients: ↓ hemispheres bilaterally, ↓ CC isthmus, ↓ right cerebellum and ↑ left VV Continuous AP use was associated with lesser VVLL alterations over time
Gur et al. (1998)	20 FESZ, drug-naïve 20 Chronic SZ 17 HC (30 months)	ROI (TBV, FL, TL, CSF).	Patients: ↓ left FL HC: ↓ TL FESZ versus chronic SZ: ↓ FL e ↑ TL AP dose was correlated with ↓ FL and TL
Keshavan et al. (1998)	15 FESZ, drug-naïve 12 HC (1 year)	ROI (STG, cerebellum)	Patients: reversion of STG volume reductions seen at baseline
Lieberman et al. (2001)	51 FESZ or SZAFF 13 HC (1–6 years)	ROI (TCV, caudate nucleus, VV, VVLL, anterior hippocampus)	Poor outcome patients: ↑ VV e ↑ hippocampus Good outcome patients: ↑ TCV HC: ↓ TCV and hippocampus Overall patients group: ↑ caudate volume No association between treatment duration and TCV, caudate or hippocampal volumes
Wood et al. (2001)	30 FEP (1.9 years) 12 Chronic SZ (2.3 years) 26 controls (2.2 years)	ROI (TBV, ICV, TL, hippocampus)	Both patient groups: ↓ TBV (similar rates FEP versus chronic SZ) No medication effect was observed

Table 1 (continued)

Study	Sample (mean follow-up interval)	Image acquisition and/or analysis methods* (brain regions evaluated)	Main results (changes over time)
Puri et al. (2001)	24 FESZ 12 HC (8 months)	ROI (TBV, VVLL)	No differences between patients and controls in mean VV, but greater than expected variation (both increases and decreases) in VV was observed in FESZ over time
Cahn et al. (2002)	34 FESZ 36 HC (1 year)	ROI (TBV, global GM/WM, VVLL, cerebellum)	Patients: ↓ TBV and GM volume, ↑ VVLL. The decrease in global GM volume significantly correlated with outcome and, independent of that, with higher cumulative dosage of AP
Ho et al. (2003)	73 SZ patients FEP=41 Previous contact=32 23 HC (3 years)	ROI (TBV, VVLL, FL, TL, PL, cerebellum, CSF)	Patients: ↑ CSF, ↓ frontal WM Poor versus good outcome SZ: ↑ VVLL Progressive ↓ frontal WM and ↑ frontal CSF were associated with greater negative symptom severity No medication effect was observed in any region
Kasai et al. (2003a, b)	13 FESZ 22 HC (2003a) 14 HC (2003b) (1.5 years)	ROI (anterior and posterior STG, anterior and posterior AHC, HG, PT)	SZ patients versus both FEP of affective type (n=15) and HC: ↓ left HG, left PT and left STG (more pronounced in its posterior portion) These results were not associated with AP use or symptom severity

Table 1 (continued)

Study	Sample (mean follow-up interval)	Image acquisition and/or analysis methods* (brain regions evaluated)	Main results (changes over time)
DeLisi et al. (2004)	26 FESZ 10 HC (10 years)	ROI (hemispheres, VVLL)	Patients: ↑ VVLL Greater ↑ VVLL over time was correlated with better, not worse, outcome at the 10th year of follow-up with regard to the presence of symptoms No association with AP use or poor outcome was observed
Bachmann et al. (2004)	14 FESZ 13 HC (scanned only at baseline) (14 months)	ROI (hemispheres, FL, TL, CSF, VVLL)	Patients: ↓ frontal WM and temporal GM bilaterally. ↑ CSF
Dickey et al. (2004)	12 FEP 15 HC (1.5 years)	ROI (prefrontal cortex)	No differences in the rate of prefrontal volume decreases were observed over time between patients and controls
Zipursky et al. (2004)	10 FESZ 9 HC (5 years)	ROI (VVLL, global/lobar GM and WM, CSF)	No between-group differences were observed in any region
DeLisi and Hoff (2005)	27 FESZ 10 HC (10 years)	ROI (TL, STG)	No between-group differences were observed in TL or STG volume over time

Table 1 (continued)

Study	Sample (mean follow-up interval)	Image acquisition and/or analysis methods* (brain regions evaluated)	Main results (changes over time)
Whitworth et al. (2005)	Mixed group of 21 FEP and 17 chronic SZ 20 HC (2–4 years)	ROI (hemispheres, TBV, VVLL, AHC)	Patients: ↑ VVLL and ↓ AHC both at baseline and at follow-up relative to controls, but no between-group differences regarding mean annual volume changes in the measured regions SZ showed higher between-subject variability in VVLL change No correlation with illness duration, PANSS scores, or level of functioning was observed
Price et al. (2006)	16 FESZ 12 HC (3.7 years)	Magnetization transfer imaging	WM deficits were observed at baseline in SZ relative to controls, but no progression was observed over time No cortical differences were detected between the groups at baseline or follow-up
Théberge et al. (2007)	16 FESZ, drug-naive 16 HC (30 months)	VBM	Patients: ↓ left STG and left caudate head
Nakamura et al. (2007)	17 FESZ 26 HC (1.5 years)	ROI (total cortical/ lobar GM, LLVV, sulcal CSF)	SZ patients: ↓ frontal and temporal cortical GM, ↑ LLVV and sulcal CSF Poorer outcome was associated with ↓ cortical GM and ↑ LLVV No association was observed with AP use

Table 1 (continued)

Study	Sample (mean follow-up interval)	Image acquisition and/or analysis methods* (brain regions evaluated)	Main results (changes over time)
Whitford et al. (2007a, b)	25 FESZ 26 HC (2–3 years)	Tensor-based morphometry	Patients: longitudinal ↓ GM in fronto-parietal cortex, and ↓ WM in the middle and inferior temporal cortex bilaterally
van Haren et al. (2007)	96 mixed FEP and Chronic SZ 113 HC (5 years)	VBM	Patients: ↓ left SFG, STG, right caudate nucleus, and right thalamus. Increased number of hospitalizations was associated with excessive ↓ left SFG, whereas a higher cumulative dose of clozapine and olanzapine during the scan interval was related to lesser volume decreases in this area
van Haren et al. (2008b)	96 mixed FEP and chronic SZ 113 HC (5 years)	ROI (TBV, ICV, total GM and WM, FL, TL, PL, OL, cerebellum, third ventricle, VVLL)	Patients showed a different trajectory of brain volume change relative to controls: before the age of 45 years, ↓ TBV/GM and ↑ VVLL were excessive in SZ relative to HC, representing approximately the first 20 years of illness. SZ versus HC: ↑ third ventricle volume across the whole age span. Poor- versus good-outcome SZ: greater ↓ TBV during the follow-up interval
Koo et al. (2008)	17 FESZ 18 HC (1.5 years)	ROI (cingulate gyrus: subgenual, affective, cognitive, and posterior subregions)	Patients: progressive ↓ GM in the subgenual, affective, cognitive, and posterior cingulate subregions

Table 1 (continued)

Study	Sample (mean follow-up interval)	Image acquisition and/or analysis methods* (brain regions evaluated)	Main results (changes over time)
Sun et al. (in press)	16 FESZ 14 HC (2 years)	Cortical pattern matching	Similar brain surface contraction patterns in patients and controls, but exaggerated in magnitude in the SZ subjects, across the entire brain surface.
Schaufelberger et al. (in revision)	39 FESZ 52 epidemiological controls (1 year)	VBM	No differences in the GM volume or ventricle-brain-ratio change between FEP subjects and controls were observed over time
			SZ showed GM in the left STG and the right hippocampus relative to controls
			Continuous AP exposure was associated with greater ventricle-brain-ratio increase over time, while a remitting course was related to reversal of baseline regional GM volume deficits in the TL

Abbreviations: ↑, increase; ↓, reduction; AHC, amygdala–hippocampal complex; AP, antipsychotic; CC, corpus callosum; CSF, cerebrospinal fluid; FEP, first-episode psychosis; FESZ, first-episode schizophrenia; FL, frontal lobe; GM, gray matter; HC, healthy controls; HG, Heschl gyrus; ICV, intracranial volume; OL, occipital lobe; PANSS, positive and negative syndrome scale; PL, parietal lobe; PT, planum temporale; ROI, region of interest; SFG, superior frontal gyrus; STG, superior temporal gyrus; SZ, schizophrenia/schizophreniform patients; SZAFF, schizoaffective disorder patients; TBV, total brain volume; TCV, total cortical volume; TL, temporal lobe; VBM, voxel-based morphometry; VV, ventricular volume; VVLL, lateral ventricles; WM, white matter.

*Whole-brain morphometric MRI acquisition protocols were employed in all studies reported in the table as using ROI- or VBM-based image analysis methods.

schizophrenia patients and 113 healthy individuals (with an age range of 16–56 years), found that the trajectory of brain volume changes over time was different in patients relative to controls. Instead of the curved trajectory that was found for cerebral gray matter volume change in healthy individuals (which replicated findings reported in several imaging studies of normal aging), schizophrenia patients showed a linear pattern of brain volume decrease over time. In addition, excessive brain volume loss in patients (particularly in the gray matter compartment) and lateral ventricle enlargement were limited to the first 20 years of the illness, i.e., before the age of 45 years. From this age onward, the total cerebral and gray matter volumes decreased in schizophrenia subjects and controls to a similar extent. Before the age of 32 years, the progressive loss of gray matter was accompanied by increases in white matter volumes in schizophrenia subjects. These patients also showed an excessive third ventricle volume increase over time, across the entire age span investigated. These results suggest that schizophrenia may be associated with maturational abnormalities in early adulthood, which corroborates the notion of schizophrenia as a neurodevelopmental condition (van Haren et al., 2008b).

However, it is important to highlight that not all longitudinal morphometric MRI investigations in the early stages of schizophrenia have reported volume loss over time in brain structures of key relevance to the disorder (see Table 1). For instance, several of the morphometric MRI studies that found reductions in temporal lobe structures at the first psychotic episode failed to demonstrate progression of these deficits over time (Gur et al., 1998; Lieberman et al., 2001, Wood et al., 2001; Whitworth et al., 2005; Schaufelberger et al., submitted for publication). Moreover, a number of MRI studies also failed to find longitudinal ventricular enlargement in schizophrenia patients compared to controls (Lieberman et al., 2001; Puri et al., 2001; Zipursky et al., 2004; Whitworth et al., 2005).

The lack of overall agreement across the longitudinal MRI studies of psychosis reported to date could be explained, at least partially, by the recruitment of schizophrenia groups of modest size in some studies and by the selection of healthy controls that may not be representative of the overall population from which psychosis subjects come from.

In the context of our epidemiological research program on first-episode psychosis, we have recently completed a follow-up investigation that is, to the best of our knowledge, the first population-based longitudinal MRI study of such disorder (Schaufelberger et al., in revision). This study included 80 schizophrenia patients and 52 nonpsychotic controls. After a mean follow-up period of 15 months, we found no differences either in the rate of change of gray matter volumes or in ventricle size between first-episode psychosis subjects and controls. These negative findings did not provide support to the hypothesis of progressive brain volumetric reductions in the initial stages of schizophrenia after the onset of psychosis. The use of epidemiological methods to identify and assess cases directly from the community, living in a circumscribed geographical region, is likely to reduce selection biases by ensuring that all individuals enrolled in the study have similar levels of exposure to environmental factors within the general population (Wacholder, 1995; Lee et al., 2007). Also, this approach may have yielded the identification of cases more representative of the overall population of schizophrenia individuals than previous MRI studies that evaluated patients recruited in in-patient hospital settings and/or specialized psychiatric services, an approach that is likely to miss cases of better prognosis. Indeed, in a number of previous longitudinal MRI studies of first-episode psychosis, all subjects initially diagnosed as suffering from schizophreniform disorder were diagnosed with schizophrenia at follow-up (van Haren et al., 2007); this rate is not consistent with findings from clinical studies, which indicate that a substantial proportion of patients with schizophreniform disorder present complete symptom remission at follow-up (Addington et al., 2006; Haahr et al., 2008). Thus our data may indicate that when representative, population-based FEP samples are recruited for longitudinal MRI studies, there is less compelling evidence of overall progression of brain volume deficits associated with schizophrenia over the first years of the disease course.

Are There State-Dependent Brain Structural Abnormalities in Schizophreniform Psychosis?

Given the preponderance of the view that brain volume deficits progress over time in schizophrenia, very little attention has been given to the possibility that some brain morphological abnormalities could be state-dependent and reversible after symptom remission, at least in a subset of patients with schizophrenia-related disorders. In one previous longitudinal MRI study, a small sample of first-episode schizophrenia subjects ($n = 11$) displayed reversal of volume decrements in the superior temporal gyrus 1 year after the disease onset (Keshavan et al., 1998). This pattern of results was interpreted as reflecting reversal of neuronal damage (for instance, induced by cortisol hyperactivity or other sources of oxidative stress) after stabilization of the illness (Keshavan et al., 1998).

In our population-based longitudinal MRI study of psychosis, we found that relative to healthy controls, patients with schizophrenia/schizophreniform disorder ($n = 39$) showed a greater degree of gray matter preservation in the left superior temporal cortex and the right hippocampus. When we dichotomized patients according to their functional outcome based on DSM-IV criteria, we found that such findings of increased gray matter in temporal lobe regions were confined to the subgroup of subjects with schizophrenia-spectrum psychosis with good prognosis, which represented 25% of our sample (Schaufelberger et al., in revision). Our results provide indication that brain volumetric abnormalities associated with some forms of schizophrenia may be associated with the acute phase of illness and may to some extent 'normalize' with symptom improvement, remission, or recovery. It is important to highlight that the remitted first-episode schizophrenia patients who showed significant volume increments over time included only a minority of subjects who were continuously treated with antipsychotics over the follow-up period. Thus, our data support a view that schizophrenia-related neuropathological processes may be potentially reversible with symptom remission in some cases, regardless of antipsychotic treatment.

Brain Abnormalities Associated with the Conversion from Prodromal States to Psychosis

Recent structural MRI studies of subjects at risk for the development of schizophrenia have contributed to the evaluation of brain abnormalities that may be present before the onset of illness and during the transition to first-episode psychosis (see Cannon, this volume). These studies have employed either of two designs, investigating respectively individuals at increased genetic risk for schizophrenia (first-degree relatives of patients with schizophrenia) (Lawrie et al., 2008) or *ultra-high risk* (UHR) subjects (people suffering from sub-syndromal psychotic symptoms, the so-called at-risk mental state (ARMS)) (Wood et al., 2008).

The largest morphometric MRI study of subjects at high risk for schizophrenia due to genetic reasons (i.e., two or more close relatives with schizophrenia) was carried out in Scotland (the Edinburgh High-Risk Study). In an initial evaluation using ROI-based analysis methods, high-risk individuals ($n=147$) were found to display reduced volumes of the amygdala–hippocampus complex and thalamus bilaterally, in a degree that was intermediate between that of healthy controls ($n=36$) and first-episode schizophrenia subjects ($n=34$) (Lawrie et al., 2001). A further VBM investigation with this same sample (except for the exclusion of one high-risk subject) revealed bilateral gray matter density reductions in the anterior cingulate gyrus of high-risk individuals compared to controls, whereas first-episode schizophrenia patients showed a distinct pattern of gray matter reductions in fronto-temporal regions (Job et al., 2003). A subsequent longitudinal evaluation with repeated MRI scanning revealed no significant differences in gray matter density changes between 65 high-risk individuals and 19 healthy controls over a period of approximately 2 years (Job et al., 2005). Also, no significant baseline differences in gray matter volumes were observed between those high-risk individuals who later developed schizophrenia ($n=8$) and those who did not. However, the individuals who later converted to schizophrenia displayed a different pattern of gray matter reduction in the left uncus and fusiform gyrus, and also in the right cerebellar cortex compared to those high-risk subjects who had psychotic symptoms but did not convert to schizophrenia ($n=18$) (Job et al., 2005). The same group has also shown that those high-risk subjects who subsequently developed schizophrenia already presented with abnormal patterns of prefrontal cortical folding at baseline, based on an index of gyrification (Harris et al., 2007). Cortical folding patterns are known to reflect neurodevelopment processes in the frontal cortex, and abnormalities in gyrification indices have previously been demonstrated in schizophrenia patients investigated with morphometric MRI (Sallet et al., 2003).

The largest data set of UHR subjects investigated with MRI to date has been acquired in Melbourne (Wood et al., 2008). These authors assessed patterns of cross-sectional and longitudinal structural brain changes in up to 100 UHR subjects during the transition to psychosis. Firstly, in a VBM study, UHR subjects who later developed psychosis ($n=23$) were found to display, relative to those individuals who did not ($n=52$), reduced gray matter volumes in the right medial temporal, lateral temporal, and inferior frontal cortices, as well as in the cingulate gyrus bilaterally at baseline (Pantelis et al., 2003). Twenty-one UHR subjects were rescanned after at least 1-year of follow-up; a subsample of 10 converters presented regional gray matter reductions affecting the cingulate, parahippocampal, and orbitofrontal cortices, whereas longitudinal volume changes were restricted to the cerebellum in non-converters (Pantelis et al., 2003). Later, in collaboration with researchers in the United States, the same research group used DBM-based methods and a 1-year longitudinal MRI design to evaluate UHR subjects who converted to psychosis ($n=11$–12) compared to both healthy controls and non-converting UHR subjects ($n=20$–23) (see Cannon, this volume). These studies demonstrated a greater degree of right prefrontal contraction specifically in the UHR subjects who converted to psychosis (Sun et al., 2009). Also, regional brain volume measurements in the same sample revealed gray matter reductions bilaterally in the superior temporal gyrus (Takahashi et al., 2009) and insula (Takahashi et al., in press) in the UHR subjects who converted to psychosis at the 1-year follow-up. These authors discuss the role of stress at the psychosis onset and a possible disturbance in the hypothalamus-pituitary-adrenal axis underlying such structural brain changes, and this proposition is supported by findings of volumetric decrements in the pituitary in the UHR subjects who later developed psychosis (Wood et al., 2008).

Also recently, Borgwardt et al. (2007, 2008) reported cross-sectional ($n=35$) and longitudinal ($n=20$) MRI findings in ARMS subjects. At baseline, those subjects who later developed psychosis ($n=12$) had less gray matter than subjects who did not ($n=23$) in the right insula, inferior frontal cortex, and superior temporal gyrus (Borgwardt et al., 2007). After 3 years of follow-up, 10 converters showed progression of gray matter decreases in the frontal, temporal, and parietal cortices, as well as in the cerebellum, while no longitudinal gray matter differences were found in the 10 non-converting subjects (Borgwardt et al., 2008).

The morphometric MRI studies mentioned above, by describing localized abnormalities of volume and shape in subjects at high risk for psychosis, favor the notion of neurodevelopmental brain abnormalities in association with the genetic liability to develop schizophrenia. Also, the results of these studies suggest strongly that regional structural brain abnormalities present in subjects at high risk for psychosis may show a dynamic pattern of progression over time, particularly during the transition to psychosis in those subjects who do develop full-blown schizophrenia (see Cannon, this volume).

Progressive Brain Abnormalities in Schizophrenia: Evidence from Studies Using Other MRI-Based Techniques

Most of the above structural MRI studies of schizophrenia have privileged the investigation of abnormalities in the gray matter compartment of the brain. Recently, however, there has been considerable interest in the in vivo assessment of structural white matter pathology in schizophrenia. Such interest stems mainly from postmortem findings suggesting the existence of glial cell and myelinization deficits associated with the disorder, as well as functional imaging evidence indicating cortico-subcortical functional dysconnectivity underlying psychotic symptoms (Bartzokis, 2002; Davis et al., 2003; Konrad and Winterer, 2008).

Recently, diffusion tensor imaging (DTI) techniques have afforded significant advances in the study of white matter tissue in the brain in vivo. This MRI-based methodology, by quantifying the diffusion of water in brain tissue and the anisotropy of this diffusion movement, enables the evaluation of integrity of white matter fiber tracts (Jones, 2008). The field of DTI studies of schizophrenia is rapidly evolving and there have been consistent findings of decreased fractional anisotropy or increased diffusivity within the prefrontal and temporal lobes, as well as abnormalities within the fiber bundles connecting these regions (Kyriakopoulos et al., 2008; McIntosh et al., 2008). These results have been confirmed by one recent meta-analysis (Ellison-Wright and Bullmore, 2009). Such DTI-based findings have been detected in some (Price et al., 2007, 2008; Cheung et al., 2008), but not all (Peters et al., 2008), samples of first-episode schizophrenia subjects and it has been suggested that white matter abnormalities would be less widespread in the early stages of the illness than in chronic schizophrenia (Price et al., 2005; Friedman et al., 2008).

Magnetic resonance spectroscopy (MRS) provides a noninvasive tool to investigate a wide variety of metabolites in the living human brain. In recent studies comparing schizophrenia patients relative to healthy controls, the compounds most often investigated have been proton-containing metabolites such as N-acetyl aspartate (NAA), creatine (Cr), choline (Cho), myoinositol, glutamine, glutamate, glutathione, and gamma-aminobutyric acid (GABA) (Keshavan et al., 2000; Gur et al., 2007), assessed using ^{1}H-MRS. Reduced NAA concentrations (indicative of neural loss) in the prefrontal cortex and hippocampus have been consistently demonstrated in schizophrenia patients. These abnormalities have been correlated with increased illness duration and are also associated with findings of cortical atrophy, cognitive impairment, and more severe negative symptoms (Keshavan et al., 2000; Gur et al., 2007).

Only three longitudinal MRS studies have been conducted to date, evaluating, respectively, individuals with schizophrenia at an early stage of their illness (Bustillo et al., 2002), at-risk individuals (Jessen et al., 2006), and patients presenting with their first psychotic episode (Théberge et al., 2007). Bustillo et al. (2002) studied 10 schizophrenia subjects minimally treated with antipsychotics (less than 3 weeks' lifetime exposure) and 10 healthy controls with ^{1}H-MRS. These authors found no differences in frontal or occipital NAA between patients and controls at baseline, but showed reduced frontal NAA in the schizophrenia group after 1 year of treatment, which was not correlated with symptom improvement. In a follow-up study of individuals at risk for the development of schizophrenia, Jessen et al. (2006) observed, at baseline, a significant reduction of the metabolic NAA/Cr and NAA/Cho ratios in the left frontal lobe and of NAA/Cr in the anterior cingulate gyrus in both at-risk and schizophrenia groups compared with healthy controls. Those at-risk individuals who converted to schizophrenia had a higher Cho/Cr and a lower NAA/Cho ratio in the anterior cingulate gyrus compared with non-converters. Thus, contradicting the previous work from Bustillo et al. (2002), these findings suggest that NAA reduction in the prefrontal and anterior cingulate gyrus may represent an endophenotype for the development of schizophrenia, whereas elevated Cho in the anterior cingulate gyrus may be a predictor of conversion to schizophrenia in at-risk individuals. Finally, Théberge et al. (2007) combined structural MRI and MRS in the evaluation of first-episode schizophrenia subjects over a 30-month period and found elevated levels of glutamine in the anterior cingulate gyrus and thalamus of never-treated patients at baseline and decreased glutamine in the thalamus after 30 months. The reduced level of thalamic glutamine correlated with temporal and parietal gray matter loss over time, suggesting that this finding may relate to neurodegeneration (Théberge et al., 2007).

The Influence of Antipsychotic Treatment on the Progression of Brain Abnormalities in Schizophrenia

Given that most longitudinal MRI studies of schizophrenia to date have been carried out on samples continuously exposed to antipsychotic drugs, it is difficult to tease out the contribution of medication effects to the findings of progressive brain abnormalities often detected in association with the disorder.

In several longitudinal MRI studies reporting progressive brain volume changes in first-episode psychosis, no significant correlations were found between the cumulative antipsychotic exposure and global or regional gray matter volumes (Wood et al., 2001; Ho et al., 2003; Kasai et al., 2003a, b; DeLisi et al., 2004; Nakamura et al., 2007). Such negative findings have been taken as indicative that the progression of brain volume deficits over time in schizophrenia subjects is not confounded by the effects of continued antipsychotic exposure. In other studies, however, cumulative antipsychotic exposure has been directly correlated with global gray matter reductions (Cahn et al., 2002) as well as with frontal and temporal lobe volumes decrements after 30 months of follow-up (Gur et al., 1998, Théberge et al., 2007).

Many MRI studies have indicated that, after short-term use, antipsychotic drugs induce evident changes in brain morphology, which may differ depending on whether typical or atypical agents are used. The use of typical antipsychotics has consistently been reported to cause volume increases in the caudate nucleus (Chakos et al., 1994; Keshavan et al., 1994; Wright et al., 2000; Lieberman et al., 2005; van Haren et al., 2007), while volume decrements in the basal ganglia (Chakos et al., 1995; Westmoreland Corson et al., 1999; Scheepers et al., 2001) and the thalamus (Wood et al., 2001; Khorram et al., 2006) have been reported in patients who shift from typical to atypical antipsychotic treatment. In a recent population-based study of first-episode psychosis, Dazzan et al. (2005) compared three groups of subjects (drug-free, and patients on typical or atypical antipsychotic treatment) and showed that both typical and atypical antipsychotics are associated with brain changes: typical antipsychotics were found to affect more extensively the basal ganglia (leading to enlargement of the putamen) and cortical areas (reducing the volumes of the lobulus paracentralis, anterior cingulate gyrus, superior and medial frontal gyri, superior and middle temporal gyri, insula, and precuneus), whereas atypical agents were particularly associated with enlargement of the thalamus (after a mean duration of antipsychotic exposure of nearly 2 months).

Given the above evidence, it cannot be ruled out that the continued use of antipsychotic agents could modify the trajectory of brain structural volumes in psychosis over time and thus confound the results of longitudinal MRI studies of psychosis. Also, because there are different rates of exposure to typical versus atypical antipsychotics across such longitudinal MRI studies, it is possible that the lack of overall agreement across separate investigations could be explained, at least partially, by different patterns of brain changes induced by typical or atypical antipsychotics (Lieberman et al., 2005; van Haren et al., 2007, 2008b; Thompson et al., 2009). Such differences may be related to the distinct pharmacological profiles of typical and atypical antipsychotics, consequently with different functional and neurochemical effects on the brain (Davis et al., 2005; Théberge et al., 2007; Schlagenhauf et al., 2008).

Some authors have suggested that antipsychotic drugs could have protective brain effects, thus halting further progression of neuropathological processes over the course of schizophrenia (DeLisi et al., 1997; Lieberman et al., 2001; Chakos et al., 2005). In recent prospective morphometric MRI studies, trends have emerged indicating that atypical, but not typical, drugs could exert such protective effects. In a 5-year follow-up MRI study of a mixed group of both first-episode and chronic schizophrenia individuals, van Haren et al. (2007, 2008b) investigated a significant proportion of patients who were shifted from typical to atypical antipsychotic over the course of the study. These authors found that a higher cumulative dose of clozapine and olanzapine during the inter-scanning interval was related to lesser volume decreases in superior frontal gray matter (a region in which the progression of gray matter density loss was directly related to the number of repeated psychotic episodes). They argued that such effects could be related either to protective neuronal effects of clozapine–olanzapine or to a release from the deleterious effects of typical antipsychotics. In one other longitudinal MRI study in which a large sample of first-episode psychosis individuals were randomly allocated to receive haloperidol or olanzapine, Lieberman et al. (2005) found that haloperidol-treated patients exhibited significant decreases in gray matter volume, mainly affecting the frontal lobe, whereas olanzapine-treated patients did not, after up to 26 months of follow-up. Interestingly, most of the gray matter decline in the haloperidol-treated group appeared to occur during the first 12 weeks of treatment. More recently, Thompson et al. (2009) prospectively followed up a group of 36 first-episode schizophrenia patients who were randomized to receive haloperidol ($n=15$) or olanzapine treatment ($n=21$) and whose brain abnormalities were mapped progressively with MRI at baseline, and after 3, 6, and 12 months. Using a DBM-based approach, the authors found that haloperidol-treated (but not olanzapine-treated) patients displayed a rapidly advancing parietal-to-frontal trajectory of cortical decreases, similar to the pattern of changes that characterize the normal cortical maturation in adulthood, but greatly intensified. In the haloperidol-treated group after 12 months, this pattern of cortical loss advanced in the frontal cortex even after symptom remission (Thompson et al., 2009).

On the other hand, findings from other research groups have failed to support the hypothesis of protective effects of atypical antipsychotic agents on brain morphology in schizophrenia subjects. In one recent study (Crespo-Facorro et al., 2008), patients with first-episode non-affective psychosis were assigned to receive low-dose haloperidol ($n=18$), risperidone ($n=16$), or olanzapine ($n=18$) treatment and were prospectively followed up with MRI scanning for 1 year, together with 25 healthy controls. After 1 year, brain volume effects were similar across the groups studied, suggesting no differences in the brain structural effects of the three antipsychotic agents. Only patients treated with risperidone showed a significant increase in lateral ventricles over time, while those exposed to either of the atypical drugs (olanzapine or risperidone) exhibited a significant decrease in caudate nucleus volume after 1 year. In a 3-year follow-up study, Molina et al. (2007) showed that olanzapine use was associated with frontal and parietal gray matter reductions in schizophrenia patients. Findings of an absence of brain protective effects of atypical antipsychotics are consistent with recent animal studies, which have revealed that the use of either typical and atypical antipsychotics may produce time-dependent alterations in neurotrophin receptors in rats (Terry et al., 2007a, b) and may be associated with smaller gray matter volume and lower glial cell number in the brains of monkeys (Konopaske et al., 2007, 2008).

Finally, Saijo et al. (2001), in a prospective study evaluating chronically ill patients with a 10-year interval between MRI scans, found no significant correlation between ventricular enlargement and daily dosage of antipsychotic medication. Other longitudinal MRI studies in which chronic schizophrenia subjects were shifted from typical to atypical antipsychotic treatment have failed to find significant differences in the volume of hippocampus (Panenka et al., 2007), caudate nucleus, frontal and temporal gray matter, global white matter, and cerebral ventricles (McClure et al., 2008). These results suggest that schizophrenia patients in a chronic phase of their illness would be less vulnerable to antipsychotic effects on brain morphology.

Taken together, the above studies do not yet allow us to draw any definitive conclusions about the effects of antipsychotic medication on brain morphology in schizophrenia subjects over the course of illness. All of the MRI studies mentioned above were conducted in samples of patients with psychotic disorders, which are associated with complex brain abnormalities per se. The most consistent findings suggest that the potential of antipsychotic agents in influencing brain morphology is greater at the earlier phases of schizophrenia, when positive symptoms and the most prominent changes in cerebral tissue density associated with the course of psychosis are also thought to occur. Also, other classes of drugs that are often used in the clinical management of psychotic disorders, such as mood stabilizers, have also been suggested to produce brain changes (Nakamura et al., 2007), and few studies of psychotic disorders have weighted the effects of these medications in their results.

Our own longitudinal MRI study of first-episode psychosis, conducted in Brazil, investigated schizophrenia patients in a setting in which treatment strategies may differ substantially from those observed in the high-income countries-dominated literature (Schaufelberger et al., in revision). The evaluation of treatment was naturalistic, with patients looking for treatment in the available care facilities in the community and they did not take part in any standard treatment protocol. Rates of adherence to treatment varied, and a proportion of our schizophrenia subjects remained predominantly untreated over the 15 months of follow-up: from the 39 patients diagnosed with first-episode schizophrenia or schizophreniform disorder, 25 patients were on drug treatment at follow-up MRI scanning (13 with typicals, 11 with atypicals, and 1 with both), while 14 had not been exposed to treatment or had their medication interrupted during the follow-up period. When progression of brain volume changes were compared between the medicated and predominantly unmedicated schizophrenia subgroups, we found that continuous antipsychotic exposure was associated with greater increases in lateral ventricle volumes over time. This suggests that antipsychotic exposure may have influenced the progression of lateral ventricle enlargement in medicated patients. However, it should be noted that there was also a direct association between lack of treatment and illness remission in our study, and it is possible that the ventricle size distinctions between these subgroups would have been influenced by differences in illness outcome, rather than solely reflecting direct effects of medication.

Novel Approaches: Association Between Gene Polymorphisms and Brain Structural Abnormalities in Schizophrenia

It is unfortunate that, for a long period of time, the fields of neuroimaging and molecular genetic research into schizophrenia remained relatively isolated from each other. This panorama has been changing rapidly in recent years, and a number of genomic neuroimaging studies investigating the association between allelic variations and brain morphometric indices, as assessed with MRI, are providing exciting data that may further inform etiological theories for schizophrenia (see Meyer Lindenberg, this volume). Specifically, neurodevelopmental hypotheses for schizophrenia gain support if associations are detected between brain abnormalities in key brain regions and polymorphisms of genes known to be implicated in early stages of brain development.

A series of recent studies of this kind have been conducted investigating the association between brain volume deficits and polymorphisms of the gene encoding BDNF (Szeszko et al., 2005; Agartz et al., 2006; Varnäs et al., 2008). This trophic protein has a relevant role in modulating neuroplasticity in mature neurons, but it is also known to be critical to developmental processes during embryonic life. In the largest of these MRI studies, Ho et al. (2006) found, in a cohort of 293 schizophrenia-spectrum disorder subjects, that carriers of the BDNF prodomain single nucleotide polymorphism resulting in a valine (Val)-to-methionine (Met) substitution presented with lower volumes of the occipital, temporal, and parietal lobe gray matter (Ho et al., 2006). More recently, Varnäs et al. (2008) described associations between prefrontal cortical volumes and various BDNF gene polymorphisms both in healthy volunteers and in schizophrenia patients, with greater statistical significance in the latter subjects (Varnäs et al., 2008). In addition to these cross-sectional MRI studies, there has been evidence that Met allele-carrying first-episode schizophrenia patients display greater progression of gray matter deficits in the prefrontal cortex and ventricle enlargement than Val homozygous patients over the three initial years of disease course; these findings suggest that progressive brain volume deficits in schizophrenia may be related to altered neuroplastic effects of BDNF in adult life (Ho et al., 2007).

There is a wide range of polymorphisms of other genes implicated in brain development that deserve testing for associations with structural brain changes in schizophrenia (see Dias-Neto et al., this volume). In a recent cross-sectional study carried out in Sao Paulo, Brazil, Gregório et al. (2009) investigated the relationship between MRI-based structural brain indices and 32 polymorphisms located in 30 genes related to neurogenesis and brain development in 25 patients with schizophrenia, with correction for multiple comparisons. Ventricle enlargement was associated with an allelic variation of the gene that encodes reelin, a protease that guides neuronal migration during embryonic life, while a polymorphism of the gene that encodes protocadherin 12, relevant to axonal guidance and synaptic specificity, was associated with reduced cortical folding in the schizophrenia group (Gregório et al., 2009). Several additional reports are rapidly appearing in the literature describing associations between structural brain changes and variations of neurodevelopment-related genes in schizophrenia samples, such as neuregulin-1 gene variants and reduced hipocampal volumes (Gruber et al., 2009) or enlarged ventricles (Mata et al., 2009); and AKT1 gene variants and abnormal prefrontal volumes (Tan et al., 2009), among others.

Concluding Remarks

In synthesis, the bulk of findings from the studies reviewed in this chapter indicate that the dichotomy of neurodevelopmental against neurodegenerative hypotheses for schizophrenia is oversimplistic. Instead, the combined evidence from recent postmortem neuropathological and in vivo neuroimaging studies support an integrative model for schizophrenia. According to such view, superimposed to brain abnormalities originated in early neurodevelopmental stages, deviations in the dynamic processes of brain changes across the span of adult life may occur, either during the transition to psychosis or after the onset of full-blown schizophrenia. Within this framework, schizophrenia should be seen as a dynamic, but not a neurodegenerative, brain disease, exhibiting a combination of early neurodevelopment abnormalities and late brain changes, related to maturational abnormalities during adulthood and/or other processes (DeLisi, 1997; Waddington et al., 1998; Woods, 1998; Keshavan, 1999; Tsuang et al., 2001; van Haren et al., 2008b).

Specifically with regard to the in vivo structural MRI literature to date, the variability of results is not surprising given the complex and heterogeneous clinical features of schizophrenia, and the interpretation of these findings stands as a considerable challenge. The MRI studies reviewed herein confirm the view that, at least in some forms of schizophrenia, there are remote brain abnormalities that are most probably of neurodevelopmental origin. Some of these changes have been found to progress over time, either during the transition from prodromal to full-blown psychotic stages or over the course of the illness after the first psychotic break (particularly in cases of worse prognosis). However, it remains possible that progressive patterns of brain tissue loss and increases in lateral ventricles may not be universally present in all forms of schizophrenia-related disorders. In more benign forms of schizophrenia-spectrum disorders, brain abnormalities in the same key brain structures affected in more severe schizophrenia cases might be state dependent, reversing after symptom remission.

In consistency with the findings of postmortem studies, the in vivo brain structural deficits associated with schizophrenia have been interpreted as reflecting neurochemical/neuropil abnormalities and/or changes in maturational brain processes, rather than neuronal degeneration. Stress-related reductions in dendritic spines, via the effects of corticotrophin-releasing hormone, have also been implicated in the pathology of schizophrenia and could influence the dynamic brain structural changes seen at the illness onset and during psychotic relapses. Other factors possibly related to late brain structural changes in schizophrenia include disease-related reductions in neurotrophic factor signaling, mitochondrial dysfunction, and decreased anti-apoptotic signaling. However, it is important to bear in mind that the use of antipsychotic medication remains a very important confounding factor when interpreting the results of the longitudinal MRI studies of schizophrenia that have found decreases in gray matter and increases in ventricular volume over time.

Finally, investigations of genes with important roles in brain development and maturation, as well as in synapse plasticity and functioning (e.g., reelin, neuregulin, dysbindin, BDNF, and myelin and oligodendrocyte-related genes), have also given support to hypotheses of a relationship between early and late neurodevelopmental abnormalities in schizophrenia leading to a misconnection of multiple brain areas (Davis et al. 2003, Harrison and Weinberger, 2005; Buckley et al. 2007, Konrad and Winterer, 2008). As reviewed in this chapter, associations between some of these gene variations and brain structural abnormalities in schizophrenia, as assessed with MRI, have recently emerged in the literature. Further studies of schizophrenia samples evaluating associations between neurodevelopment-related gene variants and patterns of progression of brain abnormalities as assessed in longitudinal MRI studies are eagerly awaited.

References

Addington, J., Chaves, A. & Addington, D. Diagnostic stability over one year in first-episode psychosis. Schizophrenia Research 86(1–3): 71–75, 2006.
Agartz, I., Sedvall, G.C., Terenius, L., Kulle, B., Frigessi, A., Hall, H. & Jönsson, E.G. BDNF gene variants and brain morphology in schizophrenia. American Journal of Medical Genetics Part B (Neuropsychiatric Genetics) 141B(5): 513–523, 2006.

Allen, L.S. & Gorski, R.A. Sexual dimorphism of the anterior commissure and massa intermedia of the human brain. Journal of Comparative Neurology 312(1): 97–104, 1991.

Arnold, S.E. & Rioux, L. Challenges, status, and opportunities for studying developmental neuropathology in adult schizophrenia. Schizophrenia Bulletin 27(3): 395–416, 2001.

Arnold, S.E., Trojanowski, J.Q., Gur, R.E., Blackwell, P., Han, L.Y, Choi, C. Absence of neurodegeneration and neural injury in the cerebral cortex in a sample of elderly patients with schizophrenia. Archives of General Psychiatry 55(3): 225–232, 1998.

Bachmann, S., Bottmer, C., Pantel, J., Schröder, J., Amann, M., Essig, M. & Schad, L.R. MRI-morphometric changes in first-episode schizophrenic patients at 14 months follow-up. Schizophrenia Research 67(2–3): 301–303, 2004.

Bartzokis, G. Schizophrenia: Breakdown in the well regulated lifelong process of brain development and maturation. Neuropsychopharmacology 27(4): 672–683, 2002.

Bogerts, B. The neuropathology of schizophrenic diseases: historical aspects and present knowledge. European Archives of Psychiatry and Clinical Neuroscience 249 (Suppl 4): 2–13, 1999.

Borgwardt, S.J., McGuire, P.K., Aston, J., Gscwandtener, U., Pflüger, M., Stielitz, R., Radue, E., Riecher-Rössler, A. Reductions of the frontal, temporal and parietal volume associated with the onset of psychosis. Schizophrenia Research 106: 108–114, 2008.

Borgwardt, S.J., Riecher-Rössler A., Dazzan, P., Chitnis, X., Aston, J. Drewe, M., Gschwandtner, U., Haller, S., Pflüger, M., Rechsteiner, E., DSouza, M., Sieglitz, R.D., Radü, E.W., McGuire P.K., Regional gray matter volume abnormalities in the at risk mental state. Biological Psychiatry 61(10): 1148–1156, 2007.

Brisch, R., Bernstein, H.G., Krell, D., Stauch, R., Trübner, K., Dobrowolny, H., Kropf, S., Bielau, H., Bogerts, B. Volumetric analysis of septal region in schizophrenia and affective disorder. European Archives of Psychiatry and Clinical Neuroscience 257(3): 140–148, 2007.

Buckley, P.F., Mahadik, S., Pillai, A., Terry, A. Neurotrophins and schizophrenia. Schizophrenia Research 94(1–3): 1–11, 2007.

Bustillo, J.R., Lauriello, J., Rowland, L.M., Thomson, L.M., Petropoulos, H., Hammond, R., Hart, B. & Brooks, W.M. Longitudinal follow-up of neurochemical changes during the first year of antipsychotic treatment in schizophrenia patients with minimal previous medication exposure. Schizophrenia Research 58(2–3): 313–321, 2002.

Cahn, W., Hulshoff Pol, H.E., Bongers, M., Schnack, H.G., Mandl, R.C., Van Haren, N.E., Durston, S., Koning, H., Van Der Linden, J.A. & Kahn, R.S. Brain morphology in antipsychotic-naïve schizophrenia: a study of multiple brain structures. British Journal of Psychiatry 43(Suppl): s66–s72, 2002.

Cahn, W., Hulshoff Pol, H.E., Lems, E.B., Van Haren, N.E., Schnack, H.G., Van Der Linden, J.A., Schothorst, P.F., Van Engeland, H. & Kahn, R.S. Brain volume changes in first-episode schizophrenia: a 1-year follow-up study. Archives of General Psychiatry 59(11): 1002–1010, 2002.

Carpenter, M.B. & Sutin, J. Human Neuroanatomy (8th ed.). Williams & Wilkins, Baltimore, pp. 52–54, 1983.

Chakos, M.H., Lieberman, J.A., Alvir, J., Bilder, R. & Ashtari, M. Caudate nuclei volumes in schizophrenic patients treated with typical antipsychotics or clozapine. Lancet 345(8947): 456–457, 1995.

Chakos, M.H., Lieberman, J.A., Bilder, R.M., Borenstein, M., Lerner, G., Bogerts, B., Wu, H., Kinon, B. & Ashtari, M. Increase in caudate nuclei volumes of first-episode schizophrenic patients taking antipsychotic drugs. American Journal of Psychiatry 151(10): 1430–1436, 1994.

Chakos, M.H., Schobel, S.A., Gu, H., Gerig, G., Bradford, D., Charles, C. & Lieberman, J.A. Duration of illness and treatment effects on hippocampal volume in male patients with schizophrenia. British Journal of Psychiatry 186: 26–31, 2005.

Chen, Y., Dubé, C.M., Rice, C.J., Baram, T.Z. Rapid loss of dendritic spines after stress involves derangement of spine dynamics by corticotropin-releasing hormone. Journal of Neuroscience 28(11): 2903–2911, 2008.

Cheung, V., Cheung, C., McAlonan, G.M., Deng, Y., Wong, J.G., Yip, L., Tai, K.S., Khong, P.L., Sham, P. & Chua, S.E. A diffusion tensor imaging study of structural dysconnectivity in never-medicated, first-episode schizophrenia. Psychological Medicine 38(6): 877–885, 2008.

Crespo-Facorro, B., Roiz-Santiáñez, R., Pérez-Iglesias, R., Pelayo-Terán, J.M., Rodríguez-Sánchez, J.M., Tordesillas-Gutiérrez, D., Ramírez, M., Martínez, O., Gutiérrez, A., De Lucas, E.M. & Vázquez-Barquero, J.L. Effect of antipsychotic drugs on brain morphometry. A randomized controlled one-year follow-up study of haloperidol, risperidone and olanzapine. Progress in Neuropsychopharmacology & Biological Psychiatry 32(8): 1936–1943, 2008.

Davis, C.E., Jeste, D.V. & Eyler, L.T. Review of longitudinal functional neuroimaging studies of drug treatments in patients with schizophrenia. Schizophrenia Research 78(1): 45–60, 2005.

Davis, K.L., Stewart, D.G., Friedman, J.I., Buchsbaum, M., Harvey, P.D., Hof, P.R., Buxbaum, J., Haroutunian, V. White matter changes in schizophrenia: evidence for myelin-related dysfunction. Archives of General Psychiatry 60(5): 443–456, 2003.

Dazzan, P., Morgan, K.D., Orr, K., Hutchinson, G., Chitnis, X., Suckling, J., Fearon, P., McGuire, P.K., Mallett, R.M., Jones, P.B., Leff, J. & Murray, R.M. Different effects of typical and atypical antipsychotics on grey matter in first episode psychosis: the AESOP study. Neuropsychopharmacology 30: 765–774, 2005.

De Souza Crippa, J.A., Zuardi, A.W., Busatto, G.F., Sanches, R.F., Santos, A.C., Araújo, D., Amaro, E., Hallak, J.E., Ng, V. & McGuire, P.K. Cavum septum pellucidum and adhesio interthalamica in schizophrenia: an MRI study. European Psychiatry 21(5): 291–299, 2006.

DeLisi, LE. Is schizophrenia a lifetime disorder of brain plasticity, growth and aging? Schizophrenia Research 23(2): 119–129, 1997.

DeLisi, L.E. The concept of progressive brain change in schizophrenia: implications for understanding schizophrenia. Schizophrenia Bulletin 34(2): 312–321, 2008.

DeLisi, L.E. & Hoff, A.L. Failure to find progressive temporal lobe volume decreases 10 years subsequent to a first episode of schizophrenia. Psychiatry Research 138(3): 265–268, 2005.

DeLisi, L.E., Hoff, A.L., Kushner, M. & Degreef, G. Increased prevalence of cavum septum pellucidum in schizophrenia. Psychiatry Research 50(3): 193–199, 1993.

DeLisi, L.E., Sakuma, M., Maurizio, A.M., Relja, M. & Hoff, A.L. Cerebral ventricular change over the first 10 years after the onset of schizophrenia. Psychiatry Research 130(1): 57–70, 2004.

DeLisi, L.E., Sakuma, M., Tew, W., Kushner, M., Hoff, A.L. & Grimson, R. Schizophrenia as a chronic active brain process: a study of progressive brain structural change subsequent to the onset of schizophrenia. Psychiatry Research 74(3): 129–140, 1997.

Dickey, C.C., McCarley, R.W., Xu, M.L., Seidman, L.J., Voglmaier, M.M., Niznikiewicz, M.A., Connor, E. & Shenton, M.E. MRI abnormalities of the hippocampus and cavum septi pellucidi in females with schizotypal personality disorder. Schizophrenia Research 89(1–3): 49–58, 2007.

Dickey, C.C., Salisbury, D.F., Nagy, A.I., Hirayasu, Y., Lee, C.U., McCarley, R.W. & Shenton, M.E. Follow-up MRI study of prefrontal volumes in first-episode psychotic patients. Schizophrenia Research 71(2–3): 349–351, 2004.

Ellison-Wright, I. & Bullmore, E. Meta-analysis of diffusion tensor imaging studies in schizophrenia. Schizophrenia Research 108(1–3): 3–10, 2009.

Ellison-Wright, I., Glahn, D.C., Laird, A.R., Thelen, S.M. & Bullmore, E. The anatomy of first-episode and chronic schizophrenia: an anatomical likelihood estimation meta-analysis. American Journal of Psychiatry 165: 1015–1023, 2008.

Ettinger, U., Picchioni, M., Landau, S., Matsumoto, K., Van Haren, N.E., Marshall, N., Hall, M.H., Schulze, K., Toulopoulou, T., Davies, N., Ribchester, T., McGuire, P.K. & Murray, R.M. Magnetic resonance imaging of the thalamus and adhesio interthalamica in twins with schizophrenia. Archives of General Psychiatry 64(4): 401–409, 2007.

Filipović, B., Kovacević, S., Stojicić, M., Prostran, M. & Filipović, B. Morphological differences among cavum septi pellucidi obtained in patients with schizophrenia and healthy individuals: forensic implications. A post-mortem study. Psychiatry and Clinical Neurosciences 59(1): 106–108, 2005.

Flashman, L.A., Roth, R.M., Pixley, H.S., Cleavinger, H.B., Mcallister, T.W., Vidaver, R. & Saykin, A.J. Cavum septum pellucidum in schizophrenia: clinical and neuropsychological correlates. Psychiatry Research 154(2): 147–155, 2007.

Friedman, J.I., Tang, C., Carpenter, D., Buchsbaum, M., Schmeider, J., Flanagan, L., Golembo, S., Kanellopoulo, I., Ng, J., Hof, P.R., Harvey, P.D., Tsopelas, N.D., Stewart, D., Davis, K.L. Diffusion tensor imaging findings in first-episode and chronic schizophrenia patients. American Journal of Psychiatry 165(8): 1024–1032, 2008.

Fukuzako, H. & Kodama, S. Cavum septum pellucidum in schizophrenia. Biological Psychiatry 43(6): 467, 1998.

Galarza, M., Merlo, A.B., Ingratta, A., Albanese, E.F. & Albanese, A.M. Cavum septum pellucidum and its increased prevalence in schizophrenia: a neuroembryological classification. Journal of Neuropsychiatry and Clinical Neurosciences 16(1): 41–46, 2004.

Glantz, L.A, Gilmore, J.H., Lieberman, J.A. & Jarskoq, L.F. Apoptotic mechanisms and the synaptic pathology of schizophrenia. Schizophrenia Research 81(1): 47–63, 2006.

Good, C.D., Johnsrude, I.S., Ashburner, J., Henson, R.N., Friston, K.J. & Frackowiak, R.S. A voxel-based morphometric study of ageing in 465 normal adult human brains. Neuroimage 14: 21–36, 2001.

Gregório, S.P., Sallet, P.C., Do, K.A., Lin, E., Gattaz, W.F. & Dias-Neto, E. Polymorphisms in genes involved in neurodevelopment may be associated with altered brain morphology in schizophrenia: preliminary evidence. Psychiatry Research 165(1–2): 1–9, 2009.

Gruber, O., Falkai, P., Schneider-Axmann, T., Schwab, S.G., Wagner, M. & Maier, W. Neuregulin-1 haplotype HAP(ICE) is associated with lower hippocampal volumes in schizophrenic patients and in non-affected family members. Journal of Psychiatric Research 43(1): 1–6, 2008.

Gur, R.E., Cowell, P., Turetsky, B.I., Gallacher, F., Cannon, T., Bilker, W. & Gur R.C. A follow-up magnetic resonance imaging study of schizophrenia. Relationship of neuroanatomical changes to clinical and neurobehavioral measures. Archives of General Psychiatry 55(2): 145–152, 1998.

Gur, R.E., Keshavan, M.S. & Lawrie, S.M. Deconstructing psychosis with human brain imaging. Schizophrenia Bulletin 33: 921–931, 2007.

Haahr, U., Friis, S., Larsen, T.K., Melle, I., Johannessen, J.O., Opjordsmoen, S., Simonsen, E., Rund, B.R., Vaglum, P. & Mcglashan, T. First-episode psychosis: diagnostic stability over one and two years. Psychopathology 41(5): 322–329, 2008.

Hagino, H., Suzuki, M., Kurokawa, K., Mori, K., Nohara, S., Takahashi, T., Yamashita, I., Yotsutsuji, T., Kurachi, M. & Seto, H. Magnetic resonance imaging study of the cavum septi pellucidi in patients with schizophrenia. American Journal of Psychiatry 158(10): 1717–1719, 2001.

Harris, J.M., Moorhead, T.W., Miller, P., Mcintosh, A.M., Bonnici, H.M., Owens, D.G., Johnstone, E.C. & Lawrie, S.M. Increased prefrontal gyrification in a large high-risk cohort characterizes those who develop schizophrenia and reflects abnormal prefrontal development. Biological Psychiatry 62(7): 722–729, 2007.

Harrison, P.J. The neuropathology of schizophrenia. A critical review of the data and their interpretation. Brain 122(4): 593–624, 1999.

Harrison, P.J. The hippocampus in schizophrenia: a review of the neuropathological evidence and its pathophysiological implications. Psychopharmacology (Berl) 174(1): 151–162, 2004.

Harrison, P.J. & Weinberger, D.R. Schizophrenia genes, gene expression and neuropathology: on the matter of their convergence. Molecular Psychiatry 10(1): 40–68, 2005.

Ho, B.C., Andreasen, N.C., Dawson, J.D. & Wassink, T.H. Association between brain-derived neurotrophic factor Val66Met gene polymorphism and progressive brain volume changes in schizophrenia. American Journal of Psychiatry 164(12): 1890–1899, 2007.

Ho, B.C., Andreasen, N.C., Nopoulos, P., Arndt, S., Magnotta, V. & Flaum, M. Progressive structural brain abnormalities and their relationship to clinical outcome: a longitudinal magnetic resonance imaging study early in schizophrenia. Archives of General Psychiatry 60(6): 585–594, 2003.

Ho, B.C., Milev, P., O'leary, D.S., Librant, A., Andreasen, N.C. & Wassink, T.H. Cognitive and magnetic resonance imaging brain morphometric correlates of brain derived neurotrophic factor Val66Met gene polymorphism in patients with schizophrenia and healthy volunteers. Archives of General Psychiatry 63(7): 731–740, 2006.

Honea, R., Crow, T.J., Passingham, D. & Mackay, C.E. Regional deficits in brain volume in schizophrenia: a meta-analysis of voxel-based morphometry studies. American Journal of Psychiatry 162(12): 2233–2245, 2005.

Hopper, K. & Wanderling, J. Revisiting the developed versus developing country distinction in course and outcome in schizophrenia: results from ISoS, the WHO collaborative followup project. International Study of Schizophrenia. Schizophrenia Bulletin 26(4): 835–846, 2000.

Hulshoff Pol, H.E. & Kahn, R.S. What happens after the first episode? A review of progressive brain changes in chronically ill patients with schizophrenia. Schizophrenia Bulletin 34(2): 354–366, 2008.

Jessen, F., Scherk, H., Träber, F., Theyson, S., Berning, J., Tepest, R., Falkai, P., Schild, H.H., Maier, W., Wagner, M. & Block, W. Proton magnetic resonance spectroscopy in subjects at risk for schizophrenia. Schizophrenia Research 87(1–3): 81–88, 2006.

Job, D.E., Whalley, H.C., Johnstone, E.C. & Lawrie, S.M. Grey matter changes over time in high risk subjects developing schizophrenia. NeuroImage 25: 1023–1030, 2005.

Job, D.E., Whallety, H.C., McConnell, S., Glabus, M. Johnstone, E.C. & Lawrie, S.M. Structural gray matter differences between first-episode schizophrenics and normal controls using voxel-based morphometry. NeuroImage 17(2): 880–889, 2002.

Job, D.E., Whalley, H.C., McConnell, S., Glabus, M., Johnstone, E.C. & Lawrie, S.M. Voxel-based morphometry of grey matter densities in subjects at high risk of schizophrenia. Schizophrenia Research 64(1): 1–13, 2003.

Jones, D.K. Studying connections in the living human brain with diffusion MRI. Cortex 44: 936–952, 2008.

Kasai, K., Iwanami, A., Yamasue, H., Kuroki, N., Nakagome, K. & Fukuda, M. Neuroanatomy and neurophysiology in schizophrenia. Neuroscience Research 43(2): 93–110, 2002.

Kasai, K., McCarley, R.W., Salisbury, D.F., et al. Cavum septi pellucidi in first-episode schizophrenia and first-episode affective psychosis: an MRI study. Schizophrenia Research 71(1): 65–76, 2004.

Kasai, K., Shenton, M.E., Salisbury, D.F., Hirayasu, Y., Lee, C.U., Ciszewski, A.A., Yurgelun-Todd, D., Kikinis, R., Jolesz, F.A. & McCarley, R.W. Progressive decrease of left superior temporal gyrus gray matter volume in patients with first-episode schizophrenia. American Journal of Psychiatry 160(1): 156–164, 2003b.

Kasai, K., Shenton, M.E., Salisbury, D.F., Hirayasu, Y., Onitsuka, T., Spencer, M.H., Yurgelun-Todd, D.A., Kikinis, R., Jolesz, F.A. & McCarley, R.W. Progressive decrease of left Heschl gyrus and planum temporale gray matter volume in first-episode schizophrenia: a longitudinal magnetic resonance imaging study. Archives of General Psychiatry 60(8): 766–775, 2003a.

Keshavan, M.S. Development, disease and degeneration in schizophrenia: a unitary pathophysiological model. Journal of Psychiatry Research 33(6): 513–521, 1999.

Keshavan, M.S., Anderson, S. & Pettegrew, J.W. Is schizophrenia due to excessive synaptic pruning in the prefrontal cortex? The Feinberg hypothesis revisited. Journal of Psychiatry Research 28(3): 239–265, 1994.

Keshavan, M.S., Bagwell, W.W., Haas, G.L., Sweeney, J.A., Schooler, N.R. & Pettegrew, J.W. Changes in caudate volume with neuroleptic treatment. Lancet 344(8934): 1434, 1994.

Keshavan, M.S., Haas, G.L., Kahn, C.E., Aguilar, E., Dick, E.L., Schooler, N.R., Sweeney, J.A. & Pettegrew, J.W. Superior temporal gyrus and the course of early schizophrenia: progressive, static, or reversible? Journal of Psychiatry Research 32(3–4): 161–167, 1998.

Keshavan, M.S., Stanley, J.A. & Pettegrew, J.W. Magnetic resonance spectroscopy in schizophrenia: methodological issues and findings – part II. Biological Psychiatry 48(5): 369–380, 2000.

Khorram, B., Lang, D.J., Kopala, L.C., Vandorpe, R.A., Rui, Q., Goghari, V.M., Smith, G.N. & Honer, W.G. Reduced thalamic volume in patients with chronic schizophrenia after switching from typical antipsychotic medications to olanzapine. American Journal of Psychiatry 163(11): 2005–2007, 2006.

Konopaske, G.T., Dorph-Petersen, K.A., Pierri, J.N., Wu, Q., Sampson, A.R. & Lewis, D.A. Effect of chronic exposure to antipsychotic medication on cell numbers in the parietal cortex of macaque monkeys. Neuropsychopharmacology 32(6): 1216–1223, 2007.

Konopaske, G.T., Dorph-Petersen, K.A., Sweet, R.A., Pierri, J.N., Zhang, W., Sampson, A.R. & Lewis, D.A. Effect of chronic antipsychotic exposure on astrocyte and oligodendrocyte numbers in macaque monkeys. Biological Psychiatry 63(8): 759–765, 2008.

Konrad, A. & Winterer, G. Disturbed structural connectivity in schizophrenia – primary factor in pathology or epiphenomenon? Schizophrenia Bulletin 34(1): 72–92, 2008.

Koo, M.S., Levitt, J.J., Salisbury, D.F., Nakamura, M., Shenton, M.E. & McCarley, R.W. A cross-sectional and longitudinal magnetic resonance imaging study of cingulated gyrus gray matter volume abnormalities in first-episode schizophrenia and first-episode affective psychosis. Archives of General Psychiatry 65(7): 746–760, 2008.

Kuhnley, E.J., White, D.H. & Granoff, A.L. Psychiatric presentation of an arachnoid cyst. Journal of Clinical Psychiatry 42(4): 167–168, 1981.

Kwon, J.S., Shenton, M.E., Hirayasu, Y., Salisbury, D.F., Fischer, I.A., Dickey, C.C., Yurgelun-Todd, D., Tohen, M., Kikinis, R., Jolesz, F.A. & McCarley, R.W. MRI study of cavum septi pellucidi in schizophrenia, affective disorder, and schizotypal personality disorder. American Journal of Psychiatry 155(4): 509–515, 1998.

Kyriakopoulos, M., Bargiotas, T., Barker, G.J. & Frangou, S. Diffusion tensor imaging in schizophrenia. European Psychiatry 23(4): 255–273, 2008.

Lawrie, S.M., Mcintosh, A.M., Hall, J., Owens, D.G. & Johnstone, E.C. Brain structure and function changes during the development of schizophrenia: the evidence from studies of subjects at increased genetic risk. Schizophrenia Bulletin 34(2): 330–340, 2008.

Lawrie, S.M., Whalley, H.C., Abukmeil, S.S., Kestelman, J.N., Donnelly, L., Miller, P., Best, J.J., Owens, D.G. & Johnstone, E.C. Brain structure, genetic liability, and psychotic symptoms in subjects at high risk of developing schizophrenia. Biological Psychiatry 49(10): 811–823, 2001.

Lee, W., Bindman, J., Ford, T., Glozier, N., Moran, P., Stewart, R. & Hotopf, M. Bias in psychiatric case–control studies: literature survey. British Journal of Psychiatry 190: 204–209, 2007.

Lencz T., Cornblatt, B. & Bilder, R.M. Neurodevelopmental models of schizophrenia: pathophysiologic synthesis and directions for intervention research. Psychopharmacology Bulletin 35(1): 95–125, 2001.

Lewis, D.A. Development of the prefrontal cortex during adolescence: insights into vulnerable neural circuits in schizophrenia. Neuropsychopharmacology 16(6): 385–398, 1997.

Lewis, S.W., Reveley, M.A., David, A.S. & Ron, M.A. Agenesis of the corpus callosum and schizophrenia: a case report. Psychological Medicine 18(2): 341–347, 1988.

Lieberman, J., Chakos, M., Wu, H., Alvir, J., Hoffman, E., Robinson, D. & Bilder, R. Longitudinal study of brain morphology in first episode schizophrenia. Biological Psychiatry 49(6): 487–499, 2001.

Lieberman, J.A., Tollefson, G.D., Charles, C., Zipursky, R., Sharma, T., Kahn, R.S., Keefe, R.S., Green, A.I., Gur, R.E., Mcevoy, J., Perkins, D., Hamer, R.M., Gu, H. & Tohen, M.; HGDH Study Group. Antipsychotic drug effects on brain morphology in first-episode psychosis. Archives of General Psychiatry 62(4): 361–370, 2005.

Malobabic, S., Puskas, L. & Blagotic, M. Size and position of the human adhaesio interthalamica. Gegenbaurs Morphologisches Jahrbuch 133(1): 175–180, 1987.

Mata, I., Perez-Iglesias, R., Roiz-Santiañez, R., Tordesillas-Gutierrez, D., Gonzalez-Mandly, A., Vazquez-Barquero, J.L. & Crespo-Facorro, B. A neuregulin 1 variant is associated with increased lateral ventricle volume in patients with first-episode schizophrenia. Biological Psychiatry 65(6): 535–540, 2009.

McClure, R.K., Carew, K., Greeter, S., Maushauer, E., Steen, G. & Weinberger, D.R. Absence of regional brain volume change in schizophrenia associated with short-term atypical antipsychotic treatment. Schizophrenia Research 98(1–3): 29–39, 2008.

Mcintosh, A.M., Maniega, S.M., Lymer, G.K., Mckirdy, J., Hall, J., Sussmann, J.E., Bastin, M.E., Clayden, J.D., Johnstone, E.C. & Lawrie, S.M. White matter tractography in bipolar disorder and schizophrenia. Biological Psychiatry 64(12): 1088–1092, 2008.

Meisenzahl, E.M., Frodl, T., Zetzsche, T., Leinsinger, G., Heiss, D., Maag, K., Hegerl, U., Hahn, K. & Möller, H.J. Adhesio interthalamica in male patients with schizophrenia. American Journal of Psychiatry 157(5): 823–825, 2000.

Meisenzahl, E.M., Frodl, T., Zetzsche, T., Leinsinger, G., Maag, K., Hegerl, U., Hahn, K. & Möller, H.J. Investigation of a possible diencephalic pathology in schizophrenia. Psychiatry Research 115(3): 127–135, 2002.

Molina, V., Reig, S., Sanz, J., Palomo, T., Benito, C., Sánchez, J., Pascau, J. & Desco, M. Changes in cortical volume with olanzapine in chronic schizophrenia. Pharmacopsychiatry 40(4): 135–139, 2007.

Morgan, K.D., Dazzan, P., Orr, K.G., Hutchinson, G., Chitnis, X., Suckling, J., Lythgoe, D., Pollock, S.J., Rossell, S., Shapleske, J., Fearon, P., Morgan, C., David, A., McGuire, P.K., Jones, P.B., Leff, J. & Murray, R.M. Grey matter abnormalities in first-episode schizophrenia and affective psychosis. British Journal of Psychiatry Supplement 51: s111–s116, 2007.

Murray, R.M. & Fearon, P. The developmental "risk factor" model of schizophrenia. Journal of Psychiatry Research 33(6): 497–499, 1999.

Murray, R.M. & Lewis, S.W. Is schizophrenia a neurodevelopmental disorder? British Medical Journal 295(6600): 681–682, 1987.

Nakamura, M., Salisbury, D.F., Hirayasu, Y., Bouix, S., Pohl, K.M., Yoshida, T., Koo, M.S., Shenton, M.E. & McCarley, R.W. Neocortical gray matter volume in first-episode schizophrenia and first-episode affective psychosis: a cross-sectional and longitudinal MRI study. Biological Psychiatry 62(7): 773–783, 2007.

Nopoulos, P., Krie, A. & Andreasen, N.C. Enlarged cavum septi pellucidi in patients with schizophrenia: clinical and cognitive correlates. Journal of Neuropsychiatry and Clinical Neurosciences 12(3): 344–349, 2000.

Nopoulos, P., Swayze, V. & Andreasen, N.C. Pattern of brain morphology in patients with schizophrenia and large cavum septi pellucidi. Journal of Neuropsychiatry and Clinical Neurosciences 8(2): 147–152, 1996.

Nopoulos, P., Swayze, V., Flaum, M., Ehrhardt, J.C., Yuh, W.T. & Andreasen, N.C. Cavum septi pellucidi in normals and patients with schizophrenia as detected by magnetic resonance imaging, Biological Psychiatry 41(11): 1102–1108, 1997.

Nopoulos, P.C., Giedd, J.N., Andreasen, N.C. & Rapoport, J.L. Frequency and severity of enlarged cavum septi pellucidi in childhood-onset schizophrenia. American Journal of Psychiatry 155(8): 1074–1079, 1998.

Nopoulos, P.C., Rideout, D., Crespo-Facorro, B. & Andreasen, N.C. Sex differences in the absence of massa intermedia in patients with schizophrenia versus healthy controls. Schizophrenia Research 48(2–3): 177–185, 2001.

Panenka, W.J., Khorram, B., Barr, A.M., Smith, G.N., Lang, D.J., Kopala, L.C., Vandorpe, R.A. & Honer, W.G. A longitudinal study on the effects of typical versus atypical antipsychotic drugs on hippocampal volume in schizophrenia. Schizophrenia Research 94(1–3): 288–292, 2007.

Pantelis, C., Velakoulis, D., McGorry, P.D., Wood, S.J., Suckling, J., Philips, L.J., Yung, A.R., Bullmore, E.T, Brewer, W., Soulsby, B., Desmond, P. & McGuire, P.K. Neuroanatomical abnormalities before and after onset of psychosis: a cross-sectional and longitudinal MRI comparison. Lancet 361: 281–288, 2003.

Pantelis, C., Yücel, M., Wood, S.J., Velakoulis, D., Sun, D., Berger, G., Stuart, G.W., Yung, A., Phillips, L. & McGorry, P.D. Structural brain imaging evidence for multiple pathological processes at different stages of brain development in schizophrenia. Schizophrenia Bulletin 31(3): 672–696, 2005.

Peters, B.D., de Haan, L., Dekker, N., Blaas, J., Becker, H.E., Dingemans, P.M., Akkerman, E.M., Majoie, C.B., Van Ameslvoort, T., Den Heeten, G.J. & Linzen, D.H. White matter fibertracking in first-episode schizophrenia, schizoaffective patients and subjects at ultra-high risk of psychosis. Neuropsychobiology 58(1): 19–28, 2008.

Price, G., Bagary, M.S., Cercignani, M., Altmann, D.R. & Ron, M.A. The corpus callosum in first episode schizophrenia: a diffusion tensor imaging study. Journal of Neurology, Neurosurgery and Psychiatry 76(4): 585–587, 2005.

Price, G., Cercignani, M., Bagary, M.S., Barnes, T.R., Barker, G.J., Joyce, E.M. & Ron, M.A. A volumetric MRI and magnetization transfer imaging follow-up study of patients with first-episode schizophrenia. Schizophrenia Research 87(1–3): 100–108, 2006.

Price, G., Cercignani, M., Parker, G.J., Altmann, D.R., Barnes, T.R., Barker, G.J., Joyce, E.M. & Ron, M.A. Abnormal brain connectivity in first-episode psychosis: a diffusion MRI tractography study of the corpus callosum. NeuroImage 35(2): 458–466, 2007.

Price, G., Cercignani, M., Parker, G.J., Altmann D.R, Barnes, T.R. Barker, G.J. Joyce, E.M. & Ron, M.A. White matter tracts in first-episode psychosis: a DTI tractography study of the uncinate fasciculus. Neuroimage 39(3): 949–955, 2008.

Puri, B.K., Hutton, S.B., Saeed, N., Oatridge, A., Hajnal, J.V., Duncan, L., Chapman, M.J., Barnes, T.R., Bydder, G.M. & Joyce, E.M. A serial longitudinal quantitative MRI study of cerebral changes in first-episode schizophrenia using image segmentation and subvoxel registration. Psychiatry Research 106(2): 141–150, 2001.

Rajarethinam, R., Miedler, J., DeQuardo, J., Smet, C.I., Brunberg, J., Kirbat, R., Tandon, R. Prevalence of cavum septum pellucidum in schizophrenia studied with MRI. Schizophrenia Research 48(2–3): 201–205, 2001.

Rajarethinam, R., Sohi, J., Arfken, C. & Keshavan, M.S. No difference in the prevalence of cavum septum pellucidum (CSP) between first-episode schizophrenia patients, offspring of schizophrenia patients and healthy controls. Schizophrenia Research 103(1–3): 22–25, 2008.

Rakic, P. & Yakovlev, P.I. Development of the corpus callosum and cavum septi in man. Journal of Comparative Neurology 132(1): 45–72, 1968.

Reveley, A.M. & Reveley, M.A. Aqueduct stenosis and schizophrenia. Journal of Neurology, Neurosurgery and Psychiatry 46(1): 18–22, 1983.

Rosales, R.K., Lemay, M.J. & Yakovlev, P.I. The development and involution of massa intermedia with regard to age and sex. Journal of Neuropathology & Experimental Neurology 27(1): 166, 1968.

Saijo, T., Abe, T., Someya, Y., Sassa, T., Sudo, Y., Suhara, T., Shuno, T., Asai, K. & Okubo, Y. Ten year progressive ventricular enlargement in schizophrenia: an MRI morphometrical study. Psychiatry and Clinical Neuroscience 55(1): 41–47, 2001.

Sallet, P.C., Elkis, H., Alves, T.M., Oliveira, J.R., Sassi, E., Campi DE Castro, C., Busatto, G.F. & Gattaz WF. Reduced cortical folding in schizophrenia: an MRI morphometric study. American Journal of Psychiatry 160(9): 1606–1613, 2003.

Schaufelberger M.S., Duran F.L. Lappin, J.M. Scazufca M. Amaro, E. JR., Leite, C.C., de Castro C.C., Murray, R.M., McGuire P.K., Menezes, P.R. & Busatto, G.F. Grey matter abnormalities in Brazilians with first-episode psychosis. British Journal of Psychiatry Supplement 51: s117–s122, 2007.

Schaufelberger, M.S., Lappin, J.M., Duran, F.L.S., Rosa, P.G.P., Uchida, R.R., Santos, L.C., Murray, R.M., McGuire, P.K., Scazufca, M., Menezes, P.R. & Busatto, G.F. Lack of progression of brain abnormalities in first-episode psychosis: a longitudinal MRI study over 15 months. Submitted for publication.

Scheepers, F.E., De Wied, C.C., Hulshoff Pol, H.E., Van De, F.W., Van Der Linden, J.A. & Kahn, R.S. The effect of clozapine on caudate nucleus volume in schizophrenic patients previously treated with typical antipsychotics. Neuropsychopharmacology 24(1): 47–54, 2001.

Schlagenhauf, F., Wüstenberg, T., Schmack, K., Dinges, M., Wrase, J., Koslowski, M., Kienast, T., Bauer, M., Gallinat, J., Juckel, G. & Heinz, A. Switching schizophrenia patients from typical neuroleptics to olanzapine: effects on BOLD response during attention and working memory. European Neuropsychopharmacology 18(8): 589–599, 2008.

Selemon, L.D. & Goldman-Rakic, P.S. The reduced neuropil hypothesis: a circuit based model of schizophrenia. Biological Psychiatry 45(1): 17–25, 1999.

Shenton, M.E., Dickey, C.C., Frumin, M. & McCarley, R.W. A review of MRI findings in schizophrenia. Schizophrenia Research 49(1–2): 1–52, 2001.

Shunk H. Congenital dilatations of the septi pellucidum. Radiology 81: 610–618, 1963.

Snyder, P.J., Bogerts, B., Wu, H., Bilder, R.M., Deoras, K.S. & Lieberman, J.A. Absence of the adhesio interthalamica as a marker of early developmental neuropathology in schizophrenia: an MRI and postmortem histologic study. Journal of Neuroimaging 8(3): 159–163, 1998.

Steen, R.G., Mull, C., McClure R., Hamer R.M. & Lieberman, J.A. Brain volume in first-episode schizophrenia: systematic review and meta-analysis of magnetic resonance imaging studies. British Journal of Psychiatry 188: 510–518, 2006.

Sun, D., Phillips, L., Velakoulis, D., Yung, A., McGorry, P.D., Wood, S.J., Van Erp, T.G., Thompson, P.M., Toga, A.W., Cannon, T.D. & Pantelis, C. Progressive brain structural changes mapped as psychosis develops in "at risk" individuals. Schizophrenia Research 108(1–3): 85–92, 2009.

Sun, D., Stuart, G.W., Jenkinson, M., Wood, S.J., McGorry, P.D., Velakoulis, D., Van Erp, T.G., Thompson, P.M., Toga, A.W., Smith, D.J., Cannon, T.D. & Pantelis, C. Brain surface contraction mapped in first-episode schizophrenia: a longitudinal magnetic resonance imaging study. Molecular Psychiatry 14(10): 976–986, 2009.

Szeszko, P.R., Lipsky, R., Mentschel, C., Robinson, D., Gunduz-Bruce, H., Sevy, S., Ashtari, M., Napolitano, B., Bilder, R.M., Kane, J.M., Goldman, D. & Malhotra, A.K. Brain-derived neurotrophic factor val66met polymorphism and volume of the hippocampal formation. Molecular Psychiatry 10(7): 631–636, 2005.

Takahashi, T., Suzuki, M., Hagino, H., Niu, L., Zhou, S.Y., Nakamura, K., Tanino, R., Kawasaki, Y., Seto, H. & Karachi, M. Prevalence of large cavum septi pellucidi and its relation to the medial temporal lobe structures in schizophrenia spectrum. Progress in Neuropsychopharmacology & Biological Psychiatry 31(6): 1235–1241, 2007.

Takahashi, T., Suzuki, M., Nakamura, K., Tanino, R., Zhou, S.Y., Hagino, H., Niu, L., Kawasaki, Y., Seto, H. & Kurachi, M. Association between absence of the adhesio interthalamica and amygdala volume in schizophrenia. Psychiatry Research 162(2): 101–111, 2008.

Takahashi, T., Wood, S.J., Yung, A.R., Phillips, L.J., Soulsby, B., McGorry, P.D., Tanino, R., Zhou, S.Y., Suzuki, M., Velakoulis, D. & Pantelis, C. Insular cortex gray matter changes in individuals at ultra-high-risk of developing psychosis. Schizophrenia Research 111(1–3): 94–102, 2009.

Takahashi, T., Wood, S.J., Yung, A.R., Soulsby, B., McGorry, P.D., Suzuki, M., Kawasaki, Y., Phillips, L.J., Velakoulis, D. & Pantelis, C. Progressive gray matter reduction of the superior temporal gyrus during transition to psychosis. Archives of General Psychiatry 66(4): 366–376, 2009.

Tan, H.Y., Nicodemus, K.K., Chen, Q., Li, Z., Brooke, J.K., Honea, R., Kolachana, B.S., Straub, R.E., Meyer-Lindenberg, A., Sei, Y., Mattay, V.S., Callicott, J.H. & Weinberger, D.R. Genetic variation in AKT1 is linked to dopamine-associated prefrontal cortical structure and function in humans. Journal of Clinical Investigations 118(6): 2200–2208, 2008.

Terry, A.V. Jr., Gearhart, D.A., Warner, S., Hohnadel, E.J., Middlemore, M.L., Zhang, G., Bartlett, M.G. & Mahadik, S.P. Protracted effects of chronic oral haloperidol and risperidone on nerve growth factor, cholinergic neurons, and spatial reference learning in rats. Neuroscience 150(2): 413–424, 2007b.

Terry, A.V. Jr., Gearhart, D.A., Warner, S.E., Zhang, G., Bartlett, M.G., Middlemore, M.L., Beck, W.D. Jr., Mahadik, S.P. & Waller, J.L. Oral haloperidol or risperidone treatment in rats: temporal effects on nerve growth factor receptors, cholinergic neurons, and memory performance. Neuroscience 146(3): 1316–1332, 2007a.

Théberge, J., Williamson, K.E., Aoyama, N., Drost, D.J., Manchanda, R., Malla, A.K., Northcott, S., Menon, R.S., Neufeld, R.W., Rajakumar, N., Pavlosky, W., Densmore, M., Schaefer, B. & Williamson, P.C. Longitudinal grey-matter and glutamatergic losses in first-episode schizophrenia. British Journal of Psychiatry 191: 325–334, 2007.

Thompson, P.M., Bartzokis, G., Hayashi, K.M., Klunder, A.D., Lu, P.H., Edwards, N., Hong, M.S., Yu, M., Geaga, J.A., Toga, A.W., Charles, C., Perkins, D.O., Mcevoy, J., Hamer, R.M., Tohen, M., Tollefson, G.D., Lieberman, J.A. & the HGDH Study Group. Time-lapse mapping of cortical changes in schizophrenia with different treatments. Cerebral Cortex 19(5): 1107–1123, 2009

Tsuang, M.T., Stone, W.S. & Faraone, S.V. Genes, environment and schizophrenia. British Journal of Psychiatry Supplement 40: s18–s24, 2001.

Uematsu, M. & Kaiya, H. Midsagittal cortical pathomorphology of schizophrenia: a magnetic resonance imaging study. Psychiatry Research 30(1): 11–20, 1989.

Van Haren, N.E., Cahn, W., Hulshoff Pol, H.E. & Kahn RS. Schizophrenia as a progressive brain disease. European Psychiatry 23(4): 245–254, 2008a.

Van Haren, N.E., Hulshoff Pol, H.E., Schnack, H.G., Cahn, W., Brans, R., Carati, I., Rais, M. & Kahn RS. Progressive brain volume loss in schizophrenia over the course of the illness: evidence of maturational abnormalities in early adulthood. Biological Psychiatry 63(1): 106–113, 2008b.

Van Haren, N.E., Hulshoff Pol, H.E., Schnack, H.G., Cahn, W., Mandl, R.C., Collins, D.L., Evans, A.C. & Kahn, R.S. Focal gray matter changes in schizophrenia across the course of the illness: a 5-year follow-up study. Neuropsychopharmacology 32(10): 2057–2066, 2007.

Varnäs, K., Lawyer, G., Jönsson, E.G., Kulle, B., Nesvåg, R., Hall, H., Terenius, L. & Agartz, I. Brain-derived neurotrophic factor polymorphisms and frontal cortex morphology in schizophrenia. Psychiatric Genetics 18(4): 177–183, 2008.

Vita A., De Peri, L., Silenzi, C. & Dieci, M. Brain morphology in first-episode schizophrenia: a meta-analysis of quantitative magnetic resonance imaging studies. Schizophrenia Research 82(1): 75–88, 2006.

Wacholder, S. Design issues in case–control studies. Statistical Methods in Medical Research 4: 293–309, 1995.

Waddington, J.L., Lane, A., Scully, P.J., Larkin, C. & OCallaghan, E. Neurodevelopmental and neuroprogressive processes in schizophrenia. Antithetical or complementary over a lifetime trajectory of disease? Psychiatry Clinics of North America 21(1): 123–149, 1998.

Wang, L., Mamah, D., Harms, M.P., Karnik, M., Price, J.L., Gado, M.H., Thompson, P.A., Barch, D.M., Miller, M.I. & Csernansky, J.G. Progressive deformation of deep brain nuclei and hippocampal–amygdala formation in schizophrenia. Biological Psychiatry 64(12): 1060–1068, 2008.

Weinberger, D.R. Implications of normal brain development for the pathogenesis of schizophrenia. Archives of General Psychiatry 44(7): 660–669, 1987.

Westmoreland Corson, P.W., Nopoulos, P., Miller, D.D., Arndt, S. & Andreasen, N.C. Change in basal ganglia volume over 2 years in patients with schizophrenia: typical versus atypical neuroleptics. American Journal of Psychiatry 156(8): 1200–1204, 1999.

Whitford, T.J., Farrow, T.F., Rennie, C.J., Grieve, S.M., Gomes, L., Brennan, J., Harris, A.W. & Williams, L.M. Longitudinal changes in neuroanatomy and neural activity in early schizophrenia. Neuroreport 18(5): 435–439, 2007a.

Whitford, T.J., Grieve, S.M., Farrow, T.F., Gomes, L., Brennan, J., Harris, A.W., Gordon, E. & Williams, L.M. Volumetric white matter abnormalities in first-episode schizophrenia: a longitudinal, tensor-based morphometry study. American Journal of Psychiatry 164(7): 1082–1089, 2007b.

Whitworth, A.B., Kemmler, G., Honeder, M., Kremser, C., Felber, S., Hausmann, A., Walch, T., Wanko, C., Weiss, E.M., Stuppaeck, C.H. & Fleischhacker, W.W. Longitudinal volumetric MRI study in first- and multiple-episode male schizophrenia patients. Psychiatry Research 140(3): 225–237, 2005.

Wood, S.J., Pantelis, C., Velakoulis, D., Yucel, M., Fornito, A., McGorry, P.D. Progressive changes in the development toward schizophrenia: studies in subjects at increased symptomatic risk. Schizophrenia Bulletin 34(2): 322–329, 2008.

Wood, S.J., Velakoulis, D., Smith, D.J., Bond, D., Stuart, G.W., McGorry, P.D., Brewer, W.J., Bridle, N., Eritaia, J., Desmond, P., Singh, B., Copolov, D. & Pantelis, C. A longitudinal study of hippocampal volume in first episode psychosis and chronic schizophrenia. Schizophrenia Research 52(1–2): 37–46, 2001.

Woods, B.T. Is schizophrenia a progressive neurodevelopmental disorder? Toward a unitary pathogenetic mechanism. American Journal of Psychiatry 155(12): 1661–1670, 1998.

Wright, I.C., Rabe-Hesketh, S., Woodruff, P.W., David, A.S., Murray, R.M. & Bullmore, E.T. Meta-analysis of regional brain volumes in schizophrenia. American Journal of Psychiatry 157(1): 16–25, 2000.

Yoon, U., Lee, J.M., Kwon, J.S., Kim, H.P., Shin, Y.W., Ha, T.H., Kim, I.Y., Chang, K.H. & Kim, S.I. An MRI study of structural variations in schizophrenia using deformation field morphometry. Psychiatry Research 146(2): 171–177, 2006.

Zipursky, R.B., Christensen, B.K. & Mikulis, D.J. Stable deficits in gray matter volumes following a first episode of schizophrenia. Schizophrenia Research 71(2–3): 515–516, 2004.

The Neuropathology of Schizophrenia: Central Role for the Hippocampus?

Peter Falkai, Eleni Parlapani, Oliver Gruber, and Andrea Schmitt

The Neurodevelopmental Hypothesis of Schizophrenia

A change in conceptual thinking about the pathogenesis of schizophrenia has occurred over the past decades. It is now hypothesized that the disorder has its origin on brain developmental neuropathology. The so-called neurodevelopmental hypothesis proposes that schizophrenia is related to adverse conditions leading to abnormal brain development during the pre- or postnatal period. This consequently leads to long-term changes in brain structure and brain malfunction, predisposing in term to functional deficits and to symptoms that respond to antidopaminergic drugs (Weinberger 1996).

Studies on what are called "minor physical abnormalities" provided weak evidence, reflected through intrauterine abnormal development (Green et al. 1989). Data referred to minor facial abnormalities (Lane et al. 1997) and small head circumference at birth (McNeil et al. 1993). Because these structures are derived from the same tissue and form at the same time during development as the brain, the observations suggested that normal development of both brain and associated structures is disrupted in schizophrenia patients.

Further evidence supporting the hypothesis came from a prospective epidemiological study of British birth cohorts, reporting that patients with schizophrenia were already neurologically, cognitively and socially impaired during childhood (Jones et al. 1994). Premorbid educational and intellectual deficits hinted at impairment before the onset of the diagnostic syndrome (Aylward et al. 1984).

Furthermore, there is enough evidence for macroscopical brain changes in schizophrenia (Harrison and Weinberger 2005). Studies using brain imaging techniques reported brain-structural abnormalities in first-episode drug-naive patients, while atrophy rates up to 5–10% were described in the fronto-temporo-limbic

P. Falkai (✉)
Department of Psychiatry and Psychotherapy, University of Goettingen, von Siebold Str. 5, 37075 Goettingen, Germany
e-mail: pfalkai@gwdg.de

W.F. Gattaz, G. Busatto (eds.), *Advances in Schizophrenia Research 2009*,
DOI 10.1007/978-1-4419-0913-8_7, © Springer Science+Business Media, LLC 2010

network (Wright et al. 2000, Shenton et al. 2001). Other studies addressed the formation of normal cerebral asymmetries. Because the formation of major cortical asymmetries is complete by the middle of the third trimester of gestation, abnormalities of such asymmetries directly implicated a disruption of the normal developmental processes. Initial studies reported anomalous lateralization of the sylvian fissures (Falkai et al. 1992) and other aspects of the temporal cortex (Crow et al. 1989).

Further investigation of abnormal cytoarchitecture in limbic cortices was most compelling with relevance to neurodevelopment (Jakob and Beckmann 1986). Additional studies revealed reduced number and smaller neuron size in layer II of the entorhinal cortex (ERC) in schizophrenia (Falkai et al. 1988, Arnold et al. 1995). Abnormal dispersion of pre-alpha-cell clusters in layer II of the ERC was also reported, suggesting migrational disturbances in schizophrenia (Falkai et al. 2000, Kovalenko et al. 2003), although other studies could not replicate this finding (Bernstein et al. 1998). A migration failure during neurodevelopment would disturb normal neocortical–hippocampal communication. Supportive evidence for a developmental failure of the normal inside-out neuronal migratory gradient was also reported in the superior frontal gyrus (Akbarian et al. 1993a), cingulate cortex (Benes et al. 1991a) and lateral temporal neocortex (Akbarian et al. 1993b).

Support for the neurodevelopmental origin of schizophrenia would provide the absence of evidence for a progressive or degenerative disorder. Progression of ventricular enlargement in first-onset patients was not observed in a 7-year follow-up study (Jaskiw et al. 1994). This finding indicated that the lesion was present early in the course of the disorder, preceded the symptoms and demonstrated a static encephalopathy. Evidence for an ongoing degenerative process, indicated by the presence of reactive gliosis, is inconsistent in schizophrenia. One early study found gliosis in 70% of brains from patients but in less than 5% of controls in several brain regions (Stevens 1982), while other authors reported progressive changes in brain regions over the duration of the illness (Kaplan et al. 1990). Still, the weight of evidence from most recent studies did not support an ongoing degenerative process, indicated by a lack of gliosis in brains of schizophrenia patients (Benes et al. 1991, Falkai et al. 1999). Additionally, well-conducted studies using routine stains and immunohistochemical methods showed that even elderly schizophrenia patients with cognitive impairment did not exhibit features of any dementing disorder (Baldessarini et al. 1997).

The Aetiology of Schizophrenia: Implication of Genetic and Environmental Factors

A question arises as to the factors that lead to the aforementioned structural brain abnormalities, namely, what causes them. The "complex" nature of schizophrenia cannot be easily explained as the result of a single genetic or environmental component. Genetic susceptibility plays an important role and genetic research in this field has a 100-year-old history (Maier et al. 2003). In a twin-based study, heritability was estimated at 83% (Cannon et al. 1998). On the other hand, genetically identical monozygotic twins show a concordance of much lower than 100%. This suggests that other factors must also contribute to the aetiology of the disorder. What makes monozygotic twins discordant for schizophrenia remains largely a question, although the recent implication of epigenetics in the aetiopathogenesis of the disorder offered an explanation (Crow 2007).

It seems that it is not schizophrenia per se that is inherited but rather a susceptibility to it, since environmental factors are important in disease manifestation. Such risk factors include prenatal and perinatal effects. Maternal viral infections during the first (Brown et al. 2004) and second trimester of gestation (Adams et al. 1993), stress, malnutrition (Brown et al. 1996), diabetes mellitus and smoking during pregnancy increased manifestation of schizophrenia in the offspring. Additionally, obstetric complications associated with hypoxia increased not only the risk of developing schizophrenia, but also associated with early onset of the disorder and reductions of hippocampal volumes (McNeil et al. 2000, Van Erp et al. 2002).

Susceptibility Genes for Schizophrenia

Regarding the genetic component of aetiopathogenesis, it is now clearly established that schizophrenia is polygenic. This non-mendelian pattern of familial transmission is defined by an additive effect of multiple genes, each one with only a modest contribution, called "disposition genes" (Maier et al. 2003). Except for polygenic, genetic architecture in schizophrenia is heterogeneous, since no particular constellation of genes is characteristic of all patients. The same causative alleles may have a variable phenotype, depending on genetic background (Harrison and Weinberger 2005).

Current strategies investigating the genetic susceptibility for schizophrenia include cytogenic, linkage and association studies. Chromosomal regions that associated with schizophrenia are 1q, 2q, 5p, 5q, 6p, 6q, 8p, 10p, 13q, 15q and 22q. Putative susceptibility genes include dysbindin 1 (*DTNBP1*), catechol-*O*-methyltransferase (*COMT*), disrupted-in-schizophrenia-1 (*DISC1*), regulator of G-protein signalling-4 (*RGS4*), metabotropic glutamate receptor-3 (*GRM3*), G72 and d-amino acid oxidase (*DAAO*) genes (Harrison and Weinberger 2005).

Neuregulin 1 Gene and Its Effects on Brain–Hippocampal Function

Genome-wide linkage studies and meta-analyses of whole-genome linkage scans identified neuregulin-1 (*NRG1*) gene, located on chromosome 8p12, as a strong candidate for schizophrenia. A core at-risk *NRG1* haplotype (HAP_{ICE}) consisting of two microsatellite markers and five single nucleotide polymorphisms (SNPs) was first reported in an Icelandic population (Stefansson et al. 2002). Association of this haplotype with schizophrenia was replicated in a Scottish, a Northern European, a Chinese and a Portuguese population (for review see Schmitt et al., 2008a). While one meta-analysis confirmed association of the original risk haplotype with schizophrenia (Li et al. 2006), two further meta-analyses reported only a non-significant association of the SNP8NRG221533 polymorphism with schizophrenia (Munafo et al. 2006, 2008), presumably because of heterogeneity of distinct populations. Except for the originally reported Icelandic haplotype, other *NRG1* haplotypes as well as alleles of individual SNPs and microsatellites were shown to significantly associate with schizophrenia (for review see Schmitt et al., 2008a).

NRG1 is an essential gene. The pan-*NRG1* knockout mice display severe developmental abnormalities in the nervous system. Unfortunately, early mortality of these mice does not allow more detailed observation of the essential role of *NRG1* in nervous system development. Mice heterozygous for two different mutations in the *NRG1* gene display a hyperactivity similar to the one observed in mice with mutations that impair glutamatergic or enhance dopaminergic neurotransmission (Falls 2003).

NRGs stimulate intracellular signalling pathways, leading to different cellular responses such as cell apoptosis, migration, differentiation, adhesion and stimulation or inhibition of proliferation. Specifically, they are involved in the differentiation and survival of Schwann cells and oligodendrocytes (Falls 2003), promoting myelination. There is supportive evidence for the essential role of NRGs in oligodendrocyte lineage development as well as in the migration of CNS neuronal precursors along radial glia cells. NRGs are involved in brain synaptic plasticity and regulate the expression of N-methyl-D-aspartate (NMDA), gamma-aminobutyric acid (GABA) receptors, as well as the function of ion channels. An in vitro study reported that neuregulins increased $\alpha 7$ nicotinic acetylcholine receptors and enhanced excitatory synaptic transmission in GABAergic interneurons of the hippocampus (for review see Schmitt et al., 2008a).

A study reported increased *NRG1* isoform type I mRNA expression in the hippocampus of schizophrenia patients and interaction with the genotype SNP8NRG221132 (Law et al. 2006). However, our recent postmortem study showed alterations of *NRG1* isoform expression in the prefrontal cortex but not in hippocampus (Parlapani et al. 2008). The effect of genotype findings on *NRG1* expression and the implication of altered *NRG1* expression in the pathophysiology of schizophrenia remain speculative and require further investigation. Still, there is evidence of concrete effects on hippocampal function. *NRG1* is highly expressed in CA3 pyramidal neurons projecting to CA1, accumulates at various central synapses including the hippocampal CA1 molecular layer (Chaudhury et al. 2003, Law et al. 2004a) and was shown to regulate synaptic plasticity in the hippocampus by reversing long-term potentiation at Schaffer collateral to CA1 synapses in an activity- and time-dependent manner (Kwon et al. 2005) and by inducing hippocampal neurite extension and arborization (Gerecke et al. 2004).

A functional magnetic resonance imaging study showed an association of the NRG1 risk genotype SNP8NRG243177 with psychotic symptoms and decreased prefrontal, temporal activation and premorbid IQ (Hall et al. 2006). The risk allele SNP8NRG243177 was linked with reduced spatial working memory capacity also in healthy probands. In addition, SNP8NRG221132 and rs6994992 predicted lower expression of $\alpha 7$ nicotinic acetylcholine receptor mRNA in the prefrontal cortex, which might in turn contribute to impairments of working memory (for review see Schmitt et al., 2008). Reduced prepulse inhibition (PPI) of an acoustic startle in carriers of a missense mutation on rs3924999 hinted at an association between this schizophrenia-related endophenotype and a potentially functional variant of the NRG1 gene (Hong et al. 2008). Finally, SNP8NRG221533 associated with defective white matter microstructure, as indicated by decreased fractional anisotropy primarily in subcortical white matter of the frontal lobe (Winterer et al. 2008), while a recent study reported an association between the *NRG1* HAP$_{ICE}$ haplotype and lower hippocampal volumes in schizophrenia patients, as well as in their first-degree relatives (Gruber et al. 2008). Altogether, genetic risk factors for schizophrenia might affect a neuronal network, with hippocampus being one key region.

Animal Models for Examining the Central Role of Hippocampus in Schizophrenia and the Neurodevelopmental Hypothesis

The hypothesis that early abnormal brain development contributes to the aetiology of schizophrenia is difficult to investigate in humans because of the inability to predict which individuals will develop the disorder. For this reason, animal models were developed to test many of the possible environmental risk factors, such as nutritional deprivation, viral infection and lesioning of hippocampal pathways.

It was hypothesized that perinatal lesion of the hippocampus is disrupting development of the widespread cortical and subcortical circuitry, in which the hippocampus participates (Lipska 2004). Interrupting neural pathways via hippocampal lesions in neonatal rats resulted in abnormal connectivity of hippocampal projection sites throughout the brain and formed an animal model of neurodevelopmental abnormalities of pathways. The lesions involved regions of the hippocampus that directly project to the prefrontal cortex, namely, the ventral hippocampus and the ventral subiculum. These regions correspond to the anterior hippocampus in humans, a region that showed anatomical abnormalities in schizophrenia. These animal models are of great interest, since various functional and structural changes in the hippocampus were consistently implicated in human schizophrenia (Weinberger 1999).

Ventral hippocampal lesions at postnatal day 7 in rat pups resulted in a lack of alteration to behaviour until the rats reached puberty at around day 56 but, following this, animals demonstrated hyperactivity and elevated responses to stress (Lipska et al. 1993). Treatment with clozapine ameliorated some of these behavioural alterations. Other studies of neonatally lesioned animals reported altered or impaired social interaction (Sams-Dodd et al. 1997, Becker et al. 1999).

Recent investigations demonstrated that adult rats with neonatal hippocampal lesions showed enhanced sensitivity to drugs of abuse such as amphetamine (Wan et al. 1996) and deficits in reward mechanisms (Le Pen et al. 2002). Additionally, neonatal hippocampal lesions resulted in deficits of radial arm maze choice accuracy, an assessment of spatial learning and working memory. This effect was present from before puberty and persisted to adulthood (Chambers et al. 1996). Impaired working memory after lesion of the ventral hippocampus was confirmed elsewhere (Lipska et al. 2002a). Finally, neonatal hippocampal lesioning resulted in the disruption of PPI of an acoustic startle similar to that observed in schizophrenia (Lipska et al. 1995), as well as disruption of latent inhibition (Grecksch et al. 1999).

In a further series of studies, it was hypothesized that also transient inactivation of the ventral hippocampus during a critical period of development may be sufficient to disrupt normal maturation of the prefrontal cortex and perhaps other interconnected late-maturing regions (Lipska et al. 2002). Transient disconnection in the CA1 and CA2 hippocampus areas might have long-lasting consequences for neurogenesis in the dentate gyrus. The overall characteristics of behavioural changes and their temporal pattern were reminiscent of the disturbances associated with the permanent excitotoxic lesion of the ventral hippocampus produced at the same neonatal age (Lipska and Weinberger 2000). Altogether, the aforementioned data suggested that a transient loss of ventral hippocampal function during a critical time in maturation of intracortical connections permanently changed the development of prefronto-temporal neural circuits mediating certain dopamine- and NMDA-related behaviours.

It is noteworthy that early postnatal damage of the hippocampal region in non-human primates altered development of the dorsal prefrontal cortex and its regulation of subcortical dopamine function, phenomena similar to those described in schizophrenia patients (Bertolino et al. 1997).

Animal models provided a unique opportunity to explore schizophrenia. Neonatal damage to the rat hippocampus reproduced a broad spectrum of schizophrenia-related phenomena and established the neurobiological plausibility of early damage with a delayed impact on neural functions implicated in schizophrenia. It is though important to recognize that any animal model of a complex disorder is unlikely to be able to produce deficits that emulate every aspect of altered brain structure, neurochemistry and function.

Neuropathological Findings of Hippocampus in Schizophrenia

The evidence for involvement of hippocampus in the pathophysiology of schizophrenia is increasing. Neuroimaging studies reported reduced hippocampal volume in schizophrenia (Shenton et al. 2001), specifically in first-episode patients (Bogerts et al. 1990, Hirayasu et al. 1998, Velakoulis et al. 1999), as well as in at-risk and unaffected relatives of schizophrenia patients (Seidman et al. 2002).

Reduced hippocampal volume, as well as its relationship to cognitive impairment, is considered a promising endophenotype for schizophrenia.

It is not clear which hippocampal region contributes to this volume reduction. Significantly reduced anterior hippocampal formation volume (Pegues et al. 2003) with no differences in volumes of either the posterior formation or amygdala was reported in antipsychotic-naive patients with first-episode schizophrenia. This finding suggested that volumetric abnormalities of the hippocampus–amygdala complex might be specific to the anterior hippocampal formation in patients experiencing a first episode of schizophrenia and were consistent with the hypothesis regarding abnormal frontolimbic connectivity as central in the pathophysiology of the disorder (Szeszko et al. 2003). However, other structural magnetic resonance imaging (MRI) studies reported reduced volume of the posterior part of the hippocampus (Velakoulis et al. 2001, Yamasue et al. 2004, Rametti et al. 2007). Finally, there was some evidence that volume differences of the hippocampal formation in schizophrenia are due to white matter abnormalities (Colter et al. 1987), hinting at a disconnection of either the intrinsic hippocampal fibre pathways or the extrinsic afferent and efferent projections.

Altogether, comprehensive reviews of the morphometric literature have concluded that the hippocampus is smaller in schizophrenia. Specifically, a meta-analysis reported a 5–10% bilateral hippocampal volume reduction in schizophrenia when compared with the normal brain (Wright et al. 2000). The findings of volume reduction, specifically in first-episode patients, argue against a degenerative process, although the finding of a slow progression of hippocampal volume reduction throughout the disease process could be interpreted as evidence for the deleterious effect of the disease process or the treatment. The finding of subtle hippocampal volume loss was confirmed in postmortem studies and linked to abnormalities in interneurons and neuropil (Arnold 1997).

Except for reduced hippocampal volume, shape distortion and deformities were observed (Casanova and Rothberg 2002). Other studies reported low N-acetyl-aspartate (NAA, a marker of neuronal integrity) signal intensity or concentration in hippocampus (Nasrallah et al. 1994). These results provided evidence for a developmental lesion or for subtle cell loss. Also unaffected first-degree relatives of patients showed decreased NAA levels (Callicott et al. 1998). Additionally, lower regional cerebral glucose metabolic rate was reported in the hippocampus in schizophrenia (Nordahl et al. 1996).

In functional MRI studies, decreased activation of the posterior part of the hippocampus was related to smooth pursuit eye movement deficits (Tregellas et al. 2004) and impaired verbal learning in schizophrenia (Eyler et al. 2008). Neurophysiological data, including verbal memory as a primary deficit present early in the course of schizophrenia, implicated the left temporal–hippocampal system in the pathophysiology of the disorder (Saykin et al. 1994).

At the microscopical level, quantitative studies of the hippocampus described reduced density of interneurons, mainly of parvalbumin-immunoreactive cells, without alterations of pyramidal neurons (Benes et al. 1998, Zhang et al. 2002). Other studies revealed however a reduced number of pyramidal neurons in the hippocampus (Falkai and Bogerts 1986), ERC (Falkai et al. 1988) as well as reduced density of pyramidal neurons in CA3 and CA4 areas (Jeste and Lohr 1989). One study reported however increased neuronal density in the hippocampus of patients (Zaidel et al. 1997a).

Other investigations revealed smaller neuron size in layer II of the ERC and the hippocampus in schizophrenia (Benes et al. 1991, Arnold et al. 1995). Except for smaller size, hippocampal pyramidal neurons showed an altered shape, being thinner and more elongated compared to controls (Zaidel et al. 1997). Despite the replication, smaller hippocampal neuronal size is a not wholly established feature of schizophrenia (Benes et al. 1998, Highley et al. 2003).

Laminar gradient abnormalities were also reported (Akbarian et al. 1993). Altered hippocampal pyramidal cell alignment (Conrad et al. 1991) and disorientation (Kovelman and Scheibel 1984) were observed in the hippocampus of schizophrenia patients. However, these findings were again not supported by later studies (Christison et al. 1989, Arnold et al. 1995).

Additionally, it was shown that hippocampal neuron populations had fewer dendritic spines and reduced dendritic arborizations (Rosoklija et al. 2000). This observation was supported by studies detecting molecular markers such as microtubule-associated protein 2 (MAP2) and spinophilin (Arnold et al. 1991, Law et al. 2004). MAP, which is involved in neuronal cytoarchitectural development, was altered unilaterally in the subiculum and hippocampal CA1 neurons in brains of schizophrenia patients, suggesting an altered cytoskeletal assembly (Cotter et al. 1997).

Evidence for reduced presynaptic markers was also reported. A more consistent finding within the hippocampus is abnormal synaptic connectivity, as shown by decreased expression of the presynaptic proteins synapsin, synaptophysin and synaptosomal-associated protein (SNAP-25). These results have been recently reviewed (Harrison and Eastwood 2001).

Results from Design-Based Stereological Investigations

To date, two design-based stereological estimates of total cell numbers in the hippocampus reported no differences between schizophrenia patients and controls. However, one study investigated only the total number of neurons (Heckers et al. 1991), while the second study failed to discriminate between different cell types and included both schizophrenia and schizoaffective patients (Walker et al. 2002). Thus, the differentiation of neuronal and glial cell types using stereological methods has not been investigated until recently.

In our recent design-based stereology study (Schmitt et al. 2008), we examined serial postmortem sections of the posterior hippocampus from 10 schizophrenia patients and 10 matched controls. We quantified separately the number of astrocytes, oligodendrocytes and neurons (pyramidal cells and interneurons together) in all hippocampal subregions (CA1, CA2/3, CA4 and subiculum).

Neither the mean density nor the mean number of astrocytes was significantly different between patients and controls in any of the investigated subregions. Still, an age effect on density and number of astrocytes was observed. The increasing number of astrocytes in the ageing brain might serve as internal validity control in future stereological investigations. Furthermore, no significant differences with respect to the mean volumes, densities and numbers of neurons were detected between patients and controls. We observed, however, significant effects of diagnosis on the mean numbers of oligodendrocytes. Schizophrenia patients showed namely a significantly reduced mean number of oligodendrocytes in CA4 subregion on both sides of the hippocampus (Schmitt et al. 2008).

Oligodendrocytes are involved in the myelination process of axons during development. Myelination of projections in the frontal and temporal lobes, including the posterior part of the hippocampus, peaks at late adolescence and early adulthood, occurring in close temporal proximity with the onset of schizophrenia (Benes 1989, Benes et al. 1994).

At the microscopical level, ultrastructural investigations revealed atrophy of axons and swelling of periaxonal processes in the hippocampus (Uranova et al. 2007). Additionally, one of the most pronounced decreases in expression of oligodendrocyte-related proteins was reported in the hippocampus of patients with schizophrenia (Katsel et al. 2005, Dracheva et al. 2006). The microarray data together with our aforementioned light microscopical findings are supported by in vivo MRI studies providing macroscopical evidence for hippocampal white matter abnormalities in schizophrenia (Colter et al. 1987), as well as by diffusion tensor imaging (DTI) studies of white matter tracts of the fornix and posterior hippocampus, showing decreased fractional anisotropy and supporting the hypothesis of functional disconnectivity in schizophrenia (Zhou et al. 2008).

Microarray and quantitative RT-PCR studies (Hakak et al. 2001, Aston et al. 2004, Katsel et al. 2005) confirm the implication of oligodendrocyte and myelin in the pathogenesis of schizophrenia by revealing downregulation of multiple oligodendrocyte and/or myelin-related genes in different brain areas in schizophrenia. Additionally, the decreased hippocampal oligodendrocyte number in the CA4 subregion points to the same direction as the decrease in the mean number of oligodendrocytes detected in the prefrontal cortex (Hof et al. 2002), anterior cingulate cortex (Stark et al. 2004) and thalamus (Byne et al. 2006) of patients.

Despite growing evidence for oligodendrocyte and myelin deficits, pathology that is characteristic of a demyelination process was not observed in schizophrenia. It appears that myelin deficits reflect a defective developmental myelination process. Altogether, evidence for "neurodegeneration without gliosis" exists; namely, the pathological processes in schizophrenia could be interpreted as an arrest of the developmental process of myelination, possibly due to decreased oligodendroglia number or reduced oligodendrocyte function.

Numerous lines of inquiry implicate "miswiring" and disconnectivity among different brain regions as a central abnormality in schizophrenia. The substrates of this aberrant communication remain largely unknown; however, abnormalities in signal propagation might contribute and one of the processes critical to rapid impulse conduction is myelination. Decreased signal propagation because of distorted myelination could lead to brain's functional asynchrony (Davis et al. 2003), with severe consequences, for example, in the performance of memory tasks (Talamini et al. 2005).

Cognitive function such as verbal declarative memory correlated with fractional anisotropy in the hippocampus of schizophrenia patients (Lim et al. 2006). Disruption of hippocampal connectivity could result not only in cognitive deficits but also in clinical negative symptoms. This is attributed to the fact that neuronal fibres traversing the limbic pathways from the posterior hippocampus connect to prefrontal regions and pathways involved in higher cognition (Goldman-Rakic et al. 1984).

Resume: Hippocampus Is Involved in a Neuronal Network That Is Relevant for the Pathophysiology of Schizophrenia

Based on the first pathological study of dementia praecox, Alzheimer (1897) and Kraepelin (1919) proposed that prefrontal abnormalities play a primary role in the pathogenesis of schizophrenia. Since then, the prefrontal cortex theory of schizophrenia dominated the field of schizophrenia research. The hippocampus is a later arrival among the brain regions implicated in the pathophysiology of schizophrenia. Initial theories of hippocampal and limbic system dysfunction in schizophrenia were built on the idea that the anatomy and behavioural affiliations of the medial temporal lobe are well suited to explain some of the abnormalities seen in schizophrenia. However, it was not until 1985 (Bogerts et al. 1985) that the first evidence for a hippocampal involvement in schizophrenia was reported. Since then, many studies have provided compelling data, consistent with the hypothesis that schizophrenia is associated with a disturbance of the structural and functional hippocampal integrity. The relatively precise and well-understood circuitry of the hippocampal formation serves studies investigating neural connectivity, a concept that became central to the pathophysiological theories of schizophrenia (Friston and Frith 1995, Andreasen 1999).

Still, there are many questions that remain unanswered. The time course of hippocampal volume changes and dysfunction in the disease process is particularly important. Could these predict the expression, onset or course of the disorder? If so, could hippocampal volume changes be used to detect patients at risk and could they be controlled over time in order to stage the disease process? Could they be regarded as an endophenotype for schizophrenia? Furthermore, what would be the relevance of hippocampal volume changes for the expression of cognitive deficits? Most importantly, what are the consequences regarding prevention of relapse or effective medical treatment? Future studies are called to elucidate further aspects of the hippocampal pathology and establish its exact role in schizophrenia.

References

Adams, W., Kendell, R.E., Hare, E.H., & Munk-Jorgensen, P. (1993) Epidemiological evidence that maternal influenza contributes to the aetiology of schizophrenia. An analysis of Scottish, English, and Danish data. Br J Psychiatry 163: 522–534

Akbarian, S., Bunney, W.E. JR., Potkin, S.G., Wigal, S.B., Hagman, J.O., Sandman, C.A., & Jones, E.G. (1993a) Altered distribution of nicotinamide-adenine dinucleotide phosphate-diaphorase cells in frontal lobe of schizophrenics implies disturbances of cortical development. Arch Gen Psychiatry 50: 169–177

Akbarian, S., Vinuela, A., Kim, J.J., Potkin, S.G., Bunney, W.E. Jr., & Jones, E.G. (1993b) Distorted distribution of nicotinamide-adenine dinucleotide phosphate-diaphorase neurons in temporal lobe of schizophrenics implies anomalous cortical development. Arch Gen Psychiatry 50: 178–187

Andreasen, N.C. (1999) A unitary model of schizophrenia: Bleuler's "fragmented phrene" as schizencephaly. Arch Gen Psychiatry 56: 781–78

Arnold, S.E. (1997) The medial temporal lobe in schizophrenia. J Neuropsychiatry Clin Neurosci 9: 460–470

Arnold, S.E., Franz, B.R., Gur, R.C., Gur, R.E., Shapiro, R.M., Moberg, P.J., & Trojanowski, J.Q. (1995) Smaller neuron size in schizophrenia in hippocampal subfields that mediate cortical–hippocampal interactions. Am J Psychiatry 152: 738–748

Arnold, S.E., Lee, V.M., Gur, R.E., & Trojanowski, J.Q. (1991) Abnormal expression of two microtubule-associated proteins (MAP2 and MAP5) in specific subfields of the hippocampal formation in schizophrenia. Proc Natl Acad Sci USA 88: 10850–10854

Aston, C., Jiang, L., & Sokolov, B.P. (2004) Microarray analysis of postmortem temporal cortex from patients with schizophrenia. J Neurosci Res 77: 858–866

Aylward, E., Walker, E., & Bettes, B. (1984) Intelligence in schizophrenia: meta-analysis of the research. Schizophr Bull 10: 430–459

Baldessarini, R.J., Hegarty, J.D., Bird, E.D., & Benes, F.M. (1997) Meta-analysis of postmortem studies of Alzheimer's disease-like neuropathology in schizophrenia. Am J Psychiatry 154: 861–863

Becker, A., Grecksch, G., Bernstein, H.G., Hollt, V., & Bogerts, B. (1999) Social behaviour in rats lesioned with ibotenic acid in the hippocampus: quantitative and qualitative analysis. Psychopharmacology (Berl) 144: 333–338

Benes, F.M. (1989) Myelination of cortical-hippocampal relays during late adolescence. Schizophr Bull 15: 585–593

Benes, F.M., Kwok, E.W., Vincent, S.L., & Todtenkopf, M.S. (1998) A reduction of nonpyramidal cells in sector CA2 of schizophrenics and manic depressives. Biol Psychiatry 44: 88–97

Benes, F.M., Mcsparren, J., Bird, E.D., Sangiovanni, J.P., & Vincent, S.L. (1991a) Deficits in small interneurons in prefrontal and cingulate cortices of schizophrenic and schizoaffective patients. Arch Gen Psychiatry 48: 996–1001

Benes, F.M., Sorensen, I., & Bird, E.D. (1991b) Reduced neuronal size in posterior hippocampus of schizophrenic patients. Schizophr Bull 17: 597–608

Benes, F.M., Turtle, M., Khan, Y., & Farol, P. (1994) Myelination of a key relay zone in the hippocampal formation occurs in the human brain during childhood, adolescence, and adulthood. Arch Gen Psychiatry 51: 477–484

Bernstein, H.G., Krell, D., Baumann, B., Danos, P., Falkai, P., Diekmann, S., Henning, H., & Bogerts, B. (1998) Morphometric studies of the entorhinal cortex in neuropsychiatric patients and controls: clusters of heterotopically displaced lamina II neurons are not indicative of schizophrenia. Schizophr Res 33: 125–132

Bertolino, A., Saunders, R.C., Mattay, V.S., Bachevalier, J., Frank, J.A., & Weinberger, D.R. (1997) Altered development of prefrontal neurons in rhesus monkeys with neonatal mesial temporo-limbic lesions: a proton magnetic resonance spectroscopic imaging study. Cereb Cortex 7: 740–748

Bogerts, B., Ashtari, M., Degreef, G., Alvir, J.M., Bilder, R.M., & Lieberman, J.A. (1990) Reduced temporal limbic structure volumes on magnetic resonance images in first episode schizophrenia. Psychiatry Res 35: 1–13

Bogerts, B., Meertz, E., & Schonfeldt-Bausch, R. (1985) Basal ganglia and limbic system pathology in schizophrenia. A morphometric study of brain volume and shrinkage. Arch Gen Psychiatry 42: 784–791

Brown, A.S., Begg, M.D., Gravenstein, S., Schaefer, C.A., Wyatt, R.J., Bresnahan, M., Babulas, V.P., & Susser, E.S. (2004) Serologic evidence of prenatal influenza in the etiology of schizophrenia. Arch Gen Psychiatry 61: 774–780

Brown, A.S., Susser, E.S., Butler, P.D., Richardson Andrews, R., Kaufmann, C.A., & Gorman, J.M. (1996) Neurobiological plausibility of prenatal nutritional deprivation as a risk factor for schizophrenia. J Nerv Ment Dis 184: 71–85

Byne, W., Kidkardnee, S., Tatusov, A., Yiannoulos, G., Buchsbaum, M.S. & Haroutunian, V. (2006) Schizophrenia-associated reduction of neuronal and oligodendrocyte numbers in the anterior principal thalamic nucleus. Schizophr Res 85: 245–253

Callicott, J.H., Egan, M.F., Bertolino, A., Mattay, V.S., Langheim, F.J., Frank, J.A., & Weinberger, D.R. (1998) Hippocampal N-acetyl aspartate in unaffected siblings of patients with schizophrenia: a possible intermediate neurobiological phenotype. Biol Psychiatry 44: 941–950

Cannon, T.D., Kaprio, J., Lonnqvist, J., Huttunen, M., & Koskenvuo, M. (1998) The genetic epidemiology of schizophrenia in a Finnish twin cohort. A population-based modeling study. Arch Gen Psychiatry 55: 67–74

Casanova, M.F., & Rothberg B. (2002) Shape distortion of the hippocampus: a possible explanation of the pyramidal cell disarray reported in schizophrenia. Schizophr Res 55: 19–24

Chambers, R.A., Moore, J., Mcevoy, J.P., & Levin, E.D. (1996) Cognitive effects of neonatal hippocampal lesions in a rat model of schizophrenia. Neuropsychopharmacology 15: 587–594

Chaudhury, A.R., Gerecke, K.M., Wyss, J.M., Morgan, D.G., Gordon, M.N., & Carroll, S.L. (2003) Neuregulin-1 and erbB4 immunoreactivity is associated with neuritic plaques in Alzheimer disease brain and in a transgenic model of Alzheimer disease. J Neuropathol Exp Neurol 62: 42–54

Christison, G.W., Casanova, M.F., Weinberger, D.R., Rawlings, R., & Kleinman, J.E. (1989) A quantitative investigation of hippocampal pyramidal cell size, shape, and variability of orientation in schizophrenia. Arch Gen Psychiatry 46: 1027–1032

Colter, N., Battal, S., Crow, T.J., Johnstone, E.C., Brown, R., & Bruton, C. (1987) White matter reduction in the parahippocampal gyrus of patients with schizophrenia. Arch Gen Psychiatry 44: 1023

Conrad, A.J., Abebe, T., Austin, R., Forsythe, S., & Scheibel, A.B. (1991) Hippocampal pyramidal cell disarray in schizophrenia as a bilateral phenomenon. Arch Gen Psychiatry 48: 413–417

Cotter, D., Kerwin, R., Doshi, B., Martin, C.S., & Everall, I.P. (1997) Alterations in hippocampal non-phosphorylated MAP2 protein expression in schizophrenia. Brain Res 765: 238–46

Crow, T.J. (2007) How and why genetic linkage has not solved the problem of psychosis: review and hypothesis. Am J Psychiatry 164: 13–21

Crow, T.J., Ball, J., Bloom, S. R., Brown, R., Bruton, C.J., Colter, N., Frith, C.D., Johnstone, E.C., Owens, D.G., & Roberts, G.W. (1989) Schizophrenia as an anomaly of development of cerebral asymmetry. A postmortem study and a proposal concerning the genetic basis of the disease. Arch Gen Psychiatry 46: 1145–1150

Davis, K.L., Stewart, D.G., Friedman, J.I., Buchsbaum, M., Harvey, P.D., Hof, P.R., Buxbaum, J., & Haroutunian, V. (2003) White matter changes in schizophrenia: evidence for myelin-related dysfunction. Arch Gen Psychiatry 60: 443–456

Dracheva, S., Davis, K.L., Chin, B., Woo, D.A., Schmeidler, J., & Haroutunian, V. (2006) Myelin-associated mRNA and protein expression deficits in the anterior cingulate cortex and hippocampus in elderly schizophrenia patients. Neurobiol Dis 21: 531–540

Eyler, L.T., Jeste, D.V., & Brown, G.G. (2008) Brain response abnormalities during verbal learning among patients with schizophrenia. Psychiatry Res 162: 11–25

Falkai, P., & Bogerts B. (1986) Cell loss in the hippocampus of schizophrenics. Eur Arch Psychiatry Neurol Sci 236: 154–161

Falkai, P., Bogerts, B., Greve, B., Pfeiffer, U., Machus, B., Folsch-Reetz, B., Majtenyi, C., & Ovary, I. (1992) Loss of sylvian fissure asymmetry in schizophrenia. A quantitative post mortem study. Schizophr Res 7: 23–32

Falkai, P., Bogerts, B., & Rozumek, M. (1988) Limbic pathology in schizophrenia: the entorhinal region – a morphometric study. Biol Psychiatry 24: 515–521

Falkai, P., Honer, W.G., David, S., Bogerts, B., Majtenyi, C., & Bayer, T.A. (1999) No evidence for astrogliosis in brains of schizophrenic patients. A post-mortem study. Neuropathol Appl Neurobiol 25: 48–53

Falkai, P., Schneider-Axmann, T., & Honer, W.G. (2000) Entorhinal cortex pre-alpha cell clusters in schizophrenia: quantitative evidence of a developmental abnormality. Biol Psychiatry 47: 937–943

Falls, D.L. (2003) Neuregulins: functions, forms, and signaling strategies. Exp Cell Res 284: 14–30

Friston, K.J., & Frith C.D. (1995) Schizophrenia: a disconnection syndrome? Clin Neurosci 3: 89–97

Gerecke, K.M., Wyss, J.M., & Carroll, S.L. (2004) Neuregulin-1beta induces neurite extension and arborization in cultured hippocampal neurons. Mol Cell Neurosci 27: 379–393

Goldman-Rakic, P.S., Selemon, L.D., & Schwartz, M.L. (1984) Dual pathways connecting the dorsolateral prefrontal cortex with the hippocampal formation and parahippocampal cortex in the rhesus monkey. Neuroscience 12: 719–743

Grecksch, G., Bernstein, H.G., Becker, A., Hollt, V., & Bogerts, B. (1999) Disruption of latent inhibition in rats with postnatal hippocampal lesions. Neuropsychopharmacology 20: 525–532

Green, M.F., Satz, P., Gaier, D.J., Ganzell, S., & Kharabi, F. (1989) Minor physical anomalies in schizophrenia. Schizophr Bull 15: 91–99

Gruber, O., Falkai, P., Schneider-Axmann, T., Schwab, S.G., Wagner, M., & Maier, W. (2008) Neuregulin-1 haplotype HAP(ICE) is associated with lower hippocampal volumes in schizophrenic patients and in non-affected family members. J Psychiatr Res 19: 19

Hakak, Y., Walker, J.R., Li, C., Wong, W.H., Davis, K.L., Buxbaum, J.D., Haroutunian, V., & Fienberg, A.A. (2001) Genome-wide expression analysis reveals dysregulation of myelination-related genes in chronic schizophrenia. Proc Natl Acad Sci USA 98: 4746–4751

Hall, J., Whalley, H.C., Job, D.E., Baig, B.J., Mcintosh, A.M., Evans, K.L., Thomson, P.A., Porteous, D.J., Cunningham-Owens, D.G., Johnstone, E.C., & Lawrie, S.M. (2006) A neuregulin 1 variant associated with abnormal cortical function and psychotic symptoms. Nat Neurosci 9: 1477–1478

Harrison, P.J., & Eastwood S.L. (2001) Neuropathological studies of synaptic connectivity in the hippocampal formation in schizophrenia. Hippocampus 11: 508–519

Harrison, P.J., & Weinberger D.R. (2005) Schizophrenia genes, gene expression, and neuropathology: on the matter of their convergence. Mol Psychiatry 10: 40–68

Heckers, S., Heinsen, H., Geiger, B., & Beckmann, H. (1991) Hippocampal neuron number in schizophrenia. A stereological study. Arch Gen Psychiatry 48: 1002–1008

Highley, J.R., Walker, M.A., McDonald, B., Crow, T.J., & Esiri, M.M. (2003) Size of hippocampal pyramidal neurons in schizophrenia. Br J Psychiatry 183: 414–417

Hirayasu, Y., Shenton, M.E., Salisbury, D.F., Dickey, C.C., Fischer, I.A., Mazzoni, P., Kisler, T., Arakaki, H., Kwon, J.S., Anderson, J.E., Yurgelun-Todd, D., Tohen, M., & Mccarley, R.W. (1998) Lower left temporal lobe MRI volumes in patients with first-episode schizophrenia compared with psychotic patients with first-episode affective disorder and normal subjects. Am J Psychiatry 155: 1384–1391

Hof, P.R., Haroutunian, V., Copland, C., Davis, K.L., & Buxbaum, J.D. (2002) Molecular and cellular evidence for an oligodendrocyte abnormality in schizophrenia. Neurochem Res 27: 1193–1200

Hong, L.E., Wonodi, I., Stine, O.C., Mitchell, B.D., Thaker, G.K. (2008) Evidence of missense mutations on the neuregulin 1 gene affecting function of prepulse inhibition. Biol Psychiatry 63: 17–23

Jakob, H., & Beckmann H. (1986) Prenatal developmental disturbances in the limbic allocortex in schizophrenics. J Neural Transm 65: 303–326

Jaskiw, G.E., Juliano, D. M., Goldberg, T.E., Hertzman, M., Urow-Hamell, E., & Weinberger, D.R. (1994) Cerebral ventricular enlargement in schizophreniform disorder does not progress. A seven year follow-up study. Schizophr Res 14: 23–28

Jeste, D.V., & Lohr J.B. (1989) Hippocampal pathologic findings in schizophrenia. A morphometric study. Arch Gen Psychiatry 46: 1019–1024

Jones, P., Rodgers, B., Murray, R., & Marmot, M. (1994) Child development risk factors for adult schizophrenia in the British 1946 birth cohort. Lancet 344: 1398–1402

Kaplan, M.J., Lazoff, M., Kelly, K., Lukin, R., & Garver, D.L. (1990) Enlargement of cerebral third ventricle in psychotic patients with delayed response to neuroleptics. Biol Psychiatry 27: 205–214

Katsel, P., Davis, K.L., & Haroutunian, V. (2005) Variations in myelin and oligodendrocyte-related gene expression across multiple brain regions in schizophrenia: a gene ontology study. Schizophr Res 79: 157–173

Kovalenko, S., Bergmann, A., Schneider-Axmann, T., Ovary, I., Majtenyi, K., Havas, L., Honer, W.G., Bogerts, B., & Falkai, P. (2003) Regio entorhinalis in schizophrenia: more evidence for migrational disturbances and suggestions for a new biological hypothesis. Pharmacopsychiatry 36: S158–161

Kovelman, J.A., & Scheibel A.B. (1984) A neurohistological correlate of schizophrenia. Biol Psychiatry 19: 1601–1621

Kwon, O.B., Longart, M., Vullhorst, D., Hoffman, D.A., & Buonanno, A. (2005) Neuregulin-1 reverses long-term potentiation at CA1 hippocampal synapses. J Neurosci 25: 9378–9383

Lane, A., Kinsella, A., Murphy, P., Byrne, M., Keenan, J., Colgan, K., Cassidy, B., Sheppard, N., Horgan, R., Waddington, J.L., Larkin, C., & O'callaghan, E. (1997) The anthropometric assessment of dysmorphic features in schizophrenia as an index of its developmental origins. Psychol Med 27: 1155–1164

Law, A.J., Lipska, B.K., Weickert, C.S., Hyde, T.M., Straub, R.E., Hashimoto, R., Harrison, P.J., Kleinman, J.E., & Weinberger, D.R. (2006) Neuregulin 1 transcripts are differentially expressed in schizophrenia and regulated by 5' SNPs associated with the disease. Proc Natl Acad Sci USA 103: 6747–6752

Law, A.J., Shannon Weickert, C., Hyde, T.M., Kleinman, J.E., & Harrison, P.J. (2004a) Neuregulin-1 (NRG-1) mRNA and protein in the adult human brain. Neuroscience 127: 125–136

Law, A.J., Weickert, C.S., Hyde, T.M., Kleinman, J.E., & Harrison, P.J. (2004b) Reduced spinophilin but not microtubule-associated protein 2 expression in the hippocampal formation in schizophrenia and mood disorders: molecular evidence for a pathology of dendritic spines. Am J Psychiatry 161: 1848–1855

Le Pen, G., Gaudet, L., Mortas, P., Mory, R., & Moreau, J.L. (2002) Deficits in reward sensitivity in a neurodevelopmental rat model of schizophrenia. Psychopharmacology (Berl) 161: 434–441

Li, D., Collier, D.A., & He, L. (2006) Meta-analysis shows strong positive association of the neuregulin 1 (NRG1) gene with schizophrenia. Hum Mol Genet 15: 1995–2002

Lim, K.O., Ardekani, B.A., Nierenberg, J., Butler, P.D., Javitt, D.C., & Hoptman, M.J. (2006) Voxelwise correlational analyses of white matter integrity in multiple cognitive domains in schizophrenia. Am J Psychiatry 163: 2008–2010

Lipska, B.K. (2004) Using animal models to test a neurodevelopmental hypothesis of schizophrenia. J Psychiatry Neurosci 29: 282–286

Lipska, B.K., Aultman, J.M., Verma, A., Weinberger, D.R., & Moghaddam, B. (2002a) Neonatal damage of the ventral hippocampus impairs working memory in the rat. Neuropsychopharmacology 27: 47–54

Lipska, B.K., Halim, N.D., Segal, P.N., & Weinberger, D.R. (2002b) Effects of reversible inactivation of the neonatal ventral hippocampus on behavior in the adult rat. J Neurosci 22: 2835–2842

Lipska, B.K., Jaskiw, G.E., & Weinberger, D.R. (1993) Postpubertal emergence of hyperresponsiveness to stress and to amphetamine after neonatal excitotoxic hippocampal damage: a potential animal model of schizophrenia. Neuropsychopharmacology 9: 67–75

Lipska, B.K., Swerdlow, N.R., Geyer, M.A., Jaskiw, G.E., Braff, D.L., & Weinberger, D.R. (1995) Neonatal excitotoxic hippocampal damage in rats causes post-pubertal changes in prepulse inhibition of startle and its disruption by apomorphine. Psychopharmacology (Berl) 122: 35–43

Lipska, B.K., & Weinberger D.R. (2000) To model a psychiatric disorder in animals: schizophrenia as a reality test. Neuropsychopharmacology 23: 223–239

Maier, W., Zobel, A., & Rietschel, M. (2003) Genetics of schizophrenia and affective disorders. Pharmacopsychiatry 36: S195–202

McNeil, T.F., Cantor-Graae, E., Nordstrom, L.G., & Rosenlund, T. (1993) Head circumference in "preschizophrenic" and control neonates. Br J Psychiatry 162: 517–523

McNeil, T.F., Cantor-Graae, E., & Weinberger, D.R. (2000) Relationship of obstetric complications and differences in size of brain structures in monozygotic twin pairs discordant for schizophrenia. Am J Psychiatry 157: 203–212

Munafo, M.R., Attwood, A.S., & Flint, J. (2008) Neuregulin 1 genotype and schizophrenia. Schizophr Bull 34: 9–12

Munafo, M.R., Thiselton, D.L., Clark, T.G., & Flint, J. (2006) Association of the NRG1 gene and schizophrenia: a meta-analysis. Mol Psychiatry 11: 539–546

Nasrallah, H.A., Skinner, T.E., Schmalbrock, P., & Robitaille, P.M. (1994) Proton magnetic resonance spectroscopy (1H MRS) of the hippocampal formation in schizophrenia: a pilot study. Br J Psychiatry 165: 481–485

Nordahl, T.E., Kusubov, N., Carter, C., Salamat, S., Cummings, A.M., O'SHORA-Celaya, L., Eberling, J., Robertson, L., Huesman, R.H., Jagust, W., & Budinger, T.F. (1996) Temporal lobe metabolic differences in medication-free outpatients with schizophrenia via the PET-600. Neuropsychopharmacology 15: 541–554

Parlapani, E., Schmitt, A., Wirths, O., Bauer, M., Sommer, C., Rueb, U., Skowronek, M.H., Treutlein, J., Petroianu, G.A., Rietschel, M., & Falkai, P. (2008) Gene expression of neuregulin-1 isoforms in different brain regions of elderly schizophrenia patients. World J Biol Psychiatry 7: 1–8

Pegues, M.P., Rogers, L.J., Amend, D., Vinogradov, S., & Deicken, R.F. (2003) Anterior hippocampal volume reduction in male patients with schizophrenia. Schizophr Res 60: 105–115

Rametti, G., Segarra, N., Junque, C., Bargallo, N., Caldu, X., Ibarretxe, N., & Bernardo, M. (2007) Left posterior hippocampal density reduction using VBM and stereological MRI procedures in schizophrenia. Schizophr Res 961–3: 62–71

Rosoklija, G., Toomayan, G., Ellis, S.P., Keilp, J., Mann, J.J., Latov, N., Hays, A.P., & Dwork, A.J. (2000) Structural abnormalities of subicular dendrites in subjects with schizophrenia and mood disorders: preliminary findings. Arch Gen Psychiatry 57: 349–356

Sams-Dodd, F., Lipska, B.K., & Weinberger, D.R. (1997) Neonatal lesions of the rat ventral hippocampus result in hyperlocomotion and deficits in social behaviour in adulthood Psychopharmacology (Berl) 132: 303–310

Saykin, A.J., Shtasel, D.L., Gur, R.E., Kester, D.B., Mozley, L.H., Stafiniak, P., & Gur, R.C. (1994) Neuropsychological deficits in neuroleptic naive patients with first-episode schizophrenia. Arch Gen Psychiatry 51: 124–131

Schmitt, A., Parlapani, E., Gruber, O., Wobrock, T., & Falkai, P. (2008a) Impact of neuregulin-1 on the pathophysiology of schizophrenia in human post-mortem studies. Eur Arch Psychiatry Clin Neurosci 258: 35–39

Schmitt, A., Steyskal, C., Bernstein, H.G., Schneider-Axmann, T., Parlapani, E., Schaeffer, E.L., Gattaz, W.F., Bogerts, B., Schmitz, C., & Falkai, P. (2008b) Stereologic investigation of the posterior part of the hippocampus in schizophrenia. Acta Neuropathol 6: 6

Seidman, L.J., Faraone, S.V., Goldstein, J.M., Kremen, W.S., Horton, N.J., Makris, N., Toomey, R., Kennedy, D., Caviness, V.S., & Tsuang, M.T. (2002) Left hippocampal volume as a vulnerability indicator for schizophrenia: a magnetic resonance imaging morphometric study of nonpsychotic first-degree relatives. Arch Gen Psychiatry 59: 839–849

Shenton, M.E., Dickey, C.C., Frumin, M., & Mccarley, R.W. (2001) A review of MRI findings in schizophrenia. Schizophr Res 49: 1–52

Stark, A.K., Uylings, H.B., Sanz-Arigita, E., & Pakkenberg, B. (2004) Glial cell loss in the anterior cingulate cortex, a subregion of the prefrontal cortex, in subjects with schizophrenia. Am J Psychiatry 161: 882–888

Stefansson, H., Sigurdsson, E., Steinthorsdottir, V., Bjornsdottir, S., Sigmundsson, T., Ghosh, S., Brynjolfsson, J., Gunnarsdottir, S., Ivarsson, O., Chou, T.T., Hjaltason, O., et al. (2002) Neuregulin 1 and susceptibility to schizophrenia. Am J Hum Genet 71: 877–892

Stevens, J.R. (1982) Neuropathology of schizophrenia. Arch Gen Psychiatry 39: 1131–1139

Szeszko, P.R., Goldberg, E., Gunduz-Bruce, H., Ashtari, M., Robinson, D., Malhotra, A.K., Lencz, T., Bates, J., Crandall, D.T., Kane, J.M., & Bilder, R.M. (2003) Smaller anterior hippocampal formation volume in antipsychotic-naive patients with first-episode schizophrenia. Am J Psychiatry 160: 2190–2197

Talamini, L.M., Meeter, M., Elvevag, B., Murre, J.M., & Goldberg, T.E. (2005) Reduced parahippocampal connectivity produces schizophrenia-like memory deficits in simulated neural circuits with reduced parahippocampal connectivity. Arch Gen Psychiatry 62: 485–493

Tregellas, J.R., Tanabe, J.L., Miller, D.E., Ross, R.G., Olincy, A., & Freedman, R. (2004) Neurobiology of smooth pursuit eye movement deficits in schizophrenia: an fMRI study. Am J Psychiatry 161: 315–321

Uranova, N.A., Vostrikov, V.M., Vikhreva, O.V., Zimina, I.S., Kolomeets, N.S., & Orlovskaya, D.D. (2007) The role of oligodendrocyte pathology in schizophrenia. Int J Neuropsychopharmacol 10: 537–545

Van Erp, T.G., Saleh, P.A., Rosso, I.M., Huttunen, M., Lonnqvist, J., Pirkola, T., Salonen, O., Valanne, L., Poutanen, V.P., Standertskjold-Nordenstam, C.G., & Cannon, T.D. (2002) Contributions of genetic risk and fetal hypoxia to hippocampal volume in patients with schizophrenia or schizoaffective disorder, their unaffected siblings, and healthy unrelated volunteers. Am J Psychiatry 159: 1514–1520

Velakoulis, D., Pantelis, C., Mcgorry, P.D., Dudgeon, P., Brewer, W., Cook, M., Desmond, P., Bridle, N., Tierney, P., Murrie, V., Singh, B., & Copolov, D. (1999) Hippocampal volume in first-episode psychoses and chronic schizophrenia: a high-resolution magnetic resonance imaging study. Arch Gen Psychiatry 56: 133–141

Velakoulis, D., Stuart, G.W., Wood, S.J., Smith, D.J., Brewer, W.J., Desmond, P., Singh, B., Copolov, D., & Pantelis, C. (2001) Selective bilateral hippocampal volume loss in chronic schizophrenia. Biol Psychiatry 50: 531–539

Walker, M.A., Highley, J.R., Esiri, M.M., Mcdonald, B., Roberts, H.C., Evans, S.P., & Crow, T.J. (2002) Estimated neuronal populations and volumes of the hippocampus and its subfields in schizophrenia. Am J Psychiatry 159: 821–828

Wan, R.Q., Giovanni, A., Kafka, S.H., & Corbett, R. (1996) Neonatal hippocampal lesions induced hyperresponsiveness to amphetamine: behavioral and in vivo microdialysis studies. Behav Brain Res 78: 211–223

Weinberger, D.R. (1996) On the plausibility of "the neurodevelopmental hypothesis" of schizophrenia. Neuropsychopharmacology 14: 1S–11S

Weinberger, D.R. (1999)Cell biology of the hippocampal formation in schizophrenia. Biol Psychiatry 45: 395–402

Winterer, G., Konrad, A., Vucurevic, G., Musso, F., Stoeter, P., & Dahmen, N. (2008) Association of 5' end neuregulin-1 (NRG1) gene variation with subcortical medial frontal microstructure in humans. Neuroimage 40: 712–718

Wright, I.C., Rabe-Hesketh, S., Woodruff, P.W., David, A.S., Murray, R.M., & Bullmore, E.T. (2000) Meta-analysis of regional brain volumes in schizophrenia. Am J Psychiatry 157: 16–25

Yamasue, H., Iwanami, A., Hirayasu, Y., Yamada, H., Abe, O., Kuroki, N., Fukuda, R., Tsujii, K., Aoki, S., Ohtomo, K., Kato, N., & Kasai, K. (2004) Localized volume reduction in prefrontal, temporolimbic, and paralimbic regions in schizophrenia: an MRI parcellation study. Psychiatry Res 131: 195–207

Zaidel, D.W., Esiri, M.M., & Harrison, P.J. (1997a) The hippocampus in schizophrenia: lateralized increase in neuronal density and altered cytoarchitectural asymmetry. Psychol Med 27: 703–713

Zaidel, D.W., Esiri, M.M., & Harrison, P.J. (1997b) Size, shape, and orientation of neurons in the left and right hippocampus: investigation of normal asymmetries and alterations in schizophrenia. Am J Psychiatry 154: 812–818

Zhang, Z., Sun, J., & Reynolds, G.P. (2002) A selective reduction in the relative density of parvalbumin-immunoreactive neurons in the hippocampus in schizophrenia patients. Chin Med J (Engl) 115: 819–823

Zhou, Y., Shu, N., Liu, Y., Song, M., Hao, Y., Liu, H., Yu, C., Liu, Z., & Jiang, T. (2008) Altered resting-state functional connectivity and anatomical connectivity of hippocampus in schizophrenia. Schizophr Res 100: 120–132

Molecular Neuroimaging, Pathophysiological Mechanisms, and Drug Discovery

Philip McGuire

Introduction

This chapter aims to review recent neuroimaging studies that have investigated the relationship between neurochemical dysfunction in psychosis and alterations in regional brain structure and function. It will focus on studies in subjects with an at-risk mental state (ARMS), who have a very high risk of developing psychosis within 1–2 years (Yung et al. 1998). Research in this population provides a powerful means of investigating the mechanisms underlying the onset of psychosis, as the same individuals can be studied before and after the onset of illness. Moreover, as most of the subjects are medication naïve, the results are not confounded by the effects of antipsychotic treatment.

Dopamine Dysfunction in Psychosis

A series of PET and SPET studies have shown that schizophrenia is associated with increased capacity for dopamine synthesis, as measured by the striatal uptake of 18-FDopa, and with increased synaptic release of dopamine in the striatum in response to the experimental administration of amphetamine (reviewed in Howes et al. 2007). However, the stage of schizophrenia when dopamine dysfunction is first evident is unclear. We addressed this issue by using PET to study 18-FDopa uptake in subjects with an ARMS. The subjects were recruited through OASIS (Outreach And Support In South London; Broome et al. 2005), a specialised clinical service for this group in South London. They were compared with healthy controls and a group of patients with first-episode psychosis. This revealed that striatal dopamine function was not only elevated in patients who had recently developed psychosis but also increased in subjects who were not psychotic, but at high risk (Howes et al. 2009). The findings were localised to the associative subdivision of the striatum, which is functionally

P. McGuire (✉)
Section of Neuroimaging, Institute of Psychiatry, London
e-mail: p.mcguire@iop.kcl.ac.uk

W.F. Gattaz, G. Busatto (eds.), *Advances in Schizophrenia Research 2009*,
DOI 10.1007/978-1-4419-0913-8_8, © Springer Science+Business Media, LLC 2010

connected to the prefrontal cortex (McGuire et al. 1991). Within the ARMS sample, the magnitude of the elevation in dopamine function was directly correlated with the severity of prodromal symptoms and with the degree to which performance was impaired on a verbal fluency task. The latter is consistent with the involvement of the associative striatum, as verbal fluency is a task of executive functions, which are normally mediated in prefrontal cortex.

We then sought to examine the relationship between striatal dopamine dysfunction and cognitive dysfunction more directly. In these studies, we used both 18-FDopa PET and functional MRI in the same individuals. We then investigated the extent to which striatal dopamine dysfunction was related to alterations in cortical activation during the performance of cognitive tasks. When performing a verbal fluency paradigm, subjects with an ARMS showed greater activation in prefrontal cortex during the task than controls. The severity of this change in prefrontal function was positively correlated with the elevation in striatal dopamine function (Fusar-Poli et al. 2008). When performing the N-back working memory task, ARMS subjects showed less prefrontal activation than controls. Again, the severity of the alteration in prefrontal activation was correlated with the degree to which striatal dopamine function was elevated in the ARMS group (Fusar-Poli et al. 2009b). Prefrontal activation during the N-back task and striatal dopamine function were also correlated in controls, but the direction of the correlation was negative, the opposite to that in the ARMS sample. This may reflect a shift in the position of ARMS subjects on the putative inverted U-shaped curve that denotes the relationship between dopamine activity and prefrontal efficiency (Williams and Castner 2006).

Glutamate Dysfunction in Psychosis

The glutamate model of psychosis proposes that altered NDMA receptor function is a critical factor in the disorder (Olney and Farber 1995; Goff and Coyle 2001). While there is great interest in the development of SPET and PET tracers for the NMDA receptor (Pilowsky et al. 2006), at present, no radiotracer that is widely accepted as being specific for this receptor in man is available. However, glutamate function can be assessed in vivo using magnetic resonance spectroscopy (MRS), which provides measures of glutamate and glutamine levels in selected regions of interest. Application of this technique in schizophrenia suggests that glutamate levels are increased in the anterior cingulate cortex and the thalamus (Theberge et al. 2002, 2003). In order to investigate the stage of psychosis at which glutamate dysfunction develops, we used MRS in subjects with an ARMS. This revealed that the ARMS was associated with a reduction in thalamic glutamate levels but an increase in anterior cingulated glutamine levels (Stone et al. 2009). Furthermore, concurrent volumetric MRI in the same subjects indicated that the severity of the reduction in thalamic glutamate in the ARMS group was correlated with reductions in grey matter volume in the medial temporal, lateral temporal, and prefrontal cortex (Stone et al. 2009). These observations suggest that glutamatergic dysfunction predates the onset of psychosis and might underlie some of the reductions in regional cortical grey matter volume that occur in psychotic disorders. Glutamate can have neurotoxic effects through its action on NMDA receptors (Deutsch et al. 2001), and altered glutamate function might thus contribute to longitudinal changes in grey matter volume that occur when ARMS subjects develop psychosis (Pantelis et al. 2003; Borgwardt et al. 2008). Longitudinal neuroimaging studies of dopamine and glutamate function in the ARMS are ongoing and the results may clarify the role of alterations in these neurochemical systems in the onset of psychosis.

Endocannabinoids and Psychosis

Cannabis is the world's most widely used illicit drug and its use in healthy people can induce acute psychotic symptoms and impair performance on tasks of memory and executive functions (McGuire et al. 1994; Ranganathan and D'Souza 2006). In the longer term, regular cannabis use, particularly when it begins in adolescence, appears to significantly increase the risk of the subsequent incidence of psychotic disorders (Moore et al. 2007). Regular use can also lead to long-term impairments in memory function (Solowij et al. 2002). While there is thus considerable evidence linking cannabis use with psychosis, how cannabis acts on the brain to produce these effects is less clear. Neuroimaging provides a way to examine this in vivo.

The cannabis plant contains over 60 cannabinoids. The major psychoactive constituent is delta-9-tetrahydrocanabinol (THC), which is thought to be responsible for most of the psychotropic effects of cannabis. It can induce acute psychotic symptoms, anxiety, and impair verbal learning (Ranganathan and D'Souza 2006). The other major ingredient of cannabis is cannabidiol (CBD), which has anxiolytic effects, may have antipsychotic actions, and does not appear to impair cognitive performance (Zuardi et al. 2006). We investigated the effects of these cannabinoids by combining their experimental administration with functional MRI. In healthy volunteers, THC induced acute psychotic symptoms and altered hippocampal activation during a verbal learning task. Moreover, its effect on psychotic symptoms was directly correlated with its effect on activation in the striatum, suggesting that this effect may be mediated via this region, consistent with evidence that THC may induce striatal dopamine release (Bhattacharyya et al. 2009a). In contrast, CBD modulated activation in the amygdala and cingulate cortex during the visual processing of fearful faces, which provoke anxiety (Fusar-Poli et al. 2009a). The magnitude of its effect on amygdalar function was correlated with its concurrent effect on skin conductance, a measure of autonomic arousal. These data suggest that the anxiolytic effects of CBD are mediated in limbic brain areas. When the effects of THC and CBD were compared with each other in the same subjects, they often had opposite effects on activation relative to those of placebo. For example, during a verbal learning task, THC attenuated activation in the striatum, whereas CBD was associated with striatal activation. These data are consistent with behavioural evidence that pre-treatment with CBD can abolish the acute effects of THC on psychotic symptoms (Bhattacharyya et al. 2009b) and reports that CBD may have an antipsychotic effect in patients with schizophrenia (Zuardi et al. 2006).

Implications for Drug Development

These studies indicate that dopamine, glutamate, and endocannabinoids may all play a role in the pathophysiology of psychosis and that alterations in neurochemical function are evident well before the clinical expression of psychosis. Moreover, these changes appear to be associated with some of the neurocognitive and structural imaging abnormalities that are features of psychosis.

Evidence that dopamine dysfunction is elevated in the ARMS is consistent with reports that antipsychotic medication can ameliorate attenuated psychotic symptoms in the ARMS (Ruhrmann et al. 2007; Woods et al. 2007) and may reduce the risk of transition to psychosis (McGorry et al. 2002; McGlashan et al. 2007). Our findings of altered glutamate levels in the ARMS support the glutamate model of psychosis and suggest that drugs that act on the glutamate system may be useful in the treatment of psychosis. A recent report suggests that a new compound that acts on mGlu2/3 receptors is an effective antipsychotic in schizophrenia (Patil et al. 2007). Our data on the opposite effects of CBD to THC are consistent with evidence that CBD may have antipsychotic effects in schizophrenia (Zuardi et al. 2006) and suggest that cannabinoids may have therapeutic applications (Robson 2001). The presence of neurochemical changes in the ARMS suggests that drugs which act on dopamine, glutamate, and the endocannabinoid system may be particularly useful if administered before the first episode of psychosis, when the underlying pathophysiological processes may still be active (McGuire et al. 2008).

References

Bhattacharyya, S., Fusar-Poli, P., Borgwardt, S., Martin-Santos, R., Nosarti, C., O'carroll, C., Allen, P., Seal, M., Fletcher, P., Crippa, J., Mechelli, A., Atakan, Z., McGuire, P. (2009a) Delta-9-tetrahydrocannabinol modulates medial temporal and striatal function in humans: a neural basis for the effects of cannabis on learning & psychosis. Archives of General Psychiatry 66: 442–451

Bhattacharyya, S., Morrison, P., Fusar-Poli, P., Martin-Santos, R., Borgwardt, S., Winton-Brown, T., Nosarti, C., O'carroll, C., Seal, M., Allen, P., Mehta, M., Giampietro, V., Kapur, S., Murray, R., Zuardi, A., Crippa, J., Atakan, Z., McGuire, P. (2009b) Opposite effects of delta-9-tetrahydrocannabinol and cannabidiol on human brain function and psychopathology. Neuropsychopharmacology (in press)

Borgwardt, S., McGuire, P., Aston, J., Gschwandtner, U., Pfluger, M., Stieglitz, R., Radue, E.W., Reicher-Rossler, A. (2008) Reductions in frontal temporal and parietal volume associated with the onset of psychosis. Schizophrenia Research 106: 108–114

Broome, M.R., Woolley, J.B., Johns, L.C., Valmaggia, L.R., Tabraham, P., Gafoor, R., Bramon, E., McGuire, P.K. (2005) Outreach and support in south London (OASIS): Implementation of a clinical service for prodromal psychosis and the at risk mental state. European Psychiatry 20: 5–6, 372–378

Deutsch, S.I., Rosse, R.B., Schwartz, B.L., Mastropaolo, J. (2001) A revised excitotoxic hypothesis of schizophrenia: therapeutic implications. Clinical Neuropharmacology 24: 43–49

Fusar-Poli, P., Howes, O., Allen, P., Broome, M., Valli, I., Montgomery, A., Grasby, P., McGuire, P. (2008) Dopaminergicmodulation of prefrontal functioning in subjects at clinical risk for psychosis: a combined pet–fmri study. Schizophrenia Research 102: 30

Fusar-Poli, P., Crippa, J., Bhattacharyya, S., Borgwardt, S., Allen, P, Martin-Santos, R., Seal, M., Surguladze, S., O'carroll, C., Atakan, Z., McGuire, P. (2009a) Distinct effects of Δ9-tetrahydrocannabinol and cannabidiol on neural activation during emotional processing. Archives of General Psychiatry 66: 95–105

Fusar-Poli, P., Howes, O., Allen, P., Broome, M., Valli, I., Montgomery, A., Grasby, P., McGuire, P. (2009b) Altered prefrontal structure and function predicts elevated striatal dopamine function in subjects at high risk of psychosis. Altered prefrontal activation directly related to striatal dopamine dysfunction in people with prodromal symptoms of schizophrenia. *Molecular Psychiatry* (In Press)

Goff, D.C., Coyle, J.T. (2001) The emerging role of glutamate in the pathophysiology and treatment of schizophrenia. American Journal of Psychiatry 158: 1367–1377

Howes, O., Montgomery, A., Asselin, M.C., Murray, R.M., Grasby, P., McGuire, P. (2007) Molecular imaging studies of the striatal dopamineric system and prediction in the prodromal phase of psychosis. British Journal of Psychiatry 191: 13–18

Howes, O., Montgomery, A., Asselin, M.C., Murray, R., Bramon-Bosch, E., Valmaggia, L., Johns, L., Broome, M., Grasby, P., McGuire, P. (2009) Elevated striatal dopamine function linked to prodromal signs of schizophrenia. Archives of General Psychiatry 66: 13–20

McGlashan, T., Zipursky, R.B., Perkins, D., Addington, J., Miller, T., Woods, S.W., Hawkins K.A., Hoffman, R.E., Preda, A., Epstein, I., Addington, D., Lindborg, S., Trzaskoma, Q., Tohen, M., Breier, A. (2006) Randomized, double-blind trial of olanzapine versus placebo in patients prodromally symptomatic for psychosis. American J Psychiatry 163: 790–799

McGorry, P.D. Yung A.R., Phillips L.J., Yuen H.P., Francey S., Cosgrave E.M., et al. (2002) Randomized controlled trial of interventions designed to reduce the risk of progression to first-episode psychosis in a clinical sample with subthreshold symptoms. Archives of General Psychiatry 59: 921–928

McGuire, P.K., Bates, J., Goldman-Rakic, P.S. (1991) Interhemispheric integration II: Symmetry and convergence of the corticostriatal connections of the left and right principal sulcus (PS) and the left and right supplementary motor area (SMA) in the rhesus monkey. Cerebral Cortex 1: 408–417

McGuire, P.K., Jones, P., Bebbington, P., Toone, B.K., Lewis, S.W., Murray, R.M. (1994) Cannabis and acute psychosis. Schizophrenia Research 13: 161–168

McGuire, P., Howes, O., Stone, J., Fusar-Poli, P. (2008) Functional neuroimaging as a tool for drug development in schizophrenia. Trends in Pharmacological Sciences 29: 91–98

Moore, T.H., Zammit, S., Lingford-Hughes, A., et al. (2007) Cannabis use and risk of psychotic or affective mental health outcomes: a systematic review. Lancet Jul 28; 370 (9584): 319–328

Olney, J.W., Farber, N.B. (1995) Glutamate receptor dysfunction and schizophrenia. Archives of General Psychiatry 52: 998–1007

Pantelis, C., Velakoulis, D., McGorry, P., Wood, S., Suckling, J., Phillips, L., Yung, A., Bullmore, E., Brewer, W., Soulsby, B., Desmond, P., McGuire, P.K. (2003) Neuroanatomical abnormalities in people who develop psychosis. Lancet 361: 281–288

Patil, S.T., Zhang, L., Marteny, F., Lowe, S., Jackson, K., Andreev, B., Avedisova, A., Bardenstein, L., Gurovich, I., Morozova, M., Mosolov, S., Neznanov, N., Reznik, A., Smulevich, A., Tochilov, V., Johnson, B., Monn, J., Schoepp, D. (2007) Activation of mGlu2/3 receptors as a new approach to treat schizophrenia: a randomised Phase 2 clinical trial. Nature Medicine 13: 1102–1107

Pilowsky, L.S., Bressan, R.A., Stone, J.M., Erlandsson, K., Mulligan, R.S., Krystal, J.H., et al. (2006) First in vivo evidence of an NMDA receptor deficit in medication-free schizophrenic patients. Molecular Psychiatry 11: 118–119

Ranganathan, M., D'Souza, D.C. (2006) The acute effects of cannabinoids on memory in humans: a review. Psychopharmacology (Berl) 188(4): 425–444

Robson, P. (2001) Therapeutic aspects of cannabis and cannabinoids. British Journal of Psychiatry 178: 107–115

Ruhrmann, S., Bechdolf, A., Kühn, K., Wagner, M., Schultze-Lutter, F., Janssen, B., Maurer, K., Häfner, H., Gaebel, W., Möller, H., Maier, W., Klosterkötter, J. (2007) Acute effects of treatment for prodromal symptoms for people putatively in a late initial prodromal state of psychosis. British Journal of Psychiatry 191: s88–s95

Solowij, N., Stephens, R.S., Roffman, R.A., et al. (2002) Cognitive functioning of long-term heavy cannabis users seeking treatment. JAMA 287(9): 1123–1131, Mar 6, 2002

Stone, J., Day, F., Tsagaraki, H., Valli, I., McLean, M., Lythgoe, D., O'Gorman, M., Barker, G., McGuire, P. (2009) Glutamate dysfunction in people with prodromal symptoms of psychosis: relationship to gray matter volume. Biological Psychiatry 66: 533–539

Theberge, J., Bartha, R., Drost, D.J., Menon, R.S., Malla, A., Takhar, J., et al. (2002) Glutamate and glutamine measured with 4.0 T proton MRS in never-treated patients with schizophrenia and healthy volunteers. American Journal of Psychiatry 159: 1944–1946

Theberge, J., Al-Semaan, Y., Williamson, P.C., Menon, R.S., Neufeld, R.W., Rajakumar, N., et al. (2003) Glutamate and glutamine in the anterior cingulate and thalamus of medicated patients with chronic schizophrenia and healthy comparison subjects measured with 4.0-T proton MRS. American Journal of Psychiatry 160: 2231–2233

Williams, G.V., Castner, S.A. (2006) Under the curve: critical issues for elucidating D1 receptor function in working memory. Neuroscience 139(1): 263–276

Woods, S.W., Tully, E.M., Walsh, B.C., Hawkins, K.A., Callahan, J.L., Cohen, S.J., Mathalon, D.H., Miller, T.H., McGlashan, T.H. (2007) Aripiprazole in the treatment of the psychosis prodrome: an open-label pilot study. British Journal of Psychiatry 191: s96–s101

Yung, A.R., Phillips, L.J., McGorry, P.D., McFarlane, C.A., Francey, S., Harrigan, S., Patton, G.C., Jackson, H.J. (1998) Prediction of psychosis – a step towards indicated prevention in schizophrenia. British Journal of Psychiatry 172: 14–20

Zuardi, A.W., Crippa, J.A., Hallak, J.E., Moreira, A., Guimaraes, F.S. (2006) Cannabidiol, a Cannabis sativa constituent, as an antipsychotic drug. Brazilian Journal of Medical and Biological Research 39(4): 421–429

Part III
Genetics

Animal Models of Schizophrenia: Focus on Hippocampal Disruption of Dopamine System Regulation

Anthony A. Grace

Introduction

For the past 40 years, the dominant hypothesis of schizophrenia has centered on a disruption of dopamine (DA) signaling. This is based on a variety of evidence, including the finding that drugs that release DA will cause psychosis in normal individuals and exacerbate the positive symptoms of schizophrenia in patients (Angrist et al., 1974, 1980), and drugs that are effective antipsychotic drugs block DA receptors (Carlsson and Lindqvist, 1963) and are given at doses that are selective for D2 receptor blockade (Seeman et al., 1976; Kapur and Remington, 2001). However, a careful analysis of this information suggests that a simple hyperdopaminergic state may not adequately explain schizophrenia pathophysiology. Thus, amphetamine will mimic a paranoid psychosis; however, it does so when given at doses that increase DA turnover 20- to 30-fold (Carboni et al., 1989), whereas the baseline level of DA metabolites in untreated schizophrenia patients is not substantially different from normal individuals (Bowers, 1974; Post et al., 1975; Berger et al., 1980). Furthermore, while antipsychotic drugs will maximally bind DA receptors (Seeman, 2002), produce behavioral actions (Janssen et al., 1965), and block the effects of DA agonists (Randrup and Munkvad, 1965; Del Rio and Fuentes, 1969) within minutes of administration, it takes time for the drugs to reach maximal efficacy (Johnstone et al., 1978; Pickar et al., 1984, 1986). These data suggest that the DA system itself is normal; however, it is believed to be regulated in an abnormal manner (Grace, 1991, 2000; Bertolino et al., 1999). Thus, although basal DA levels are comparatively normal, studies show that low doses of amphetamine will cause significantly higher levels of DA release in schizophrenia patients when tested using raclopride displacement, and the level of increased DA release is proportional to the propensity of the amphetamine to worsen psychosis (Laruelle et al., 1996). Therefore, recent research has focused on identifying the source of

A.A. Grace (✉)
Departments of Neuroscience, Psychiatry and Psychology, A210 Langley Hall, University of Pittsburgh, Pittsburgh, PA 15260, USA
e-mail: graceaa@pitt.edu

W.F. Gattaz, G. Busatto (eds.), *Advances in Schizophrenia Research 2009*,
DOI 10.1007/978-1-4419-0913-8_9, © Springer Science+Business Media, LLC 2010

DA system disruption and the development of novel therapeutic agents to address this deficit.

Glutamate and the Developmental Model of Schizophrenia

There has been an emerging shift in concepts regarding the pathophysiology of schizophrenia. Much of this began with the recognition that drugs that alter glutamate transmission, such as phencyclidine (PCP) and ketamine, can effectively mimic psychosis in humans (Javitt and Zukin, 1991; Lahti et al., 1995); moreover, they can produce a symptom-specific, long-duration exacerbation of schizophrenia in patients to an extent that the patients cannot distinguish it from a relapse. This has occurred with emerging evidence for disrupted function in glutamatergic cortical structures, such as the prefrontal cortex (Weinberger and Berman, 1996; Goldman-Rakic, 1999; Weinberger et al., 2001), and the focus on disruptions of working memory in schizophrenia patients. Thus, in control patients, there is an activation of the dorsolateral PFC during working memory tasks (Berman et al., 1995), whereas in schizophrenia patients there is a failure to activate the dorsolateral PFC that is associated with a failure to perform working memory tasks (Weinberger and Berman, 1996; Manoach, 2003). The hippocampus has also attracted substantial attention, given early evidence of a pathology within this structure (Heckers et al., 1991; Shenton et al., 1992; Arnold, 1997).

The relevance of alterations in function in the hippocampus and PFC has become more ingrained with the concept that schizophrenia is a developmentally determined disorder, with the emergent pathophysiology centered around limbic cortical system dysfunction. The first evidence that drove this line of thinking was by Lipska and Weinberger who, drawing from studies demonstrating decreased hippocampal volume in the afflicted monozygotic twin discordant for schizophrenia (Goldberg et al., 1994), demonstrated that a neonatal lesion of the ventral hippocampal region of a rat can recapitulate many of the symptom states, including hypersensitivity to amphetamine, observed in the schizophrenia patient (Lipska et al., 1993). This has given rise to a number of models based on disrupted development, ranging from early life stress through genetic manipulations.

This developmental disruption approach has engendered a wide array of approaches to study the etiology and pathophysiology of schizophrenia. Of course, schizophrenia patients at the first break do not show a "hole" in their hippocampus, as is present with the neonatal ventral hippocampal lesion. However, other models that take advantage of developmental disruption have also identified dysfunctions in the hippocampus. One model in particular utilizes administration of a DNA methylating mitotoxin, methyl azoxymethanol acetate (MAM; Johnston et al., 1981). It has been known for some time that risk factors presented to pregnant women during the second trimester lead to a higher incidence of schizophrenia births (Pilowsky et al., 1993; McDonald and Murray, 2000). Using this as a guide, MAM was administered to pregnant rats on gestation day 17, which was functionally equivalent to the human second trimester and is a time when limbic cortical regions are developing (Moore and Grace, 1997; Grace and Moore, 1998; Moore et al., 2006). When examined as adults, MAM-treated rats demonstrated a number of pathologies consistent with what one would expect for an animal model of schizophrenia, including thinning of limbic cortical structures with an increase in cell packing density, indicative of a loss in neuropil rather than cell loss (Moore et al., 2006), which is consistent with what is reported in schizophrenia patients (Harrison, 1999). The rats also exhibit deficits in executive function (Gourevitch et al., 2004; Moore et al., 2006), disrupted social interactions (Talamini et al., 1999), and sensory gating abnormalities, such as prepulse inhibition of startle (Talamini et al., 2000; Moore et al., 2006) and latent inhibition (Lodge et al., 2009). Moreover, there are alterations in responses to drugs similar to that reported in schizophrenia patients, including hyperresponsivity to amphetamine in the postpubertal rat but not prepubertally (Flagstad et al., 2004; Moore et al., 2006) and a heightened response to PCP (Moore et al., 2006). Given this identification, we proceeded to examine the types of functional alterations that are present neurophysiologically in the MAM-treated adult rat.

Hippocampal Dysfunction and Dopamine System Dysregulation

Studies show that neurons in the nucleus accumbens (NAc; O'Donnell and Grace, 1995) and the medial prefrontal cortex (mPFC; West et al., 2002) exhibit bistable membrane potential states, in which the membrane potential is driven from a hyperpolarized, nonfiring state to a depolarized state. Only NAc neurons in the depolarized state can fire action potentials. In general, a stimulus arriving in the hyperpolarized or "down" state will not cause the neuron to fire; however, if it arrives when the neuron is in the "up" state, the NAc neuron is more likely to fire an action potential and transmit information. Therefore, the transition between these two states serves as a type of gating of information flow. Studies indicate that the determinant of these up–down states is input from the ventral subiculum of the hippocampus (vSub). If the vSub input is blocked, NAc neurons fail to show these state transitions (O'Donnell and Grace, 1995). This is believed to be essential in the gating of information flow in the NAc. The vSub itself is believed to play an important role in gating information related to context (Jarrard, 1995; Maren, 1999; Sharp, 1999; Fanselow, 2000; Maren and Quirk, 2004). The ability to interpret a stimulus based on context is an important mechanism in information processing. Thus, stimuli can have very different interpretations based on context. For example, say the stimulus is someone pointing at you. How this stimulus is interpreted will have very different meanings in different contexts. A friend pointing to you in a party may be interpreted in a friendly manner as a way of introduction; however, pointing to someone in a police lineup has a very different connotation. A functioning vSub is believed to be essential in evaluating context. Moreover, schizophrenia patients are known to be deficient in contextual references (Cho et al., 2005; Weiss et al., 2006).

In the MAM-treated rat, we found that the up–down states of neurons in the NAc and the mPFC are disrupted (Moore et al., 2006). Specifically, particularly in the NAc, the neurons do not make transitions between the up and down states; instead, most neurons appear to be tonically in the "up" or transmissive state. As a result, the neurons should be reactive to all stimuli without any contextual filtering or interpretation. A result could be that the individual would be bombarded with sensory input with no ability to focus on important stimuli within a relevant context, but instead interpret all stimuli as salient, self-referential, potentially threatening, and requiring a response. Interestingly, administration of PCP to a rat also eliminates up–down state transitions in NAc neurons (O'Donnell and Grace, 1998), thereby mimicking this disruption in contextual processing.

The above data demonstrate that the vSub is altered in the MAM-treated rat, in that it appears to be driving NAc neurons into a constant "up" state. Moreover, we have demonstrated that MAM-treated rats show a hyperresponsive DA system. Studies of schizophrenia patients suggest that the activity within the hippocampus is correlated with a psychotic state (Krieckhaus et al., 1992; Venables, 1992; Silbersweig et al., 1995), which should indicate a DA-dependent action. However, the vSub does not project directly to the ventral tegmental area (VTA) DA neurons. How would changes in the vSub affect DA neuron activity? We found that nonspecific activation of the vSub will produce a unique action on VTA DA neurons. Specifically, if the vSub is activated by injection of the glutamatergic agonist NMDA, the result is an increase in the number of DA neurons firing. In the normal state, the population of DA neurons exists either in a spontaneously firing mode or in a condition in which the neurons are hyperpolarized and inactive. The neurons are held in the hyperpolarized, inactive state due to a potent GABAergic inhibition arising from the ventral pallidum. Upon activation of the vSub, the vSub provides a powerful glutamatergic excitation of the NAc, which in turn inhibits the ventral pallidum and releases VTA DA neurons from inhibition (Figure 1). Only DA neurons that are in a spontaneously firing state can respond to external stimuli by emitting a burst of action potentials, burst firing being the behaviorally salient output of the DA system (Schultz, 1998).

The vSub therefore exerts a unique influence on the DA system; by controlling the number of DA neurons active, it provides the "gain" of the DA system to a signal. Thus, if an external signal arrives at the VTA and most of the DA neurons are not active, the number driven to a burst firing state is also small as is the DA signal reaching postsynaptic sites. However, if the vSub causes most of the DA neurons to be active, then the same stimulus will cause a much greater DA output (Lodge and Grace, 2006). This can be seen as a function of context; in a benign context, the vSub would not be providing a strong drive to the DA neurons and a stimulus will not create a large response from the DA neuron population. However, if the environment is highly threatening or potentially highly rewarding, requiring a heightened state of vigilance, the vSub would cause more of the neurons to be active, thereby amplifying the resultant DA signal generated to the external event.

Of course, to be effective, the vSub activity must be matched effectively to the context; a constant state of vSub overdrive would cause the subject to be unable

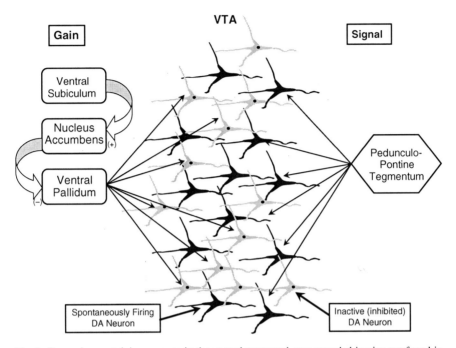

Fig. 1 Dopamine-containing neurons in the ventral tegmental area recorded in vivo are found in several activity states. First, the neurons can be either in a spontaneously firing state (black neurons) or in an inhibited, nonfiring state (gray neurons). Whether a DA neuron is firing or not is controlled by the ventral subiculum of the hippocampus. Thus, in the basal state, a powerful GABAergic input from the ventral pallidum keeps subsets of DA neurons hyperpolarized and nonfiring. If the ventral subiculum is activated, it will increase glutamatergic excitation of the nucleus accumbens, which in turn will inhibit the ventral pallidum and remove inhibition from DA neurons, causing them to begin to fire spontaneously. In addition to being in an active or inactive state, DA neurons are known to fire in bursts. Studies show that burst firing is the behaviorally relevant output of the DA neurons, since DA neurons in animals exposed to salient stimuli respond by firing a burst of action potentials. Burst firing is driven primarily by the pedunculopontine tegmentum. However, for the pedunculopontine tegmentum to drive burst firing, the DA neuron must first be spontaneously firing. Thus, only neurons that the ventral subiculum allows to fire spontaneously can be driven to fire in bursts. Increased activity in the ventral subiculum would cause more neurons to be spontaneously active; therefore, the pedunculopontine can drive a larger number of neurons to fire in bursts. As a consequence, the pedunculopontine-driven burst is the "signal," with the amplitude of the signal (i.e., the "gain" of the signal) being determined by the ventral subiculum

to screen out stimuli effectively independent of the environmental context. Indeed, studies in schizophrenia patients have revealed that the anterior hippocampus, which is the primate homolog of the vSub, is hyperactive in schizophrenia subjects (Nordahl et al., 1996; Heckers et al., 1998; Kegeles et al., 2000; Medoff et al., 2001; Meyer-Lindenberg et al., 2005; Lahti et al., 2006; Weiss et al., 2006). Postmortem histological studies suggest that a source of this hyperactivity may be related to the loss of a class of GABAergic inhibitory neurons, specifically those containing the peptide parvalbumin (Lewis et al., 2001; Zhang and Reynolds, 2002; Hashimoto et al., 2003; Lewis et al., 2004). This condition is remarkably similar to what is also observed in the MAM-treated rat. Thus, in MAM-treated rats, the vSub demonstrates hyperactivity compared to controls. Moreover, this hyperactivity is correlated with an increase in the number of VTA DA neurons firing spontaneously 2 (Figure 2); essentially the same condition is found when the vSub is activated by NMDA (Floresco et al., 2001, 2003). Importantly, both the increase in VTA DA neuron firing and the behavioral hyperresponsivity to amphetamine are reversed by inactivation of the vSub. Therefore, hyperactivity in the vSub of MAM-treated rats causes an interference in contextual gating and a hyperresponsive state of the VTA DA neurons, which should lead to an abnormally large release of DA in the striatum. Inactivation of the vSub both restores DA neuron firing to normal and reverses behavioral hyperresponsiveness to amphetamine, returning the behaviorally activating effects of amphetamine to that of control rats.

What is the source of vSub hyperactivity in the MAM model? Our studies show that there is a selective loss of parvalbumin interneuron staining specifically within the vSub and the mPFC of MAM-treated rats, essentially the same as that reported in schizophrenia patients. Parvalbumin interneurons within the vSub and mPFC have

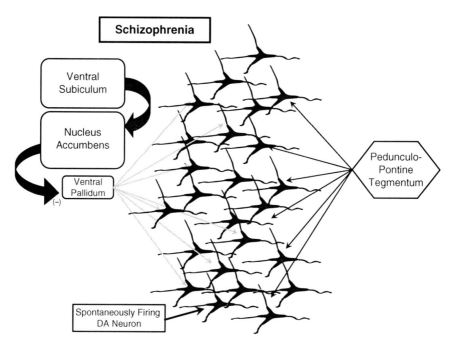

Fig. 2 In the case of schizophrenia, evidence suggests that the hippocampus subiculum is overdriven, potentially due to parvalbumin interneuron loss. As a consequence, the overactive ventral subiculum would provide a powerful drive of the nucleus accumbens, which in turn would potently inhibit the ventral pallidum. This would remove ventral pallidal inhibition of DA neurons, causing the entire population to become spontaneously active. As a consequence, any signal coming from the pedunculopontine tegmentum would produce a maximal DA output into striatal targets

been shown to play a specific role in the organization of activity within these regions. Specifically, parvalbumin interneurons have been shown to be necessary for the generation of gamma rhythms (Vida et al., 2006; Bartos et al., 2007; Fuchs et al., 2007; Tukker et al., 2007). Gamma rhythms are believed to be a required component of signal recognition in cortical structures (Buzsaki and Draguhn, 2004). Studies have shown a disruption of gamma signaling in schizophrenia patients (Gonzalez-Hernandez et al., 2003; Gallinat et al., 2004; Cho et al., 2005; Basar-Eroglu et al., 2007). We have examined gamma signaling using a behavioral conditioning model. In this model, tones are paired with a footshock. In a normal animal, following pairing the tone will elicit the activation of gamma signaling in the mPFC and the vSub. However, in the MAM animal, although they learn the association behaviorally, this is not accompanied by tone-activated gamma signaling (Lodge et al., 2009). Moreover, the loss of gamma signaling correlates with those regions showing deficits in parvalbumin interneurons. Thus, a model arises in which a signaling deficit is present in the vSub–mPFC circuit involving a loss of parvalbumin interneurons. As a result, the normal up–down state transitions and stimulus-evoked gamma activity are disrupted and instead replaced by a nonspecific, high-frequency overdrive of the NAc. The result is a drive of the NAc into a permanent up state preventing contextual organization of information flow and an overdrive of the VTA DA neurons to cause them to be hyperresponsive to stimuli.

Amphetamine, Stress, and the Hippocampus

The contextual disruption of schizophrenia therefore may be directly related to interneuron loss and hyperactivity within the vSub. Interestingly, there are other conditions that exhibit a contextual component and that result in a hyper-dopaminergic state not unlike that observed in schizophrenia. This relates to amphetamine sensitization and stress, which, remarkably, are both risk factors for schizophrenia (Benes, 1997; Tsuang, 2000). When amphetamine is administered repeatedly to a rat, a phenomenon known as sensitization occurs, in which there is an increase in the behavioral response to amphetamine (Segal and Mandell, 1974; Post and Rose, 1976), which is accompanied by an increase in amphetamine-induced DA release (Pierce and Kalivas, 1997). Moreover, the sensitization itself is context-dependent, in that the behavioral response is maximally augmented when the animal is tested in the same environmental context in which it was treated (Vezina et al., 1989; Badiani et al., 2000; Crombag et al., 2000). We found that administration of amphetamine for 5 days followed by 5 days withdrawal, which induces robust behavioral sensitization, elicits the same response in the DA system as observed in the MAM-treated rats – i.e., an increase in the number of DA neurons firing spontaneously (Lodge and Grace, 2008). This is accompanied by an increase in vSub neuron firing. Moreover, if the vSub is inactivated, DA neuron activity is restored to baseline, and the behavioral sensitization to amphetamine is reversed to the pretreatment response (Lodge and Grace, 2008).

Another risk factor for schizophrenia is stress. It is also context-dependent, in that animals show the greatest behavioral reaction to stressful stimuli when they are tested in the environment in which the stressor occurred (Kalivas and Stewart, 1991). Moreover, stress will cross-sensitize with amphetamine. Thus, a 2-h period of restraint stress of a rat will cause the animal to show hyperresponsivity to amphetamine given as long as 24 h after the restraint (Pacchioni et al., 2002). Stress can activate a number of regions within the brain. Two regions in particular have shown strong activation and functional relevance to stress: the amygdala and the noradrenergic system. Thus, stressors are known to activate amygdala neuron firing in rats (LeDoux, 2000; Rosenkranz and Grace, 2002) as well as increase metabolic activity in the amygdala of human subjects during imaging studies (Bremner et al., 1999; Rauch et al., 2000; Drevets, 2003). The noradrenergic system is also known to play a powerful role in stress. Therefore, stressors cause a potent activation of noradrenergic neuron firing (Abercrombie and Jacobs, 1987) and an increase in norepinephrine metabolites (Thierry et al., 1968; Abercrombie et al., 1988; Shanks et al., 1991; Serova et al., 1999). Furthermore, the amygdala and the noradrenergic neurons are potently interconnected. Interestingly, both the amygdala and the noradrenergic system will produce a powerful activation of the vSub (Lipski and Grace, 2008). Our recent studies show that stress will activate the same circuits that we found are involved in schizophrenia and amphetamine sensitization. Thus, a 2-h period of restraint will increase the number of DA neurons firing, an effect that can be reversed by inactivation of the vSub. Therefore, each of these variables, namely amphetamine sensitization, stress, and an animal model of schizophrenia, is characterized by DA hyperresponsivity mediated by an increase in the number of DA neurons that can respond to stimuli. Moreover, all are context-dependent phenomena that can be reversed by inactivation of a hyperactive vSub. Such results provide important insight into the role of context in guiding behavior and the type of disrupted behavior that can result when the normal modulation of contextual responses is altered within the vSub.

Stress as an Etiological Factor in the Development of Schizophrenia

Stress itself may also be an etiological factor in the pathogenesis of schizophrenia. It is known that schizophrenia symptoms emerge in late adolescence/early adulthood. However, the genetic predisposition and risk are present presumably from birth. What happens during this intervening period that could lead to the onset of the first psychotic break later in life? There have been several studies of high-risk individuals that have focused on evaluating the changes that take place during this premorbid phase. In general, evidence suggests that those at risk for schizophrenia often show deficits in executive functioning during this early period (Morey et al., 2005; Lencz et al., 2006; Pukrop et al., 2006; Chung et al., 2008). Such a deficit could point to disturbances in PFC function. Moreover, studies in high-risk individuals have revealed several other alterations. Thus, Johnstone et al. (2002) have shown that in the population of children at risk for developing schizophrenia, those that convert showed significantly higher stress responses. Furthermore, there is evidence of increased hypothalamic-pituitary axis (Garner et al., 2005) and hippocampal (Phillips et al., 2002; Pantelis et al., 2003) alterations at the first break stage. Such a confluence of data could point to a common pathophysiological risk in developing schizophrenia.

The mPFC in particular was found to play an important role in regulating stress responsivity. Thus, activation of the mPFC will attenuate stress responses in the amygdala (Rosenkranz and Grace, 2003; Rosenkranz et al., 2003), an area known to be activated in anxiety states (LeDoux, 2000). Furthermore, an involvement of the mPFC has been shown to be important in "immunizing" a system to known sources of stress (Amat et al., 2006). Thus, a deficit in mPFC function could cause an individual to show abnormally high stress reactivity, as reported by Johnstone and colleagues. Stress itself can produce multiple deleterious actions within the brain. One brain region that has shown a high potential for stress-related damage is the hippocampus (Sapolsky et al., 1990; Magarinos and McEwen, 1995; Conrad et al., 1999; Sapolsky, 2000). Thus, deficits in the regulation of stress could lead to increased glucocorticoid release and hippocampal drive, which, in turn, could be a source of hippocampal damage (Grace, 2004; Thompson et al., 2004). When combined with other risk factors, such as cannabis use (that will alter the ability of the mPFC to respond appropriately to learned stressors; (Laviolette et al., 2006)) and social stress, it could lead to hippocampal damage and the hyperactive vSub state proposed above. If such a cascade of events does indeed take place, this would suggest that an intervention that can treat the abnormal stress responsivity in these high-risk children may actually circumvent the transition to psychosis (Figure 3) (Grace, 2004; Thompson et al., 2004).

Conclusion

In summary, there is an association between the disruption of vSub activity, contextual gating, and DA system overdrive in the MAM-treated rodent model of schizophrenia, which appears to parallel what is happening in the brain of schizophrenia patients. Currently, the DA hyperresponsivity of schizophrenia is treated by blocking DA receptors in postsynaptic regions, leading to attenuation of DA signaling and driving VTA DA neurons into an inactive state of depolarization blockade (Bunney and Grace, 1978; Chiodo and Bunney, 1983; White and Wang, 1983; Grace et al., 1997). Indeed, inactivating DA neuron firing via depolarization block should reverse what is proposed here as a deficit in DA signaling – i.e., decreasing the number of spontaneously active DA neurons. However, the model proposed here provides a different, potentially more effective target – i.e., restoration of interneuron function within the vSub and the mPFC. By restoring functionality to the GABA neuron system, we should be able to pharmacologically target the actual deficit that drives the hyperdopaminergic state and potentially other deficit states (e.g., cognitive, negative symptoms) of the schizophrenia patient.

Stress-induced Hippocampal Pathology:

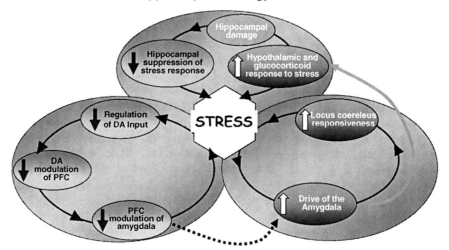

Stress from multiple factors, whether due to genetic predisposition, maternal insult, or fetal stress, may predispose an individual to stress-induced damage of the hippocampal interneurons, leading to the onset of schizophrenia in the adult

Fig. 3 Stress is a known risk factor in the development and in the exacerbation of schizophrenia. Furthermore, individuals at risk for schizophrenia are reported to be hyperresponsive to stressors. One factor that limits the effects of stress in the brain is the prefrontal cortex. Thus, the prefrontal cortex can limit the ability of the amygdala to respond to stress. However, if the prefrontal cortex is dysfunctional, this would release its regulatory control over the stress system. As a consequence, there would be an activation of a positive feedback loop in which stress would drive amygdala activity, which in turn would increase locus coeruleus noradrenergic potentiation of the stress response, leading to hippocampal damage and further exacerbation of stress. The hippocampus is known to be susceptible to stress-induced damage. Therefore, in an individual with a premorbid dysfunctional prefrontal cortex, the unregulated stress response could lead to hippocampal damage and hyperactivity, thereby driving the fall into the psychotic state

References

Abercrombie ED, Jacobs BL (1987) Single-unit response of noradrenergic neurons in the locus coeruleus of freely moving cats. I. Acutely presented stressful and nonstressful stimuli. Journal of Neuroscience 7:2837–2843.

Abercrombie ED, Keller RW, Jr, Zigmond MJ (1988) Characterization of hippocampal norepinephrine release as measured by microdialysis perfusion: pharmacological and behavioral studies. Neuroscience 27:897–904.

Amat J, Paul E, Zarza C, Watkins LR, Maier SF (2006) Previous experience with behavioral control over stress blocks the behavioral and dorsal raphe nucleus activating effects of later uncontrollable stress: role of the ventral medial prefrontal cortex. Journal of Neuroscience 26: 13264–13272.

Angrist B, Rotrosen J, Gershon S (1980) Differential effects of amphetamine and neuroleptics on negative vs. positive symptoms in schizophrenia. Psychopharmacology 72:17–19.

Angrist B, Sathananthan G, Wilk S, Gershon S (1974) Amphetamine psychosis: behavioral and biochemical aspects. Journal of Psychiatric Research 11:13–23.

Arnold SE (1997) The medial temporal lobe in schizophrenia. Journal of Neuropsychiatry & Clinical Neurosciences 9:460–470.

Badiani A, Oates MM, Fraioli S, Browman KE, Ostrander MM, Xue CJ, Wolf ME, Robinson TE (2000) Environmental modulation of the response to amphetamine: dissociation between changes in behavior and changes in dopamine and glutamate overflow in the rat striatal complex. Psychopharmacology (Berl) 151:166–174.

Bartos M, Vida I, Jonas P (2007) Synaptic mechanisms of synchronized gamma oscillations in inhibitory interneuron networks. Nature Reviews Neuroscience 8:45–56.

Basar-Eroglu C, Brand A, Hildebrandt H, Karolina Kedzior K, Mathes B, Schmiedt C (2007) Working memory related gamma oscillations in schizophrenia patients. International Journal of Psychophysiology 64:39–45.

Benes FM (1997) The role of stress and dopamine–GABA interactions in the vulnerability for schizophrenia. Journal of Psychiatric Research 31:257–275.

Berger PA, Faull KF, Kilkowski J, Anderson PJ, Kraemer H, Davis KL, Barchas JD (1980) CSF monoamine metabolites in depression and schizophrenia. American Journal of Psychiatry 137:174–180.

Berman KF, Ostrem JL, Randolph C, Gold J, Goldberg TE, Coppola R, Carson RE, Herscovitch P, Weinberger DR (1995) Physiological activation of a cortical network during performance of the Wisconsin Card Sorting Test: a positron emission tomography study. Neuropsychologia 33:1027–1046.

Bertolino A, Knable MB, Saunders RC, Callicot JH, Kolachana B, Mattay VS, Bachevalier J, Frank JA, Egan M, Weinberger DR (1999) The relationship between dorsolateral prefrontal N-acetylaspartate measures and striatal dopamine activity in schizophrenia. Biological Psychiatry 45:660–667.

Bowers MB (1974) Central dopamine turnover in schizophrenic syndromes. Archives of General Psychiatry 31:50–54.

Bremner JD, Staib LH, Kaloupek D, Southwick SM, Soufer R, Charney DS (1999) Neural correlates of exposure to traumatic pictures and sound in Vietnam combat veterans with and without posttraumatic stress disorder: a positron emission tomography study. Biological Psychiatry 45:806–816.

Bunney BS, Grace AA (1978) Acute and chronic haloperidol treatment: comparison of effects on nigral dopaminergic cell activity. Life Sciences 23:1715–1727.

Buzsaki G, Draguhn A (2004) Neuronal oscillations in cortical networks. Science 304: 1926–1929.

Carboni E, Imperato A, Perezzani L, Di Chiara G (1989) Amphetamine, cocaine, phencyclidine and nomifensine increase extracellular dopamine concentrations preferentially in the nucleus accumbens of freely moving rats. Neuroscience 28:653–661.

Carlsson A, Lindqvist M (1963) Effect of chlorpromazine or haloperidol on formation of 3-methoxytyramine and normetanephrine in mouse brain. Acta Pharmacologica et Toxicologica 20:140–144.

Chiodo LA, Bunney BS (1983) Typical and atypical neuroleptics: differential effects of chronic administration on the activity of A9 and A10 midbrain dopaminergic neurons. Journal of Neuroscience 3:1607–1619.

Cho RY, Konecky RO, Carter CS (2005) Impairments in gamma band syncrhonization and context processing in schizophrenia. Schizophrenia Bulletin 31:450–451.

Chung YS, Kang DH, Shin NY, Yoo SY, Kwon JS (2008) Deficit of theory of mind in individuals at ultra-high-risk for schizophrenia. Schizophrenia Research 99:111–118.

Conrad CD, LeDoux JE, Magarinos AM, McEwen BS (1999) Repeated restraint stress facilitates fear conditioning independently of causing hippocampal CA3 dendritic atrophy. Behavioral Neuroscience 113:902–913.

Crombag HS, Badiani A, Maren S, Robinson TE (2000) The role of contextual versus discrete drug-associated cues in promoting the induction of psychomotor sensitization to intravenous amphetamine. Behavioural Brain Research 116:1–22.

Del Rio J, Fuentes JA (1969) Further studies on the antagonism of stereotyped behaviour induced by amphetamine. European Journal of Pharmacology 8:73–78.

Drevets WC (2003) Neuroimaging abnormalities in the amygdala in mood disorders. Annals of the New York Academy of Sciences 985:420–444.

Fanselow MS (2000) Contextual fear, gestalt memories, and the hippocampus. Behavioural Brain Research 110:73–81.

Flagstad P, Mork A, Glenthoj BY, van Beek J, Michael-Titus AT, Didriksen M (2004) Disruption of neurogenesis on gestational day 17 in the rat causes behavioral changes relevant to positive and negative schizophrenia symptoms and alters amphetamine-induced dopamine release in nucleus accumbens. Neuropsychopharmacology 29:2052–2064.

Floresco SB, Todd CL, Grace AA (2001) Glutamatergic afferents from the hippocampus to the nucleus accumbens regulate activity of ventral tegmental area dopamine neurons. Journal of Neuroscience 21:4915–4922.

Floresco SB, West AR, Ash B, Moore H, Grace AA (2003) Afferent modulation of dopamine neuron firing differentially regulates tonic and phasic dopamine transmission. Nature Neuroscience 6:968–973.

Fuchs EC, Zivkovic AR, Cunningham MO, Middleton S, Lebeau FE, Bannerman DM, Rozov A, Whittington MA, Traub RD, Rawlins JN, Monyer H (2007) Recruitment of parvalbumin-positive interneurons determines hippocampal function and associated behavior. Neuron 53:591–604.

Gallinat J, Winterer G, Herrmann CS, Senkowski D (2004) Reduced oscillatory gamma-band responses in unmedicated schizophrenic patients indicate impaired frontal network processing. Clinical Neurophysiology 115:1863–1874.

Garner B, Pariante CM, Wood SJ, Velakoulis D, Phillips L, Soulsby B, Brewer WJ, Smith DJ, Dazzan P, Berger GE, Yung AR, van den Buuse M, Murray R, McGorry PD, Pantelis C (2005) Pituitary volume predicts future transition to psychosis in individuals at ultra-high risk of developing psychosis. Biological Psychiatry 58:417–423.

Goldberg TE, Torrey EF, Berman KF, Weinberger DR (1994) Relations between neuropsychological performance and brain morphological and physiological measures in monozygotic twins discordant for schizophrenia. Psychiatry Research 55:51–61.

Goldman-Rakic PS (1999) The physiological approach: functional architecture of working memory and disordered cognition in schizophrenia. Biological Psychiatry 46:650–661.

Gonzalez-Hernandez JA, Cedeno I, Pita-Alcorta C, Galan L, Aubert E, Figueredo-Rodriguez P (2003) Induced oscillations and the distributed cortical sources during the Wisconsin card sorting test performance in schizophrenic patients: new clues to neural connectivity. International Journal of Psychophysiology 48:11–24.

Gourevitch R, Rocher C, Le Pen G, Krebs MO, Jay TM (2004) Working memory deficits in adult rats after prenatal disruption of neurogenesis. Behavioral Pharmacology 15:287–292.

Grace AA (1991) Phasic versus tonic dopamine release and the modulation of dopamine system responsivity: a hypothesis for the etiology of schizophrenia. Neuroscience 41:1–24.

Grace AA (2000) Gating of information flow within the limbic system and the pathophysiology of schizophrenia. Brain Research – Brain Research Reviews 31:330–341.

Grace AA (2004) Developmental dysregulation of the dopamine system and the pathophysiology of schizophrenia. In: Keshavan MS, Kennedy, JL, Murray, RM, (eds) Neurodevelopment and Schizophrenia, pp 273–294. Cambridge, UK: Cambridge University Press.

Grace AA, Bunney BS, Moore H, Todd CL (1997) Dopamine-cell depolarization block as a model for the therapeutic actions of antipsychotic drugs. Trends in Neurosciences 20:31–37.

Grace AA, Moore H (1998) Regulation of information flow in the nucleus accumbens: a model for the pathophysiology of schizophrenia. In: Lenzenweger MF, Dworkin RH, (eds) Origins and Development of Schizophrenia: Advances in Experimental Psychopathology, pp 123–157. Washington, DC: American Psychological Association Press.

Harrison PJ (1999) The neuropathology of schizophrenia. A critical review of the data and their interpretation. Brain 122(Pt 4):593–624.

Hashimoto T, Volk DW, Eggan SM, Mirnics K, Pierri JN, Sun Z, Sampson AR, Lewis DA (2003) Gene expression deficits in a subclass of GABA neurons in the prefrontal cortex of subjects with schizophrenia. Journal of Neuroscience 23:6315–6326.

Heckers S, Heinsen H, Geiger B, Beckmann H (1991) Hippocampal neuron number in schizophrenia. A stereological study. Archives of General Psychiatry 48:1002–1008.

Heckers S, Rauch SL, Goff D, Savage CR, Schacter DL, Fischman AJ, Alpert NM (1998) Impaired recruitment of the hippocampus during conscious recollection in schizophrenia. Nature Neuroscience 1:318–323.

Janssen PA, Niemegeers CJ, Schellekens KH (1965) Is it possible to predict the clinical effects of neuroleptic drugs (Major Tranquillizers) from animal data? I. "Neuroleptic Activity Spectra" for rats. Arzneimittelforschung 15:104–117.

Jarrard LE (1995) What does the hippocampus really do? Behavioural Brain Research 71:1–10.

Javitt DC, Zukin SR (1991) Recent advances in the phencyclidine model of schizophrenia. American Journal of Psychiatry 148:1301–1308.

Johnston MV, Carman AB, Coyle JT (1981) Effects of fetal treatment with methylazoxymethanol acetate at various gestational dates on the neurochemistry of the adult neocortex of the rat. Journal of Neurochemistry 36:124–128.

Johnstone EC, Crow TJ, Frith CD, Carney MWP, Price JS (1978) Mechanism of the antipsychotic effect in the treatment of acute schizophrenia. Lancet April 22:848–851.

Johnstone EC, Lawrie SM, Cosway R (2002) What does the Edinburgh High-Risk Study tell us about schizophrenia? American Journal of Medical Genetics (Neuropsychiatric Genetics) 114:906–912.

Kalivas PW, Stewart J (1991) Dopamine transmission in the initiation and expression of drug- and stress-induced sensitization of motor activity. Brain Research Brain Research Reviews 16: 223–244.

Kapur S, Remington G (2001) Dopamine D(2) receptors and their role in atypical antipsychotic action: still necessary and may even be sufficient. Biological Psychiatry 50:873–883.

Kegeles LS, Shungu DC, Anjilvel S, Chan S, Ellis SP, Xanthopoulos E, Malaspina D, Gorman JM, Mann JJ, Laruelle M, Kaufmann CA (2000) Hippocampal pathology in schizophrenia: magnetic resonance imaging and spectroscopy studies. Psychiatry Research 98: 163–175.

Krieckhaus EE, Donahoe JW, Morgan MA (1992) Paranoid schizophrenia may be caused by dopamine hyperactivity of CA1 hippocampus. Biological Psychiatry 31:560–570.

Lahti AC, Holcomb HH, Medoff DR, Tamminga CA (1995) Ketamine activates psychosis and alters limbic blood flow in schizophrenia. Neuroreport 6:869–872.

Lahti AC, Weiler MA, Holcomb HH, Tamminga CA, Carpenter WT, McMahon R (2006) Correlations between rCBF and symptoms in two independent cohorts of drug-free patients with schizophrenia. Neuropsychopharmacology 31:221–230.

Laruelle M, Abi-Dargham A, Van Dyck CH, Gil R, D'Souza CD, Erdos J, McCance E, Rosenblatt W, Fingado C, Zoghbi SS, Baldwin RM, Seibyl JP, Krystal JH, Charney DS, Innis RB (1996) Single photon emission computerized tomography imaging of amphetamine-induced dopamine release in drug-free schizophrenic subjects. Proceedings of the National Academy of Science 93:9235–9240.

Laviolette SR, Grace AA, Laviolette SR, Grace AA (2006) Cannabinoids potentiate emotional learning plasticity in neurons of the medial prefrontal cortex through basolateral amygdala inputs. Journal of Neuroscience 26:6458–6468.

LeDoux JE (2000) Emotion circuits in the brain. Annual Review of Neuroscience 23:155–184.

Lencz T, Smith CW, McLaughlin D, Auther A, Nakayama E, Hovey L, Cornblatt BA (2006) Generalized and specific neurocognitive deficits in prodromal schizophrenia. Biological Psychiatry 59:863–871.

Lewis DA, Cruz DA, Melchitzky DS, Pierri JN (2001) Lamina-specific deficits in parvalbumin-immunoreactive varicosities in the prefrontal cortex of subjects with schizophrenia: evidence for fewer projections from the thalamus. American Journal of Psychiatry 158:1411–1422.

Lewis DA, Volk DW, Hashimoto T (2004) Selective alterations in prefrontal cortical GABA neuro-transmission in schizophrenia: a novel target for the treatment of working memory dysfunction. Psychopharmacology (Berl) 174:143–150.

Lipska BK, Jaskiw GE, Weinberger DR (1993) Postpubertal emergence of hyperresponsiveness to stress and to amphetamine after neonatal excitotoxic hippocampal damage: a potential animal model of schizophrenia. Neuropsychopharmacology 9:67–75.

Lipski WJ, Grace AA (2008) Neurons in the ventral subiculum are activated by noxious stimuli and are modulated by noradrenergic afferents. Program No 1951, 2008 Neuroscience Meeting Planner Washington, DC; Society for Neuroscience, 2008 Online.

Lodge DJ, Behrens MM, Grace AA (2009) A loss of parvalbumin-containing interneurons is associated with diminished oscillatory activity in an animal model of schizophrenia. Journal of Neuroscience (Online) 29:2344–2354.

Lodge DJ, Grace AA (2006) The hippocampus modulates dopamine neuron responsivity by regulating the intensity of phasic neuron activation. Neuopsychopharmacology 31:1356–1361.

Lodge DJ, Grace AA (2008) Amphetamine activation of hippocampal drive of mesolimbic dopamine neurons: a mechanism of behavioral sensitization. Journal of Neuroscience 28: 7876–7882.

Magarinos AM, McEwen BS (1995) Stress-induced atrophy of apical dendrites of hippocampal CA3c neurons: involvement of glucocorticoid secretion and excitatory amino acid receptors. Neuroscience 69:89–98.

Manoach DS (2003) Prefrontal cortex dysfunction during working memory performance in schizophrenia: reconciling discrepant findings. Schizophrenia Research 60:285–298.

Maren S (1999) Neurotoxic or electrolytic lesions of the ventral subiculum produce deficits in the acquisition and expression of Pavlovian fear conditioning in rats. Behavioural Neuroscience 113:283–290.

Maren S, Quirk GJ (2004) Neuronal signalling of fear memory. Nature Reviews in Neuroscience 5:844–852.

McDonald C, Murray RM (2000) Early and late environmental risk factors for schizophrenia. Brain Research Brain Research Reviews 31:130–137.

Medoff DR, Holcomb HH, Lahti AC, Tamminga CA (2001) Probing the human hippocampus using rCBF: contrasts in schizophrenia. Hippocampus 11:543–550.

Meyer-Lindenberg AS, Olsen RK, Kohn PD, Brown T, Egan MF, Weinberger DR, Berman KF (2005) Regionally specific disturbance of dorsolateral prefrontal–hippocampal functional connectivity in schizophrenia. Archives of General Psychiatry 62:379–386.

Moore H, Grace AA (1997) Anatomical changes in limbic structures produced by methylazoxymethanol acetate (MAM) during brain development are associated with changes in physiological interactions among afferents to the nucleus accumbens. Society for Neuroscience Abstracts 23:2378.

Moore H, Jentsch JD, Ghajarnia M, Geyer MA, Grace AA (2006) A neurobehavioral systems analysis of adult rats exposed to methylazoxymethanol acetate on E17: implications for the neuropathology of schizophrenia. Biological Psychiatry 60:253–264.

Morey RA, Inan S, Mitchell TV, Perkins DO, Lieberman JA, Belger A (2005) Imaging frontostriatal function in ultra-high-risk, early, and chronic schizophrenia during executive processing. Archives of General Psychiatry 62:254–262.

Nordahl TE, Kusubov N, Carter C, Salamat S, Cummings AM, O'Shora-Celaya L, Eberling J, Robertson L, Huesman RH, Jagust W, Budinger TF (1996) Temporal lobe metabolic differences in medication-free outpatients with schizophrenia via the PET-600. Neuropsychopharmacology 15:541–554.

O'Donnell P, Grace AA (1995) Synaptic interactions among excitatory afferents to nucleus accumbens neurons: hippocampal gating of prefrontal cortical input. Journal of Neuroscience 15:3622–3639.

O'Donnell P, Grace AA (1998) Phencyclidine interferes with the hippocampal gating of nucleus accumbens neuronal activity in vivo. Neuroscience 87:823–830.

Pacchioni AM, Gioino G, Assis A, Cancela LM (2002) A single exposure to restraint stress induces behavioral and neurochemical sensitization to stimulating effects of amphetamine: involvement of NMDA receptors. Annals of the New York Academy of Sciences 965:233–246.

Pantelis C, Velakoulis D, McGorry PD, Wood SJ, Suckling J, Phillips LJ, Yung AR, Bullmore ET, Brewer W, Soulsby B, Desmond P, McGuire PK (2003) Neuroanatomical abnormalities before and after onset of psychosis: a cross-sectional and longitudinal MRI comparison. Lancet 361:281–288.

Phillips LJ, Velakoulis D, Pantelis C, Wood S, Yuen HP, Yung AR, Desmond P, Brewer W, McGorry PD (2002) Non-reduction in hippocampal volume is associated with higher risk of psychosis. Schizophrenia Research 58:145–158.

Pickar D, Labarca R, Doran AR, Wolkowitz OM, Roy A, Breier A, Linnoila M, Paul SM (1986) Longitudinal measurement of plasma homovanillic acid levels in schizophrenic patients. Archives of General Psychiatry 43:669–676.

Pickar D, Labarca R, Linnoila M, Roy A, Hommer D, Everett D, Paul SM (1984) Neuroleptic-induced decrease in plasma homovanillic acid and antipsychotic activity in schizophrenic patients. Science 225:954–957.

Pierce RC, Kalivas PW (1997) A circuitry model of the expression of behavioral sensitization to amphetamine-like psychostimulants. Brain Research Brain Research Reviews 25: 192–216.

Pilowsky LS, Kerwin RW, Murray RM (1993) Schizophrenia: a neurodevelopmental perspective. Neuropsychopharmacology 9:83–91.

Post RM, Fink E, Carpenter WT, Jr, Goodwin FK (1975) Cerebrospinal fluid amine metabolites in acute schizophrenia. Archives of General Psychiatry 32:1063–1069.

Post RM, Rose H (1976) Increasing effects of repetitive cocaine administration in the rat. Nature 260:731–732.

Pukrop R, Schultze-Lutter F, Ruhrmann S, Brockhaus-Dumke A, Tendolkar I, Bechdolf A, Matuschek E, Klosterkotter J (2006) Neurocognitive functioning in subjects at risk for a first episode of psychosis compared with first- and multiple-episode schizophrenia. Journal of Clinical and Experimental Neuropsychology 28:1388–1407.

Randrup A, Munkvad I (1965) Special antagonism of amphetamine-induced abnormal behaviour. Inhibition of stereotyped activity with increase of some normal activities. Psychopharmacologia 7:416–422.

Rauch SL, Whalen PJ, Shin LM, McInerney SC, Macklin ML, Lasko NB, Orr SP, Pitman RK (2000) Exaggerated amygdala response to masked facial stimuli in posttraumatic stress disorder: a functional MRI study. Biological Psychiatry 47:769–776.

Rosenkranz JA, Grace AA (2002) Dopamine-mediated modulation of odour-evoked amygdala potentials during pavlovian conditioning. Nature 417:282–287.

Rosenkranz JA, Grace AA (2003) Affective conditioning in the basolateral amygdala of anesthetized rats is modulated by dopamine and prefrontal cortical inputs. Annals of the New York Academy of Sciences 985:488–491.

Rosenkranz JA, Moore H, Grace AA (2003) The prefrontal cortex regulates lateral amygdala neuronal plasticity and responses to previously conditioned stimuli. Journal of Neuroscience 23:11054–11064.

Sapolsky RM (2000) Glucocorticoids and hippocampal atrophy in neuropsychiatric disorders. Archives of General Psychiatry 57:925–935.

Sapolsky RM, Uno H, Rebert CS, Finch CE (1990) Hippocampal damage associated with prolonged glucocorticoid exposure in primates. Journal of Neuroscience 10:2897–2902.

Schultz W (1998) The phasic reward signal of primate dopamine neurons. Advances in Pharmacology 42:686–690.

Seeman P (2002) Atypical antipsychotics: mechanism of action. Canadian Journal of Psychiatry 47:27–38.

Seeman P, Lee T, Chau-Wong M, Wong K (1976) Antipsychotic drug doses and neuroleptic/dopamine receptors. Nature 261:717–719.

Segal DS, Mandell AJ (1974) Long-term administration of d-amphetamine: progressive augmentation of motor activity and stereotypy. Pharmacology Biochemistry and Behavior 2: 249–255.

Serova LI, Nankova BB, Feng Z, Hong JS, Hutt M, Sabban EL (1999) Heightened transcription for enzymes involved in norepinephrine biosynthesis in the rat locus coeruleus by immobilization stress. Biological Psychiatry 45:853–862.

Shanks N, Zalcman S, Zacharko RM, Anisman H (1991) Alterations of central norepinephrine, dopamine and serotonin in several strains of mice following acute stressor exposure. Pharmacology, Biochemistry & Behavior 38:69–75.

Sharp PE (1999) Complimentary roles for hippocampal versus subicular/entorhinal place cells in coding place, context, and events. Hippocampus 9:432–443.

Shenton ME, Kikinis R, Jolesz FA, Pollak SD, LeMay M, Wible CG, Hokama H, Martin J, Metcalf D, Coleman M, et al. (1992) Abnormalities of the left temporal lobe and thought disorder in schizophrenia. A quantitative magnetic resonance imaging study. New Engl Journal of Medicine 327:604–612.

Silbersweig DA, Stern E, Frith C, Cahill C, Holmes A, Grootoonk S, Seaward J, McKenna P, Chua SE, Schnorr L, et al. (1995) A functional neuroanatomy of hallucinations in schizophrenia. Nature 378:176–179.

Talamini LM, Ellenbroek B, Koch T, Korf J (2000) Impaired sensory gating and attention in rats with developmental abnormalities of the mesocortex. Implications for schizophrenia. Annals of the New York Academy of Sciences 911:486–494.

Talamini LM, Koch T, Luiten PG, Koolhaas JM, Korf J (1999) Interruptions of early cortical development affect limbic association areas and social behaviour in rats; possible relevance for neurodevelopmental disorders. Brain Research 847:105–120.

Thierry AM, Javoy F, Glowinski J, Kety SS (1968) Effects of stress on the metabolism of norepinephrine, dopamine and serotonin in the central nervous system of the rat. I. Modifications of norepinephrine turnover. Journal of Pharmacology & Experimental Therapeutics 163: 163–171.

Thompson JL, Pogue-Geile MF, Grace AA (2004) The interactions among developmental pathology, dopamine, and stress as a model for the age of onset of schizophrenia symptomatology. Schizophrenia Bulletin 30:875–900.

Tsuang M (2000) Schizophrenia: genes and environment. Biological Psychiatry 47:210–220.

Tukker JJ, Fuentealba P, Hartwich K, Somogyi P, Klausberger T (2007) Cell type-specific tuning of hippocampal interneuron firing during gamma oscillations in vivo. Journal of Neuroscience 27:8184–8189.

Venables PH (1992) Hippocampal function and schizophrenia. Experimental psychological evidence. Annals of the New York Academy of Sciences 658:111–127.

Vezina P, Giovino AA, Wise RA, Stewart J (1989) Environment-specific cross-sensitization between the locomotor activating effects of morphine and amphetamine. Pharmacology Biochemistry and Behaviour 32:581–584.

Vida I, Bartos M, Jonas P (2006) Shunting inhibition improves robustness of gamma oscillations in hippocampal interneuron networks by homogenizing firing rates. Neuron 49: 107–117.

Weinberger DR, Berman KF (1996) Prefrontal function in schizophrenia: confounds and controversies. Philosophical Transactions of the Royal Society of London – Series B: Biological Sciences 351:1495–1503.

Weinberger DR, Egan MF, Bertolino A, Callicott JH, Mattay VS, Lipska BK, Berman KF, Goldberg TE (2001) Prefrontal neurons and the genetics of schizophrenia. Biological Psychiatry 50:825–844.

Weiss AP, Goff D, Schacter DL, Ditman T, Freudenreich O, Henderson D, Heckers S (2006) Fronto-hippocampal function during temporal context monitoring in schizophrenia. Biological Psychiatry 60:1268–1277.

West AR, Moore H, Grace AA (2002) Direct examination of local regulation of membrane activity in striatal and prefrontal cortical neurons in vivo using simultaneous intracellular recording and microdialysis. Journal of Pharmacology & Experimental Therapeutics 301: 867–877.

White FJ, Wang RY (1983) Differential effects of classical and atypical antipsychotic drugs on A9 and A10 dopamine neurons. Science 221:1054–1057.

Zhang ZJ, Reynolds GP (2002) A selective decrease in the relative density of parvalbumin-immunoreactive neurons in the hippocampus in schizophrenia. Schizophrenia Research 55:1–10.

Genetic and Proteomic Studies in Schizophrenia

Emmanuel Dias-Neto, Daniel Martins-de-Souza, Elida P.B. Ojopi,
and Wagner F. Gattaz

Introduction

Schizophrenia (SCZ), as most other common human diseases, is a result of a complex interaction network of endogenous and exogenous factors. In SCZ, the genetic components are among the most important elements of this network: several types of DNA alterations may occur, resulting in gene expression and proteome variations that, independently or in concert, will lead to physiological imbalances that trigger the disease. Unfortunately, despite the tremendous efforts and significant contributions made by dozens of research groups around the world, most of the putative SCZ biomarkers revealed showed no consistent results when challenged with distinct sample sets.

This lack of progress in understanding the genetic aspects of SCZ – which also forms the basis of the assorted treatment response – is mainly due to the genetic heterogeneity seen in patients and to the multifaceted set of interconnected systems that conduct to the establishment of the disease. These interconnected systems include relevant and poorly characterized environmental players (such as urbanicity, lifestyle, social status, migration, drug abuse, and many forms of stress) and a number of converging metabolic pathways, each containing a large number of genes and regulatory noncoding RNA molecules. In diseased subjects, alterations in DNA segments containing relevant transcripts may occur at many levels including single or multiple base mutations/polymorphisms, methylation, or copy-number variations at DNA level; alterations in mRNA processing or posttranscriptional regulation, as well as mRNA stability and other factors that ultimately will lead to protein fluctuations. Furthermore, posttranslational protein modifications and altered enzyme activities as well as disturbances in the concentration of cellular metabolites might be a leading guide to the disease. Thus, at a population level, large series of alterations might be involved in the disorder, but in a given affected individual it is likely

E. Dias-Neto (✉)
Laboratory of Neuroscience (LIM-27) Institute of Psychiatry, Faculty of Medicine - University of
São Paulo - Brazil
e-mail: emmanuel@usp.br

W.F. Gattaz, G. Busatto (eds.), *Advances in Schizophrenia Research 2009*,
DOI 10.1007/978-1-4419-0913-8_10, © Springer Science+Business Media, LLC 2010

that a few of these genes mediate the development of the disease. As a consequence, the disruption of a metabolic pathway may occur by alterations on any of its various gene components; and distinct individuals may have different gene alterations that will lead to the same phenotype. The identification of statistically significant associations between these alterations and the disease requires numerous genomic loci to be investigated in a large number of samples.

In the last decades, due to technical restrictions, the studies have tended to be limited to few genes usually restricted to a small number of pathways. It is our belief that the over-simplification of the problem, together with technical limitations in the investigation of larger genomic regions in many samples, has certainly hampered the progress toward the deeper understanding of the basis of this disease.

RNAs and proteins are the central classes of biomarkers that can be directly influenced by endogenous alterations such as DNA variations and mutations, as well as influenced by exogenous alterations. Besides, RNA categories – such as regulatory noncoding RNAs – are emerging as biomarkers due to its dramatic influences over the proteome. To date, many potential RNA and proteins biomarkers to SCZ have already been described and a few have already been validated in a considerable set of individual samples.

Together, genome, transcriptome, and proteome analysis may provide a complete molecular basis that can shed light on the molecular basis of SCZ and can grant potential biomarkers derived from different and complementary approaches. In this chapter, we will discuss and contrast with the literature some of the studies involving DNA alterations, large-scale gene expression, and proteomics, which we have conducted in the last few years in the Laboratory of Neurosciences (LIM-27) at the Institute and Department of Psychiatry at the Faculdade de Medicina of Universidade de São Paulo (USP).

DNA Studies

Schizophrenia and DNA Polymorphisms: Association Studies

Due to the complexity of SCZ and the intricacies of the human genome and transcriptome, the search for the genetic glitches behind SCZ has become mired in findings that could not always be confirmed by subsequent studies. As many genes are involved, "small-effect" genetic alterations are likely to be implicated in the disease pathogenesis, but their effect can only be seen after a large number of individuals has been studied. When the disease tissues (i.e., brains) need to be investigated, the collection of a large sample size imposes a serious limitation.

An approach to reduce this limitation is to evaluate alternative samples, such as peripheral blood cells of affected individuals, which potentially carry DNA alterations with important consequences over the establishment of the disease. The potential importance of DNA markers, together with the higher feasibility of collecting blood samples, has made quite popular the study of genetic polymorphisms, with >2,300 papers (as of February 1, 2009) found in PubMed using "polymorphism" and "schizophrenia" as keywords. Unfortunately, the largest part of these studies could not be replicated in distinct samples, and most have focused on the same very few genes (posing a limitation for a broader view of the many actors playing roles in this disease).

The approach undertaken in our laboratory for the study of DNA polymorphisms in SCZ was to select pathways related to processes that are related to the disease and to pinpoint genes associated with these processes that are mapped to genomic regions relevant to the disease. Bioinformatics databases such as the Gene Ontology Project (The gene ontology consortium, 2000 – www.geneontology.org). As several lines of evidence point SCZ as a neurodevelopmental disorder (McCarley et al., 1999; Harrison, 1999; Shenton et al., 2001) that may also include adult neurogenesis as a main event (Duan et al., 2007), neurogenesis-related genes are plausible candidates to be involved in the etiology of SCZ. Thus, neurogenesis was the first pathway we selected. Among the genes to be investigated, we have chosen those containing new or already described DNA polymorphisms, including single nucleotide polymorphisms (SNPs) or insertion/deletion (indels) events, with a major emphasis on DNA alterations that were likely to have functional consequences, based on their location (such as regulatory or coding regions) or intrinsic characteristics (for instance, creating/abolishing promoter or regulatory regions or altering amino acids on the encoded protein). Most of the DNA variations investigated here were never studied before for any human disease. The list of genes and polymorphisms selected for SCZ association studies is presented in Table 1, and some examples of our findings using this strategy will be given in the next pages.

One of the first genes evaluated in our studies was *NOGO* (Neurite Outgrowth inhibitor), which maps to a relevant region for SCZ (DeLisi et al., 2002) and encodes for a myelin-associated protein that is important for shaping the neuronal circuitry (Fournier et al., 2001; Meier et al., 2003). Before we started our study, a polymorphism in the 3'-untranslated region of the *NOGO* transcript, consisting of the insertion of three nucleotides (CAA), has been described to be associated with SCZ in a limited sample set (81 patients and 61 controls; Novak et al., 2002). In order to evaluate this association in a larger and better paired sample set, we evaluated this same polymorphism over 725 samples (Gregório et al., 2005). Instead of indicating associations with SCZ, this trinucleotide insertion demonstrated a remarkably biased distribution in ethnical groups, which was in agreement with a subsequent paper by Covault et al. (2004).

To continue the search for gene alterations associated with SCZ, we investigated some genes of the Notch signaling pathway, which has a remarkable importance in neurodevelopment (reviewed in Shimizu et al., 2002). Neurophysiologic processes that involve Notch include bilateral symmetry regulation, cell fate determination, and neural stem cell proliferation and differentiation (Hrabe de Angelis et al., 1997; Apelqvist et al., 1999; Kiernan et al., 2001; Kim and Hebrok, 2001; De Bellard et al., 2002; Przemeck et al., 2003). In general, Notch activity leads to inhibition of cell differentiation signaling, which preserves responsive progenitors, thus conserving the cell diversity potential (Kopan and Turner, 1996). The expression of Notch pathway molecules in post-mitotic neurons seems to be important for the plasticity of the

Table 1 List of neurogenesis-related genes and polymorphisms mapped to genomic regions relevant to SCZ selected for analysis (adapted from Gregório et al., 2009)

Gene symbol	Gene description	Function in neurogenesis	Genomic mapping	Polymorphism	dbSNP code (only for SNPs)
ADAM15	A Disintegrin And Metalloproteinase domain 15	Cell adhesion, neurogenesis	1q21.3	SNP C/A (THR191LYS)	rs6427128
ADAM22	A Disintegrin And Metalloproteinase domain 22	Cell adhesion, neurogenesis	7q21	SNP C/G (ARG81PRO)	rs2279542
ADAM28	A Disintegrin And Metalloproteinase domain 28	Cell adhesion, neurogenesis	8p21.2	SNP A/G (ILE684MET)	rs7829965
ADAMTS4	A Disintegrin And Metalloproteinase with Thrombospondin type 1 motif, 4	Cell adhesion, neurogenesis	1q21-q23	SNP G/A (ARG626GLN)	rs4233367
AKT1	v-akt murine thymoma viral oncogene homolog 1	Neurogenesis	14q32.32	SNP1: C/T (intron 5) SNP2: C/T (intergenic)	SNP1: rs3730358 SNP2: rs2498784
ASCL1	Achaete-scute complex-like 1	Essential for the development of 5-HT neurons	12q22–23	Microsatellite (poly-glutamine repeat)	N/A
ASPM	ASP (abnormal spindle)-like, microcephaly associated	Cell cortex development	1q31	SNP A/C (ILE2657LEU)	rs3762271
BDNF	Brain-Derived Neurotrophic Factor	Neurodevelopment, maintenance, synaptic remodeling, neuroprotection	11p13	SNP G/A (VAL66MET)	rs6265
FLNB	Filamin B, beta	Neural cytoarchitecture	3p14.3	SNP A/G (ASN1157ASP)	rs1131356
FZD3	Frizzled homolog 3	WNT proteins receptor, involved in CNS development	8p21	SNP C/T (promoter region)	rs7836920

Table 1 (continued)

Gene symbol	Gene description	Function in neurogenesis	Polymorphism	Genomic mapping	dbSNP code (only for SNPs)
JAG2	Jagged 2	Notch protein ligand	SNP G/A (GLU502LYS)	14q32	rs1057744
MAP1B	Microtubule-associated protein 1B	Axonal development	SNP G/A (VAL468ILE)	5q13	rs1866374
NEFH	Neurofilament, heavy polypeptide 200kDA	Neurofilaments	SNP C/A (ALA805GLU)	22q12.2	rs165602
NOGO/RTN4	Reticulon 4	Modulator of neurite growth	CAA 3'UTR insertion	2p14–p13	N.A.
NOTCH2	Notch homolog 2	Cell differentiation during development of tissues, neuritogenesis, body symmetry regulator	SNP T/C (ILE197THR)	1p13–p11	rs8002
NOTCH3	Notch homolog 3	Cell differentiation during development of tissues	SNP T/C (VAL2223ALA)	19p13.2–p13.1	rs1044009
NRG1	Neuregulin 1	Modulation of synaptic plasticity; activation of neurotransmitter expression	SNP A/G (GLN38ARG)	8p21–p12	rs3924333
NRP1	Neuropilin 1	Semaphorin ligand	SNP A/G (ILE733VAL)	10p12	rs2228638
NUDT6 / FGF2	Nudix (nucleoside diphosphate linked moiety X)-type	Neuroectodermal development	SNP G/A (Arg209Gln)	4q26	rs1048201
NUMB	Numb Homolog	Neuronal cell fate decisions	SNP C/A (THR232ASN)	14q23	rs1050477
NUMBL	Numb homolog-like	Neuronal cell fate decisions	Microsatellite (poly-glutamine repeat)	19q13.13–q13.2	N/A
PCDH3a	Protocadherin alpha 3	Definition of synaptic specificity of the neuronal network	SNP T332G (promoter region)	5q31	rs3756340

Table 1 (continued)

Gene symbol	Gene description	Function in neurogenesis	Genomic mapping	Polymorphism	dbSNP code (only for SNPs)
PCDH12	Protocadherin 12	Definition of synaptic specificity of the neuronal network	5q31	SNP G/A (SER640ASN)	rs164515
PCDHB11	Protocadherin beta 11	Definition of synaptic specificity of the neuronal network	5q31	SNP G/A (ARG7HIS)	rs917535
PCDH α CLUSTER	Protocadherin a cluster (PCDHa8 to PCDHa10)	Definition of synaptic specificity of the neuronal network	5q31	16.7 Kb deletion	N.A.
PPT1 *RELN*	Palmitoyl-protein thioesterase 1 Reelin	Synaptic modulation Neural migration and signalization	1p32 7Q22	SNP C/T (THR134ILE) SNP C/G (VAL997LEU)	rs1800205 rs362691
SEMA3D	Semaphorin 3D	Axonal growth and synaptic connectivity maintenance	7q21.12	SNP C/A (GLN340LYS)	rs7800072
SEMA6C	Semaphorin 6C	Axonal growth and synaptic connectivity maintenance	1q21.2	SNP C/A (PRO455THR)	rs4971007
SIM1	Single-minded homolog 1	Synaptic modulation	6q16.3–q21	SNP1: T/C (VAL371ALA) SNP2: A/C (THR352PRO)	SNP1: rs3734355 SNP2: 3734354
SMPD1	Sphingomyelin Phosphodiesterase 1	Sphingomyelin processing	11p15.4–p15.1	SNP G/A (GLY/ARG)	N.A.
WIF1 *WNT7A*	WNT Inhibitory Factor 1 Wingless-type MMTV integration site family, member 7A	WNT protein inhibitor Tissue development and maintenance, cell fate, synaptogenesis	12q13.13 3p25	SNP G/A (ALA27VAL) SNP G/C (2nd Intron)	N.A. N.A.

mature brain as well as for the formation of long-term memory (reviewed in Costa et al., 2005). Evidence indicates that Notch participates in the regulation of neurite growth and branching, growth and retraction of synapses, and adult neurogenesis, processes that are the basis of the plastic rearrangements of the neuronal circuitry. Important members of the Notch pathway are located in genomic regions that have previously been linked to SCZ such as *NOTCH2* (1p13–p11), *NUMB* (14q24.3), and *NUMBL* (19q13.13–q13.2) (Bailer et al., 2000; Chiu et al., 2002; Lewis et al., 2003; MacGregor et al., 2004).

In this study we investigated, in patients with SCZ and matched controls, the polymorphic status of selected non-synonymous DNA alterations located in *NOTCH2* and *NOTCH3*, together with other members of the Notch pathway (*JAGGED2*, *ASCL1*, *NUMB*, and *NUMBL*), with the hypothesis that potentially functional polymorphisms in these genes would impact neurogenesis and may confer liability to SCZ. A complete analysis of the whole sample set was performed for all polymorphisms in 200 DNA samples derived from schizophrenic patients and 200 paired controls, both groups from Brazil. The most promising finding was replicated in an unrelated set of 684 Danish DNA samples, including cases and controls. Our findings, derived from a total of 1,084 subjects from Brazil and Denmark, suggested the allele with 18 CAG repeats in *NUMBL* ($p=0.003$, $x^2=8.88$, OR=1.30, 95% CI: 1.09–1.56) as well as the 18/18 CAG genotype ($p=0.002$, $x^2=9.46$, OR=1.46, 95% CI: 1.15–1.87) to be associated with SCZ in sample sets (Gregório et al., 2006).

DNA Polymorphisms and Brain Morphometry Alterations: Genetic Brain Imaging in Schizophrenia

As neurodevelopment alterations may be the basis of well-known structural brain abnormalities that are present at early phases of psychosis, recent studies have focused on the analysis of DNA alterations that could be associated with SCZ-related brain morphology alterations. A recent example is the study of alterations in the Neuregulin-1 gene (*NRG1*), which encodes a signaling protein that mediates cell–cell interactions and plays a critical role in the development and plasticity of the CNS. Mata et al. (2009) have examined whether variations in this gene could influence brain volumes in first-episode SCZ subjects and found an allele significantly associated with increased lateral ventricle volume.

In the same line, we also reasoned that genetic variations in our neurodevelopment-related genes (mapped to relevant genomic regions for SCZ) might correlate with brain morphometry. We investigated this possibility using our set of 32 DNA polymorphisms, located in 30 genes related to neurogenesis and brain development. The polymorphic status of these DNA alterations was evaluated in SCZ patients (whose brain structural data were obtained by MRI), and the possible associations between structural brain measures and DNA alterations were calculated. After stringent Bonferroni corrections, we found a relevant association of the Val997Leu polymorphism on Reelin (a protease that guides neurons in the developing brain and underlies neurotransmission and synaptic plasticity in adults) and the enlargement of left and right brain ventricles. A putative association was also found between PCDH12, a cell adhesion molecule involved in axonal guidance and synaptic specificity, and cortical folding (asymmetry coefficient of gyrification index). Although our results are preliminary, due to the small number of individuals analyzed, such an approach could reveal new candidate genes implicated in anomalous neurodevelopment in SCZ (Gregório et al., 2009).

The results presented here suggest that gene alterations may be important for the development of SCZ. However, a complete picture of the importance of genetic variations will only be attained after the analysis of large, multiethnical groups, and the inclusion of a careful analysis of multi-locus effects is increasingly being recognized. Nowadays, whole genome association (WGA) studies are slowly substituting the analysis of single polymorphisms and may even replace traditional linkage studies. Other classes of genomic alterations are being demonstrated and include the recent emergence of structural genomic polymorphisms named "copy-number variation" or CNVs. CNVs constitute a substantial fraction of total genetic variability found in humans and may involve duplications and deletions of genome blocks that can result in many characteristics, including inherited or sporadic neuropsychiatric diseases. The importance of CNVs in modulating human disease is increasingly being recognized and its impact in SCZ seems to be remarkable, as demonstrated by recent publications (Stefansson et al. 2009; Kirov et al., 2009).

Gene and Protein Expression Studies in Schizophrenia

In contrast with many other "brain diseases" such as Alzheimer's or Parkinson's, SCZ lacks a clear unifying pathology at a system, tissue, or cellular level. Despite the family aggregation of SCZ, its underlying genetic etiology is complex. Linkage studies have often identified nonoverlapping regions of interest and regularly failed to replicate many risk chromosomal regions (Pulver, 2000). This suggests the involvement of multiple genes in the disease, some of which may represent common genetic alterations, each conferring a minor increase in disorder susceptibility (Sobell et al., 2002). The idea of a polygenic origin of the disease is reinforced by studies in SCZ postmortem brains, revealing altered expression of several genes and proteins (Hakak et al., 2001; Mirnics et al., 2000).

Alterations in gene expression could derive from a number of factors including DNA polymorphisms (SNPs or CNVs), promoter methylation, or chromatin conformational alterations, to name a few. Structural variations may lead to fluctuations in the expression of regulatory microRNAs (regulators of RNA stability and potent regulators of translation), alterations in gene splicing isoforms, and variations in the expression of relevant genes and their transcription factors. All these will ultimately affect the proteome and contribute to establish phenotypes. The capability of

studying the brain, the "diseased tissue" in SCZ, opens the possibility of understanding gene and protein expression patterns, which form the basis of complex
regulatory patterns of SCZ and other diseases.

The cumulative effects of genetic and environmental factors related to brain function and development may result in SCZ. The genetic components involved are
likely to be a sum of series of alterations in genes of "small effect," being most
adequately studied collectively by large-scale projects. The vast majority of large-
scale expression profiling studies of human brain tissues has been performed with
cDNA microarrays, which allow a fast, simultaneous, and sensitive analysis of a
large number of biological samples for the concurrent expression of thousands of
genes. Through the use of these arrays, global gene expression analysis was used
as valuable tool to obtain major insights into diagnosis, progression, prognosis,
and response to therapy for a number of human diseases. Recent developments of
microarray technology allowed the investigation of larger fractions of the transcriptome, increasing the cDNA arrays' accuracy and reducing its costs, permitting their
use as a common tool in the search of markers of human diseases. In SCZ, cDNA
microarrays have been used for gene expression analysis in diverse brain areas such
as the prefrontal (Tkachev et al., 2003; Polesskaya et al., 2003; Middleton et al.,
2002; Hakak et al., 2001; Johnston-Wilson et al., 2000; Mirnics et al., 2000; Volk
et al., 2000), entohinal (Hemby et al., 2002), and temporal (Aston et al., 2004;
Vawter et al., 2001) brain cortices.

Gene expression alterations have been demonstrated for several putative SCZ
susceptibility genes after comparing diseased and control brains. Examples of more
consistent alterations identified are *DTNBP1* (Weickert et al., 2008, 2004; Talbot
et al., 2004), *G72* (DAOA; Korostishevsky et al., 2004), *NRG1* (Law et al., 2006;
Hashimoto et al., 2004), and *RGS4* (Bowden et al., 2007; Erdely et al., 2006).
However, maybe more important than individual genes, the accumulation of transcriptome analysis in SCZ has demonstrated the consistent alteration of specific
pathways such as synaptic function (Hemby et al., 2002; Vawter et al., 2002; Mirnics et al., 2000), energy metabolism (Altar et al., 2005; Prabakaran et al., 2004;
Middleton et al., 2002), and oligodendrocyte function (Sugai et al., 2004; Tkachev
et al., 2003; Hakak et al., 2001). The identification of consistent alterations in certain pathways demonstrates the power of gene expression studies. However, cDNA
microarray expression analyses have its own constraints and maybe the more important is that the genes to be studied are limited to those that are present on the array.
This, together with the inadequacy of the method to provide absolute quantification
results, makes other approaches attractive to complement large-scale gene expression analyses.

Serial Analysis of Gene Expression in Schizophrenia

After our collaborations with Dr. Andrea Schmitt, from the Central Institute of Mental Health, in Mannheim, Germany, we received brain samples from SCZ patients

and matched controls. With these samples, we were able to investigate transcriptome and proteome alterations in the disease. For transcriptome studies, instead of using "closed" platforms such as cDNA microarrays, we undertook an alternative approach, based on the generation, sequencing, and quantification of short nucleotide tags derived from human transcripts. The approach undertaken here was first described by Velculescu et al. (1995) and it is named serial analysis of gene expression (SAGE). Since its inception, SAGE has become one of the leading functional genomics methodologies and a number of groups in academia and industry have demonstrated the utility of SAGE for novel gene and pathway discovery, for biomarker identification, and for gene expression profiling of numerous disease and normal conditions in multiple species. SAGE provides a statistical description of the mRNA population present in a cell without prior selection of the genes to be studied, and this constitutes its major advantage when compared to microarrays. The use of this open platform allows hypothesis-free expression profiling of SCZ tissue and thus has the potential to highlight previously unexplored molecular processes in the disorder.

To perform SAGE in our samples, we prepared two library pools from the right hemisphere of the prefrontal cortex. One pool was prepared from patient's samples (four females, four males, average 72.6 years old) and a second pool was made from controls (three females, three males, average 73.2 years old). After sequencing, we produced a total of 51,661 SCZ-derived tags (SCZ tags) and 46,134 controls tags (CN tags). These tags were enough to cover >10,000 genes, and at the cutoff of $P \leq 0.001$, 169 appeared to be differentially expressed between cases and controls. Twenty tags (representing 14 genes) were only seen among the SCZ set, whereas 21 were present only in the control set, strongly suggesting the corresponding genes to be differentially regulated in the disease. Overall, the data suggest an upregulation trend in SCZ brains compared to non-SCZ controls, as 107 of the 169 (63.3%) differentially expressed tags were significantly more abundant in the diseased samples. Among the gene tags identified in our SAGE study, we observed transcripts encoding proteins related to a number of important pathways such as calcium-binding proteins, synthesis and excretion of bioamines, signal transduction, cell proliferation and differentiation, and others. The limitations of our study include the presence of confounding factors (such as different postmortem intervals and the use of psychoactive drugs by the patients), the relatively small sample size, and the gene expression evaluation in pooled samples. Whereas the importance of certain genes in individual samples can still be confirmed by a careful analysis of each gene in a higher sample size, the other limitations are common to most other transcriptome or proteome studies in SCZ. However, the ability of our results (derived from a totally distinct technical approach) to corroborate diverse pathways and genes previously identified by others not only reinforces the validity of our own findings (including the putative new markers observed here) but also confirms the importance of some physiological routes in the pathology of this disease. We are currently validating the most relevant findings in individual samples by quantitative RT-PCR analysis and the data will be published elsewhere.

Proteomic Studies

The study of RNA and proteins poses distinct technical challenges but also offers complementary sources of potentially useful disease markers. In terms of stability, both RNA and proteins are labile and can be easily degraded in the postmortem interval. However, differently from proteins, the analysis of RNA benefits from extremely sensitive and less-expensive techniques that allow the study of single molecules permitting the study of the whole universe of molecules present in a tissue. All these molecules can be precisely quantified and sequenced in a good number of samples, using equipments easily available nowadays. In most cases, however, RNAs are intermediates between DNA and the proteins, which are the real biological effectors. Thus, the encounter of a certain RNA marker is not enough evidence of the involvement of the gene in the disease. Due to post-transcriptional regulatory events, high RNA levels do not necessarily indicate high protein levels and vice versa. On the other hand, even the most advanced proteome approaches available today do not allow the precise detection and quantification of all proteins present in a sample, and for most proteomic approaches the set of proteins studied is limited to the small fraction of the proteome that contains proteins with adequate solubility and higher abundance. In summary, RNA analysis is more precise and sensitive, but the proteomic information however is technically more limited, providing more direct and biologically relevant markers. A collection of some of the most relevant papers published on SCZ transcriptome and proteome, as well as the brain regions and platforms used in the study, is presented in Table 2.

Shotgun Proteomics

Shotgun peptide sequencing was the main technique used in our study of SCZ proteins. Also known as shotgun proteomics, this is a mass-spectrometry-based strategy that allows a comprehensive analysis of complex protein mixtures, which was developed as a new strategy to overcome the limitations of two-dimensional gel electrophoresis (2DE), the most traditional method used in proteome studies, and to provide a better representation of the proteome (Link et al., 1999). Traditionally, shotgun approaches are combined with quantitative methods based on differential labeling of proteins with stable isotopes, like Isotope-Coded Affinity Tags (ICAT) (Gygi et al., 1999), Global Internal Standard Technology (GIST) (Goodlett et al., 2001), Isobaric Tags for Relative and Absolute Quantification (iTRAQ) (Ross et al., 2004), and Isotope-coded protein label (ICPL) (Schmidt et al., 2005). Nowadays, metabolic labeling (Ong et al., 2002; Gruhler et al., 2005) is considered a powerful approach to support enhanced quantification methods. Shotgun proteomics is based on the digestion of a complex protein mixture with the help of specific enzymes followed by the separation of the resulting peptides by multidimensional chromatographic techniques and subsequent analysis by mass spectrometry (MS).

Table 2 Analysis of gene and proteome expression of *postmortem* SCZ brain tissue

Brain region	Transcriptome reference	Subjects	Methodology	Proteome reference	Subjects	Methodology
Dorso-lateral prefrontal cortex (BA46)	(1) Mirnics et al. (2000)	(1) 11 SCZ; 11 controls	(1) Microarray	(1) Martins-de-Souza et al. (2008a)	(1) 9 SCZ; 7 controls	(1) 2DE
	(2) Hakak et al. (2001)	(2) 12 SCZ; 12 controls	(2) Microarray	(2) Martins-de-Souza et al. (2009a)	(2) 9 SCZ; 7 controls	(2) Shotgun
	(3) Vawter et al. (2001)	(3) 8 SCZ; 3 Controls	(3) Microarray			
	(4) Middleton et al. (2002)	(4) 10 SCZ; 10 controls	(4) Microarray			
	(5) Mimmack et al. (2002)	(5) 10 SCZ; 10 controls	(5) Microarray			
	(6) Vawter et al. (2002)	(6) 15 SCZ; 15 controls	(6) Microarray			
	(7) Tkachev et al. (2003)	(7) 15 SCZ; 15 controls	(7) Microarray			
	(8) Katsel et al. (2005)	(8) 16 SCZ; 14 controls	(8) Microarray			
	(9) Arion et al. (2007)	(9) 12 SCZ; 12 controls	(9) Microarray			
Cerebellum	Vawter et al. (2001)	5 SCZ; 3 unmedicated SCZ; 3 Controls	Microarray	–	–	–
Middle temporal gyrus (BA21)	(1) Vawter et al. (2001)	(1) 5 medicated SCZ 3 unmedicated SCZ 3 Controls	(1) Microarray	–	–	–
	(2) Katsel et al. (2005)	(2) 16 SCZ: 14 controls	(2) Microarray			

Table 2 (continued)

Brain region	Transcriptome reference	Subjects	Methodology	Proteome reference	Subjects	Methodology
Prefrontal cortex (BA9)	(1) Vawter et al. (2002) (2) Tkachev et al. (2003)	(1) 15 SCZ; 15 controls (2) 15 SCZ; 15 controls	(1) Microarray (2) Microarray	(1) Prabakaran et al. (2004) (2) Pennington et al. (2008) (3) Behan et al. (2008)	(1) 54 SCZ; 50 controls (2) 35 SCZ; 35 controls (3) 30 SCZ; 30 controls	(1) 2DE-DIGE (2) 2DE (3) 2DE and Shotgun
Temporal cortex (middle temporal gyrus - BA21)	Aston et al. (2004)	12 SCZ; 14 controls	Microarray	–	–	–
Frontal cortex (BA10)	Katsel et al. (2005)	16 SCZ; 14 controls	Microarray	Johnston-Wilson et al. (2000)	24 SCZ; 19 controls	2DE
Superior frontal gyrus (BA8)						
Insular cortex (BA44)						
Anterior cingulate (BA32)						
Posterior cingulate (BA:23/31)						
Parietal (BA7)	Katsel et al. (2005)	16 SCZ; 14 controls	Microarray	–	–	–
Inferior temporal gyrus (BA20)						
Superior temporal gyrus (BA22)						
Parahippocampal gyrus (BA:36/28)						
Occipital (BA17)						
Hippocampus						
Caudate nucleus						
Caudate putamen						

Table 2 (continued)

Brain region	Transcriptome reference	Subjects	Methodology	Proteome reference	Subjects	Methodology
I- Cingulate gyrus (Brodmann area 24/32) II- Hippocampus III- Caudate nucleus IV- Caudate putamen	Dracheva et al. (2006)	I- 30 SCZ; 25 Controls II- 24 SCZ; 21 Controls III- 23 SCZ; 20 Controls IV- 24 SCZ; 19 Controls	qPCR	—	—	—
Anterior cingulate cortex (BA24)	(1) Katsel et al. (2005) (2) McCullumsmith et al. (2007)	(1) 16 SCZ; 14 controls (2) 41 SCZ; 34 Controls	(1) Microarray (2) in situ hybridization	(1) Clark et al. (2006) (2) Beasley et al. (2006)	(1) 10 SCZ; 10 controls (2) 15 SCZ; 15 controls	(1) 2DE (2) 2DE
Genus of the corpus callosum	—	—	—	Sivagnanasundaram et al. (2007)	10 SCZ; 10 controls	2DE
Anterior temporal lobe (BA38)	—	—	—	Martins-de-Souza et al. (2009b)	5 SCZ; 4 controls	Shotgun
Wernicke's area (BA22p)	—	—	—	Martins-de-Souza et al. (2009c)	9 SCZ; 7 controls	2DE

Abbreviations: 2DE, two-dimensional gel electrophoresis; DIGE, differential in gel electrophoresis.

Protein identification is performed by database search with algorithms that assign experimental peptide molecular masses with those included in the protein sequence databases (Haas et al., 2006). Unlike 2DE, the shotgun technology has the ability to achieve a comprehensive representation of many protein classes, including extremely acidic and basic proteins as well as very hydrophobic and less abundant proteins. There are uncountable possibilities to develop a shotgun approach, combining all the different chromatography and electrophoretic steps (Martins-de-Souza et al., 2008b).

In the next pages we will present a synthesis of our findings using shotgun proteomics and 2DE, highlighting our most relevant markers and comparing our data with the literature. The results are presented according to the most suited metabolic pathway that encompasses the putative markers identified here and evidence reinforcement, given by gene-expression studies, will be presented.

Alterations in Oligodendrocyte Metabolism

The formation and maintenance of the myelin sheath in the axons of neurons in the central nervous system is the main function of the oligodendrocytes, which constitute approximately half the cells around the soma of large neurons in the human cortex (Polak et al. 1982). Myelin is a basic protein that surrounds the axons of many neurons forming an electrically insulating phospholipid layer that facilitates the propagation of the axonal electric signal. The role of oligodendrocytes in SCZ has emerged recently mainly after a combination of evidences derived from histological observations (Uranova et al. 2001), imaging and transcriptional (microarray-based) studies, deviating SCZ from the dopaminergic hypotheses (reviewed in Segal et al., 2007).

Hakak et al. (2001), using cDNA microarrays for the analysis of pooled dorsolateral prefrontal cortex samples (DLPFC) of controls and medicated chronic SCZ patients, opened the series of studies that revealed the dysregulation of oligodendrocytes metabolism. The findings from Hakak et al. were subsequently reinforced by a number of other papers (Tkachev et al. 2003; Aston et al. 2004; Katsel et al. 2005; Arion et al. 2007), including the validation of some genes by real-time quantitative PCR (qPCR) (Dracheva et al. 2006) or in situ hybridization (McCullumsmith et al. 2007). The demonstration of oligodendrocyte dysfunction in SCZ, using proteomics, was inaugurated by Prabakaran et al. (2004) analyzing the SCZ prefrontal cortex (PFC). Some of the findings on the altered regulation of specific mRNAs were subsequently confirmed by proteomics and include 2′,3′-cyclic nucleotide 3′ phosphodiesterase (CNP), myelin oligodendrocyte glycoprotein (MOG), myelin basic protein (MBP), transferrin (TF) (Table 3) that we also consistently found downregulated in our SCZ proteomics studies in DLPFC and anterior temporal lobe (Martins-de-Souza et al., 2008a, 2009a, b).

It is interesting to note that the final steps of the prefrontal cortex myelinization occur in adolescence, when SCZ onset is more common. Moreover, demyelinization diseases, such as metachromatic leukodystrophy, present schizophrenic-like psychoses (Hyde et al. 1992). Probably, as mentioned by Hakak et al. (2001), alterations

Table 3 Oligodendrocyte-related genes and proteins presenting altered expression in SCZ brain tissues

Gene symbol	Gene name	Gene expression alteration previously described by	Confirmed by Proteomics
MBP	Myelin Basic Protein	Tkachev et al. (2003)	Martins-de-Souza et al., 2008a Martins-de-Souza et al., 2009b
CNP	2′,3′-cyclic nucleotide 3′ phosphodiesterase	Hakak et al. (2001) Tkachev et al. (2003) Aston et al. (2004) Katsel et al. (2005) Dracheva et al. (2006) McCullumsmith et al. (2007)	Prabakaran et al. 2004 Martins-de-Souza et al., 2009a Martins-de-Souza et al., 2009b
MAG	Myelin-associated glycoprotein	Hakak et al. (2001) Tkachev et al. (2003) Aston et al. (2004) Katsel et al. (2005) Aberg et al. (2006b) Dracheva et al. (2006) McCullumsmith et al. (2007)	–
ERBB3	v-erb-b2 erythroblastic leukemia viral oncogene	Hakak et al. (2001) Tkachev et al. (2003) Aston et al. (2004) Katsel et al. (2005)	–
TF	Transferrin	Hakak et al. (2001) Tkachev et al. (2003) Katsel et al. (2005) Aberg et al. (2006b) McCullumsmith et al. (2007) Arion et al. (2007)	Prabakaran et al. 2004 Clark et al., 2006 Pennington et al., 2008 Martins-de-Souza et al., 2008a

Table 3 (continued)

Gene symbol	Gene name	Gene expression alteration previously described by	Confirmed by Proteomics
GSN	Gelsolin	Hakak et al. (2001) Katsel et al. (2005)	Prabakaran et al. 2004
MAL	T-lymphocyte maturation-associated protein	Hakak et al. (2001) Aston et al. (2004) Katsel et al. (2005)	–
CLDN11	Claudin 11; Oligodendrocyte specific protein	Tkachev et al. (2003) Katsel et al. (2005) Dracheva et al. (2006)	–
MOG	Myelin oligodendrocyte glycoprotein	Tkachev et al. (2003) Katsel et al. (2005) Arion et al. (2007)	Martins-de-Souza et al. (2009a) Martins-de-Souza et al. (2009b)
PLP	Proteolipid protein	Tkachev et al. (2003) Aston et al. (2004) Aberg et al. (2006b)	–
PLLP/ TM4SF11	Plasmolipin or Transmembrane 4 superfamily 11	Aston et al. (2004) Katsel et al. (2005)	–
QKI	Quaking homolog	Aberg et al. (2006a) McCullumsmith et al. (2007)	–

in oligodendrocyte–axon interactions may underlie cytoarchitectural changes found in SCZ. Clinical and physiological evidences, together with data from transcriptome and proteome large-scale studies from different brain regions, showed significant alterations in the expression of myelinization pathways and put oligodendrocytes as central players in SCZ.

Alterations in Calcium Homeostasis

The conversion of electrical pulses into chemical signals requires a precise control of calcium (Ca^{2+}) levels in the central nervous system. After the depolarization of presynaptic membranes, Ca^{2+} ions enter the neurons through voltage-gated channels and this sudden increase in the intracellular Ca^{2+} concentration triggers the synaptic vesicles to fuse with the presynaptic membrane, releasing neurotransmitters into the synaptic cleft. The tight regulation of Ca^{2+} involves extracellular and intracellular compartments of the central nervous system, including transport mechanisms across the blood–brain barrier and cellular membranes, extensive binding by proteins and other macromolecules, and ion sequestration within a variety of intracellular organelles.

Ca^{2+} plays a central role in SCZ dopamine hypothesis since it regulates the function D1 and D2 dopamine receptors (Bergson et al., 2003). In our transcriptome and proteome studies, we found alterations in a series of Ca^{2+}-related proteins including some of the most important regulators of this ion. It is worth mentioning the observation of reduced levels of calcineurin (CALN or PPP3CA) in our SAGE and proteomic data from two distinct brain areas. Calcineurin is the major Ca^{2+}/calmodulin-binding protein; it has pivotal functions in neuronal metabolism (Malenka, 1994; Liu et al., 1994) and is a regulator of dopaminergic (Greengard, 2001) and glutamatergic (Zeng et al., 2001) neurotransmission, both frequently compromised in SCZ (Seeman, 1987; Carlsson et al., 2001). More interestingly, calcineurin knockout mice subjected to a comprehensive behavioral test battery displayed strikingly similar phenotypes to those described for SCZ (Miyakawa et al., 2003). Other Ca^{2+}-related proteins found altered in our studies include calmodulin (CALM), plasma membrane calcium-transporting ATPase 4 (PMCA-4), and Visinin-like protein 1 (VILIP-1), which are sensors and maintainers of Ca^{2+} homeostasis in the cell, whose alterations can lead to abnormal brain Ca^{2+} concentrations that may increase Ca^{2+}-dependent phospholipase A2 (PLA2) activity and account for the accelerated phospholipid turnover and reduced dopaminergic activity previously observed in the SCZ frontal lobe (Gattaz et al., 1990; Gattaz and Brunner, 1996).

Alterations in Energy Metabolism

Neuronal activity is an energetically demanding process. Any sensible alterations of the sophisticated and complex mitochondria's network system, which involves different and sensible regulated biochemical pathways such as Krebs cycle and oxidative phosphorylation, could lead to an overall energetic dysregulation. The role of the energy metabolism in neuronal plasticity and synapse (reviewed in Ben-Shachar and Laifenfeld 2004) and evidences of oxidative damage in SCZ brains (reviewed in Yao et al. 2001) strongly suggest that SCZ has an important energetic component in its pathogenesis. It was hypothesized that the energy metabolism dysfunction in SCZ could be related to the hyperdopaminergic states observed in SCZ patients. Probably, the excess of dopamine-oxidized metabolites in SCZ tissues can lead to an oxidative stress, which consequently inhibits the mitochondrial respiratory system (Ben-Shachar et al. 2004).

Large-scale transcriptome and proteome analysis consensually showed the dysregulation of energy metabolism in SCZ (Vawter et al., 2001; Middleton et al., 2002; Johnston-Wilson et al., 2000; Prabakaran et al. 2004; Clark et al. 2006). Our proteomics studies showed that most of differentially expressed proteins identified play roles in energy metabolism, such as hexokinase brain form, creatine kinase, aldolase C, and gamma-enolase (Martins-de-Souza et al., 2008a, 2009a, b, c), in agreement with other proteomics reports (Johnston-Wilson et al., 2000; Prabakaran et al., 2004; Clark et al., 2006; Sivagnanasundaram et al. 2007; Pennington et al. 2008) (Table 4).

Summary and Conclusions

It is more and more clear that the study of complex conditions, such as SCZ, requires more comprehensive methods. Multidisciplinary approaches involving the study of DNA, RNA, and proteins derived from large and heterogeneous populations of affected individuals and matched controls have to be accompanied by imaging studies, detailed clinical records to group patients by endophenotypes, and careful patient and family interviews to collect data related to environmental influences such as immigration, stress, and use of recreational drugs. The task is complex not only because it involves many distinct features but also due to the organizational complexity of the molecules studied, the large number of patients required, and is further challenged by the availability of adequate samples (including the hunt for diseased tissue samples hard to obtain such as those from drug-naïve subjects or tissues adequate for RNA and protein analysis) and the absence of proper animal models of SCZ.

SCZ research urges to discover peculiar molecules that could not only be used as tools for SCZ diagnosis but also serve as molecular signs toward the understanding of its pathogenesis. Beyond the diagnose biomarkers, the dynamic nature of the transcriptome and proteome can reveal the complexity of gene and protein expression regulation, contributing to the understanding of important clinical aspects such as the comprehension of the disease establishment, determination of acute and chronic phases, endophenotypes, and response to treatment.

Table 4 Energy metabolism-related genes and proteins revealed as differentially expressed in transcriptome and proteome studies of SCZ brain tissue

Gene symbol	Gene name	Transcriptome studies	Proteome studies
MDH	Malate dehydrogenase	Middleton et al. (2002)	Martins-de-Souza et al. (2008a)
ATP5A1	ATP synthase, H+ transporting, mitochondrial F1 complex, alpha subunit isoform b	Middleton et al. (2002) Altar et al. (2005)	Martins-de-Souza et al. (2008a) Martins-de-Souza et al. (2009c)
ATP6V1A	ATPase, H+ transporting, lysosomal 70kD, V1 subunit A, isoform 1	Altar et al. (2005)	Pennington et al. (2008) Behan et al. (2008) Martins-de-Souza et al. (2008a) Martins-de-Souza et al. (2009a)
ALDOC	Fructose bisphosphate aldolase C		Johnston-Wilson et al. (2000) Prabakaran et al. (2004) Clark et al. (2006) Martins-de-Souza et al. (2009b) Martins-de-Souza et al. (2008a) Martins-de-Souza et al. (2009c)
CA2	Carbonic Anhydrase 2		Johnston-Wilson et al. (2000) Beasley et al. (2006) Martins-de-Souza et al. (2009b)
CKB	Creatine kinase, B chain		Prabakaran et al. (2004) Clark et al. (2006) Beasley et al. (2006) Sivagnanasundaram et al. (2007) Behan et al. (2008) Martins-de-Souza et al. (2009a) Martins-de-Souza et al. (2009c)
ENO2	Gamma enolase (2-phospho-D-glycerate hydro-lyase)		Prabakaran et al. (2004) Sivagnanasundaram et al. (2007) Pennington et al. (2008) Martins-de-Souza et al. (2009c)
ACO2	Aconitate hydratase, mitochondrial precursor (Aconitase)		Prabakaran et al. (2004) Beasley et al. (2006) Martins-de-Souza et al. (2008b) Martins-de-Souza et al. (2009c)
HK1	Hexokinase brain form		Prabakaran et al. (2004) Martins-de-Souza et al. (2009b) Martins-de-Souza et al. (2009a)
GAPDH	Glyceraldehyde-3-phosphate dehydrogenase		Prabakaran et al. (2004) Martins-de-Souza et al. (2009c)
PGAM1	Phosphoglycerate mutase 1		Prabakaran et al. (2004) Martins-de-Souza et al. (2009c)
TPI1	Triosephosphate isomerase		Prabakaran et al. (2004) Martins-de-Souza et al. (2009c)

Acknowledgments The authors thank ABADHS (Associação Beneficente Alzira Denise Hertzog Silva), FAPESP (Fundação de Amparo à Pesquisa do Estado de São Paulo – Brazil), CNPq (Conselho Nacional de Pesquisas), and DAAD (Deutscher Akademischer Austauschdienst) for their fundamental support to our research.

References

Aberg, K., Saetre, P., Lindholm, E., Ekholm, B., Pettersson, U., Adolfsson, R. & Jazin, E. Human QKI, a new candidate gene for schizophrenia involved in myelination. Am J Med Genet B Neuropsychiatr Genet 141: 84–90, 2006a.

Aberg, K., Saetre, P., Jareborg, N. & Jazin, E. Human QKI, a potential regulator of mRNA expression of human oligodendrocyte-related genes involved in schizophrenia. Proc Natl Acad Sci USA 103: 7482–7487, 2006b.

Altar, C.A., Jurata, L.W., Charles, V., Lemire, A., Liu, P., Bukhman, Y., Young, T.A., Bullard, J., Yokoe, H., Webster, M.J., Knable, M.B. & Brockman, J.A. Deficient hippocampal neuron expression of proteasome, ubiquitin, and mitochondrial genes in multiple schizophrenia cohorts. Biol Psychiatry 58: 85–96, 2005.

Apelqvist, A., Li, H., Sommer, L., Beatus, P., Anderson, D.J., Honjo, T., Hrabe De Angelis, M., Lendahl, U. & Edlund, H. Notch signalling controls pancreatic cell differentiation. Nature 400: 877–881, 1999.

Arion, D., Unger, T. & Lewis, D.A. Molecular evidence for increased expression of genes related to immune and chaperone function in the prefrontal cortex in schizophrenia. Biol Psychiatry 62: 711–721, 2007.

Aston, C., Jiang, L. & Sokolov, B.P. Microarray analysis of postmortem temporal cortex from patients with schizophrenia. J Neurosci Res 77: 858–866, 2004.

Bailer, U., Leisch, F., Meszaros, K., Lenzinger, E., Willinger, U., Strobl, R., Gebhardt, C., Gerhard, E., Fuchs, K., Sieghart, W., Kasper, S., Hornik, K. & Aschauer, H.N. Genome scan for susceptibility loci for schizophrenia. Neuropsychobiology 42: 175–182, 2000.

Beasley, C.L., Pennington, K., Behan, A., Wait, R., Dunn, M.J. & Cotter, D. Proteomic analysis of the anterior cingulate cortex in the major psychiatric disorders: Evidence for disease-associated changes. Proteomics 6: 3414–3425, 2006.

Behan, A., Byrne, C., Dunn, M.J., Cagney, G. & Cotter, D.R. Proteomic analysis of membrane microdomain-associated proteins in the dorsolateral prefrontal cortex in schizophrenia and bipolar disorder reveals alterations in LAMP, STXBP1 and BASP1 protein expression. Mol Psychiatry 2008 Feb 12. [Epub ahead of print]

Ben-Shachar, D. & Laifenfeld, D. Mitochondria, synaptic plasticity, and schizophrenia. Int Rev Neurobiol 59: 273–296, 2004.

Ben-Shachar, D., Zuk, R., Gazawi, H. & Ljubuncic, P. Dopamine toxicity involves mitochondrial complex I inhibition: Implications to dopamine-related neuropsychiatric disorders. Biochem Pharmacol 67: 1965–1974, 2004.

Bergson, C., Levenson, R., Goldman-Rakic, P.S. & Lidow, M.S. Dopamine receptor-interacting proteins: The Ca(2+) connection in dopamine signaling. Trends Pharmacol Sci 24: 486–492, 2003.

Bowden, N.A., Scott, R.J. & Tooney, P.A. Altered expression of regulator of G-protein signalling 4 (RGS4) mRNA in the superior temporal gyrus in schizophrenia. Schizophr Res 89: 165–168, 2007.

Carlsson, A., Waters, N., Holm-Waters, S., Tedroff, J., Nilsson, M. & Carlsson, M.L. Interactions between monoamines, glutamate, and GABA in schizophrenia: New evidence. Annu Rev Pharmacol Toxicol 41: 237–260, 2001.

Chiu, Y.F., Mcgrath, J.A., Thornquist, M.H., Wolyniec, P.S., Nestadt, G., Swartz, K.L., Lasseter, V.K., Liang, K.Y. & Pulver, A.E. Genetic heterogeneity in schizophrenia II: Conditional analyses of affected schizophrenia sibling pairs provide evidence for an interaction between markers on chromosome 8p and 14q. Mol Psychiatry 7: 658–664, 2002.

Clark, D., Dedova, I., Cordwell, S. & Matsumoto, I. A proteome analysis of the anterior cingulate cortex gray matter in schizophrenia. Mol Psychiatry 11: 459–470, 2006.

Costa, R.M., Drew, C. & Silva, A.J. Notch to remember. Trends Neurosci 28: 429–435, 2005.

Covault, J., Lee, J., Jensen, K. & Kranzler, H. Nogo 3'-untranslated region CAA insertion: Failure to replicate association with schizophrenia and demonstration of marked population difference in frequency of the insertion. Brain Res Mol Brain Res 120: 197–200, 2004.

De Bellard, M.E., Ching, W., Gossler, A. & Bronner-Fraser, M. Disruption of segmental neural crest migration and ephrin expression in delta-1 null mice. Dev Biol 249: 121–130, 2002.

Delisi, L.E., Mesen, A., Rodriguez, C., Bertheau, A., Laprade, B., Llach, M., Riondet, S., Razi, K., Relja, M., Byerley, W. & Sherrington, R. Genome-wide scan for linkage to schizophrenia in a Spanish-origin cohort from Costa Rica. Am J Med Genet 114: 497–508, 2002.

Dracheva, S., Davis, K.L., Chin, B. Woo, D.A., Schmeidler, J. & Haroutunian, V. Myelin-associated mRNA and protein expression deficits in the anterior cingulate cortex and hippocampus in elderly schizophrenia patients. Neurobiol Dis 21 :531–540, 2006.

Duan, X., Chang, J.H., Ge, S., Faulkner, R.L., et al. Disrupted-in-schizophrenia 1 regulates integration of newly generated neurons in the adult brain. Cell 130: 1146–1158, 2007.

Erdely, H.A., Tamminga, C.A., Roberts, R.C. & Vogel, M.W. Regional alterations in RGS4 protein in schizophrenia. Synapse 59: 472–479, 2006.

Fournier, A.E., Grandpre, T. & Strittmatter, S.M. Identification of a receptor mediating Nogo-66 inhibition of axonal regeneration. Nature 409: 341–346, 2001.

Gattaz, W.F. & Brunner, J. Phospholipase A2 and the hypofrontality hypothesis of schizophrenia. Prostaglandins Leukot Essent Fatty Acids 55: 109–113, 1996.

Gattaz, W.F., Hubner, C.V., Nevalainen, T.J., Thuren, T. & Kinnunen, P.K. Increased serum phospholipase A2 activity in schizophrenia: A replication study. Biol Psychiatry 28: 495–501, 1990.

Goodlett, D.R., Keller, A., Watts, J.D., Newitt, R., Yi, E.C., Purvine, S., Eng, J.K., Von Haller, P., Aebersold, R., & Kolker, E. Differential stable isotope labeling of peptides for quantitation and de novo sequence derivation. Rapid Commun Mass Spectrom 15: 1214–1221, 2001.

Greengard, P. The neurobiology of slow synaptic transmission. Science 294: 1024–1030, 2001.

Gregório, S.P., Gattaz, W.F., Tavares, H., Kieling, C., Timm, S., Wang, A.G., Rasmussen, H.B., Werge, T. & Dias-Neto, E. Analysis of coding-polymorphisms in NOTCH-related genes reveals NUMBL poly-glutamine repeat to be associated with schizophrenia in Brazilian and Danish subjects. Schizophr Res 88: 275–282, 2006.

Gregório, S.P., Mury, F.B., Ojopi, E.B., Sallet, P.C., Moreno, D.H., Yacubian, J., Tavares, H., Santos, F.R., Gattaz, W.F. & Dias-Neto, E. Nogo CAA 3'UTR Insertion polymorphism is not associated with Schizophrenia nor with Bipolar Disorder. Schizophr Res 75: 5–9, 2005.

Gregório, S.P., Sallet, P.C., Do, K.A., Lin, E., Gattaz, W.F. & Dias-Neto, E. Polymorphisms in genes involved in neurodevelopment may be associated with altered brain morphology in schizophrenia: Preliminary evidence. Psychiatry Res 165: 1–9, 2009.

Gruhler, A., Olsen, J.V., Mohammed, S., Mortensen, P., Faergeman, N.J., Mann, M. & Jensen, O.N. Quantitative phosphoproteomics applied to the yeast pheromone signaling pathway. Mol Cell Proteomics 4: 310–327, 2005.

Gygi, S.P., Rist, B., Gerber, S.A., Turecek, F., Gelb, M.H. & Aebersold, R. Quantitative analysis of complex protein mixtures using isotope-coded affinity tags. Nat Biotechnol 17: 994–999, 1999.

Haas, W., Faherty, B.K., Gerber, S.A., Elias, J.E., Beausoleil, S.A., Bakalarski, C.E., LI, X., Villen, J. & Gygi S.P. Optimization and use of peptide mass measurement accuracy in shotgun proteomics. Mol Cell Proteomics 5: 1326–1337, 2006.

Hakak, Y., Walker, J.R., Li, C., Wong, W.H., Davis, K.L., Buxbaum, J.D., Haroutunian, V. & Fienberg, A.A. Genome-wide expression analysis reveals dysregulation of myelination-related genes in chronic schizophrenia. Proc Natl Acad Sci USA 98: 4746–4751, 2001.

Harrison, P.J. The neuropathology of schizophrenia. A critical review of the data and their interpretation. Brain 122: 593–624, 1999.

Hashimoto, R., Straub, R.E., Weickert, C.S., Hyde, T.M., Kleinman, J.E. & Weinberger, D.R. Expression analysis of neuregulin-1 in the dorsolateral prefrontal cortex in schizophrenia. Mol Psychiatry 9: 299–307, 2004.

Hemby, S.E., Ginsberg, S.D., Brunk, B., Arnold, S.E., Trojanowski, J.Q. & Eberwine, J.H. Gene expression profile for schizophrenia: Discrete neuron transcription patterns in the entorhinal cortex. Arch Gen Psychiatry 59: 631–640, 2002.

Hrabe De Angelis, M., Mcintyre, J. & Gossler, A. Maintenance of somite borders in mice requires the Delta homologue DII1. Nature 386: 717–721, 1997.

Hyde, T.M., Ziegler, J.C. & Weinberger, D.R. Psychiatric disturbances in metachromatic leukodystrophy. Insights into the neurobiology of psychosis. Arch Neurol 49: 401–406, 1992.

Johnston-Wilson, N.L., Sims, C.D., Hofmann, J.P., Anderson, L., Shore, A.D., Torrey, E.F. & Yolken, R.H. Disease-specific alterations in frontal cortex brain proteins in schizophrenia, bipolar disorder, and major depressive disorder. The Stanley Neuropathology Consortium. Mol Psychiatry 5: 142–149, 2000.

Katsel, P., Davis, K.L. & Haroutunian, V. Variations in myelin and oligodendrocyte-related gene expression across multiple brain regions in schizophrenia: A gene ontology study. Schizophr Res 79: 157–173, 2005.

Kiernan, A.E., Ahituv, N., Fuchs, H., Balling, R., Avraham, K.B., Steel, K.P. & Hrabe De Angelis, M. The Notch ligand Jagged1 is required for inner ear sensory development. Proc Natl Acad Sci USA 98: 3873–3878, 2001.

Kim, S.K. & Hebrok, M. Intercellular signals regulating pancreas development and function. Genes Dev 15: 111–127, 2001.

Kirov, G., Grozeva, D., Norton, N., Ivanov, D., Mantripragada, K.K., Holmans, P. International Schizophrenia Consortium; The Wellcome Trust Case Control Consortium, Craddock, N., Owen, M.J. & O'donovan, M.C. Support for the involvement of large CNVs in the pathogenesis of schizophrenia. Hum Mol Genet 2009 [Epub ahead of print]

Kopan, R. & Turner, D.L. The Notch pathway: Democracy and aristocracy in the selection of cell fate. Curr Opin Neurobiol 6: 594–601, 1996.

Korostishevsky, M., Kaganovich, M., Cholostoy, A., Ashkenazi, M., Ratner, Y., Dahary, D., Bernstein, J., Bening-Abu-Shach, U., Ben-Asher, E., Lancet, D., Ritsner, M. & Navon, R. Is the G72/G30 locus associated with schizophrenia? Single nucleotide polymorphisms, haplotypes, and gene expression analysis. Biol Psychiatry 56: 169–176, 2004.

Law, A.J., Lipska, B.K., Weickert, C.S., Hyde, T.M., Straub, R.E., Hashimoto, R., Harrison, P.J., Kleinman, J.E. & Weinberger, D.R. Neuregulin 1 transcripts are differentially expressed in schizophrenia and regulated by 5' SNPs associated with the disease. Proc Natl Acad Sci USA 103: 6747–6752, 2006.

Lewis, C.M., Levinson, D.F., Wise, L.H., Delisi, L.E., Straub, R.E., Hovatta, I., Williams, N.M., Schwab, S.G., Pulver, A.E., Faraone, S.V., Brzustowicz, L.M., Kaufmann, C.A., Garver, D.L., Gurling, H.M., Lindholm, E., Coon, H., Moises, H.W., Byerley, W., Shaw, S.H., Mesen, A., Sherrington, R., O'neill, F.A., Walsh, D., Kendler, K.S., Ekelund, J., Paunio, T., Lönnqvist, J., Peltonen, L., et al. Genome scan meta-analysis of schizophrenia and bipolar disorder, part II: Schizophrenia. Am J Human Genetics 73: 34–48, 2003.

Link, A.J., Eng, J., Schieltz, D.M., Carmack, E., Mize, G.J., Morris, D.R., Garvik, B.M. & Yates, J.R. III Direct analysis of protein complexes using mass spectrometry. Nat Biotechnol 17: 676–682, 1999.

Liu, J.P., Sim, A.T. & Robinson, P.J. Calcineurin inhibition of dynamin I GTPase activity coupled to nerve terminal depolarization. Science 265: 970–973, 1994.

Macgregor, S., Visscher, P.M., Knott, S.A., Thomson, P., Porteous, D.J., Millar, J.K. Devon, R.S., Blackwood, D. & Muir, W.J. A genome scan and follow-up study identify a bipolar disorder susceptibility locus on chromosome 1q42. Mol Psychiatry 9: 1083–1090, 2004.

Malenka, R.C. Synaptic plasticity in the hippocampus: LTP and LTD. Cell 78: 535–538, 1994.

Martins-De-Souza, D., Gattaz, W.F., Schmitt, A., Maccarrone, G., Hunyadi-Gulyás, E., Eberlin, M.N., Souza, G.H., Marangoni, S., Novello, J.C., Turck, C.W. & Dias-Neto, E. Proteomic analysis of dorsolateral prefrontal cortex indicates the involvement of cytoskeleton, oligodendrocyte, energy metabolism and new potential markers in schizophrenia. J Psychiatr Res [Epub ahead of print], 2008a.

Martins-De-Souza, D., Gattaz, W.F., Schmitt, A, Rewerts, C., Maccarrone, G., Dias-Neto, E. & Turck, C.W. Proteome analysis of human dorsolateral prefrontal cortex using shotgun mass spectrometry. J Sep Sci 31: 3122–3126, 2008b.

Martins-De-Souza, D., Gattaz, W.F., Schmitt, A., Rewerts, C., Maccarrone, G., Dias-Neto, E. & Turck, C.W. Prefrontal cortex shotgun proteome analysis reveals altered calcium homeostasis and immune system imbalance in schizophrenia. Eur Arch Psychiatry Clin Neurosci 2009 Jan 22. [Epub ahead of print], 2009a.

Martins-De-Souza, D., Gattaz, W.F., Schmitt, A., Rewerts, C., Marangoni, S., Novello, J.C., Maccarrone, G., Turck, C.W. & Dias-Neto, E. Alterations in oligodendrocyte proteins, calcium homeostasis and new potential markers in schizophrenia anterior temporal lobe are revealed by shotgun proteome analysis. J Neural Transm 116: 275–289, 2009b.

Martins-De-Souza, D., Gattaz, W.F., Schmitt, A., Novello, J.C., Turck, C.W., Marangoni, S. & Dias-Neto, E. Proteome analysis of schizophrenia patients Wernicke's area reveals an energy metabolism dysregulation. BMC Psychiatry 9:17, 2009c.

Mata, I., Perez-Iglesias, R., Roiz-Santiañez, R., Tordesillas-Gutierrez, D., Gonzalez-Mandly, A., Vazquez-Barquero, J.L. & Crespo-Facorro, B. A neuregulin 1 variant is associated with increased lateral ventricle volume in patients with first-episode schizophrenia. Biol Psychiatry 65: 535–540, 2009.

McCarley, R.W., Wible, C.G., Frumin, M., Hirayasu, Y., Levitt, J.J., Fischer, I.A. & Shenton, M.E. MRI anatomy of schizophrenia. Biol Psychiatry 45: 1099–1119, 1999.

McCullumsmith, R.E., Gupta, D., Beneyto, M., Kreger, E., Haroutunian, V., Davis, K.L., Meador-Woodruff, J.H. Expression of transcripts for myelination -related genes in the anterior cingulated cortex in schizophrenia Schizophr Res 90: 15-27, 2007.

Meier, S., Brauer, A.U., Heimrich, B., Schwab, M.E., Nitsch, R. & Savaskan, N.E. Molecular analysis of Nogo expression in the hippocampus during development and following lesion and seizure. FASEB J 17: 1153–1155, 2003.

Middleton, F.A., Mirnics, K., Pierri, J.N., Lewis, D.A. & Levitt, P. Gene expression profiling reveals alterations of specific metabolic pathways in schizophrenia. J Neurosci 22: 2718–2729, 2002.

Mimmack, M.L., Ryan, M., Baba, H., Navarro-Ruiz, J., Iritani, S., Faull, R.L., Mckenna, P.J., Jones, P.B., Arai, H., Starkey, M., Emson, P.C. & Bahn, S. Gene expression analysis in schizophrenia: Reproducible up-regulation of several members of the apolipoprotein L family located in a high-susceptibility locus for schizophrenia on chromosome 22. Proc Natl Acad Sci USA 99: 4680–4685, 2002.

Mirnics, K., Middleton, F.A., Marquez, A., Lewis, D.A. & Levitt, P. Molecular characterization of schizophrenia viewed by microarray analysis of gene expression in prefrontal cortex. Neuron 28: 53–67, 2000.

Miyakawa, T., Leiter, L.M., Gerber, D.J., Gainetdinov, R.R., Sotnikova, T.D., Zeng, H., Caron, M.G. & Tonegawa, S. Conditional calcineurin knockout mice exhibit multiple abnormal behaviors related to schizophrenia. Proc Natl Acad Sci USA 100: 8987–8992, 2003.

Novak, G., Kim, D., Seeman, P. & Tallerico, T. Schizophrenia and Nogo: Elevated mRNA in cortex, and high prevalence of a homozygous CAA insert. Brain Res Mol Brain Res 107: 183–189, 2002.

Ong, S.E., Blagoev, B., Kratchmarova, I., Kristensen, D.B., Steen, H., Pandey, A. & Mann, M. Stable isotope labeling by amino acids in cell culture, SILAC, as a simple and accurate approach to expression proteomics. Mol Cell Proteomics 1: 376–386, 2002.

Pennington, K., Beasley, C.L., Dicker, P., Fagan, A., English, J., Pariante, C.M., Wait, R., Dunn, M.J. & Cotter, D.R. Prominent synaptic and metabolic abnormalities revealed by proteomic analysis of the dorsolateral prefrontal cortex in schizophrenia and bipolar disorder. Mol Psychiatry 13: 1102–1117, 2008.

Polak, M., Haymaker, W., Johnson, J.E. & D'amelio, F. (1982) Neuroglia and their reactions. In: Haymaker W, Adams RD (Eds.) Histology and Histopathology of the Nervous System. Springfield: Charles C. Thomas, 1982.

Polesskaya, O.O., Haroutunian, V., Davis, K.L., Hernandez, I. & Sokolov, B.P. Novel putative nonprotein-coding RNA gene from 11q14 displays decreased expression in brains of patients with schizophrenia. J Neurosci Res 74: 111–122, 2003.

Prabakaran, S., Swatton, J.E., Ryan, M.M., Huffaker, S.J., Huang, J.T., Griffin, J.L., Wayland, M., Freeman, T., Dudbridge, F., Lilley, K.S., Karp, N.A., Hester, S., Tkachev, D., Mimmack, M.L., Yolken, R.H., Webster, M.J., Torrey, E.F. & Bahn, S. Mitochondrial dysfunction in schizophrenia: Evidence for compromised brain metabolism and oxidative stress. Mol Psychiatry 9: 684–697, 2004.

Przemeck, G.K., Heinzmann, U., Beckers, J. & Hrabe De Angelis, M. Node and midline defects are associated with left-right development in Delta1 mutant embryos. Development 130: 3–13, 2003.

Pulver, A.E. Search for schizophrenia susceptibility genes. Biol Psychiatry 47: 221–230, 2000.

Ross, P.L., Huang, Y.N., Marchese, J.N., Williamson, B., Parker, K., Hattan, S., Khainovski, N., Pillai, S., Dey, S., Daniels, S., Purkayastha, S., Juhasz, P., Martin, S., Bartlet-Jones, M., He, F., Jacobson, A. & Pappin, D.J. Multiplexed protein quantitation in Saccharomyces cerevisiae using amine-reactive isobaric tagging reagents. Mol Cell Proteomics 3: 1154–1169, 2004.

Schmidt, A., Kellermann, J. & Lottspeich, F. A novel strategy for quantitative proteomics using isotope-coded protein labels. Proteomics 5: 4–15, 2005.

Seeman, P. Dopamine receptors and the dopamine hypothesis of schizophrenia. Synapse 1: 133–152, 1987.

Segal, D., Koschnick, J.R., Slegers, L.H. & Hof, P.R. Oligodendrocyte pathophysiology: A new view of schizophrenia. Int J Neuropsychopharmacol 10: 503–511, 2007.

Shenton, M.E., Dickey, C.C., Frumin, M. & McCarley, R.W. A review of MRI findings in schizophrenia. Schizophr Res 49: 1–52, 2001.

Shimizu, K., Chiba, S., Saito, T., Kumano, K., Hamada, Y. & Hirai, H. Functional diversity among Notch1, Notch2, and Notch3 receptors. Biochem Biophys Res Commun 291: 775–779, 2002.

Sivagnanasundaram, S., Crossett, B., Dedova, I., Cordwell, S. & Matsumoto, I. Abnormal pathways in the genu of the corpus callosum in schizophrenia pathogenesis: A proteome study. Proteomics Clin Appl 1: 1291–1305, 2007.

Sobell, J.L., Mikesell, M.J. & Mcmurray, C.T. Genetics and etiopathophysiology of schizophrenia. Mayo Clin Proc 77: 1068–1082, 2002.

Stefansson, H., Rujescu, D., Cichon, S., Pietiläinen, O.P., Ingason, A., Steinberg, S. et al., Large recurrent microdeletions associated with schizophrenia. Nature 455: 232–236, 2009.

Sugai, T., Kawamura, M., Iritani, S., Araki, K., Makifuchi, T., Imai, C., Nakamura, R., Kakita, A., Takahashi, H. & Nawa, H. Prefrontal abnormality of schizophrenia revealed by DNA microarray: Impact on glial and neurotrophic gene expression. Ann N Y Acad Sci 1025: 84–91, 2004.

Talbot, K., Eidem, W.L., Tinsley, C.L., Benson, M.A., Thompson, E.W., Smith, R.J., Hahn, C.G., Siegel, S.J., Trojanowski, J.Q., Gur, R.E., Blake, D.J. & Arnold, S.E. Dysbindin-1 is reduced in intrinsic, glutamatergic terminals of the hippocampal formation in schizophrenia. J Clin Invest 113: 1353–1363, 2004.

Tkachev, D., Mimmack, M.L., Ryan, M.M., Wayland, M., Freeman, T., Jones, P.B., Starkey, M., Webster, M.J., Yolken, R.H. & Bahn, S. Oligodendrocyte dysfunction in schizophrenia and bipolar disorder. Lancet 362: 798–805, 2003.

Uranova, N., Orlovskaya, D., Vikhreva, O. Zimina, I., Kolomeets, N., Vostrikov, V. & Rachmanova, V. Electron microscopy of oligodendroglia in severe mental illness. Brain Res Bull 55: 597–610, 2001.

Vawter, M.P., Barret, T., Cheadle, C., Sokolov, B.P., Wood, W.H., Donovan, D.M., Webster, M., Freed, W.J. & Becker, K.G. Application of cDNA microarrays to examine gene expression differences in schizophrenia. Brain Res Bull 55: 641–650, 2001.

Vawter, M.P., Crook, J.M., Hyde, T.M., Kleinman, J.E., Weinberger, D.R., Becker, K.G. & Freed, W.J. Microarray analysis of gene expression in the prefrontal cortex in schizophrenia: A preliminary study. Schizophr Res. 58: 11–20, 2002.

Velculescu, E., Zhang, L., Volgelstein, B., & Kinzler, W. Serial analysis of gene expression. Science 270: 484–487, 1995.

Volk, D.W., Austin, M.C., Pierri, J.N., Sampson, A.R. & Lewis, D.A. Decreased glutamic acid decarboxylase67 messenger RNA expression in a subset of prefrontal cortical gamma-aminobutyric acid neurons in subjects with schizophrenia. Arch Gen Psychiatry 57: 237–245, 2000.

Weickert, C.S., Rothmond, D.A., Hyde, T.M., Kleinman, J.E. & Straub, R.E. Reduced DTNBP1 (dysbindin-1) mRNA in the hippocampal formation of schizophrenia patients. Schizophr Res 98: 105–110, 2008.

Weickert, C.S., Straub, R.E., Mcclintock, B.W., Matsumoto, M., Hashimoto, R., Hyde, T.M., Herman, M.M., Weinberger, D.R. & Kleinman, J.E. Human dysbindin (DTNBP1) gene expression in normal brain and in schizophrenic prefrontal cortex and midbrain. Arch Gen Psychiatry 61: 544–555, 2004.

Yao, J.K., Reddy, R.D. & Van Kammen, D.P. Oxidative damage and schizophrenia: An overview of the evidence and its therapeutic implications. CNS Drugs 15: 287–310, 2001.

Zeng, H., Chattarji, S., Barbarosie, M., Rondi-Reig, L., Philpot, B.D., Miyakawa, T., Bear, M.F. & Tonegawa, S. Forebrain-specific calcineurin knockout selectively impairs bidirectional synaptic plasticity and working/episodic-like memory. Cell 107: 617–629, 2001.

Neurogenetic Risk Mechanisms of Schizophrenia: An Imaging Genetics Approach

Andreas Meyer-Lindenberg

Introduction

It is now broadly recognized that schizophrenia is a largely heritable brain disorder in which interactions with the environment also play a prominent role. This means that understanding how these genetic variants work is essential to identifying the pathophysiological mechanisms of schizophrenia, which in turn is the key to finding novel treatments.

A large body of work on the neurobiology of schizophrenia provides several convenient points of departure for translational genetics. Brain structure, for example, has clearly been shown to be abnormal in the disorder, with abnormalities in gray matter volume, density, cortical thickness, white matter volume, white matter connectivity, and structural connectivity all having been described. Both the lateral and medial temporal lobes as well as the dorsolateral prefrontal cortex in particular have emerged as regions which have consistently been implicated. To nominate any of these regions as a candidate phenotype for translational genetics, it is of interest to ascertain whether that phenotype is heritable. Taking dorsolateral prefrontal cortex again as an example, our own work does not reach an unambiguous conclusion. In a recent publication, we measured cortical thickness in a large sample of patients with schizophrenia, their first-degree relatives, and controls finding pronounced reductions of thickness in prefrontal cortex with clear evidence for heritability. As healthy siblings only showed nonsignificant reductions in thickness, however, it can be argued that although heritable, thickness of cortex may not be an ideal endophenotype (Goldman et al., in press).

A much clearer picture emerges when the function of dorsolateral prefrontal cortex is being considered. Cognitive paradigms, such as the n-back task, that reliably activate this region as part of the so-called working memory network, which also include the parietal lobule and cerebellum, among others, can be used to probe

A. Meyer-Lindenberg (✉)

Central Institute of Mental Health, Zentralinstitut für Seelische Gesundheit, J5, 68159 Mannheim, Germany

e-mail: a-meyer-lindenberg@zi-mannheim.de

W.F. Gattaz, G. Busatto (eds.), *Advances in Schizophrenia Research 2009*, DOI 10.1007/978-1-4419-0913-8_11, © Springer Science+Business Media, LLC 2010 prefrontal function in schizophrenia. While the directionality of the observed abnormalities does not always agree, the overwhelming majority of studies have found functional changes at a specific locale, namely, in the BA 46/9 region of dorsolateral prefrontal cortex. Furthermore, evidence from the study of genetically high-risk individuals (in this case, siblings) does show that dorsolateral prefrontal cortex functional activation exhibits disease-related genetic risk effects (Rasetti et al., 2009). Taken together with the findings from structure, dorsolateral prefrontal cortex is clearly one of the regions where translational genetic efforts in schizophrenia should be targeted.

What underlies the observed functional abnormalities in dorsolateral prefrontal cortex? One important contribution comes from dopaminergic modulation of its functions. According to the influential model of Durstewitz et al. (2000), dopamine, acting primarily through D1 receptors and in interaction with other neurotransmitter systems, especially glutamate and GABA, modulates signal-to-noise ratio in the cortex: during working memory, the activation peak corresponding to the token of information held "in mind" is stable to disturbance when dopamine levels are optimal, whereas a suboptimal level of stimulation leads to an instable peak and an increase in task-irrelevant noise. This line of work is relevant for schizophrenia since dopamine synthesis and release have consistently been found to be disinhibited in subcortical structures, particularly striatum, and shown to be related to genetic risk. Given the difficulties of reliably measuring dopamine in cortex, data in this region are less clear. Overall, however, the balance of the evidence speaks in favor of decreased (suboptimally low) dopamine in cortex, resulting in a complex picture of subcortical disinhibition and cortical reduction in dopamine that has replaced the original "dopamine hypothesis" of schizophrenia.

While at this juncture these convergent data on regional dysfunction in dorsolateral prefrontal cortex, its structural correlates, and dopaminergic mechanisms are compelling, an important conceptual point applying to brain function in general, but resonating especially with schizophrenia research, argues/suggests that very few neural functions can be localized to a single region of the brain, implying the importance of studying distributed systems whose functional relevance can lie as much in the interconnections between brain regions and their alterations as in regional activity. More than 100 years ago, Wernicke posited that given the severity of the symptoms of psychosis, the scarce neuroanatomical findings of his time argued for an abnormality in connectivity between brain areas. Brain imaging offers a rich repertoire to study connectivity both in structure (by examining structural covariation of regional volumes – structural covariance – or more directly through diffusion tensor imaging) and in function, using methods called functional connectivity (which are based on correlations between time series measured in fMRI or PET) or effective connectivity (more elaborate techniques that usually presuppose a model of how brain regions are interconnected and proceed to give a statistical estimate of whether that model fits, and, if it fits, allow inferences about directionality of connections not possible in the functional connectivity approach). Using these approaches, a considerable strand of the recent neuroimaging literature in schizophrenia has successfully demonstrated abnormal connectivity in the disorder, amply confirming Wernicke's thesis (Stephan et al., 2006). An example from our own work is provided by studying the hippocampus, a relevant structure for schizophrenia where structural and functional regional abnormalities have been described. Considering hippocampal activation during working memory in patients with schizophrenia compared to controls, we found that patients showed reduced activation of the right dorsolateral prefrontal cortex. In both patients and controls, inverse correlations were observed between the hippocampal formation and the contralateral dorsolateral prefrontal cortex. While these did not differ between diagnostic groups during the control task, the working memory challenge revealed a specific abnormality in dorsolateral prefrontal cortex–hippocampal formation functional connectivity. Although the right dorsolateral prefrontal cortex was significantly coupled to the left hippocampal formation in both groups during the control task, this correlation was not seen in healthy subjects during working memory but persisted undiminished in patients, resulting in a significant task-by-group interaction and suggesting a regionally specific alteration of hippocampal formation–dorsolateral prefrontal cortex functional connectivity in schizophrenia that manifests as an unmodulated persistence of a hippocampal formation–dorsolateral prefrontal cortex linkage during working memory activation (Meyer-Lindenberg et al., 2005b).

In other words, circuits matter in understanding schizophrenia and, as we will argue, also in understanding neurogenetic mechanisms in this disorder. One critical circuit for schizophrenia research links dorsolateral prefrontal cortex to the dopamine-synthesizing midbrain neurons that supply dorsolateral prefrontal cortex with this important regulatory neurotransmitter, forming a feedback loop. This circuit is important because it links two well-established pathophysiological components of the disorder, dorsolateral prefrontal cortex dysfunction, and dopamine synthesis. The question therefore arises whether these two phenomena are related; and if they are, whether this particular feedback circuit is involved. In an earlier study, we were able to produce evidence for both of these assertions (Meyer-Lindenberg et al., 2002): We measured presynaptic dopaminergic function simultaneously with regional cerebral blood flow during the Wisconsin Card Sorting Test (WCST), another well-established working memory test in a small group of unmedicated schizophrenic subjects and matched controls. We show that a PET measure of dopamine synthesis in the striatum was significantly higher for patients than for controls. Patients had significantly less WCST-related activation in dorsolateral prefrontal cortex. Both of these findings were expected from the literature, but the key new contribution was that we found that the two parameters were strongly linked in patients but not in controls. This tight within-patient coupling of these values, with decreased PFC activation predicting exaggerated striatal dopamine synthesis, supported the hypothesis that prefrontal cortex dysfunction may lead to dopaminergic transmission abnormalities.

At this point, we can speculate about the link between these findings on the neural systems level and their relevance for psychopathology, particularly with regard to qualitatively abnormal experiences in psychosis such as delusions. A large body of work, starting with the seminal paper by Schultz et al. (1997), has shown the key neural correlate of salience to be a dopaminergic burst in midbrain. This finding, which emerged in the context of reward prediction (reward being a typically salient event in the environment), has become known as prediction error signaling. Clearly, the existence of such a signal is essential for adaptive learning processes, since a discrepancy between the environment and the internal expectation has to be registered first for the need to readjust these expectations (through learning and neural plasticity) to become apparent. Now, several recent papers from Paul Fletchers group in Cambridge (Corlett et al., 2007a, b; Murray et al., 2008) have shown that this salience signal is profoundly abnormal in schizophrenia, during ketamine-induced psychosis, and in subjects at risk. Specifically, patients with schizophrenia do not show normal midbrain activation for a rewarding stimulus (a finding that could contribute to the genesis of anhedonia and other negative symptoms) but, critically, show increased prediction error signals in midbrain to control stimuli where normal controls show no such activation. This implies that in schizophrenia, salience is signaled for events that have no behavioral relevance, arguing for neural mechanisms for abnormal attributions of relevance that form a fundamental aspect of the genesis of delusions. In a recent study, we have found (Dreher et al., 2008) that during reward expectation, dopamine synthesis is in fact related to dorsolateral prefrontal cortex activation and, furthermore, that the directionality of this connection is positive in young, but not older, adults. This latter finding suggests that the tuning of this dorsolateral prefrontal cortex–midbrain circuit may also be relevant for understanding why symptoms of schizophrenia emerge in the second and third decade in men, although this point requires further study.

Using these circuits as a point of departure, we now turn to results from translational genetics. At the outset it has to be stated that the genetics of schizophrenia are rather complex. While the heritability of the disease is clearly very high, decades of work using linkage and association studies have shown that there are no frequent genetic risk variants for the disorder of large individual effect. More specifically, given the currently available GWAS data, it is unlikely that a single frequent variant exists that increases disease risk by more than 20%. However, rare microdeletion variants have recently been identified that, although they may explain only up to 15% of the risk in sporadic schizophrenia, may increase disease risk up to 50-fold if present (2008b; Stefansson et al., 2008). Such sporadic microdeletions have been found in 22q11, 1q21, and several other chromosomal regions. Taking these findings together, it is clear that the high heritability of schizophrenia is not explained by single gene variants, but is likely due to gene–gene interactions (epistasis) and interactions between genes and environment (which in the twin designs usually employed to assess heritability contribute to the "genetic" variance, much of which may therefore actually be due to or influenced by environmental interactions). If these interacting variants are frequent enough (the so-called common disease – common variant hypothesis), GWAS studies are the method of choice for their detection; the first results from this approach for schizophrenia imaging genetics are discussed below. Although GWAS studies are currently not powered to study epistatic interactions, we will argue below that microdeletion findings form attractive a priori hypotheses to constrain and focus searches for epistatic genes.

In this complex setting, bringing neuroimaging in the picture to measure genetic effects on brain structure and function is an attractive approach as this promises higher penetrance of genetic effects on this biological, quantitative level than can be expected on the level of psychiatric diagnoses, which, at this point, lack biological validity. This line of reasoning has come to be called the "endophenotype" or "intermediate phenotype approach." Meta-analytic evidence does in fact support this approach by showing that imaging genetics phenotypes exhibit much higher genetic effect sizes than those observed for the same genetic variants in behavior. Nevertheless, the brain shows an unprecedented level of complexity by itself and it would be naïve to assume one-on-one mappings from genes to brain or from brain to behavior or psychiatric disorder. Instead, we are dealing with a complex and largely unknown network of interacting effects. It is, therefore, with this note of caution that we proceed toward the examination of genetic effects.

We will start by examining the effects of candidate genes in the dopaminergic system with regard to the circuits discussed above. Candidate genes have been nominated and studied through their assumed pathophysiological relevance for the disorder and usually have a somewhat inconsistent record of being associated with the psychiatric categorical disease phenotype of schizophrenia. They offer the advantage of being a focused tool to study specific neurobiological mechanisms in vivo by contributing genetic variance that can be studied across individuals using methods such as genetics. However, depending on the level of confidence that individual researchers require before they accept a genetic variant as being associated with schizophrenia, the relevance of candidate gene findings for understanding the disorder can be assessed differently. A vigorous methodological debate is ongoing over the merits, or otherwise, of candidate genes (Meyer-Lindenberg and Weinberger, 2006; Flint and Munafo, 2007). While proponents of imaging genetics (often, psychiatrists and neuroscientists) point to the substantial body of neurobiological insights this method has provided, opponents (often, geneticists) question the relevance of these findings for mental illness given that few common genetic variants have been unambiguously associated with the clinical, categorical phenotype of schizophrenia, demanding a level of statistical evidence that has been developed for genome-wide searches for disease genes. To counter this objection, imaging geneticists, including our group, have argued that at currently available sample sizes, one can expect variable associations with a "messy" clinical/behavioral phenotype such as schizophrenia with limited intrinsic validity, which not only do not invalidate but also in fact precipitate the move away from clinical entities to more biological meditating processes: intermediate phenotypes.

An excellent example for this approach is provided by catechol-*O*-methyltransferase (COMT), a major enzyme degrading cortical dopamine. Dopamine action at the synapse is terminated either by dopamine transporter reuptake, via diffusion out of the synapse, or by COMT catabolism. Since dopamine transporters are scarce in prefrontal cortex (Lewis et al., 2001), COMT is a critical determinant of prefrontal dopamine flux (Tunbridge et al., 2004, 2006). The *COMT* gene is located at 22q11.2, a region implicated in schizophrenia by linkage (O'Donovan et al., 2008) and by the 22q11.2 syndrome (Mendelian Inheritance in

Man – MIM#192430), a hemideletion associated with a strongly increased risk of schizophrenia-like illness (Murphy, 2002). A common substitution of Val by Met (at amino acid 158 of the membrane-bound form of the protein found in brain) affects the stability of the COMT protein, leading to conformational changes and a subsequent significant decrease in enzyme activity in brain and lymphocytes (Chen et al., 2004). Neuroimaging studies using a reliable activator for prefrontal cortex, the n-back working memory task, have demonstrated that this coding variant impacts on prefrontal cortex activation (Meyer-Lindenberg et al., 2001). In agreement with this, variation in COMT also modulates PFC-dependent neuropsychological performance (Goldberg et al., 2003) and the cortical response to amphetamine, which increases synaptic dopamine (Mattay et al., 2003). The latter finding suggested that COMT genotype places individuals at predictable points along the putative inverted-u-shaped curve linking prefrontal dopamine stimulation and neuronal activities, with homozygotes for the Val-encoding allele, which presumably possess less synaptic dopamine due to maximal COMT activity, positioned to the left of Met-allele carriers, who appear to be located near the optimum of that curve. Additional evidence for this finding comes from a positron emission tomography (PET) study (Meyer-Lindenberg et al., 2005a) showing that COMT genotype has an impact on prefrontal regulation of midbrain dopamine synthesis in a genotype-dependent directionality, consistent with the inverted-u-shaped model (Akil et al., 2003; Behrens et al., 2005). This suggests that the risk for schizophrenia associated with this common variant is due to reduced signal-to-noise ratio in prefrontal cortex, an idea supported by the finding that working-memory-related and working-memory-unrelated activity in the PFC are inversely coupled to midbrain dopamine synthesis and directionally dependent on COMT genotype (Meyer-Lindenberg et al., 2005a).

Importantly, understanding this circuit can be used to develop innovative personalized treatments. In a proof of concept study, Apud et al. (2007) used a COMT-inhibiting drug, tolcapone, to demonstrate genotype-dependent effects on prefrontal function and cognitive performance. They performed a randomized, double-blind, placebo-controlled crossover design in 47 normal subjects stratified by COMT (val158met) genotype, 34 of whom also underwent fMRI. They found significant drug effects on measures of executive function and verbal episodic memory and a significant drug-by-genotype interaction on the latter, such that individuals with val/val genotypes improved, whereas individuals with met/met genotypes worsened on tolcapone. Additionally, fMRI revealed a significant tolcapone-induced improvement in the efficiency of information processing in prefrontal cortex during the n-back working memory test. This study demonstrated enhancement of prefrontal cortical function in normal human subjects with a nonstimulant drug having COMT inhibitory activity. In essence, this is an approach to innovative therapy of a key functional impairment in schizophrenia that can only work as personalized therapy: as the study results show, indiscriminately giving tolcapone would be unhelpful as it would worsen one proportion of patients while helping another; however, our understanding of the genetic variant and the neural system that it impacts on will enable a genotype-based selection of individuals (carrying val alleles) who can indeed benefit.

After this evidence for mechanisms impacted by genetic variation modulating extracellular dopamine, we now turn to the postsynaptic transduction of the dopamine signal, mediated through D2 receptors. In the classical signal transduction pathway, these receptors couple through Gαi/o protein to reduce cAMP production and PKA activity. Downstream from PKA, dopamine- (dopamine-) and cAMP-regulated phosphoprotein of molecular weight 32 (DARPP-32) is a key signaling integrator that regulates an array of subsequent neurophysiological processes, including the response to neuroleptics, psychotomimeticsor drugs of abuse, and affecting striatal function and plasticity. The canonical cAMP/PKA/DARPP-32 pathway, however, is not the only molecular network to transduce dopamine signals in dopaminoceptive neurons, since D2 receptors may also signal through an AKT1/GSK-3 signaling cascade via β-arrestin 2, independently of the cAMP-associated one. We have argued (Tan et al., 2008) that it represents a novel means by which D2 receptor signaling and associated cognitive and neuropsychiatric effects could be mediated. As reviewed in Tan et al. (2008, AKT1-knockout mice show schizophrenia-associated phenotypes (abnormal prepulse inhibition of startle) and antipsychotic enhanced AKT1 signaling. AKT1 regulates the trafficking of presynaptic dopamine transporters, and decreased AKT1 protein levels have been observed in lymphoblasts and postmortem prefrontal cortices of patients with schizophrenia.

Using imaging genetics, we have examined the neural systems responsive to both variants in the gene encoding DARPP-32, PPP1R1B, and AKT1. In the former, we found, through resequencing in 298 chromosomes, a frequent PPP1R1B haplotype predicting mRNA expression of PPP1R1B isoforms in postmortem human brain that impacted on neostriatal volume, activation, and the functional connectivity of the prefrontal cortex (Meyer-Lindenberg et al., 2007). The haplotype was associated with the risk for schizophrenia in a family-based association analysis. In AKT1, a very similar prefrontal–striatal circuit was implicated (Tan et al., 2008): we found that the AKT1 genotype predicted cognitive performance linked to frontostriatal circuitry, prefrontal physiology during executive function, and frontostriatal gray matter volume on MRI. Again, the same AKT1 variant functional in imaging was associated with risk for schizophrenia.

This convergent evidence from both the canonical and the noncanonical dopamine signaling pathway identifies prefrontal–striatal interactions as a key target circuit through which the genetic risk for schizophrenia related to dopamine is transduced. These results integrate well with what is known from basic neurobiology, since the neostriatum receives excitatory glutamatergic projections from the cortex and thalamus, integrates them with monoaminergic inputs, and sends them via the globus pallidus and substantia nigra pars reticulata to the thalamus, which projects back to prefrontal cortex (Alexander et al., 1986). These parallel processing loops are critical for the integration of sensorimotor, cognitive, and emotional information (Alexander et al., 1986). Lesions to the neostriatal–prefrontal system impair prefrontal-dependent cognitive functions (Dunnett et al., 2005) that are characteristic of the cognitive deficits found in schizophrenia (Pantelis et al., 1997). Prefrontal–striatal interactions have been proposed as providing a "filter" of information competing for cortical processing (Swerdlow et al., 2001), a mechanism that

could underlie cognitive symptoms and potential schizophrenia intermediate phenotypes such as abnormal pre-pulse inhibition of startle (Swerdlow et al., 2001).

These results should suffice to illustrate the power of the candidate gene approach
in understanding the genetic risk architecture of schizophrenia. In the remainder
of this paper, we will discuss current strategies to go beyond the elucidation of
single-gene single-variant effects, a move that is necessitated by the genetic considerations which, above all, stress the relevance of epistasis and gene–environment
interactions.

An illustrative example of epistasis is again provided by *COMT*, where the evidence supports the existence of multiple variants within the gene: in a large sample
of Israelis of Ashkenazi descent (O'Donovan et al., 2008) a haplotype, combining the Val/Met polymorphism, (rs4680), with two common SNPs at other loci, one
upstream in intron 1 (rs737865) and the other in a 3′-untranslated region (rs165599),
was highly associated with schizophrenia and with differentially affected expression of rs4680 alleles in human brain tissue (Bray et al., 2003), suggesting the
presence of a *cis*-acting functional locus within *COMT* interacting with Val/Met.
A population study found that this three-marker haplotype is markedly heterogeneous in populations worldwide (Palmatier et al., 2004) despite the relatively constant prevalence of schizophrenia and suggested relevance of another possible *cis*
functional variant (rs2097603) linked upstream in the P2 promoter driving transcription of the predominant form of *COMT* in the brain (MB-*COMT*). This variant
also affects COMT activity in lymphocytes and postmortem brain tissue (Chen et
al., 2004). Thus, *COMT* may contain at least three functional polymorphisms that
impact differentially on its biological actions and confound its clinical associations.
The combinatorial possibilities of diplotypes based on varying alleles at these three
sites are difficult to model in preclinical systems, but imaging offers unique potential to identify the functional affects of these combinations. Work in our laboratory
using a method adapted from haplotype regression demonstrates interacting effects
of these functional variants on prefrontal function (Meyer-Lindenberg et al., 2006).
The combined effects of these loci are not linear, consistent with predictions based
on the inverted-u-shaped function described above. Confirmatory convergent evidence comes from a study of executive cognition finding similar nonlinear effects
of these haplotypes on working memory performance (Diaz-Asper et al., 2008).

Staying in the dopamine system, a second example for epistasis is provided by
RGS4, encoding a regulatory protein in the canonical dopamine signal transduction pathway described above. By itself, a genetic variant in RGS4 linked to the
risk for schizophrenia impacted (rs951436) on dorsolateral–frontoparietal and fron-
totemporal activation and network coupling during working memory and resulted in
regionally specific reductions in gray and white matter structural volumes in individuals carrying the A (risk) allele (Buckholtz et al., 2007b). These findings now
afford the opportunity to study epistatic interactions of COMT and RGS4, influencing both the amount of extracellular dopamine available and the mechanisms by
which dopamine is postsynaptically transduced. Confirming the circuit hypothesis
outlined above, we found clear evidence for such epistasis not only in dorsolateral
prefrontal cortex but, importantly, also in striatum, recapitulating the biochemical

interactions in the neural circuitry modulated by genetic variants (Buckholtz et al., 2007a).

While we have focused on dopaminergic variants for ease of exposition, it is important to stress that dopamine is not the only neurotransmitter relevant for schizophrenia. In particular, glutamate, the most abundant excitatory neurotransmitter in cortex, has been hypothesized to play a major role in schizophrenia. Several risk genes in the dopaminergic system have been described. Of note, GRM3, encoding a metabotropic glutamate receptor localized on astroglia, has been implicated in the risk for schizophrenia. Genetic risk variants for GRM3 have been shown to modulate hippocampal function and episodic memory. Given the neurophysiological data summarized above showing an interaction of dopaminergic and glutamatergic neurotransmission in regulating the signal-to-noise ratio during cortical activity during working memory, it appears an attractive hypothesis that risk variants in GRM3 and COMT, influencing glutamate and dopamine availability, respectively, would show epistasis in dorsolateral prefrontal cortex during a working memory probe. This is exactly the result reported by Tan et al. (2007) in the NIMH sibling study genetic sample, where the GRM3 genotype associated with suboptimal glutamatergic signaling was significantly associated with inefficient prefrontal engagement and altered prefrontal–parietal coupling against the background of COMT Val-homozygous genotype. Conversely, COMT Met-homozygous background mediated against the effect of GRM3 genotype. This finding has potential therapeutic implications since a partial agonist at this receptor (as well as the GRM2 receptor) has shown evidence for antipsychotic efficacy when tested against the established atypical antipsychotic olanzapine (Patil et al. 2007).

These three examples illustrate the power of imaging genetics to elucidate epistatic interactions through parsing their neural impact. Several further studies of epistasis relevant for schizophrenia have appeared (Tan et al., 2008). One problem with this line of research is that current samples are in danger of being underpowered, at least when more than one interacting variant is considered. Based on meta-analytic evidence, current recommendations for sample sizes for imaging genetics, considering frequent variants, are on the order of 60–80 subjects (Meyer-Lindenberg and Weinberger, 2006; Munafo et al., 2009); the needed number for epistasis can be expected to be considerably above that, although the studies cited above have successfully obtained evidence for epistasis with sample sizes in the mid-100s.

In addition to these candidate gene studies, considerable further advances can be expected from data identifying variants with genome-wide significance. From these studies, as mentioned above, two kinds of variants have been identified: rare microdeletions under negative selection that carry a multifold higher risk for psychosis; and, in the recently published paper by O'Donovan et al. (2008), the first common variant with genome-wide support for risk for psychosis (a brad definition was used that also included bipolar I disorder), located in an assumed regulatory protein, ZNF804A, on chromsome 2.

Considering the microdeletions first, it will be of great interest to study the neural circuits that they impact upon. This is going to be difficult given their relative rarity. Currently available data suggest that several of these variants (certainly 22q11, associated with velocardiofacial syndrome) cause complex neurodevelopmental phenotypes that go beyond the realm of schizophrenia proper also impacting on general intelligence and neurocognition and may be associated with other axis I disorders ranging from ADHD to autism (Karayiorgou and Gogos, 2004; Brunetti-Pierri et al., 2008). These "new" microdeletions would then join the array of other neurogenetic disorders that increase risk for schizophrenia, such as Klinefelters syndrome or hyperprolactinemia. Nevertheless, parsing these symptom clusters on the neural systems level is likely to advance the field, especially if circuits impaired by several or all of these microdeletions (that then would have a very high probability of being relevant for the neurogenetics of schizophrenia) can be delineated. A second useful aspect of these data meriting its study is the proposal that microdeletions form an a priori regional hypothesis, in the genetic realm, for the presence of epistasis: a parsimonious explanation of the finding that these but not many other sporadic microdeletions show a schizophrenia risk phenotype could be that several risk genes for the disorder happen to be situated in spatial proximity in these regions. A first hint that this idea might be true comes from studying the gene immediately adjacent to COMT in the 22q11 region, PRODH, encoding proline oxidase (POX) (Kempf et al., 2008). In a family-based sample, we found that functional polymorphisms in PRODH were associated with schizophrenia, with protective and risk alleles having opposite effects on POX activity. Using a multimodal imaging genetics approach, we then showed that haplotypes constructed from these risk and protective functional polymorphisms had dissociable correlations with structure, function, and connectivity of striatum and prefrontal cortex. In particular, the schizophrenia risk haplotype was associated with decreased striatal volume and increased striatal–frontal functional connectivity, while the protective haplotype was associated with decreased striatal–frontal functional connectivity. In summary, PRODH, although biochemically clearly distinct in action from the dopaminergic system, impacts on a similar critical circuit relevant for schizophrenia also modulated by COMT, therefore providing neural systems-level evidence for a target for a "double genetic hit" for epistasis when both genes are hemideleted. In this context, it is intriguing to note that in the PRODH knockout mouse model, the most dysregulated gene in an expression screen was in fact COMT (Paterlini et al., 2005).

Finally, considering the first genome-wide significant psychosis variant, we have recently completed the first study investigating the impact of this SNP on brain function during working memory and an emotional face matching task (Esslinger et al., accepted for publication). Intriguingly, we found no difference in activation, but a pronounced impact on functional coupling of the dorsolateral prefrontal cortex, which was reduced toward contralateral dorsolateral prefrontal cortex and to ipsilateral subregions of lateral prefrontal cortex. Conversely, healthy carriers of the risk variant showed a gene-load-dependent inability to uncouple hippocampus from dorsolateral prefrontal cortex during working memory, exactly mirroring the finding in patients with manifest disease summarized above. It appears, then, that this variant acts primarily on connectivity, through a mechanism that is presently unknown but might involve neurodevelopmental alterations. Of interest, the same variant strongly increased coupling of amygdala to several regions of the extended limbic system. Since amygdala interactions in the context of emotional face matching are unlikely to be related to heritable risk for schizophrenia (Rasetti et al., 2009), we have proposed that this might contribute to the risk of this variant related to bipolar I disorder, supporting a genetic dysconnectivity hypothesis across the Kraepelinian divide.

In summary, I have given an overview of the state of the art and current major lines of development in imaging genetics of schizophrenia, moving from candidate genes to epistatic interactions and genome-wide significant risk variants. It is likely that in the years until the next Search for the Causes of Schizophrenia, the combination of large-scale genome-wide searches for schizophrenia risk genes will further fuel our understanding of these risk mechanisms and provide further targets for treatment development. Soon, it will be desirable to reverse the direction of inference and (a) search for genes directly using neural intermediate phenotypes in combination with GWAS and other -omics markers and (b) use these systems-level markers to tackle the problem of a biologically valid subclassification of "the schizophrenias" either by a fully dimensional approach or through the identification (though reverse phenotyping) of clinical subsyndromes consistently associated with an identifiable unitary biology, at least on the neural systems level. A second major frontier that is being explored by international consortia such as the EU-GEI (2008a) is gene–environment interactions in schizophrenia; recent work from our own group has begun to investigate neural mechanisms underlying social–behavioral risk factors such as social status.

References

Akil M, Kolachana BS, Rothmond DA, Hyde TM, Weinberger DR, Kleinman JE (2003) Catechol-O-methyltransferase genotype and dopamine regulation in the human brain. J Neurosci 23:2008–2013.

Alexander GE, DeLong MR, Strick PL (1986) Parallel organization of functionally segregated circuits linking basal ganglia and cortex. Annu Rev Neurosci 9:357–381.

Apud JA, Mattay V, Chen J, Kolachana BS, Callicott JH, Rasetti R, Alce G, Iudicello JE, Akbar N, Egan MF, Goldberg TE, Weinberger DR (2007) Tolcapone improves cognition and cortical information processing in normal human subjects. Neuropsychopharmacology 32:1011–1020.

Behrens BA, Nolte I, Bouguecha A, Kammler M, Halbritter U, Besdo S, Meyer-Lindenberg A (2005) [Measurement of the elastic properties of the cancellous bone in the femoral head of the dog]. Berl Munch Tierarztl Wochenschr 118:160–163.

Bray NJ, Buckland PR, Williams NM, Williams HJ, Norton N, Owen MJ, O'Donovan MC (2003) A haplotype implicated in schizophrenia susceptibility is associated with reduced COMT expression in human brain. Am J Hum Genet 73:152–161.

Brunetti-Pierri N, Berg JS, Scaglia F, Belmont J, Bacino CA, Sahoo T, Lalani SR, Graham B, Lee B, Shinawi M, Shen J, Kang SH, Pursley A, Lotze T, Kennedy G, Lansky-Shafer S, Weaver C, Roeder ER, Grebe TA, Arnold GL, Hutchison T, Reimschisel T, Amato S, Geraghty MT, Innis JW, Obersztyn E, Nowakowska B, Rosengren SS, Bader PI, Grange DK, Naqvi S, Garnica AD, Bernes SM, Fong CT, Summers A, Walters WD, Lupski JR, Stankiewicz P, Cheung SW, Patel A (2008) Recurrent reciprocal 1q21.1 deletions and duplications associated with microcephaly or macrocephaly and developmental and behavioral abnormalities. Nat Genet 40:1466–1471.

Buckholtz JW, Sust S, Tan HY, Mattay VS, Straub RE, Meyer-Lindenberg A, Weinberger DR, Callicott JH (2007a) fMRI evidence for functional epistasis between COMT and RGS4. Mol Psychiatry 12: 893–895, 885.

Buckholtz JW, Meyer-Lindenberg A, Honea RA, Straub RE, Pezawas L, Egan MF, Vakkalanka R, Kolachana B, Verchinski BA, Sust S, Mattay VS, Weinberger DR, Callicott JH (2007b) Allelic variation in RGS4 impacts functional and structural connectivity in the human brain. J Neurosci 27: 1584–1593.

Chen J, Lipska BK, Halim N, Ma QD, Matsumoto M, Melhem S, Kolachana BS, Hyde TM, Herman MM, Apud J, Egan MF, Kleinman JE, Weinberger DR (2004) Functional analysis of genetic variation in catechol-O-methyltransferase (COMT): effects on mRNA, protein, and enzyme activity in postmortem human brain. Am J Hum Genet 75:807–821.

Corlett PR, Honey GD, Fletcher PC (2007a) From prediction error to psychosis: ketamine as a pharmacological model of delusions. J Psychopharmacol 21: 238–252.

Corlett PR, Murray GK, Honey GD, Aitken MR, Shanks DR, Robbins TW, Bullmore ET, Dickinson A, Fletcher PC (2007b) Disrupted prediction-error signal in psychosis: evidence for an associative account of delusions. Brain 130: 2387–2400.

Diaz-Asper CM, Goldberg TE, Kolachana BS, Straub RE, Egan MF, Weinberger DR (2008) Genetic variation in catechol-O-methyltransferase: effects on working memory in schizophrenic patients, their siblings, and healthy controls. Biol Psychiatry 63:72–79.

Dreher JC, Meyer-Lindenberg A, Kohn P, Berman KF (2008) Age-related changes in midbrain dopaminergic regulation of the human reward system. Proc Natl Acad Sci USA 105: 15106–15111.

Dunnett SB, Meldrum A, Muir JL (2005) Frontal-striatal disconnection disrupts cognitive performance of the frontal-type in the rat. Neuroscience 135:1055–1065.

Durstewitz D, Seamans JK, Sejnowski TJ (2000) Dopamine-mediated stabilization of delay-period activity in a network model of prefrontal cortex. J Neurophysiol 83:1733–1750.

Esslinger C, Walter H, Kirsch P, Erk S, Schnell K, Arnold C, Haddad L, Mier D, Opitz von Boberfeld C, Raab K, Witt SH, Rietschel M, Cichon S, Meyer-Lindenberg A, Rietschel M CA, Meyer-Lindenberg A (2009) Neural mechanisms of a genome-wide significant psychosis variant. Science 324(5927): 605.

European Network of Schizophrenia Networks for the Study of Gene- Environment Interactions (2008a) Schizophrenia aetiology: do gene-environment interactions hold the key? Schizophr Res 102:21–26.

Flint J, Munafo MR (2007) The endophenotype concept in psychiatric genetics. Psychol Med 37:163–180.

Goldberg TE, Egan MF, Gscheidle T, Coppola R, Weickert T, Kolachana BS, Goldman D, Weinberger DR (2003) Executive subprocesses in working memory: relationship to catechol-O-methyltransferase Val158Met genotype and schizophrenia. Arch Gen Psychiatry 60:889–896.

Goldman A, Pezawas L, Mattay V, Fischl B, Verchinski B, Chen Q, Weinberger DR, Meyer-Lindenberg A (2009) Widespread reductions of cortical thickness in schizophrenia and evidence for heritability. Arch Gen Psychiatry 66(5) 467–477.

International Schizophrenia Consortium (2008b) Rare chromosomal deletions and duplications increase risk of schizophrenia. Nature 455:237–241.

Karayiorgou M, Gogos JA (2004) The molecular genetics of the 22q11-associated schizophrenia. Brain Res Mol Brain Res 132:95–104.

Kempf L, Nicodemus KK, Kolachana B, Vakkalanka R, Verchinski BA, Egan MF, Straub RE, Mattay VA, Callicott JH, Weinberger DR, Meyer-Lindenberg A (2008) Functional polymorphisms in PRODH are associated with risk and protection for schizophrenia and fronto-striatal structure and function. PLoS Genet 4:e1000252.

Lewis DA, Melchitzky DS, Sesack SR, Whitehead RE, Auh S, Sampson A (2001) Dopamine transporter immunoreactivity in monkey cerebral cortex: regional, laminar, and ultrastructural localization. J Comp Neurol 432:119–136.

Mattay VS, Goldberg TE, Fera F, Hariri AR, Tessitore A, Egan MF, Kolachana B, Callicott JH, Weinberger DR (2003) Catechol O-methyltransferase val158-met genotype and individual variation in the brain response to amphetamine. Proc Natl Acad Sci USA 100: 6186–6191.

Meyer-Lindenberg A, Weinberger DR (2006) Intermediate phenotypes and genetic mechanisms of psychiatric disorders. Nat Rev Neurosci 7:818-827.

Meyer-Lindenberg A, Poline JB, Kohn PD, Holt JL, Egan MF, Weinberger DR, Berman KF (2001) Evidence for abnormal cortical functional connectivity during working memory in schizophrenia. Am J Psychiatry 158:1809–1817.

Meyer-Lindenberg A, Miletich RS, Kohn PD, Esposito G, Carson RE, Quarantelli M, Weinberger DR, Berman KF (2002) Reduced prefrontal activity predicts exaggerated striatal dopaminergic function in schizophrenia. Nat Neurosci 5:267–271.

Meyer-Lindenberg A, Kohn PD, Kolachana B, Kippenhan S, McInerney-Leo A, Nussbaum R, Weinberger DR, Berman KF (2005a) Midbrain dopamine and prefrontal function in humans: interaction and modulation by COMT genotype. Nat Neurosci 8: 594–596.

Meyer-Lindenberg A, Nichols T, Callicott JH, Ding J, Kolachana B, Buckholtz J, Mattay VS, Egan M, Weinberger DR (2006) Impact of complex genetic variation in COMT on human brain function. Mol Psychiatry 11(9): 867–877.

Meyer-Lindenberg A, Straub RE, Lipska BK, Verchinski BA, Goldberg T, Callicott JH, Egan MF, Huffaker SS, Mattay VS, Kolachana B, Kleinman JE, Weinberger DR (2007) Genetic evidence implicating DARPP-32 in human frontostriatal structure, function, and cognition. J Clin Invest 117:672–682.

Meyer-Lindenberg AS, Olsen RK, Kohn PD, Brown T, Egan MF, Weinberger DR, Berman KF (2005b) Regionally specific disturbance of dorsolateral prefrontal-hippocampal functional connectivity in schizophrenia. Arch Gen Psychiatry 62: 379–386.

Munafo MR, Freimer NB, Ng W, Ophoff R, Veijola J, Miettunen J, Jarvelin MR, Taanila A, Flint J (2009) 5-HTTLPR genotype and anxiety-related personality traits: a meta-analysis and new data. Am J Med Genet B Neuropsychiatr Genet 150B:271–281.

Murphy KC (2002) Schizophrenia and velo-cardio-facial syndrome. Lancet 359:426–430.

Murray GK, Corlett PR, Clark L, Pessiglione M, Blackwell AD, Honey G, Jones PB, Bullmore ET, Robbins TW, Fletcher PC (2008) Substantia nigra/ventral tegmental reward prediction error disruption in psychosis. Mol Psychiatry 13:239, 267–276.

O'Donovan MC, Craddock N, Norton N, Williams H, Peirce T, Moskvina V, Nikolov I, Hamshere M, Carroll L, Georgieva L, Dwyer S, Holmans P, Marchini JL, Spencer CC, Howie B, Leung HT, Hartmann AM, Moller HJ, Morris DW, Shi Y, Feng G, Hoffmann P, Propping P, Vasilescu C, Maier W, Rietschel M, Zammit S, Schumacher J, Quinn EM, Schulze TG, Williams NM, Giegling I, Iwata N, Ikeda M, Darvasi A, Shifman S, He L, Duan J, Sanders AR, Levinson DF, Gejman PV, Gejman PV, Sanders AR, Duan J, Levinson DF, Buccola NG, Mowry BJ, Freedman R, Amin F, Black DW, Silverman JM, Byerley WF, Cloninger CR, Cichon S, Nothen MM, Gill M, Corvin A, Rujescu D, Kirov G, Owen MJ (2008) Identification of loci associated with schizophrenia by genome-wide association and follow-up. Nat Genet 40(9): 1053–1055.

Palmatier MA, Pakstis AJ, Speed W, Paschou P, Goldman D, Odunsi A, Okonofua F, Kajuna S, Karoma N, Kungulilo S, Grigorenko E, Zhukova OV, Bonne-Tamir B, Lu RB, Parnas J, Kidd JR, DeMille MM, Kidd KK (2004) COMT haplotypes suggest P2 promoter region relevance for schizophrenia. Mol Psychiatry 9:859–870.

Pantelis C, Barnes TR, Nelson HE, Tanner S, Weatherley L, Owen AM, Robbins TW (1997) Frontal-striatal cognitive deficits in patients with chronic schizophrenia. Brain 120(Pt 10): 1823–1843.

Paterlini M, Zakharenko SS, Lai WS, Qin J, Zhang H, Mukai J, Westphal KG, Olivier B, Sulzer D, Pavlidis P, Siegelbaum SA, Karayiorgou M, Gogos JA (2005) Transcriptional and behavioral interaction between 22q11.2 orthologs modulates schizophrenia-related phenotypes in mice. Nat Neurosci 8:1586–1594.

Patil ST, Zhang L, Martenyi F, Lowe SL, Jackson KA, Andreev BV, Avedisova AS, Bardenstein LM, Gurovich IY, Morozova MA, Mosolov SN, Neznanov NG, Reznik AM, Smulevich AB, Tochilov VA, Johnson BG, Monn JA, Schoepp DD (2007) Activation of mGlu2/3 receptors as a new approach to treat schizophrenia: a randomized Phase 2 clinical trial. Nat Med. 2007 13(9):1102–1107. Erratum in: Nat Med. 2007 Oct;13(10):1264.

Rasetti R, Mattay VS, Wiedholz LM, Kolachana BS, Hariri AR, Callicott JH, Meyer-Lindenberg A, Weinberger DR (2009) Evidence that altered amygdala activity in schizophrenia is related to clinical state and not genetic risk. Am J Psychiatry 166:216–225.

Schultz W, Dayan P, Montague PR (1997) A neural substrate of prediction and reward. Science 275:1593–1599.

Stefansson H, Rujescu D, Cichon S, Pietilainen OP, Ingason A, Steinberg S, Fossdal R, Sigurdsson E, Sigmundsson T, Buizer-Voskamp JE, Hansen T, Jakobsen KD, Muglia P, Francks C, Matthews PM, Gylfason A, Halldorsson BV, Gudbjartsson D, Thorgeirsson TE, Sigurdsson A, Jonasdottir A, Bjornsson A, Mattiasdottir S, Blondal T, Haraldsson M, Magnusdottir BB, Giegling I, Moller HJ, Hartmann A, Shianna KV, Ge D, Need AC, Crombie C, Fraser G, Walker N, Lonnqvist J, Suvisaari J, Tuulio-Henriksson A, Paunio T, Toulopoulou T, Bramon E, Di Forti M, Murray R, Ruggeri M, Vassos E, Tosato S, Walshe M, Li T, Vasilescu C, Muhleisen TW, Wang AG, Ullum H, Djurovic S, Melle I, Olesen J, Kiemeney LA, Franke B, Sabatti C, Freimer NB, Gulcher JR, Thorsteinsdottir U, Kong A, Andreassen OA, Ophoff RA, Georgi A, Rietschel M, Werge T, Petursson H, Goldstein DB, Nothen MM, Peltonen L, Collier DA, St Clair D, Stefansson K (2008) Large recurrent microdeletions associated with schizophrenia. Nature 455:232–236.

Stephan KE, Baldeweg T, Friston KJ (2006) Synaptic plasticity and dysconnection in schizophrenia. Biol Psychiatry 59:929–939.

Swerdlow NR, Geyer MA, Braff DL (2001) Neural circuit regulation of prepulse inhibition of startle in the rat: current knowledge and future challenges. Psychopharmacology (Berl) 156: 194–215.

Tan HY, Chen Q, Sust S, Buckholtz JW, Meyers JD, Egan MF, Mattay VS, Meyer-Lindenberg A, Weinberger DR, Callicott JH (2007) Epistasis between catechol-O-methyltransferase and type II metabotropic glutamate receptor 3 genes on working memory brain function. Proc Natl Acad Sci USA 104:12536–12541.

Tan HY, Nicodemus KK, Chen Q, Li Z, Brooke JK, Honea R, Kolachana BS, Straub RE, Meyer-Lindenberg A, Sei Y, Mattay VS, Callicott JH, Weinberger DR (2008) Genetic variation in AKT1 is linked to dopamine-associated prefrontal cortical structure and function in humans. J Clin Invest 118:2200–2208.

Tunbridge EM, Harrison PJ, Weinberger DR (2006) Catechol-o-Methyltransferase, Cognition, and Psychosis: Val(158)Met and Beyond. Biol Psychiatry 60(2): 141–151.

Tunbridge EM, Bannerman DM, Sharp T, Harrison PJ (2004) Catechol-o-methyltransferase inhibition improves set-shifting performance and elevates stimulated dopamine release in the rat prefrontal cortex. J Neurosci 24:5331–5335.

Progress in Genetic Studies of Schizophrenia

Renan P. Souza, Marco A. Romano Silva, and James L. Kennedy

Overview of the Current Status of Genetic Studies of Schizophrenia

The current interpretation of the family and twin data suggest that most of the genetic risk to schizophrenia is conferred by multiple interacting loci, each causing a small increase in risk. As schizophrenia has similar symptoms and roughly similar prevalence throughout the world, a reasonable hypothesis is that at least some loci have effects in many populations. Until recently, there have been only a few undisputed genetic associations to complex non-Mendelian human diseases (for example, the HLA locus association to diabetes), but for many diseases, the advent of genome-wide association study (GWAS) technology has recently altered this situation. GWASs to date have focused on analyzing each individual marker of the 500,000 or more markers on the microarray and presenting the p-values in one large analysis, with statistical significance thresholds adjusted for the extensive multiple testing. The current findings from the few published GWASs of schizophrenia (and bipolar disorder), along with the data from significant candidate genes that predate the GWAS era, are supportive of the hypothesis that common genetic variants contribute to schizophrenia. However, no single marker has been reported for schizophrenia that reaches genome-wide levels of significance across more than one study. The GWAS investigations published thus far include the following (with sample sizes of cases): Lencz et al. (2007) ($n = 450$); O'Donovan et al. (2008) ($n = 479$ plus replication sample); Walsh et al. (2008) ($n = 418$); International Schizophrenia Consortium (2008) ($n = 3,391$); and Stefansson et al. (2008) ($n = 1,433$). In the current reports, there are a few genes of interest since they have been relatively positive across more than one sample. One example is *ZNF804A*, a zinc finger gene that does not have a well-characterized function. In a recent study investigating this gene with brain imaging phenotypes, Esslinger et al. (2009) have shown that healthy carriers of the *ZNF804A* risk genotypes have marked alterations in the correlated

R.P. Souza (✉)
Centre for Addiction and Mental Health, Neurogenetics Section, Toronto, ON, Canada, M5T1R8
e-mail: renan_desouza@camh.net

W.F. Gattaz, G. Busatto (eds.), *Advances in Schizophrenia Research 2009*,
DOI 10.1007/978-1-4419-0913-8_12, © Springer Science+Business Media, LLC 2010

activity (coupling) of dorsolateral prefrontal cortex across hemispheres and with hippocampus, similar to the coupling abnormalities seen in functional imaging of schizophrenia patients. Thus the original effect of *ZNF804A* gene variants creating risk for schizophrenia diagnosis is now exhibiting validation from neuroimaging phenotypes.

It is worth pointing out that the failure of a gene to appear in any of the GWAS significant association marker lists should also be viewed with caution. There are no results showing genome-wide significance for the major candidate genes such as dysbindin (*DTNBP1*), neuregulin1 (*NRG1*), D-amino-acid oxidase activator (*DAOA*), or disrupted in schizophrenia 1 (*DISC1*). These genes showed considerable replication before the advent of GWASs and thus were among the most prominent candidates for schizophrenia. One of the more interesting outcomes of the GWASs of schizophrenia and bipolar disorder is that nearly all of the genes that show relatively strong association for schizophrenia also show significant positive results in bipolar disorder as well. This is surprising evidence in favor of a common etiology for both diseases. It is possible that these common genetic variants create vulnerability in the brain for destabilization of behavior, and then different environmental influences lead to the outcome of schizophrenia diagnosis versus bipolar.

When the details of the GWAS data for markers in and around these genes are investigated in a given schizophrenia sample, these genes typically have reached a higher significance level than expected by chance. However, only a very small portion of the disease risk is explained by these genes; thus, considerable work remains to identify the bulk of the genetic risk. It may be that complexities such as parental imprinting, gene–environment interaction, or epigenetic effects may be obscuring the full clinical impact of the risk genes. Another complexity may be the new discovery of increased chromosomal deletions and duplications in schizophrenia patients compared to healthy controls. The advent of GWAS technology allowed researchers to scan across the genome-wide data and ask: Are there regions where there is one segment of the chromosome missing, or alternatively, duplicated? The extensive nature of the scanning process makes the finding of these gaps or duplications relatively straightforward. Recent papers describing an increase in these copy number variants (CNVs) in schizophrenia and an excess of de novo CNV events in that disorder have raised the possibility of a significant contribution from rare events, some of apparently high penetrance. For example, generalizing across studies, in a comparison of 1,000 schizophrenia patients versus 1,000 controls, there may be 10–15 patients with a deletion at a site on chromosome 15q, while only 1 or 0 of the controls will have this deletion. Although it is not yet clear whether the contribution from CNVs is small or substantial, these findings can be interpreted as supporting the hypothesis that rare variants may play a highly penetrant role in a small but significant number of schizophrenia cases. The three main sites of CNVs noted thus far in schizophrenia are 1q, 15q, and (as expected) 22q.

Researchers have looked for genetic markers of schizophrenia by attempting to subdivide the disease into more homogeneous groups. This is often done by defining "alternative phenotypes" that, after genetic analysis, may lead to the discovery of one or more genes associated with that more specific phenotype. Alternative phenotypes may include neuropsychological data, ocular motor physiology, or neuroimaging data, for example.

An important alternative phenotype may be defined by a malfunctioning brain circuit or pathway. In schizophrenia, functional imaging and postmortem neuropathology implicate alterations in the dorsolateral prefrontal–basal ganglia–thalamocortical circuit in core schizophrenia. In contrast, abnormalities in the anterior cingulate–basal ganglia–thalamocortical circuit are associated with psychosis, which is shared by all schizophrenic patients whether or not they manifest deficit symptoms (Tamminga et al. 1992). For over a century, disturbed interactions between brain areas have been proposed to underlie schizophrenia. Extensive work in patients has demonstrated abnormal coupling between brain regions implicated in schizophrenia, most notably the dorsolateral prefrontal cortex and hippocampal formation, but the relevance for heritable risk was unclear (Thaker and Carpenter 2001). The new link by Esslinger et al. (2009) between the *ZNF804A* gene and coupling of the DLPFC with the hippocampus described above provides strong support for the usefulness of neuroimaging phenotypes. In general, these alternative phenotypes will be most valuable for schizophrenia researchers if they also exhibit a strong and relatively simple genetic basis.

One of the historically most studied alternative phenotypes in schizophrenia has been abnormal movement of the eyes while tracking a moving object across a screen. Holzman et al. (1973) reported an association between abnormal eye tracking and schizophrenia, and documented an increased prevalence of this feature in patients' relatives. A preliminary study has also linked abnormal eye tracking to a chromosome 6q site in schizophrenia probands (Arolt et al. 1996). Other alternative phenotypes include impairments in attention, language, and memory, as well as deficits in expression levels of the neuronal marker *N*-acetyl-aspartate in the hippocampal region. Freedman et al. (1999) used electrophysiological measurements to identify a linkage between a sensory gating defect and a locus at chromosome 15q14 in schizophrenic patients. There have been several recent replications of this linkage finding at 15q14 locus using diagnosis of schizophrenia as a phenotype. This region contains the gene encoding an α-7 nicotinic-cholinergic receptor subunit gene (*CHNRA1*), which is involved in sensory gating. Genetic studies of *CHNRA1* show fairly strong linkage to prepulse inhibition; an electrophysiological measure of sensory gating, however, the statistical association to the diagnosis of schizophrenia is not as strong. Given the recent finding of increased copy number variants in this region of 15q in schizophrenia, further investigations are warranted.

Another set of important alternate phenotypes is the response and side effects that schizophrenia patients have when administered antipsychotic medication. The genetic study of these medication effects is referred to as pharmacogenetics. Pharmacogenetics is the study of genetically determined, interindividual differences in therapeutic response to drugs and susceptibility to their adverse effects. The principal objective of pharmacogenetics is to identify and categorize the genetic factors that underlie these differences and to apply these observations in the clinic. Individualization of drug treatment to the specific patient is thus a core objective of pharmacogenetics. A priori identification of the patients who will respond well to a particular antipsychotic, or who will be at higher risk for development of adverse effects, has the potential to help clinicians to avoid lengthy ineffective medication trials and to limit the exposure of the patient to side effects. Moreover, improved predictability of treatment response early in the course of illness may result in enhanced patient compliance and willingness to seek treatment rapidly upon symptom exacerbation or recurrence. In terms of the etiology of schizophrenia, if we can identify genes involved in antipsychotic response or side effects, then the overall mechanisms of the disease as a whole may be illuminated.

Pharmacogenetics of Schizophrenia

Efficacy and side effects remain major concerns in antipsychotic management. The proportion of treatment-resistant schizophrenia has been estimated as 20–40% in schizophrenic patients, and this unfortunate situation in clinical psychiatry still remains unchanged even after the introduction of several new antipsychotic agents (Weiss et al. 1999). There are two broad reasons for treatment failure: lack of efficacy and adverse reactions. Antipsychotics may fail to generate a clinical response because of failure to reach a sustained therapeutic concentration (pharmacokinetics) or because of altered receptor binding or coupling (pharmacodynamics). In addition, differences in the pathophysiology or symptom clusters of schizophrenia, a heterogeneous and complex disease, may affect response. Hopefully, the study of specific pharmacogenetic subtypes of schizophrenia may lead to better understanding of the etiologic mechanisms of the disease in general.

Antipsychotics used to treat schizophrenia symptoms are originally categorized into two groups, typical and atypical, that differ in their ability to induce catalepsy in rodents. Some clinicians define typicals, including chlorpromazine, haloperidol, and perphenazine, as having more specific dopamine D2 receptor antagonism. Atypicals, including olanzapine, risperidone, and quetiapine, are categorized as having a different pharmacological profile from typicals. Other clinicians may differentiate between them by defining typicals as being effective in treating positive symptoms of schizophrenia but with a high propensity for developing unfavorable motor side effects such as tardive dyskinesia (TD), and atypicals as being effective in treating both positive and negative symptoms of schizophrenia but with a higher chance of developing metabolic adverse effects such as weight gain.

Molecular genetic studies into disease-related factors are usually preceded by epidemiological investigations involving twin, family, and adoption studies to determine the existence and extent of the genetic influence. Twin, family, and adoption studies of schizophrenia have provided strong evidence of a genetic contribution to the etiology of the disease; however, no similar studies exist in relation to response to antipsychotic treatment. Collections of monozygotic twins or family members concordant for disease and treatment are difficult to obtain and gathering the necessary epidemiological data has proved problematic to date. In the absence of a systematic epidemiological study, supporting evidence is limited to a number of case reports of monozygotic twins responding similarly to different antipsychotics: identical twins showing equal levels of response to treatment with the antipsychotics clozapine and olanzapine and/or presenting the same adverse reactions (for example, weight gain and agranulocytosis) (Arranz and de Leon 2007).

Most of the pharmacogenetic research to date has been conducted without formal consideration of environmental influences (stress levels, or smoking, for example). This may partly explain the difficulties encountered in correlating genetic variants with observed treatment variability and in replicating reported findings. Relating genetic variants with associated biological effects is relatively straightforward, even without considering environmental factors. However, the correlation between genetic variants and end response is less clear, especially if environmental factors are not considered in the equation. Most pharmacogenetic studies in the last two decades have used candidate gene approaches, selecting genes to be investigated from current knowledge, for the identification of response-related genes. Candidate genes involved in pharmacokinetic and pharmacodynamics processes have been investigated in a number of studies, and recent investigations have expanded to genes involved in neuronal plasticity, transport, and metabolism.

A critical issue for genetic studies is the reliability and validity of the phenotype under investigation. The two most important points for evaluation of treatment response are the instrument used to assess response and the length of the treatment. The most common phenotype has been short-term drug response, in which efficacy is assessed by changes in standardized rating scales such as the Brief Psychiatric Rating Scale (BPRS) over periods that range from 3 weeks up to a few months. The phenotype of drug-induced side effects is likely to be complex (although perhaps not as complex as the overall disease). Patients may be taking multiple medications or have comorbid illnesses that predispose them to the development of an adverse event. Pharmacogenetic studies of antipsychotic drug-induced weight gain are often conducted in patient populations with chronic schizophrenia in which previous antipsychotic drug treatment may have resulted in weight gain. This may complicate the analysis of subsequent weight gain when they take a new antipsychotic. Likewise, in some cases, the underlying illness may contribute to the development of an adverse event, and thus, the drug may not be specifically responsible for the observed event. These issues require careful consideration and should be critically evaluated during consideration of the design of pharmacogenetic studies, particularly those conducted in chronically patient groups (Malhotra et al. 2004).

Pharmacogenetics of Antipsychotic Treatment Response

Among the atypical antipsychotics, only clozapine has been reported to be effective for 30–60% of schizophrenia subjects that are refractory to typical and atypical antipsychotics (Wilson 1996). Clozapine is thought to provide antipsychotic effects through binding to dopamine as well as to several serotonin receptor subtypes although the actual mechanism of clozapine for treatment-resistant schizophrenia has not been elucidated as yet. Pharmacogenetic studies of antipsychotic drug response have focused on the atypical antipsychotic drug clozapine, perhaps because of the ease of access to blood samples from clozapine-treated patients from which to extract DNA or because the superior clozapine efficacy in treatment-resistant populations suggests that an understanding of the genetic contributions to its effects could provide novel data on the molecular basis of antipsychotic efficacy. In order to clarify this mechanism, several research groups around the world have investigated genetic factors thought to be involved in the clinical response to clozapine and these will be reviewed briefly below.

There are two treatment definitions that have been used in genetic investigations of treatment-resistant schizophrenia. Kane et al. (1988) introduced a definition (1) at least three periods of treatment in the preceding 5 years with antipsychotics (from at least two different chemical classes) at doses greater than 1,000 mg/day of chlorpromazine equivalents for a period of 6 weeks, each without significant symptomatic relief, and (2) no period of good functioning within the preceding 5 years. Inada et al. (2003) have used a definition of treatment-resistant schizophrenia that was modified from that proposed by Kane et al. (1988), which was defined based on observations of monotherapy antipsychotic treatment. Schizophrenia patients were diagnosed as having treatment-resistant schizophrenia when they had been hospitalized for more than 1 year and had been receiving antipsychotic therapy at dosages of at least 1,000 mg/day chlorpromazine equivalents for more than 1 year (Inada et al. 2003). The main reason for modifying the definition of treatment-resistant schizophrenia was that Japanese psychiatrists generally prefer use of multiple medications in routine clinical practice. If patients relapse during their antipsychotic maintenance therapy, Japanese psychiatrists often prescribe another antipsychotic agent in addition to the original one, instead of switching to it, so it is quite rare for patients in Japanese routine psychiatric practice to be diagnosed as having treatment-resistant schizophrenia as proposed by Kane et al. (1988), even when the schizophrenia is considered treatment resistant.

Treatment resistance could be considered a useful phenotype to examine in genetics of schizophrenia. Using the treatment-resistance definition of Kane et al. (1988), Mundo et al. (2005) have shown no association between the variant A2518G on the monocyte chemoattractant protein 1 (MCP-1) gene (*SCYA2*), a protein that influences the expression of cytokines, with treatment resistance in schizophrenia patients. However, significant association of *SCYA2* in allele-wise analysis has been shown with resistance to antipsychotic treatment (Mundo et al. 2005). Thus far, three reports using the sample and criteria reported by Inada et al. (2003) have been published in Asian samples. Inada et al. (2003) failed to find association of the functional polymorphism (Valine158Methionine) of the *COMT* gene with clinical manifestations and response to antipsychotics of schizophrenia patients. However, the daily neuroleptic dosage that patients received during their maintenance therapy was significantly higher in patients with homozygous methionine genotype than in the other patients, suggesting that this variant may help in the understanding of treatment-resistant features of schizophrenia. Comparing treatment-resistant and non-treatment-resistant schizophrenia patients, Ji et al. (2008a) found that a

3-bp deletion allele located in the serotonin receptor 3B (*HTR3B*) promoter region was significantly more frequent in their treatment-resistant group than the insertion allele. No significant results were found in the serotonin receptors 2A and 3A and four genes (*HTR2A*, *HTR3A*, and *HTR4*), although the daily neuroleptic dosage was significantly higher in patients with the T/T *HTR3A* genotype at marker rs1062613 (Ji et al. 2008b).

Most of the studies that have evaluated genetic components in treatment-resistant schizophrenia have not focused their analyses to compare treatment-resistant and treatment-responsive patients. The main focus has been on the pharmacogenetic component of response to clozapine in this particular group of treatment-resistant subjects. The Kane et al. (1988) treatment-resistant concept was used for most of these studies. Using a multicenter Caucasian/African-American sample, including the one described in Kane et al. (1988), Dr. Kennedy's group reported that the *HTR2A* His452Tyr variant was associated with clozapine response (Masellis et al. 1998), although other variants in the serotonergic system were not associated, such as *HTR2A* T102C, serotonin receptor 2C (*HTR2C*) Cys23Ser, and serotonin receptor 6 (*HTR6*) T267C (Masellis et al. 1995, 1998, 2001). In the same sample, Hwang et al. (2005, 2006, 2007) have reported no associations for dopamine receptor 1 (*DRD1*) and 2 (*DRD2*) gene variants in the Caucasian sample; however, the *DRD1* rs265976, *DRD2* Taq1A, *DRD2* Taq1B, and *DRD2* rs1125394 were associated with clozapine response in their African-American subsample. Souza et al. (2008) have reported no association with glycogen synthase kinase 3β (*GSK-3β*) gene variants in the Caucasian sample. Patients with allele "A" for the G308A variant of the tumor necrosis factor-alpha (*TNF-α*) gene showed significant improvement on BPRS change score after 3 and 6 months of clozapine treatment when compared with patients without allele A (Zai et al. 2006). Muller et al. (2005a) have examined the functional C825T polymorphism of the β3 subunit gene (*GNB3*) and have shown that the C/C genotype was significantly associated with relative clinical improvement as measured by BPRS change scores after 6 and 12 weeks in Caucasians.

Arranz et al. (1996, 1998b, 2000) have reported treatment response association in treatment-resistant schizophrenia patients with the *HTR2A* T102C and *HTR2A* His452Tyr, but not the *HTR2A* C516T variant, in a Caucasian European population. Furthermore, the *HTR2C* Cys23Ser was also associated with clozapine response (Sodhi et al., 1995), although this finding was not supported by Arranz et al. (2000). Two other positive results have been found for clozapine response: dopamine receptor 3 (*DRD3*) Ser9Gly and histamine receptor 2 (H2)-G1018A variants (Shaikh et al. 1996; Mancama et al. 2002). No significant associations were observed between treatment response and the following genes: *DRD2* (Arranz et al. 1998a); the variable-number tandem repeat (VNTR) in the exon III of the dopamine receptor 4 (*DRD4*) (Shaikh et al. 1993, 1995); HTTLPR; HTT VNTR; serotonin receptor 5A (*HTR5A*)-A12T and -G19C (Birkett et al. 2000); as well as the cytochrome P450 enzyme gene (*CYP2D6*) (Arranz et al. 1995).

In an ambitious study, Arranz et al. (2000) examined a relatively large number of candidate gene markers in clozapine response, both alone and in combination. They reported that most of the 19 analyzed variants by themselves were not associated with treatment response, that is, no significant associations were found for ADRA2A-G261A, ADRA2A-C1291G, ADRA1A Arg 492Cys, DRD3 Ser9Gly, histamine receptor 1 (H1) Leu449Ser, H2-G1018A, HTR3A-C178T, HTR3A-G1596A, HTR5A-A12T, HTR5A-G19C, and a HTT VNTR. However, a combination of six of these variants (HTR2A T102C, HTR2A His452Tyr, HTR2C-G330T/-C244T, HTR2C Cys23Ser, HTTLPR, and H2-G1018A) resulted in 76·7% success in the prediction of clozapine response in a discriminant function type of analysis. No other group has yet been able to complete the full analysis of these six variants; thus, the result remains unreplicated.

There have been modest treatment response associations with the HTR6 T267C marker (Yu et al. 1999) and the brain-derived neurotrophic factor (BDNF) Val66Met (Hong et al. 2003) functional variant in a Chinese Han sample. No significant associations were observed for HTR2A T102C (Lin et al. 1999), the serotonin-transporter promoter region polymorphism (HTTLPR) (Tsai et al. 2000), apolipoprotein E (APOE) ε4 (Hong et al. 2000), and α2A-adrenoceptor (ADRA2A)-C1291G (Tsai et al. 2001) variants. Hong et al. (2001a) have examined clozapine dosage as an alternative phenotype related to response, showing that a marginally higher means of clozapine dosage is needed for N-methyl-D-aspartate (NMDA) glutamate receptor 2B subunit (GRIN2B) C2664C patients than 2664T carriers.

A number of studies have evaluated genetic prediction of treatment response in patients treated with an antipsychotic other than clozapine. There have been reports of association of DRD2 with haloperidol response (Schäfer et al. 2001) and bromperidol response (Suzuki et al. 2001). The multidrug resistance gene (MDR-1) was also associated with bromperidol response (Yasui-Furukori et al. 2006). Risperidone efficacy has been associated with HTR1A (Wang et al. 2008), HTR2A (Lane et al. 2002), DRD2, COMT (Yamanouchi et al. 2003), and DRD4 (Zalsman et al. 2003) genes. Olanzapine response has been associated with 5HTR2A/2C (Ellingrod et al. 2002a), GNB-3 (Bishop et al. 2006), choline acetyltransferase (Mancama et al. 2007), and MDR-1 (Lin et al. 2006). Although many studies have reported positive associations and some of these findings have been replicated in independent samples, there is no genetic testing currently available for antipsychotic treatment response. The most promising findings thus far were in the dopaminergic and serotonergic systems but these results have not shown enough strength to be used in routine clinical care.

Pharmacogenetics of Antipsychotic-Induced Tardive Dyskinesia

The mechanisms underlying the development of dyskinesias and other movement disorders are poorly understood. TD is a potentially irreversible movement disorder caused by long-term antipsychotic exposure, characterized by involuntary athetoid, choreiform, and/or rhythmic movements affecting mostly orofacial muscles, with more severe cases involving the trunk and limbs. Prevalence data are difficult to interpret due to heterogeneous study populations and different TD assessment methodologies. Kane and Smith (1982) reviewed 56 studies from 1959 to 1979 and found TD occurrence to range from 0.5 to 65%. Yassa and Jeste (1992) reported a prevalence of 24% in 39,187 patients pooled from 76 studies. Using the Schooler and Kane (1982) criteria for TD occurrence, Woerner et al. (1991) and Muscettola et al. (1993) reported that 23.4 and 19.1%, respectively, of an antipsychotic-treated mixed population had TD.

Supersensitivity of dopamine receptors, other neurotransmitters changes, and disturbances in antioxidative protection have been proposed as possible pathophysiological mechanisms. Additionally, development of TD has been directly associated with increases in drug dosage and plasma levels, which may exacerbate the pathophysiological mechanisms. Genetics is a prominent factor in determining the risk of TD, as suggested by increased incidence of TD among relatives reported in several family studies (Yassa and Ananth 1981; Youssef et al. 1989; Muller et al. 2001). Survey of the literature reveals that genes influencing the pharmacokinetics, pharmacodynamics, and oxidative stress associated with antipsychotics have been considered for TD risk.

Genes associated with dopaminergic signaling have been one of the obvious first priority systems to analyze in association studies (Ozdemir et al. 2001). In support of the hypothesis that the dopaminergic system may play a central role in TD development, variants in the *DRD2* gene have shown association with TD (Chen et al. 1997). Other significant variants were found in the *DRD1* (Srivastava et al. 2006) and *DRD3* (Steen et al. 1997; Basile et al. 1999). The *DRD4*, *COMT*, and *DAT* genes have also been analyzed but have not shown significant results. Genes in other neurotransmission systems, most notably the serotonin system, have been investigated, including TD association analyses with *HTR2A* (Segman et al. 2001), *HTR2C* (Segman et al. 2000), *HTR6* (Ohmori et al. 2002), *HTT* (Chong et al. 2000), *TPH* (Segman et al. 2003), and *MAOA* (Matsumoto et al. 2004). Other positive findings are found across oxidative-stress genes as well as other signaling molecules, although these studies would require replications of their results.

Pharmacogenetics of the Antipsychotic-Induced Weight Gain

Weight gain is a serious problem in patients treated with antipsychotics. Evidence exists that antipsychotic drugs interact with neuroendocrine signaling pathways leading to adverse effects such as increase in appetite, obesity, hyperglycemia, and diabetes (Muller and Kennedy 2006). Extra weight is a common feature in schizophrenia patients and they show a higher body mass index than other psychiatry patients and than the general population. The weight gain induced by antipsychotics is different among drugs and across dosages, with some drugs creating from 1.5 up to 8.8 kg gain in a period of 6 months (Allison and Casey 2001). Several studies have reported greater weight gain induced by atypical drugs than typical, in particular with olanzapine and clozapine treatment.

Genetics of antipsychotic-induced weight gain is a recent field with a relatively small number of studies conducted. Wehmeier et al. (2005) and Theisen et al. (2005) have shown concordant weight gain induced by antipsychotics in monozygotic twins and sibling pairs, respectively. Most of the studies evaluating a genetic component in antipsychotic-induced weight gain have focused on genes associated with monoamine neurotransmission. On the other hand, it can be hypothesized that antipsychotics may have some peripheral effects such as metabolism control and muscle tone, modulation of caloric "burn," and lipogenesis (Basile et al. 2001). Most studies to date have analyzed the serotonergic system that has been associated with satiety and eating behavior. Overall, the serotonin increase would be associated with a reduction in feeding behavior and vice versa. Among the serotonergic genes, *HTR2C* is the one showing the most positive results (Rietschel et al. 1997). Other serotonin genes that have been studied were *HTR1A* (Basile et al. 2001), *HTR2A*, *HTR6*, and *HTT* (Hong et al. 2001b).

Exploratory studies with *DRD1*, *DRD2*, *DRD3* (Lane et al. 2006), *DRD4* (Rietschel et al. 1996), H_1, H_2 (Basile et al. 2001), SNAP-25 (Muller et al. 2005b), *CYP2D6* (Ellingrod et al. 2002b), *CYP1A2* (Basile et al. 2001), adrenergic receptors (Basile et al. 2001), leptin and its receptor (Zhang et al. 2003), neuropeptide Y paraoxonase 1 (Ruaño et al. 2007), and *GNB-3* (Tsai et al. 2004) have been reported. Overall, genetics findings in antipsychotic-induced weight gain have little replication and further analyses are required to strengthen the mentioned gene hypotheses.

Conclusions

The advent of chip-based genome-wide investigations has ushered in a new era of genetic research. However, there are no major findings emerging as yet for schizophrenia. Insertions and deletions (CNVs) appear to be developing into an important cause of relatively rare cases of schizophrenia, although their full effect on risk remains to be determined. Alternative phenotypes, particularly brain imaging, are showing great promise as helpful partners in genetic investigations of schizophrenia. Pharmacogenetic studies of antipsychotic response have begun to identify several genes that may be implicated in diverse phenotypes, such as drug efficacy, and development of drug-induced adverse events. These genes require further study as well as careful functional genomics to identify the specific molecular events that may produce clinical effects in order to contribute to future drug development strategies. Although attempts have been made at standardizing the requirements for pharmacogenetic studies, the difficulty in collecting appropriate cohorts for the study of response traits means that heterogeneity across studies is relatively high and some level of spurious findings will remain. In general, large samples are recommended for pharmacogenetic studies investigating the relevance of genetic variants. However, nothing will compensate for the necessity to confirm significant findings in independent samples that are as clinically similar as possible. It should be noted as well that a given clinical confounding factor may have a different weight of effect across different samples. Undoubtedly the introduction of pharmacogenetic tests in the clinical arena will be facilitated if they are robust enough to stand out above the variations among different clinical settings.

The development of rapid techniques for mutation screening and genotyping by using DNA array technology has greatly accelerated the throughput of measurement of single-nucleotide polymorphisms across the genome. However, it must be noted that the rate of discovery of schizophrenia-associated polymorphisms will depend on the quality of the phenotype. Prospective genotyping of schizophrenic patients for the many genes at the level of the drug target, drug metabolism, and disease pathways will contribute to individualized therapy matching the patient's unique genetic make up with an optimally effective drug. Finally, such optimization will also result in decreasing the overall direct treatment costs of schizophrenia through prescription of the right drug for the right patient and improvement of quality of life and other aspects of day-to-day functioning. Finally, it is hoped that the understanding of genetic variants that are involved in antipsychotic response or side effects will illuminate the pathologic and etiologic mechanisms in the complex syndromes that we refer to as schizophrenia.

References

Allison, D.B. & Casey, D.E. (2001) Antipsychotic-induced weight gain: a review of the literature. Journal of Clinical Psychiatry 62: 22–31

Arolt, V., Lencer, R., Nolte, A., Muller-Myhsok, B., Purmann, S., Schurmann, M., Leutelt, J., Pinnow, M., & Schwinger, E. (1996) Eye tracking dysfunction is a putative phenotypic susceptibility marker of schizophrenia and maps to a locus on chromosome 6p in families with multiple occurrence of the disease. American Journal of Medical Genetics 67: 564–579

Arranz, M.J., Dawson, E., Shaikh, S., Sham, P., Sharma, T., Aitchison, K., Crocq, M.A., Gill, M., Kerwin, R., & Collier, D.A. (1995) Cytochrome P4502D6 genotype does not determine response to clozapine. British Journal of Clinical Pharmacology 39: 417–420

Arranz, M.J., Collier, D.A., Munro, J., Sham, P., Kirov, G., Sodhi, M., Roberts, G., Price, J., & Kerwin, R.W. (1996) Analysis of a structural polymorphism in the 5-HT2A receptor and clinical response to clozapine. Neuroscience Letters 217: 177–178

Arranz, M.J., Munro, J., Sham, P., Kirov, G., Murray, R.M., Collier, D.A., & Kerwin, R.W. (1998a) Meta-analysis of studies on genetic variation in 5-HT2A receptors and clozapine response. Schizophrenia Research 32: 93–99

Arranz, M.J., Li, T., Munro, J., Liu, X., Murray, R., Collier, D.A., & Kerwin, R.W. (1998b) Lack of association between a polymorphism in the promoter region of the dopamine-2 receptor gene and clozapine response. Pharmacogenetics 8: 481–484

Arranz, M.J., Munro, J., Birkett, J., Bolonna, A., Mancama, D., Sodhi, M., Lesch, K.P., Meyer, J.F., Sham, P., Collier, D.A., Murray, R.M., & Kerwin, R.W. (2000) Pharmacogenetic prediction of clozapine response. Lancet 355: 1615–1616

Arranz, M.J. & de, L.J. (2007) Pharmacogenetics and pharmacogenomics of schizophrenia: a review of last decade of research. Molecular Psychiatry 12: 707–747

Basile, V.S., Masellis, M., Badri, F., Paterson, A.D., Meltzer, H.Y., Lieberman, J.A., Potkin, S.G., Macciardi, F., & Kennedy, J.L. (1999) Association of the MscI polymorphism of the dopamine D3 receptor gene with tardive dyskinesia in schizophrenia. Neuropsychopharmacology 21: 17–27

Basile, V.S., Masellis, M., McIntyre, R.S., Meltzer, H.Y., Lieberman, J.A., & Kennedy, J.L. (2001) Genetic dissection of atypical antipsychotic-induced weight gain: novel preliminary data on the pharmacogenetic puzzle. Journal of Clinical Psychiatry 62 Suppl 23: 45–66

Birkett, J.T., Arranz, M.J., Munro, J., Osbourn, S., Kerwin, R.W., & Collier, D.A. (2000) Association analysis of the 5-HT5A gene in depression, psychosis and antipsychotic response. Neuroreport 11: 2017–2020

Bishop, J.R., Ellingrod, V.L., Moline, J., & Miller, D. (2006) Pilot study of the G-protein beta3 subunit gene (C825T) polymorphism and clinical response to olanzapine or olanzapine-related weight gain in persons with schizophrenia. Medical Science Monitor 12: 47–50

Chen, C.H., Wei, F.C., Koong, F.J., & Hsiao, K.J. (1997) Association of TaqI A polymorphism of dopamine D2 receptor gene and tardive dyskinesia in schizophrenia. Biological Psychiatry 41: 827–829

Chong, S.A., Tan, E.C., Tan, C.H., Mahendren, R., Tay, A.H., & Chua, H.C. (2000) Tardive dyskinesia is not associated with the serotonin gene polymorphism (5-HTTLPR) in Chinese. American Journal of Medical Genetics 96: 712–715

Ellingrod, V.L., Perry, P.J., Lund, B.C., Bever-Stille, K., Fleming, F., Holman, T.L., & Miller, D. (2002a) 5HT2A and 5HT2C receptor polymorphisms and predicting clinical response to olanzapine in schizophrenia. Journal of Clinical Psychopharmacology 22: 622–624

Ellingrod, V.L., Miller, D., Schultz, S.K., Wehring, H., & Arndt, S. (2002b) CYP2D6 polymorphisms and atypical antipsychotic weight gain. Psychiatric Genetics 12: 55–58

Esslinger, C., Walter, H., Kirsch, P., Erk, S., Schnell, K., Arnold, C., Haddad, L., Mier, D., Opitz von, B.C., Raab, K., Witt, S.H., Rietschel, M., Cichon, S., & Meyer-Lindenberg, A. (2009) Neural mechanisms of a genome-wide supported psychosis variant. Science 324: 605

Freedman, R., Adler, L.E., & Leonard, S. (1999) Alternative phenotypes for the complex genetics of schizophrenia. Biological Psychiatry 45: 551–558

Holzman, P.S., Proctor, L.R., & Hughes, D.W. (1973) Eye-tracking patterns in schizophrenia. Science 181: 179–181

Hong, C.J., Yu, Y.W., Lin, C.H., Song, H.L., Lai, H.C., Yang, K.H., & Tsai, S.J. (2000) Association study of apolipoprotein E epsilon4 with clinical phenotype and clozapine response in schizophrenia. Neuropsychobiology 42: 172–174

Hong, C.J., Yu, Y.W., Lin, C.H., Cheng, C.Y., & Tsai, S.J. (2001a) Association analysis for NMDA receptor subunit 2B (GRIN2B) genetic variants and psychopathology and clozapine response in schizophrenia. Psychiatric Genetics 11: 219–222

Hong, C.J., Lin, C.H., Yu, Y.W., Yang, K.H., & Tsai, S.J. (2001b) Genetic variants of the serotonin system and weight change during clozapine treatment. Pharmacogenetics 11: 265–268

Hong, C.J., Yu, Y.W., Lin, C.H., & Tsai, S.J. (2003) An association study of a brain-derived neurotrophic factor Val66Met polymorphism and clozapine response of schizophrenic patients. Neuroscience Letters 349: 206–208

Hwang, R., Shinkai, T., De, L., V, Muller, D.J., Ni, X., Macciardi, F., Potkin, S., Lieberman, J.A., Meltzer, H.Y., & Kennedy, J.L. (2005) Association study of 12 polymorphisms spanning the dopamine D(2) receptor gene and clozapine treatment response in two treatment refractory/intolerant populations. Psychopharmacology (Berlin) 181: 179–187

Hwang, R., Shinkai, T., Deluca, V., Macciardi, F., Potkin, S., Meltzer, H.Y., & Kennedy, J.L. (2006) Dopamine D2 receptor gene variants and quantitative measures of positive and negative symptom response following clozapine treatment. European Neuropsychopharmacology 16: 248–259

Hwang, R., Shinkai, T., De, L., V, Ni, X., Potkin, S.G., Lieberman, J.A., Meltzer, H.Y., & Kennedy, J.L. (2007) Association study of four dopamine D1 receptor gene polymorphisms and clozapine treatment response. Journal of Psychopharmacology 21: 718–727

Inada, T., Nakamura, A., & Iijima, Y. (2003) Relationship between catechol-O-methyltransferase polymorphism and treatment-resistant schizophrenia. American Journal of Medical Genetics B Neuropsychiatric Genetics 120B: 35–39

International Schizophrenia Consortium (2008) Rare chromosomal deletions and duplications increase risk of schizophrenia. Nature 455: 237–241

Ji, X., Takahashi, N., Branko, A., Ishihara, R., Nagai, T., Mouri, A., Saito, S., Maeno, N., Inada, T., & Ozaki, N. (2008a) An association between serotonin receptor 3B gene (HTR3B) and treatment-resistant schizophrenia (TRS) in a Japanese population. Nagoya Journal of Medical Science 70: 11–17

Ji, X., Takahashi, N., Saito, S., Ishihara, R., Maeno, N., Inada, T., & Ozaki, N. (2008b) Relationship between three serotonin receptor subtypes (HTR3A, HTR2A and HTR4) and treatment-resistant schizophrenia in the Japanese population. Neuroscience Letters 435: 95–98

Kane, J.M. & Smith, J.M. (1982) Tardive dyskinesia: prevalence and risk factors, 1959 to 1979. Archive of General Psychiatry 39: 473–481

Kane, J., Honigfeld, G., Singer, J., & Meltzer, H. (1988) Clozapine for the treatment-resistant schizophrenic. A double-blind comparison with chlorpromazine. Archives of General Psychiatry 45: 789–796

Lane, H.Y., Chang, Y.C., Chiu, C.C., Chen, M.L., Hsieh, M.H., & Chang, W.H. (2002) Association of risperidone treatment response with a polymorphism in the 5-HT(2A) receptor gene. American of Journal Psychiatry 159: 1593–1595

Lane, H.Y., Liu, Y.C., Huang, C.L., Chang, Y.C., Wu, P.L., Lu, C.T., Chang, W.H. (2006) Risperidone-related weight gain: genetic and nongenetic predictors. J Clin Psychopharmacol 26(2): 128–34

Lencz, T., Lambert, C., Derosse, P., Burdick, K.E., Morgan, T.V., Kane, J.M., Kucherlapati, R., & Malhotra, A.K. (2007) Runs of homozygosity reveal highly penetrant recessive loci in schizophrenia. Proceedings of the National Academy of Sciences USA 104: 19942–19947

Lin, C.H., Tsai, S.J., Yu, Y.W., Song, H.L., Tu, P.C., Sim, C.B., Hsu, C.P., Yang, K.H., & Hong, C.J. (1999) No evidence for association of serotonin-2A receptor variant (102T/C) with schizophrenia or clozapine response in a Chinese population. Neuroreport 10: 57–60

Lin, Y.C., Ellingrod, V.L., Bishop, J.R., & Miller, D. (2006) The relationship between P-glycoprotein (PGP) polymorphisms and response to olanzapine treatment in schizophrenia. Therapeutic Drug Monitoring 28: 668–672

Malhotra, A.K., Murphy, G.M., Jr., & Kennedy, J.L. (2004) Pharmacogenetics of psychotropic drug response. American Journal of Psychiatry 161: 780–796

Mancama, D., Arranz, M.J., Munro, J., Osborne, S., Makoff, A., Collier, D., & Kerwin, R. (2002) Investigation of promoter variants of the histamine 1 and 2 receptors in schizophrenia and clozapine response. Neuroscience Letters 333: 207–211

Mancama, D., Mata, I., Kerwin, R.W., & Arranz, M.J. (2007) Choline acetyltransferase variants and their influence in schizophrenia and olanzapine response. American Journal of Medical Genetics B Neuropsychiatric Genetics 144B: 849–853

Masellis, M., Paterson, A.D., Badri, F., Lieberman, J.A., Meltzer, H.Y., Cavazzoni, P., & Kennedy, J.L. (1995) Genetic variation of 5-HT2A receptor and response to clozapine. Lancet 346: 1108

Masellis, M., Basile, V., Meltzer, H.Y., Lieberman, J.A., Sevy, S., Macciardi, F.M., Cola, P., Howard, A., Badri, F., Nothen, M.M., Kalow, W., & Kennedy, J.L. (1998) Serotonin subtype 2 receptor genes and clinical response to clozapine in schizophrenia patients. Neuropsychopharmacology 19: 123–132

Masellis, M., Basile, V.S., Meltzer, H.Y., Lieberman, J.A., Sevy, S., Goldman, D.A., Hamblin, M.W., Macciardi, F.M., & Kennedy, J.L. (2001) Lack of association between the T->C 267 serotonin 5-HT6 receptor gene (HTR6) polymorphism and prediction of response to clozapine in schizophrenia. Schizophrenia Research 47: 49–58

Matsumoto, C., Shinkai, T., Hori, H., Ohmori, O., & Nakamura, J. (2004) Polymorphisms of dopamine degradation enzyme (COMT and MAO) genes and tardive dyskinesia in patients with schizophrenia. Psychiatry Research 127: 1–7

Muller, D.J., Schulze, T.G., Knapp, M., Held, T., Krauss, H., Weber, T., Ahle, G., Maroldt, A., Alfter, D., Maier, W., Nothen, M.M., & Rietschel, M. (2001) Familial occurrence of tardive dyskinesia. Acta Psychiatrica Scandinavica 104: 375–379

Muller, D.J., De, L., V, Sicard, T., King, N., Hwang, R., Volavka, J., Czobor, P., Sheitman, B.B., Lindenmayer, J.P., Citrome, L., McEvoy, J.P., Lieberman, J.A., Meltzer, H.Y., & Kennedy, J.L. (2005a) Suggestive association between the C825T polymorphism of the G-protein beta3 subunit gene (GNB3) and clinical improvement with antipsychotics in schizophrenia. European Neuropsychopharmacology 15: 525–531

Muller, D.J., Klempan, T.A., De Luca, V., Sicard, T., Volavka, J., Czobor, P., Sheitman, B.B., Lindenmayer, J.P., Citrome, L., McEvoy, J.P., Lieberman, J.A., Honer, W.G., & Kennedy, J.L. (2005b) The SNAP-25 gene may be associated with clinical response and weight gain in antipsychotic treatment of schizophrenia. Neuroscience Letters 379: 81–89

Muller, D.J. & Kennedy, J.L. (2006) Genetics of antipsychotic treatment emergent weight gain in schizophrenia. Pharmacogenomics 7: 863–887

Mundo, E., Altamura, A.C., Vismara, S., Zanardini, R., Bignotti, S., Randazzo, R., Montresor, C., & Gennarelli, M. (2005) MCP-1 gene (SCYA2) and schizophrenia: a case-control association study. American Journal of Medical Genetics B Neuropsychiatric Genetics 132B: 1–4

Muscettola, G., Pampallona, S., Barbato, G., Casiello, M., & Bollini, P. (1993) Persistent tardive dyskinesia: demographic and pharmacological risk factors. Acta Psychiatrica Scandinavica 87: 29–36

O'Donovan, M.C., Craddock, N., Norton, N., Williams, H., Peirce, T., Moskvina, V., Nikolov, I., Hamshere, M., Carroll, L., Georgieva, L., Dwyer, S., Holmans, P., Marchini, J.L., Spencer, C.C., Howie, B., Leung, H.T., Hartmann, A.M., Moller, H.J., Morris, D.W., Shi, Y., Feng, G., Hoffmann, P., Propping, P., Vasilescu, C., Maier, W., Rietschel, M., Zammit, S., Schumacher, J., Quinn, E.M., Schulze, T.G., Williams, N.M., Giegling, I., Iwata, N., Ikeda, M., Darvasi, A., Shifman, S., He, L., Duan, J., Sanders, A.R., Levinson, D.F., Gejman, P.V., Cichon, S., Nothen, M.M., Gill, M., Corvin, A., Rujescu, D., Kirov, G., Owen, M.J., Buccola, N.G., Mowry, B.J., Freedman, R., Amin, F., Black, D.W., Silverman, J.M., Byerley, W.F., & Cloninger, C.R. (2008) Identification of loci associated with schizophrenia by genome-wide association and follow-up. Nature Genetics 40: 1053–1055

Ohmori, O., Shinkai, T., Hori, H., & Nakamura, J. (2002) Genetic association analysis of 5-HT(6) receptor gene polymorphism (267C/T) with tardive dyskinesia. Psychiatry Research 110: 97–102

Ozdemir, V., Basile, V.S., Masellis, M., & Kennedy, J.L. (2001) Pharmacogenetic assessment of antipsychotic-induced movement disorders: contribution of the dopamine D3 receptor and cytochrome P450 1A2 genes. Journal of Biochemical and Biophysics Methods 47: 151–157

Rietschel, M., Naber, D., Oberlander, H., Holzbach, R., Fimmers, R., Eggermann, K., Moller, H.J., Propping, P., & Nothen, M.M. (1996) Efficacy and side-effects of clozapine: testing for association with allelic variation in the dopamine D4 receptor gene. Neuropsychopharmacology 15: 491–496

Rietschel, M., Naber, D., Fimmers, R., Moller, H.J., Propping, P., & Nothen, M.M. (1997) Efficacy and side-effects of clozapine not associated with variation in the 5-HT2C receptor. Neuroreport 8: 1999–2003

Ruaño, G., Goethe, J.W., Caley, C., Woolley, S., Holford, T.R., Kocherla, M., Windemuth, A., & de Leon, J. (2007) Physiogenomic comparison of weight profiles of olanzapine- and risperidone-treated patients. Molecular Psychiatry 12: 474–482

Schäfer, M., Rujescu, D., Giegling, I., Guntermann, A., Erfurth, A., Bondy, B., & Moller, H.J. (2001) Association of short-term response to haloperidol treatment with a polymorphism in the dopamine D(2) receptor gene. American Journal of Psychiatry 158: 802–804

Schooler, N.R. & Kane, J.M. (1982) Research diagnoses for tardive dyskinesia. Archives of General Psychiatry 39: 486–487

Segman, R.H., Heresco-Levy, U., Finkel, B., Inbar, R., Neeman, T., Schlafman, M., Dorevitch, A., Yakir, A., Lerner, A., Goltser, T., Shelevoy, A., & Lerer, B. (2000) Association between the serotonin 2C receptor gene and tardive dyskinesia in chronic schizophrenia: additive contribution of 5-HT2Cser and DRD3gly alleles to susceptibility. Psychopharmacology (Berlin) 152: 408–413

Segman, R.H., Heresco-Levy, U., Finkel, B., Goltser, T., Shalem, R., Schlafman, M., Dorevitch, A., Yakir, A., Greenberg, D., Lerner, A., & Lerer, B. (2001) Association between the serotonin 2A receptor gene and tardive dyskinesia in chronic schizophrenia. Molecular Psychiatry 6: 225–229

Segman, R.H., Goltser, T., Heresco-Levy, U., Finkel, B., Shalem, R., Schlafman, M., Yakir, A., Greenberg, D., Strous, R., Lerner, A., Shelevoy, A., & Lerer, B. (2003) Association of dopaminergic and serotonergic genes with tardive dyskinesia in patients with chronic schizophrenia. Pharmacogenomics Journal 3: 277–283

Shaikh, S., Collier, D., Kerwin, R.W., Pilowsky, L.S., Gill, M., Xu, W.M., & Thornton, A. (1993) Dopamine D4 receptor subtypes and response to clozapine. Lancet 341: 116

Shaikh, S., Collier, D.A., Sham, P., Pilowsky, L., Sharma, T., Lin, L.K., Crocq, M.A., Gill, M., & Kerwin, R. (1995) Analysis of clozapine response and polymorphisms of the dopamine D4 receptor gene (DRD4) in schizophrenic patients. American Journal of Medical Genetics 60: 541–545

Shaikh, S., Collier, D.A., Sham, P.C., Ball, D., Aitchison, K., Vallada, H., Smith, I., Gill, M., & Kerwin, R.W. (1996) Allelic association between a Ser-9-Gly polymorphism in the dopamine D3 receptor gene and schizophrenia. Human Genetics 97: 714–719

Sodhi, M.S., Arranz, M.J., Curtis, D., Ball, D.M., Sham, P., Roberts, G.W., Price, J., Collier, D.A., & Kerwin, R.W. (1995) Association between clozapine response and allelic variation in the 5-HT2C receptor gene. Neuroreport 7: 169–172

Souza, R.P., Romano-Silva, M.A., Lieberman, J.A., Meltzer, H.Y., Wong, A.H., & Kennedy, J.L. (2008) Association study of GSK3 gene polymorphisms with schizophrenia and clozapine response. Psychopharmacology (Berlin) 200: 177–186

Srivastava, V., Varma, P.G., Prasad, S., Semwal, P., Nimgaonkar, V.L., Lerer, B., Deshpande, S.N., & BK, T. (2006) Genetic susceptibility to tardive dyskinesia among schizophrenia subjects: IV. Role of dopaminergic pathway gene polymorphisms. Pharmacogenetics and Genomics 16: 111–117

Steen, V.M., Lovlie, R., MacEwan, T., & McCreadie, R.G. (1997) Dopamine D3-receptor gene variant and susceptibility to tardive dyskinesia in schizophrenic patients. Molecular Psychiatry 2: 139–145

Stefansson, H., Rujescu, D., Cichon, S., Pietilainen, O.P., Ingason, A., Steinberg, S., Fossdal, R., Sigurdsson, E., Sigmundsson, T., Buizer-Voskamp, J.E., Hansen, T., Jakobsen, K.D., Muglia, P., Francks, C., Matthews, P.M., Gylfason, A., Halldorsson, B.V., Gudbjartsson, D., Thorgeirsson, T.E., Sigurdsson, A., Jonasdottir, A., Jonasdottir, A., Bjornsson, A., Mattiasdottir, S., Blondal, T., Haraldsson, M., Magnusdottir, B.B., Giegling, I., Moller, H.J., Hartmann, A., Shianna, K.V., Ge, D., Need, A.C., Crombie, C., Fraser, G., Walker, N., Lonnqvist, J., Suvisaari, J., Tuulio-Henriksson, A., Paunio, T., Toulopoulou, T., Bramon, E., Di, F.M., Murray, R., Ruggeri, M., Vassos, E., Tosato, S., Walshe, M., Li, T., Vasilescu, C., Muhleisen, T.W., Wang, A.G., Ullum, H., Djurovic, S., Melle, I., Olesen, J., Kiemeney, L.A., Franke, B., Sabatti, C., Freimer, N.B., Gulcher, J.R., Thorsteinsdottir, U., Kong, A., Andreassen, O.A., Ophoff, R.A., Georgi, A., Rietschel, M., Werge, T., Petursson, H., Goldstein, D.B., Nothen, M.M., Peltonen, L., Collier, D.A., St, Clair, D., & Stefansson, K. (2008) Large recurrent microdeletions associated with schizophrenia. Nature 455: 232–236

Suzuki, A., Kondo, T., Mihara, K., Yasui-Furukori, N., Ishida, M., Furukori, H., Kaneko, S., Inoue, Y., & Otani, K. (2001) The -141C Ins/Del polymorphism in the dopamine D2 receptor gene promoter region is associated with anxiolytic and antidepressive effects during treatment with dopamine antagonists in schizophrenic patients. Pharmacogenetics 11: 545–550

Tamminga, C.A., Thaker, G.K., Buchanan, R., Kirkpatrick, B., Alphs, L.D., Chase, T.N., & Carpenter, W.T. (1992) Limbic system abnormalities identified in schizophrenia using positron emission tomography with fluorodeoxyglucose and neocortical alterations with deficit syndrome. Archives of General Psychiatry 49: 522–530

Thaker, G.K. & Carpenter, W.T., Jr. (2001) Advances in schizophrenia. Nature Medicine 7: 667–671

Theisen, F.M., Gebhardt, S., Haberhausen, M., Heinzel-Gutenbrunner, M., Wehmeier, P.M., Krieg, J.C., Kuhnau, W., Schmidtke, J., Remschmidt, H., & Hebebrand, J. (2005) Clozapine-induced weight gain: a study in monozygotic twins and same-sex sib pairs. Psychiatric Genetics 15: 285–289

Tsai, S.J., Hong, C.J., Yu, Y.W., Lin, C.H., Song, H.L., Lai, H.C., Yang, K.H. (2000) Association study of a functional serotonin transporter gene polymorphism with schizophrenia, psychopathology and clozapine response. Schizophr Res 44(3): 177–81

Tsai, S.J., Wang, Y.C., Yu Younger, W.Y., Lin, C.H., Yang, K.H., & Hong, C.J. (2001) Association analysis of polymorphism in the promoter region of the alpha2aadrenoceptor gene with schizophrenia and clozapine response. Schizophrenia Research 49: 53–58

Tsai, S.J., Yu, Y.W., Lin, C.H., Wang, Y.C., Chen, J.Y., & Hong, C.J. (2004) Association study of adrenergic beta3 receptor (Trp64Arg) and G-protein beta3 subunit gene (C825T) polymorphisms and weight change during clozapine treatment. Neuropsychobiology 50: 37–40

Walsh, T., McClellan, J.M., McCarthy, S.E., Addington, A.M., Pierce, S.B., Cooper, G.M., Nord, A.S., Kusenda, M., Malhotra, D., Bhandari, A., Stray, S.M., Rippey, C.F., Roccanova, P., Makarov, V., Lakshmi, B., Findling, R.L., Sikich, L., Stromberg, T., Merriman, B., Gogtay, N., Butler, P., Eckstrand, K., Noory, L., Gochman, P., Long, R., Chen, Z., Davis, S., Baker, C., Eichler, E.E., Meltzer, P.S., Nelson, S.F., Singleton, A.B., Lee, M.K., Rapoport, J.L., King, M.C., & Sebat, J. (2008) Rare structural variants disrupt multiple genes in neurodevelopmental pathways in schizophrenia. Science 320: 539–543

Wang, L., Fang, C., Zhang, A., Du, J., Yu, L., Ma, J., Feng, G., Xing, Q., & He, L. (2008) The −1019 C/G polymorphism of the 5-HT(1)A receptor gene is associated with negative symptom response to risperidone treatment in schizophrenia patients. Journal of Psychopharmacology 22: 904–909

Wehmeier, P.M., Gebhardt, S., Schmidtke, J., Remschmidt, H., Hebebrand, J., & Theisen, F.M. (2005) Clozapine: weight gain in a pair of monozygotic twins concordant for schizophrenia and mild mental retardation. Psychiatry Research 133: 273–276

Weiss, E.L., Longhurst, J.G., Bowers, M.B., Jr., & Mazure, C.M. (1999) Olanzapine for treatment-refractory psychosis in patients responsive to, but intolerant of, clozapine. Journal of Clinical Psychopharmacology 19: 378–380

Wilson, W.H. (1996) Time required for initial improvement during clozapine treatment of refractory schizophrenia. American Journal of Psychiatry 153: 951–952

Woerner, M.G., Kane, J.M., Lieberman, J.A., Alvir, J., Bergmann, K.J., Borenstein, M., Schooler, N.R., Mukherjee, S., Rotrosen, J., & Rubinstein, M. (1991) The prevalence of tardive dyskinesia. Journal of Clinical Psychopharmacology 11: 34–42

Yamanouchi, Y., Iwata, N., Suzuki, T., Kitajima, T., Ikeda, M., & Ozaki, N. (2003) Effect of DRD2, 5-HT2A, and COMT genes on antipsychotic response to risperidone. Pharmacogenomics Journal 3: 356–361

Yassa, R. & Ananth, J. (1981) Familial tardive dyskinesia. American Journal of Psychiatry 138: 1618–1619

Yassa, R. & Jeste, D.V. (1992) Gender differences in tardive dyskinesia: a critical review of the literature. Schizophrenia Bulletin 18: 701–715

Yasui-Furukori, N., Saito, M., Nakagami, T., Kaneda, A., Tateishi, T., & Kaneko, S. (2006) Association between multidrug resistance 1 (MDR1) gene polymorphisms and therapeutic response to bromperidol in schizophrenic patients: a preliminary study. Progress in Neuropsychopharmacology and Biological Psychiatry 30: 286–291

Youssef, H., Lyster, G., & Youssef, F. (1989) Familial psychosis and vulnerability to tardive dyskinesia. International Clinical Psychopharmacology 4: 323–328

Yu, Y.W., Tsai, S.J., Lin, C.H., Hsu, C.P., Yang, K.H., & Hong, C.J. (1999) Serotonin-6 receptor variant (C267T) and clinical response to clozapine. Neuroreport 10: 1231–1233

Zai, G., Muller, D.J., Volavka, J., Czobor, P., Lieberman, J.A., Meltzer, H.Y., & Kennedy, J.L. (2006) Family and case-control association study of the tumor necrosis factor-alpha (TNF-alpha) gene with schizophrenia and response to antipsychotic medication. Psychopharmacology (Berlin) 188: 171–182

Zalsman, G., Frisch, A., Lev-Ran, S., Martin, A., Michaelovsky, E., Bensason, D., Gothelf, D., Nahshoni, E., Tyano, S., & Weizman, A. (2003) DRD4 exon III polymorphism and response to risperidone in Israeli adolescents with schizophrenia: a pilot pharmacogenetic study. European Neuropsychopharmacology 13: 183–185

Zhang, Z.J., Yao, Z.J., Mou, X.D., Chen, J.F., Zhu, R.X., Liu, W., Zhang, X.R., Sun, J., & Hou, G. (2003) [Association of -2548G/A functional polymorphism in the promoter region of leptin gene with antipsychotic agent-induced weight gain]. Zhonghua Yi Xue Za Zhi 83: 2119–2123

Part IV
Psychopathology, Cognition, Outcome

Prediction of Psychosis Through the Prodromal Syndrome

Tyrone D. Cannon

Introduction

Can prevention models now common to medicine be extended to psychotic disorders? Advances in early detection and intervention in cardiovascular disease, diabetes, and cancer have led to substantial reductions in morbidity and mortality and improved quality of life among individuals with these conditions (Adams et al. 2007; Berenson 2005; Parekh et al. 2006; Peters et al. 1996). The success of these programs is based on four primary factors: (1) they target disorders with relatively high prevalence; (2) risk is known to be greatest among particular demographic groups, facilitating efficiency of screening; (3) accurate and objective assessment methods exist for early detection; and (4) an array of interventions are available that scale in invasiveness with stage of illness. For the first three factors, there are ready parallels to psychotic disorders. Schizophrenia and other psychotic disorders have a worldwide prevalence of 3–5% (Kirkbride et al. 2006; Saha et al. 2005) and isolated symptoms (e.g., hearing a voice call one's name) are even more common, in the range of 20–30% (Loewy et al. 2007). Risk for onset of psychosis is clearly highest in the late adolescent to early adulthood period (Jablensky et al. 1992; Kirkbride et al. 2006). In addition, criteria for diagnosing an at-risk clinical state ('prodrome') have been developed and shown to have excellent predictive accuracy (McGlashan and Johannessen 1996; McGorry et al. 2003; Yung and McGorry 1996). However, available treatments are reactive rather than proactive, palliative rather than curative or preventive (Lieberman et al. 2005a).

The case for testing antipsychotic drugs as prophylactic measures rests entirely on their empirically proven efficacy in decreasing the severity of positive psychotic symptoms among patients with established illness. Initial applications of these

T.D. Cannon (✉)
Departments of Psychology and Psychiatry and Biobehavioral Sciences, University of California, Los Angeles, CA, USA
e-mail: cannon@psych.ucla.edu

Chapter in W.F. Gattaz & G.F. Busatto (eds.), Search for the Causes of Schizophrenia, Vol. VI, Springer Verlag, New York.

agents in studies of prodromal patients have produced discouraging results on the primary question of preventive effects (McGlashan et al. 2006; McGorry et al. 2002). Among patients with established illness whose positive symptoms respond to antipsychotics, such treatment must be continuous in order to maintain treatment gains; it is therefore not surprising that trials of antipsychotics in prodromal patients would show effects of drug on positive symptom reduction only during the active treatment phase. With no demonstrable prophylactic effects, and with little or no effect on motivational symptoms or functional disability, antipsychotic drug treatment in the prodromal phase is clearly not the "silver bullet" of psychosis prevention.

Most of the current research in the area of psychosis prevention focuses on longitudinal evaluation of individuals with a prodromal risk syndrome to improve prediction of psychosis and to elucidate the mechanisms of disease onset and progression. Clearly, the long-term goal is to facilitate application of interventions before the illness takes hold, thereby preventing the disorder and related functional disability (Hafner 1998; Keshavan et al. 2003; Malla et al. 2002; McGlashan 1999; Watanabe-Galloway and Zhang 2007) and reducing risk of suicide (Saha et al. 2007; Schwartz-Stav et al. 2006). Specification of rational preventive interventions requires knowledge of the mechanisms underlying the progression from prodromal to fully psychotic symptoms (Insel and Scolnick 2006). On the one hand, addressing this question may seem premature since we still lack definitive knowledge of the specific pathophysiological mechanisms underlying full-blown schizophrenia. It also seems possible that such processes may already be quite advanced in patients with prodromal symptoms, particularly those who will later convert to psychosis. On the other hand, there is clearly further clinical and functional deterioration as individuals move from a prodromal to fully psychotic state, suggesting that there may well be dynamic changes in neurobiological processes that drive these phenotypic effects. Overall, it would seem that the psychosis prodrome provides a unique window on the unfolding pathophysiology of illness, without the clouding effects of disease chronicity and long-term treatment that plague studies of patients with established illness. Longitudinal studies of progressive neurobiological processes in the psychosis prodrome would therefore appear to offer a useful point of contrast with similar studies of first-episode and chronic patients.

This chapter reviews research in the areas of psychosis prediction and neurobiological mechanisms of psychosis onset, with a particular focus on work done in our prodromal research center at UCLA and in collaboration with other prodromal programs in North America and Australia.

Psychosis Prodrome and Clinical Prediction Algorithm

In the past decade, it has become possible to ascertain individuals with a high likelihood of an onset of psychosis within 1–2 years based on the recent emergence of psychotic-like symptoms that are sub-psychotic in intensity. The Structured Interview for Prodromal Syndromes (SIPS) developed by McGlashan and colleagues at Yale (Miller et al. 2002, 2003) identifies three such at-risk syndromes: attenuated

positive symptoms (APS), genetic risk and deterioration (GRD), and brief inter-
mittent psychotic symptoms (BIPS). The SIPS criteria are consistent with those of
the Comprehensive Assessment of At-Risk Mental States (CAARMS), developed
by McGorry and colleagues at the University of Melbourne (Yung et al. 2005). In
studies using the SIPS or CAARMS, initial reports found a 40–50% annual rate of
conversion to psychosis (Klosterkotter et al. 2001; Miller et al. 2002; Yung et al.
1998, 2003), while more recent studies yield rates in the 20–30% range (Cornblatt
et al. 2003; Haroun et al. 2006; Lencz et al. 2003; Yung et al. 2005). The Melbourne
group reported a conversion rate of 34% in a recent sample of 104 UHR cases at
their site (Yung et al. 2006). The only other report with a sample size over 100
subjects found a conversion rate of 49.4% after long-term (9.6 years) follow-up in
a sample of 110 individuals (Klosterkotter et al. 2001) identified using the Bonn
Scale of Basic Symptoms (Gross and Huber 1985). Other reported conversion rates
of 9–76% have been noted in sample sizes of 13–40 subjects at follow-up of 1, 2,
or 3 years (Haroun et al. 2006). Existing data sets are underpowered to adequately
determine the positive predictive power of existing prodromal criteria. Additionally,
there is a great deal of variability in the assessment methods, samples, and follow-up
duration across studies (Haroun et al. 2006).

The North American Prodrome Longitudinal Study (NAPLS) was developed to
overcome these limitations. NAPLS is a consortium of eight clinical research programs, each of which is organized around the scientific goal of improving the accuracy of prospective prediction of initial psychosis by ascertaining clinical high-risk
individuals using the SIPS/SOPS system and following them longitudinally up to
3 years. Although originally developed as independent studies, the sites employed
similar ascertainment and longitudinal assessment methods and thus were able to
form a standardized protocol for mapping already acquired data into a new scheme
representing the common components across sites (Addington et al. 2007), yielding
the largest database on prospectively followed prodromal cases worldwide.

The federated NAPLS database (Addington et al. 2007) consists of 370 subjects meeting SIPS/SOPS criteria for the psychosis prodrome, of which 291 (78.6%)
completed at least one follow-up evaluation (i.e., at 6, 12, 18, or 24 months) and 79
(21.4%) were lost to follow-up. There were no differences in those who remained
and those lost to follow-up in terms of age, parental education, severity of positive
or negative symptoms, social, role, or general functioning, SIPS subdiagnosis, race,
ethnicity, year at study entry, SPD diagnosis, or presence of a first- or second-degree
relative with psychosis. The only significant effect related to attrition was that males
were overrepresented among those lost to follow-up (i.e., 75 vs. 58%).

Eighty-two of the 291 cases converted to psychosis, with a mean±SD time to
conversion of 275.5±243.7 days since the baseline evaluation (Cannon et al. 2008).
Seventy-nine of the converted cases were APS and 3 were BIPS. The remaining
209 cases were followed for an average of 575.4±258.4 days since the baseline.
The cumulative prevalence rate ± se of conversion to psychosis was 12.7 ± 1.9%
at 6 months, 21.7 ± 2.5% at 12 months, 26.8 ± 2.8% at 18 months, 32.6 ± 3.3%
at 24 months, and 35.3 ± 3.7% at 30 months. The incidence rate of conversion
(considering new cases only) shows an overall decelerating trend during the follow-
up period at a rate of 13% in the first 6 months, 9% between 7 and 12 months,

5% per 6 months epoch between 13 and 24 months, and then 2.7% between 25 and 30 months. In contrast, there were no conversions among 134 demographically matched normal controls.

Additional analyses were conducted to determine whether clinical and/or demographic features could improve prediction of psychosis among those who were 'prodromal' at baseline (Cannon et al. 2008). Of 77 potential predictor variables across 10 assessment domains, 37 were associated with conversion to psychosis at the univariate level. When multivariate analysis was applied to sets of predictors from each domain, the number of predictors meeting the cutoff for inclusion fell to 16. When the 16 predictors that survived domain-wise multivariate screening were examined in an omnibus (cross-domain) multivariate analysis, conversion to psychosis continued to be related significantly and uniquely to genetic risk for schizophrenia with recent functional deterioration ($\chi^2=10.45$, $p=0.001$), unusual thought content ($\chi^2=6.36$, $p=0.01$), suspicion–paranoia ($\chi^2=9.24$, $p=0.002$), social impairment ($\chi^2=14.98$, $p=0.0001$), and history of any drug abuse ($\chi^2=6.82$, $p=0.009$). With these terms in the model, none of the other predictors that had survived the domain-wise screening procedure were related to conversion risk, indicating that their predictive associations were redundant with the other model terms. In particular, treatment with antipsychotic drugs during the follow-up interval was not significantly associated with conversion in the cross-domain multivariate analysis ($\chi^2=0.59$, $p=0.44$).

Prediction statistics for each of the five uniquely predictive variables and their 26 possible combinations were evaluated (Cannon et al. 2008). At the univariate level, these factors have approximately equivalent PPP (i.e., 43–52%) and each is superior in this regard to the SIPS criteria alone (35%). Nevertheless, the adjunctive use of these predictors in determining risk status results in a reduction in sensitivity. Sensitivity is excellent for suspicion–paranoia and impaired social functioning (80%), moderate for genetic risk for schizophrenia with recent functional decline and unusual thought content (56–66%), and poor for history of substance abuse (29%). Among the algorithms requiring co-occurrence of two risk factors, the models including genetic risk for schizophrenia with recent functional decline and either unusual thought content or impaired social functioning have the highest PPP (69 and 60%, respectively), both substantially higher than that of the one-factor models, though sensitivity is again relatively modest (i.e., 38 and 55%, respectively). Two of the three-factor models, involving genetic risk for schizophrenia with recent functional decline, unusual thought content, and either suspicion–paranoia or impaired social functioning, result in even higher PPP (74–81%) compared with the two-factor models, with only marginal additional loss in sensitivity, and there is no further gain in prediction among any of the four-factor models or the five-factor model. An algorithm reflecting the sum of the five independent risk factors is no better in terms of PPP (i.e., 77–79%) than the best-performing three-factor model. Controlling for antipsychotic drugs during the follow-up interval did not modify the significance or the magnitude of the results. Multivariate algorithms not requiring co-occurrence of risk factors have lower PPP (i.e., 40–45%) but substantially higher sensitivity (i.e., 70–95%) compared with those above.

Importantly, these multivariate algorithms combine predictors that have been previously associated with conversion risk at the univariate level in other studies (Arseneault et al. 2004; Haroun et al. 2006; Kristensen and Cadenhead In Press; Owens et al. 2005; Rosen et al. 2006; Semple et al. 2005; Weiser et al. 2004; Yung et al. 2004), but the power of the large sample size in the NAPLS project is readily apparent in revealing particular multivariate configurations with the best prediction statistics. It is important to emphasize that although a relatively conservative statistical approach was used in our analyses, the algorithms were nevertheless derived empirically rather than confirmed through hypothesis testing and they thus require confirmation in an independent sample of equivalent or greater size. In addition, the prediction algorithms thus far identified apply to the initial diagnosis of psychosis, and further refinement is needed to resolve the considerable heterogeneity of ultimate diagnostic and functional outcomes.

Neurobiological Markers of Vulnerability and Progression in the Psychosis Prodrome

Current knowledge of the mechanisms underlying the emergence of psychosis is quite limited. However, a number of theoretical perspectives on the pathophysiology of schizophrenia have emerged that have relevance to the possible mechanisms of psychosis onset. A prominent theory holds that schizophrenia (and potentially other psychotic disorders) reflects a process of neuronal volume reduction involving principally synapses and dendrites (Feinberg 1982; Hoffman and McGlashan 1993; Hoffman and McGlashan 2001; McGlashan and Hoffman 2000; Selemon and Goldman-Rakic 1999; Weinberger 1987), resulting in reduced cortical connectivity (Ford and Mathalon 2005; Ford et al. 2002; Winder et al. 2007; Winterer et al. 2003; Wolf et al. 2007), particularly in prefrontal and superior and medial temporal lobe regions governing attention, executive, auditory language, and memory-related functions. This reduction in neuronal volume and cortical connectivity is likely to be present in some cases from birth, representing a life-long biological vulnerability, but may progress beyond a threshold critical for expression of psychotic symptoms as a function of *normal* neuromaturational events during adolescence, such as synaptic pruning (Weinberger 1987). In other cases, the reduction in neuronal volume and cortical connectivity may emerge during adolescence due to *aberrant* neurodevelopmental processes (i.e., abnormal pruning) and/or environmental insults, such as elevated cortisol leading to dendritic atrophy (Feinberg 1982; Hoffman and McGlashan 1993; McGlashan and Hoffman 2000). The contributions of early (pre- and perinatal) and later (adolescent) brain developmental processes to psychosis risk are not mutually exclusive, and both sets of processes may be operative in some cases (Cannon et al. 2003).

Markers of *Vulnerability* to Psychosis: Multiple lines of evidence suggest that disrupted synaptic plasticity and cortical connectivity are core pathophysiological processes in schizophrenia and related disorders. For example, in vivo MRI findings showing less cortical gray matter in patients with schizophrenia (Cannon et al. 2002a; Shenton et al. 2001) are thought to reflect a reduction in interneuronal neuropil, as demonstrated by postmortem evidence of decreased thickness of prefrontal cortex without a reduction in the number of cell bodies (Selemon et al. 1995, 1998). This loss of neuropil impacts directly on cellular connectivity, as supported by observations of reduced dendritic spine density on prefrontal cortical pyramidal neurons (Glantz and Lewis 2000). However, the timing of onset of these changes and their course in relation to the onset and course of psychotic symptoms are unknown. Because similar anatomical abnormalities are seen in the non-schizophrenic co-twins and siblings of patients on MRI (Cannon et al. 1998, 2002a), at least some of the neuroatomical changes are likely to be reflective of an inherited vulnerability to schizophrenia, and recent work has shown associations between prefrontal and hippocampal gray matter reductions and polymorphisms in putative schizophrenia risk genes (Buckholtz et al. 2007; Cannon et al. 2005; Harrison and Weinberger 2005; Prasad et al. 2005). Perinatal complications, particularly those associated with fetal hypoxia, also contribute to the anatomical deficits in schizophrenia (Cannon et al. 2002b; Preti 2003; Van Erp et al. 2002), suggesting that they are present to some degree early in life. Decreased gray matter in frontal regions has been observed among genetic high-risk individuals (Cannon et al. 2002a), and these deficits are more severe in those who subsequently develop prodromal symptoms (Ho 2007). Compared with healthy controls, clinically defined prodromal patients have been observed to show smaller volumes in the insula, superior temporal gyrus, cingulate, precuneus, and medial temporal lobe, and patients who later converted had less gray matter than those who did not in the insular, inferior frontal, and superior temporal cortex (Borgwardt et al. 2007). Surprisingly, in one study, larger hippocampal volumes at baseline were associated with conversion to psychosis among a prodromal group (Phillips et al. 2002). This result may reflect the instability of findings from small samples, as a subsequent report from the same investigators found normal hippocampal volumes in prodromal patients but lower hippocampal volumes in first-episode and chronic schizophrenia patients compared with controls (Velakoulis et al. 2006).

Markers of *Progression* to Psychosis: Many of the neurobiological measures associated with vulnerability to psychosis are expected to change dynamically as a consequence of normal brain maturation during late adolescence and early adulthood. At the anatomical level, cortical gray matter density on MRI declines normally during this period of development, reflecting a number of regressive processes (e.g., axon retraction, synaptic elimination) which result in decreased neuropil in brain regions implicated in the pathophysiology of schizophrenia (Huttenlocker 1979; Huttenlocker and Dabhokar 1997). It is therefore imperative to evaluate whether the rate of change observed in groups with or at risk for psychosis deviates from the pattern shown by healthy individuals during the same period of development. In fact, some of the neuroanatomical changes in schizophrenia appear to be progressive beyond that associated with normal development or aging, at least during the early phases of illness (Gur et al. 1998; Ho et al. 2003; Jacobsen et al. 1998; Lieberman et al. 2005b; Schreiber et al. 1999). Thus, while disturbances of

brain structure early in life may be necessary for the future emergence of schizophrenia (Weinberger 1987), neuromaturational events during the late adolescent–early
adult period may participate in (and be required for) psychotic symptom formation
(Feinberg 1982; Keshavan et al. 1994; Weinberger 1987). Brain structural changes
have also been reported in affective and other forms of psychosis (Strakowski et al.
2005), but whether there is ongoing excessive brain tissue loss prior to onset of
these forms of psychosis is less clear and remains controversial (Mathalon et al.
2003; Weinberger and McClure 2002).

   Studies examining longitudinal brain changes suggest that tissue loss occurs over
time in individuals at high risk of developing psychosis, but statistical power has
been limited in comparisons of rates of loss among at risk individuals who converted to psychosis relative to those who did not or to healthy controls (Job et
al. 2005; Pantelis et al. 2003). One study examined gray matter changes in UHR
subjects in a 1-year follow-up period (Pantelis et al. 2003). Both the converted
and unconverted groups showed between-scan gray matter loss in the left cerebellum, but the converted group also showed gray matter loss in a left inferior frontal
region, a left medial temporal region, and a cingulate region bilaterally. Another
study reported different patterns of gray matter loss between healthy controls and
subjects at high genetic risk (GHR) of schizophrenia during a 2-year follow-up
period (Job et al. 2005). While control subjects showed gray matter reduction in
the right gyrus rectus, GHR subjects showed gray matter reduction in the temporal lobes, the right frontal lobe, and the right parietal lobe. These studies suggest
that there is gray matter reduction in high-risk individuals, but fail to confirm that
these changes differentially affect those who convert to psychosis or schizophrenia compared to non-converters and healthy controls. However, in a subsequent
report from the latter investigators, changes in the inferior temporal gyrus over a
1.5-year follow-up interval gave a positive predictive value of 60% in relation to
psychosis conversion compared with 13% in the group overall (Job et al. 2006).
It is likely that robust between-group differences in rates of change cannot be
revealed in such small samples and that more refined image analytical methods
will be required to test for relatively subtle differences in change over 1- to 2-year
intervals.

   A key element of our strategy is the use of cortical surface modeling and pattern
matching to aggregate imaging data sets in the same anatomic reference locations
across subjects (Thompson et al. 1996b, 2000a, b). Power is greatly increased as
the residual anatomic variability is directly modeled and confounding variations are
factored out before making intersubject comparisons. Because surface models can
be used to drive deformation fields that warp one anatomy to match another, they
are often used to generate deformation fields that store information on anatomical
shape differences (deformation-based morphometry) (Grenander and Miller 1998;
Thompson et al. 1996a, 2001). Surface models are also powerful building blocks
of brain atlases. Their surface grid structure helps in building average templates of
anatomy and statistics that capture its variation. When assessing the significance
of group effects, we perform corrections for multiple comparisons using permutation (Holmes et al. 1996; Sowell et al. 1999), nonstationary Gaussian field theory

(Worsley et al. 1999), or adaptive grids whose deformation gradient matches the smoothness tensor of the residuals (Thompson et al. 2000b).

We recently applied the cortical pattern-matching algorithm to high-resolution T1-weighted MRI data sets from the University of Melbourne to investigate whether there are differential rates of change in cortical gray matter among CHR patients who convert to psychosis ($N=12$) as compared with those who do not ($N=23$) (Sun et al. 2009) and in individuals with first-episode schizophrenia ($N=16$) compared with healthy controls ($N=12$) (Sun et al. 2008). Cortical pattern matching was used in combination with surface displacement techniques capable of detecting changes at the cortical surface (contraction or expansion) at sub-voxel (<1 mm) resolution. We created maps comparing CHR patients who converted to psychosis with those who did not convert (Sun et al. 2009) and maps comparing FEZ patients with healthy controls (Sun et al. 2008). In contrast to the average rate of surface contraction in non-converters, the magnitude of which was less than 0.1 mm per annum, the converters showed greater brain surface contraction in bilateral dorsolateral prefrontal regions and occipital poles, with a maximum magnitude of 0.3 mm per annum. In the between-group comparison, prefrontal regions, especially the right superior frontal gyrus, showed the most prominent differences. Using permutation tests with p-value at 0.05, in the prodromal analysis, only the between-group difference in the right prefrontal region remained significant ($p=0.036$), while the differences in left prefrontal, left occipital, and right occipital regions showed trends toward significance ($p=0.090$, 0.051, and 0.056, respectively). No significant results appeared in other regions of interest and rates of surface expansion did not differ by group. In the FEZ analysis, surface contraction occurred in prefrontal regions in both groups, with FEZ patients showing a significantly greater rate of retraction in this region compared with controls (Sun et al. 2008).

These data build on a prior report using lower resolution T2 and proton density dual echo image data on a subset of the same prodromal subjects, in which significant within-group changes in cortical gray matter density were observed only in converters; the magnitude of these changes did not, however, differ significantly from non-converters (Pantelis et al. 2003). In our follow-up study, 2 more converted subjects and 12 more non-converters were involved in the comparison, providing additional statistical power. Furthermore, a new parameter of longitudinal brain change, i.e., brain surface contraction, with resolution at a sub-voxel level, was utilized, in contrast to the previous voxel-based morphometry analysis. In combination with the cortical pattern matching method, which provides a precise brain surface registration, the surface contraction measurement showed an advantage in detecting subtle changes. The maximum group-mean local brain surface contraction was less than 0.3 mm per annum; this suggests that the prior gray matter density measurement was limited by the image voxel resolution. Importantly, however, we have confirmed that rates of surface contraction and rates of reduction in brain tissue are highly correlated at a voxel level across most of the cortical surface, including prefrontal regions. Furthermore, in a separate study of white matter integrity, prodromal patients failed to show the normal increase in fractional anisotropy (FA) with age that was observed in the healthy adolescent control group, and lower

FA in the patient group was predictive of poorer functional outcome at follow-up (Karlsgodt et al. 2008).

While we cannot entirely rule out effects of antipsychotic or other neuroleptic medications as a source of these effects, drug treatment is not likely to be a major source of the observed changes, given that the majority of converted subjects and FEZ patients received risperidone (an atypical antipsychotic drug) after onset of psychosis, and atypical antipsychotics appear to be associated with less brain volume reduction compared with typical antipsychotics or even with volume increase (Dazzan et al. 2005; Lieberman et al. 2005b). That the pattern of structural change in the early course of schizophrenia corresponds so closely to that associated with normal development is consistent with the hypothesis that a schizophrenia-related factor interacts with normal adolescent brain developmental processes in the pathophysiology of schizophrenia. The exaggerated progressive changes seen in prodromal and FEZ patients may reflect an increased rate of synaptic pruning, resulting in excessive loss of neuronal connectivity, as predicted by the late neurodevelopmental hypothesis of the illness. Taken together, these findings suggest that regressive developmental processes active during late adolescence and early adulthood that are likely to result in reduced cellular connectivity (such as synaptic pruning and disrupted white matter development) may underlie the emergence and early course of psychotic symptoms. While the results of these studies are provocative in this regard, they are limited primarily by the small numbers of cases included (N's in the teens to twenties), by the uncontrolled nature of treatments received by the patients, and by heterogeneity of outcomes among converters.

Conclusions

Further large-scale longitudinal studies focusing on biological indicators are needed to determine whether prodromal patients who convert to psychosis show a steeper rate of change in neurobiological risk indicators compared to non-converters and healthy controls and to isolate the brain systems involved (e.g., dorsolateral prefrontal cortex, superior temporal gyrus, hippocampus) across multiple levels of analysis (anatomical, physiological, behavioral). If a steeper rate of change occurs with psychosis onset, this would suggest deviant adolescent brain maturational processes as playing a role and encourage search for molecular mechanisms underlying these changes. On the other hand, if prodromal patients who convert to psychosis show greater deviance on these measures at baseline, but not a differential rate of change over time, this would suggest that adolescent brain maturational processes are likely to be intact in those who convert, but these maturational processes may nevertheless be required for the preexisting neurobiological vulnerability to manifest in psychotic symptoms. In either case, prodromal research is likely to lead to improved theoretical specification of the biological mechanisms subserving psychosis onset, advances that will be crucial to the development of new preventive strategies targeting the specific cellular and molecular processes involved and the specific periods of development when intervention could conceivably halt or attenuate the underlying pathophysiological deterioration.

Neurobiological measures may or may not also lead to an enhancement of psychosis prediction over and above that associated with clinical and demographic risk indicators. However, even if the contribution to the prediction of psychosis contributed by biological measures is ultimately shown to overlap entirely with that of clinical and demographic measures, such knowledge would in itself be valuable. Biological measures would then be validated as predictive biomarkers in prodromal populations. Such findings, in turn, would be likely to generate future research to determine whether biological measures could be used to ascertain individuals at risk, independent of prodromal symptoms and before substantial clinical and functional deterioration has occurred. Given the heterogeneity of the prodromal population in terms of risk factors and outcomes, testing the unique predictive roles of multiple biological and clinical predictors simultaneously requires very large samples (i.e., N's in the several hundreds to thousands) and systematically acquired data, which will only be possible in multisite collaborative studies.

As noted above, the existing trials of antipsychotic drugs have essentially found no differences in conversion rates by the end of active treatment or with longer term follow-up between any of the treated groups vs. placebo (McGlashan et al. 2006; McGorry et al. 2002). Based on these considerations, it seems unlikely that any of the currently available pharmacological treatments for psychosis will have substantial prophylactic effects. Thus, without a more detailed understanding of the biological mechanisms underlying onset of psychosis, even if we could predict perfectly who in the population will develop a psychotic illness, we would lack the knowledge needed to target the specific pathways involved and our interventions will remain reactive and palliative.

At the same time, it is clear that some form of treatment needs to be offered to young people at greatest risk. That is, prodromal patients are in high distress and treatment seeking. Therefore, it is ethically necessary to provide (low-risk) psychosocial interventions to address presenting issues. Such treatments could be offered to all patients or the differential effectiveness of different psychological interventions (e.g., cognitive-behavioral therapy versus family-based therapy) could be tested in a randomized study. Psychosocial interventions appear to be well suited to address issues of motivational deficits and functional disability in the psychosis prodrome. Given our present state of knowledge regarding the mechanisms of psychosis onset, a reduction in functional disability would appear to represent a more achievable target in the short term than a reduction in psychosis incidence.

References

Adams, E.K., Breen, N., and Joski, P.J. Impact of the National Breast and Cervical Cancer Early Detection Program on mammography and pap test utilization among white, Hispanic, and African American women: 1996–2000. *Cancer*, 109(2 Suppl):348–58, 2007.

Addington, J., Cadenhead, K.S., Cannon, T.D., Cornblatt, B., McGlashan, T.H., Perkins, D.O., Seidman, L.J., Tsuang, M., Walker, E.F., Woods, S.W., and Heinssen, R. North American

Prodrome Longitudinal Study: a collaborative multisite approach to prodromal schizophrenia research. *Schizophr Bull*, 33(3):665–72, 2007.

Arseneault, L., Cannon, M., Witton, J., and Murray, R.M. Causal association between cannabis and psychosis: examination of the evidence. *Br J Psychiatry*, 184:110–7, 2004.

Berenson, G.S. Obesity – a critical issue in preventive cardiology: the Bogalusa Heart Study. *Prev Cardiol*, 8(4):234–41, quiz 242–3, 2005.

Borgwardt, S.J., Riecher-Rossler, A., Dazzan, P., Chitnis, X., Aston, J., Drewe, M., Gschwandt-ner, U., Haller, S., Pfluger, M., Rechsteiner, E., D'Souza, M., Stieglitz, R.D., Radu, E.W., and McGuire, P.K. Regional gray matter volume abnormalities in the at risk mental state. *Biol Psychiatry*, 61(10):1148–56, 2007.

Buckholtz, J.W., Meyer-Lindenberg, A., Honea, R.A., Straub, R.E., Pezawas, L., Egan, M.F., Vakkalanka, R., Kolachana, B., Verchinski, B.A., Sust, S., Mattay, V.S., Weinberger, D.R., and Callicott, J.H. Allelic variation in RGS4 impacts functional and structural connectivity in the human brain. *J Neurosci*, 27(7):1584–93, 2007.

Cannon, T.D., Cadenhead, K., Cornblatt, B., Woods, S.W., Addington, J., Walker, E., Seidman, L.J., Perkins, D., Tsuang, M., McGlashan, T., and Heinssen, R. Prediction of psychosis in youth at high clinical risk: a multisite longitudinal study in North America. *Arch Gen Psychiatry*, 65(1):28–37, 2008.

Cannon, T.D., Hennah, W., van Erp, T.G., Thompson, P.M., Lonnqvist, J., Huttunen, M., Gasperoni, T., Tuulio-Henriksson, A., Pirkola, T., Toga, A.W., Kaprio, J., Mazziotta, J., and Peltonen, L. Association of DISC1/TRAX haplotypes with schizophrenia, reduced prefrontal gray matter, and impaired short- and long-term memory. *Arch Gen Psychiatry*, 62(11):1205–13, 2005.

Cannon, T.D., Thompson, P.M., van Erp, T.G., Toga, A.W., Poutanen, V.P., Huttunen, M., Lonnqvist, J., Standerskjold-Nordenstam, C.G., Narr, K.L., Khaledy, M., Zoumalan, C.I., Dail, R., and Kaprio, J. Cortex mapping reveals regionally specific patterns of genetic and disease-specific gray-matter deficits in twins discordant for schizophrenia. *Proc Natl Acad Sci USA*, 99:3228–33, 2002a.

Cannon, T.D., van Erp, T.G., Bearden, C.E., Loewy, R., Thompson, P., Toga, A.W., Huttunen, M.O., Keshavan, M.S., Seidman, L.J., and Tsuang, M.T. Early and late neurodevelopmental influences in the prodrome to schizophrenia: contributions of genes, environment, and their interactions. *Schizophr Bull*, 29:653–69, 2003.

Cannon, T.D., van Erp, T.G., Huttunen, M., Lönnqvist, J., Salonen, O., Valanne, L., Poutanen, V.P., Standertskjöld-Nordenstam, C.G., Gur, R.E., and Yan, M. Regional gray matter, white matter, and cerebrospinal fluid distributions in schizophrenic patients, their siblings, and controls. *Arch Gen Psychiatry*, 55(12):1084–91, 1998.

Cannon, T.D., van Erp, T.G., Rosso, I.M., Huttunen, M., Lonnqvist, J., Pirkola, T., Salonen, O., Valanne, L., Poutanen, V.P., and Standertskjold-Nordenstam, C.G. Fetal hypoxia and structural brain abnormalities in schizophrenic patients, their siblings, and controls. *Arch Gen Psychiatry*, 59(1):35–41, 2002b.

Cornblatt, B.A., Lencz, T., Smith, C.W., Correll, C.U., Auther, A.M., and Nakayama, E. The schizophrenia prodrome revisited: a neurodevelopmental perspective. *Schizophr Bull*, 29(4):633–51, 2003.

Dazzan, P., Morgan, K.D., Orr, K., Hutchinson, G., Chitnis, X., Suckling, J., Fearon, P., McGuire, P.K., Mallett, R.M., Jones, P.B., Leff, J., and Murray, R.M. Different effects of typical and atypical antipsychotics on grey matter in first episode psychosis: the AESOP study. *Neuropsychopharmacology*, 30:765–74, 2005.

Feinberg, I. Schizophrenia: Caused by a fault in programmed synaptic elimination during adolescence? *J Psychiatr Res*, 17(4):319–34, 1982.

Ford, J.M., and Mathalon, D.H. Corollary discharge dysfunction in schizophrenia: can it explain auditory hallucinations? *Int J Psychophysiol*, 58(2–3):179–89, 2005.

Ford, J.M., Mathalon, D.H., Whitfield, S., Faustman, W.O., and Roth, W.T. Reduced communication between frontal and temporal lobes during talking in schizophrenia. *Biol Psychiatry*, 51(6):485–92, 2002.

Glantz, L.A., and Lewis, D.A. Decreased dendritic spine density on prefrontal cortical pyramidal neurons in schizophrenia. *Arch Gen Psychiatry*, 57(1):65–73, 2000.

Grenander, U., and Miller, M.I. Computational anatomy: an emerging discipline. *Q Appl Math*, 4:617–94, 1998.

Gross, G., and Huber, G. Psychopathology of basic stages of schizophrenia in view of formal thought disturbances. *Psychopathology*, 18(2–3):115–25, 1985.

Gur, R.E., Cowell, P., Turetsky, B.I., Gallacher, F., Cannon, T., Bilker, W., and Gur, R.C. A follow-up magnetic resonance imaging study of schizophrenia. Relationship of neuroanatomical changes to clinical and neurobehavioral measures. *Arch Gen Psychiatry*, 55:145–52, 1998.

Hafner, H. Onset and course of the first schizophrenic episode. *Kao-Hsiung i Hsueh Ko Hsueh Tsa Chih [kaohsiung Journal of Medical Sciences]*, 14(7):413–31, 1998.

Haroun, N., Dunn, L., Haroun, A., and Cadenhead, K.S. Risk and protection in prodromal schizophrenia: ethical implications for clinical practice and future research. *Schizophr Bull*, 32(1):166–78, 2006.

Harrison, P.J., and Weinberger, D.R. Schizophrenia genes, gene expression, and neuropathology: on the matter of their convergence. *Mol Psychiatry*, 10(1):40–68, image 5, 2005.

Ho, B.C. MRI brain volume abnormalities in young, nonpsychotic relatives of schizophrenia probands are associated with subsequent prodromal symptoms. *Schizophr Res*, 96(1–3):1–13, 2007.

Ho, B.C., Andreasen, N.C., Nopoulos, P., Arndt, S., Magnotta, V., and Flaum, M. Progressive structural brain abnormalities and their relationship to clinical outcome: a longitudinal magnetic resonance imaging study early in schizophrenia. *Arch Gen Psychiatry*, 60:585–94, 2003.

Hoffman, R.E., and McGlashan, T.H. Parallel distributed processing and the emergence of schizophrenic symptoms. *Schizophr Bull*, 19(1):119–40, 1993.

Hoffman, R.E., and McGlashan, T.H. Neural network models of schizophrenia. *Neuroscientist*, 7(5):441–54, 2001.

Holmes, A.P., Blair, R.C., Watson, J.D., and Ford, I. Nonparametric analysis of statistic images from functional mapping experiments. *J Cereb Blood Flow Metab*, 16(1):7–22, 1996.

Huttenlocker, P.R. Synaptic density in the human frontal cortex – developmental changes and effects of aging. *Brain Res*, 163:195–205, 1979.

Huttenlocker, P.R., and Dabhokar, A.S. Regional differences in synaptogenesis in human cerebral cortex. *J Comparative Neurol*, 387:167–78, 1997.

Insel, T.R., and Scolnick, E.M. Cure therapeutics and strategic prevention: raising the bar for mental health research. *Mol Psychiatry*, 11(1):11–7, 2006.

Jablensky, A., Sartorius, N., Ernberg, G., Anker, M., Korten, A., Cooper, J.E., Day, R., and Bertelsen, A. Schizophrenia: manifestations, incidence and course in different cultures. A World Health Organization ten-country study. *Psychol Med Monogr Suppl*, 20:1–97, 1992.

Jacobsen, L.K., Giedd, J.N., Castellanos, F.X., Vaituzis, A.C., Hamburger, S.D., Kumra, S., Lenane, M.C., and Rapoport, J.L. Progressive reduction of temporal lobe structures in childhood-onset schizophrenia. *Am J Psychiatry*, 155(5):678–85, 1998.

Job, D.E., Whalley, H.C., Johnstone, E.C., and Lawrie, S.M. Grey matter changes over time in high risk subjects developing schizophrenia. *Neuroimage*, 25:1023–30, 2005.

Job, D.E., Whalley, H.C., McIntosh, A.M., Owens, D.G.C., Johnstone, E.C., and Lawrie, S.M. Grey matter changes can improve the prediction of schizophrenia in subjects at high risk. *BMC Medicine*, 4:29, 2006.

Karlsgodt, K.H., Sun, D., Jimenez, A.M., Lutkenhoff, E.S., Willhite, R., van Erp, T.G., and Cannon, T.D. Developmental disruptions in neural connectivity in the pathophysiology of schizophrenia. *Dev Psychopathol*, 20(4):1297–327, 2008.

Keshavan, M.S., Anderson, S.A., and Pettegrew, J.W. Is schizophrenia due to excessive synaptic pruning in the prefrontal cortex? The Feinberg hypothesis revisited. *J Psychiatr Res*, 28(3):239–65, 1994.

Keshavan, M.S., Haas, G., Miewald, J., Montrose, D.M., Reddy, R., Schooler, N.R., and Sweeney, J.A. Prolonged untreated illness duration from prodromal onset predicts outcome in first episode psychoses. *Schizophr Bull*, 29(4):757–69, 2003.

Kirkbride, J.B., Fearon, P., Morgan, C., Dazzan, P., Morgan, K., Tarrant, J., Lloyd, T., Holloway, J., Hutchinson, G., Leff, J.P., Mallett, R.M., Harrison, G.L., Murray, R.M., and Jones, P.B. Heterogeneity in incidence rates of schizophrenia and other psychotic syndromes: findings from the 3-center AeSOP study. *Arch Gen Psychiatry*, 63(3):250–8, 2006.

Klosterkotter, J., Hellmich, M., Steinmeyer, E.M., and Schultze-Lutter, F. Diagnosing schizophrenia in the initial prodromal phase. *Arch Gen Psychiatry*, 58(2):158–64, 2001.

Kristensen, K., and Cadenhead, K.S. Cannabis Abuse and Risk for Psychosis in a Prodromal Sample. *Psychiatry Res*, 151(1–2):151–4, 2007.

Lencz, T., Smith, C.W., Auther, A.M., Correll, C.U., and Cornblatt, B.A. The assessment of "prodromal schizophrenia": unresolved issues and future directions. *Schizophr Bull*, 29(4):717–28, 2003.

Lieberman, J.A., Stroup, T.S., McEvoy, J.P., Swartz, M.S., Rosenheck, R.A., Perkins, D.O., Keefe, R.S., Davis, S.M., Davis, C.E., Lebowitz, B.D., Severe, J., and Hsiao, J.K. Effectiveness of antipsychotic drugs in patients with chronic schizophrenia. *N Engl J Med*, 353(12):1209–23, 2005a.

Lieberman, J.A., Tollefson, G.D., Charles, C., Zipursky, R., Sharma, T., Kahn, R.S., Keefe, R.S., Green, A.I., Gur, R.E., McEvoy, J., Perkins, D., Hamer, R.M., Gu, H., and Tohen, M. Antipsychotic drug effects on brain morphology in first-episode psychosis. *Arch Gen Psychiatry*, 62(4):361–70, 2005b.

Loewy, R.L., Johnson, J.K., and Cannon, T.D. Self-report of attenuated psychotic experiences in a college population. *Schizophr Res*, 93(1–3):144–51, 2007.

Malla, A.K., Norman, R.M., Manchanda, R., Ahmed, M.R., Scholten, D., Harricharan, R., Cortese, L., and Takhar, J. One year outcome in first episode psychosis: influence of DUP and other predictors. *Schizophr Res*, 54(3):231–42, 2002.

Mathalon, D.H., Rapoport, J.L., Davis, K.L., and Krystal, J.H. Neurotoxicity, neuroplasticity, and magnetic resonance imaging morphometry. *Arch Gen Psychiatry*, 60:846–8, 2003.

McGlashan, T.H. Duration of untreated psychosis in first-episode schizophrenia: marker or determinant of course? *Biol Psychiatry*, 46(7):899–907, 1999.

McGlashan, T.H., and Hoffman, R.E. Schizophrenia as a disorder of developmentally reduced synaptic connectivity. *Arch Gen Psychiatry*, 57:637–48, 2000.

McGlashan, T.H., and Johannessen, J.O. Early detection and intervention with schizophrenia: Rationale. *Schizophr Bull*, 22(2):201–22, 1996.

McGlashan, T.H., Zipursky, R.B., Perkins, D., Addington, J., Miller, T., Woods, S.W., Hawkins, K.A., Hoffman, R.E., Preda, A., Epstein, I., Addington, D., Lindborg, S., Trzaskoma, Q., Tohen, M., and Breier, A. Randomized double-blind clinical trial of olanzapine versus placebo in patients prodromally symptomatic for psychosis. *Am J Psychiatry*, 163:790–9, 2006.

McGorry, P.D., Yung, A.R., and Phillips, L.J. The "close-in" or ultra high-risk model: a safe and effective strategy for research and clinical intervention in prepsychotic mental disorder. *Schizophr Bull*, 29:771–90, 2003.

McGorry, P.D., Yung, A.R., Phillips, L.J., Yuen, H.P., Francey, S., Cosgrave, E.M., Germano, D., Bravin, J., McDonald, T., Blair, A., Adlard, S., and Jackson, H. Randomized controlled trial of interventions designed to reduce the risk of progression to first-episode psychosis in a clinical sample with subthreshold symptoms. *Arch Gen Psychiatry*, 59(10):921–8, 2002.

Miller, T.J., McGlashan, T.H., Rosen, J.L., Cadenhead, K., Ventura, J., McFarlane, W., Perkins, D.O., Pearlson, G.D., and Woods, S.W. Prodromal assessment with the structured interview for prodromal syndromes and the scale of prodromal symptoms: predictive validity, interrater reliability, and training to reliability. *Schizophr Bull*, 29(4):703–15, 2003.

Miller, T.J., McGlashan, T.H., Rosen, J.L., Somjee, L., Markovich, P.J., Stein, K., and Woods, S.W. Prospective diagnosis of the initial prodrome for schizophrenia based on the Structured

Interview for Prodromal Syndromes: preliminary evidence of interrater reliability and predictive validity. *Am J Psychiatry*, 159(5):863–5, 2002.

Owens, D.G., Miller, P., Lawrie, S.M., and Johnstone, E.C. Pathogenesis of schizophrenia: a psychopathological perspective. *Br J Psychiatry*, 186:386–93, 2005.

Pantelis, C., Velakoulis, D., McGorry, P.D., Wood, S.J., Suckling, J., Phillips, L.J., Yung, A.R., Bullmore, E.T., Brewer, W., Souldsby, B., Desmond, P., and McGuire, P.K. Neuroanatomical abnormalities before and after onset of psychosis: a cross-sectional and longitudinal MRI comparison. *Lancet*, 361:281–8, 2003.

Parekh, D.J., Ankerst, D.P., Higgins, B.A., Hernandez, J., Canby-Hagino, E., Brand, T., Troyer, D.A., Leach, R.J., and Thompson, I.M. External validation of the Prostate Cancer Prevention Trial risk calculator in a screened population. *Urology*, 68(6):1152–5, 2006.

Peters, A.L., Davidson, M.B., Schriger, D.L., and Hasselblad, V. A clinical approach for the diagnosis of diabetes mellitus: an analysis using glycosylated hemoglobin levels. Meta-analysis Research Group on the Diagnosis of Diabetes Using Glycated Hemoglobin Levels. *JAMA*, 276(15):1246–52, 1996.

Phillips, L.J., Velakoulis, D., Pantelis, C., Wood, S., Yuen, H.P., Yung, A.R., Desmond, P., Brewer, W., and McGorry, P.D. Non-reduction in hippocampal volume is associated with higher risk of psychosis. *Schizophr Res*, 58(2–3):145–58, 2002.

Prasad, K.M., Chowdari, K.V., Nimgaonkar, V.L., Talkowski, M.E., Lewis, D.A., and Keshavan, M.S. Genetic polymorphisms of the RGS4 and dorsolateral prefrontal cortex morphometry among first episode schizophrenia patients. *Mol Psychiatry*, 10(2):213–9, 2005.

Preti, A. Fetal hypoxia, genetic risk, and schizophrenia. *Am J Psychiatry*, 160(6):1186, author reply 1186, 2003.

Rosen, J.L., Miller, T.J., D'Andrea, J.T., McGlashan, T.H., and Woods, S.W. Comorbid diagnoses in patients meeting criteria for the schizophrenia prodrome. *Schizophr Res*, 85(1–3):124–31, 2006.

Saha, S., Chant, D., and McGrath, J. A systematic review of mortality in schizophrenia: is the differential mortality gap worsening over time? *Arch Gen Psychiatry*, 64(10):1123–31, 2007.

Saha, S., Chant, D., Welham, J., and McGrath, J. A systematic review of the prevalence of schizophrenia. *PLoS Medicine*, 2(5):e141, 2005.

Schreiber, H., Baur-Seack, K., Kronhuber, H.H., Wallner, B., Friedrich, J.M., De Winter, I.M., and Born, J. Brain morphology in adolescents at genetic risk for schizophrenia assessed by qualitative and quantitative magnetic resonance imaging. *Schizophr Res*, 40(1):81–4, 1999.

Schwartz-Stav, O., Apter, A., and Zalsman, G. Depression, suicidal behavior and insight in adolescents with schizophrenia. *Eur Child Adolesc Psychiatry*, 15(6):352–9, 2006.

Selemon, L.D., and Goldman-Rakic, P.S. The reduced neuropil hypothesis: a circuit based model of schizophrenia. *Biol Psychiatry*, 45(1):17–25, 1999.

Selemon, L.D., Rajkowska, G., and Goldman-Rakic, P.S. Abnormally high neuronal density in the schizophrenic cortex: a morphometric analysis of prefrontal area 9 and occipital area 17. *Arch Gen Psychiatry*, 52(10):805–18, 1995.

Selemon, L.D., Rajkowska, G., and Goldman-Rakic, P.S. Elevated neuronal density in prefrontal area 46 in brains from schizophrenic patients: application of a three-dimensional, stereologic counting method. *J Comparative Neurol*, 392:402–12, 1998.

Semple, D.M., McIntosh, A.M., and Lawrie, S.M. Cannabis as a risk factor for psychosis: systematic review. *J Psychopharmacol*, 19(2):187–94, 2005.

Shenton, M.E., Dickey, C.C., Frumin, M., and McCarley, R.W. A review of MRI findings in schizophrenia. *Schizophr Res*, 49(1–2):1–52, 2001.

Sowell, E.R., Thompson, P.M., Holmes, C.J., Jernigan, T.L., and Toga, A.W. In vivo evidence for post-adolescent brain maturation in frontal and striatal regions. *Nat Neurosci*, 2(10):859–61, 1999.

Strakowski, S.M., Delbello, M.P., and Adler, C.M. The functional neuroanatomy of bipolar disorder: a review of neuroimaging findings. *Mol Psychiatry*, 10:105–16, 2005.

Sun, D., Phillips, L., Velakoulis, D., Yung, A., McGorry, P.D., Wood, S.J., van Erp, T.G., Thompson, P.M., Toga, A.W., Cannon, T.D., and Pantelis, C. Progressive brain structural changes mapped as psychosis develops in 'at risk' individuals. *Schizophr Res*, 108(1–3):85–92, 2009.

Sun, D., Stuart, G.W., Jenkinson, M., Wood, S.J., McGorry, P.D., Velakoulis, D., van Erp, T.G., Thompson, P.M., Toga, A.W., Smith, D.J., Cannon, T.D., and Pantelis, C. Brain surface contraction mapped in first-episode schizophrenia: a longitudinal magnetic resonance imaging study. *Mol Psychiatry*, 2:1063–1122, 2008.

Thompson, P.M., Mega, M.S., Narr, K.L., Sowell, E.R., Blanton, R.E., and Toga, A.W. Brain image analysis and atlas construction. In: Sonka, M., ed. *SPIE Handbook of Medical Image Processing and Analysis*: SPIE press, 2000a.

Thompson, P.M., Schwartz, C., Lin, R.T., Khan, A.A., and Toga, A.W. Three-dimensional statistical analysis of sulcal variability in the human brain. *J Neurosci*, 16:4261–74, 1996a.

Thompson, P.M., Schwartz, C., and Toga, A.W. High-resolution random mesh algorithms for creating a probabilistic 3D surface atlas of the human brain. *Psychiatry Res: Neuroimaging*, 3:19-34, 1996b.

Thompson, P.M., Vidal, C., Giedd, J.N., Gochman, P., Blumenthal, J., Nicolson, R., Toga, A.W., and Rapoport, J.L. Mapping adolescent brain change reveals dynamic wave of accelerated gray matter loss in very early-onset schizophrenia. *Proc Natl Acad Sci USA*, 98(20):11650–5, 2001.

Thompson, P.M., Woods, R.P., Mega, M.S., and Toga, A.W. Mathematical/computational challenges in creating deformable and probabilistic atlases of the human brain. *Human Brain Mapp*, 9:81–92, 2000b.

Van Erp, T.G., Saleh, P.A., Rosso, I.M., Huttunen, M., Lonnqvist, J., Pirkola, T., Salonen, O., Valanne, L., Poutanen, V.P., Standertskjold-Nordenstam, C.G., and Cannon, T.D. Contributions of genetic risk and fetal hypoxia to hippocampal volume in patients with schizophrenia or schizoaffective disorder, their unaffected siblings, and healthy unrelated volunteers. *Am J Psychiatry*, 159(9):1514–20, 2002.

Velakoulis, D., Wood, S.J., Wong, M.T., McGorry, P.D., Yung, A., Phillips, L., Smith, D., Brewer, W., Proffitt, T., Desmond, P., and Pantelis, C. Hippocampal and amygdala volumes according to psychosis stage and diagnosis: a magnetic resonance imaging study of chronic schizophrenia, first-episode psychosis, and ultra-high-risk individuals. *Arch Gen Psychiatry*, 63(2):139–49, 2006.

Watanabe-Galloway, S., and Zhang, W. Analysis of U.S. trends in discharges from general hospitals for episodes of serious mental illness, 1995–2002. *Psychiatr Serv*, 58(4):496–502, 2007.

Weinberger, D.R. Implications of normal brain development for the pathogenesis of schizophrenia. *Arch Gen Psychiatry*, 44(7):660–9, 1987.

Weinberger, D.R., and McClure, R.K. Neurotoxicity, neuroplasticity, and magnetic resonance imaging morphometry: what is happening to the schizophrenic brain? *Arch Gen Psychiatry*, 59:553–8, 2002.

Weiser, M., Reichenberg, A., Grotto, I., Yasvitzky, R., Rabinowitz, J., Lubin, G., Nahon, D., Knobler, H.Y., and Davidson, M. Higher rates of cigarette smoking in male adolescents before the onset of schizophrenia: a historical-prospective cohort study. *Am J Psychiatry*, 161(7):1219–23, 2004.

Winder, R., Cortes, C.R., Reggia, J.A., and Tagamets, M.A. Functional connectivity in fMRI: A modeling approach for estimation and for relating to local circuits. *Neuroimage*, 34(3):1093–107, 2007.

Winterer, G., Smolka, M., Samochowiec, J., Ziller, M., Mahlberg, R., Gallinat, J., Rommelspacher, H.P., Herrmann, W.M., and Sander, T. Association of EEG coherence and an exonic GABA(B)R1 gene polymorphism. *Am J Med Genet B Neuropsychiatr Genet*, 117(1):51–6, 2003.

Wolf, D.H., Gur, R.C., Valdez, J.N., Loughead, J., Elliott, M.A., Gur, R.E., and Ragland, J.D. Alterations of fronto-temporal connectivity during word encoding in schizophrenia. *Psychiatry Res*, 154(3):221–32, 2007.

Worsley, K.J., Andermann, M., Koulis, T., MacDonald, D., and Evans, A.C. Detecting changes in nonisotropic images. *Hum Brain Mapp*, 8(2–3):98–101, 1999.

Yung, A.R., and McGorry, P.D. The prodromal phase of first-episode psychosis: Past and current conceptualizations. *Schizophr Bull*, 22(2):353–70, 1996.

Yung, A.R., Phillips, L.J., McGorry, P.D., McFarlane, C.A., Francey, S., Harrigan, S., Patton, G.C., and Jackson, H.J. Prediction of psychosis. A step towards indicated prevention of schizophrenia. *Br J Psychiatry*, (Supplement), 172(33):14–20, 1998.

Yung, A.R., Phillips, L.J., Yuen, H.P., Francey, S.M., McFarlane, C.A., Hallgren, M., and McGorry, P.D. Psychosis prediction: 12-month follow up of a high-risk ("prodromal") group. *Schizophr Res*, 60(1):21–32, 2003.

Yung, A.R., Phillips, L.J., Yuen, H.P., and McGorry, P.D. Risk factors for psychosis in an ultra high-risk group: psychopathology and clinical features. *Schizophr Res*, 67(2–3):131–42, 2004.

Yung, A.R., Stanford, C., Cosgrave, E., Killackey, E., Phillips, L., Nelson, B., and McGorry, P.D. Testing the Ultra High Risk (prodromal) criteria for the prediction of psychosis in a clinical sample of young people. *Schizophr Res*, 84(1):57–66, 2006.

Yung, A.R., Yuen, H.P., McGorry, P.D., Phillips, L.J., Kelly, D., Dell'Olio, M., Francey, S.M., Cosgrave, E.M., Killackey, E., Stanford, C., Godfrey, K., and Buckby, J. Mapping the onset of psychosis: the Comprehensive Assessment of At-Risk Mental States. *Aust N Z J Psychiatry*, 39(11–12):964–71, 2005.

Schizophrenia as a Cognitive Disorder: Recent Approaches to Identifying its Core Cognitive Components to Aid Treatment Development

Keith H. Nuechterlein, Michael F. Green, and Robert S. Kern

Introduction

In recent years the central role of cognitive deficits in schizophrenia has been increasingly accepted (Gold & Green, 2005; Green & Nuechterlein, 1999), so much so that the cognitive deficits have become very prominent new targets for treatment development (Gold, 2004; Hyman & Fenton, 2003). In this paper we examine factors that led to the conclusion that cognitive factors are core features of schizophrenia and then discuss recent approaches to identifying the cognitive domains and processes that offer promise as treatment targets.

Specifically, we will address the following four key issues:

(1) Why are cognitive deficits increasingly believed to be core features of schizophrenia?
(2) What are the key separable domains of cognitive functioning in schizophrenia from an empirical perspective?
(3) What partitioning of cognitive processes from cognitive neuroscience might bring us even closer to neural underpinnings?
(4) In developing treatments for cognitive deficits in schizophrenia, should we focus on separable cognitive processes or on the generalized cognitive deficit?

Issue 1: Why Are Cognitive Deficits Increasingly Believed to be Core Deficits in Schizophrenia?

Persistence over Time and Clinical State

One key reason as to why cognitive deficits are considered core features of schizophrenia is that they are persistently present over time and even across major

K.H. Nuechterlein (✉)
University of California, Los Angeles, Department of Psychiatry and Biobehavioral Sciences,
Semel Institute for Neuroscience and Human Behavior, Los Angeles, CA 90095-6968, USA
e-mail: keithn@ucla.edu

W.F. Gattaz, G. Busatto (eds.), *Advances in Schizophrenia Research 2009*,
DOI 10.1007/978-1-4419-0913-8_14, © Springer Science+Business Media, LLC 2010

changes in symptomatic states. Longitudinal studies have demonstrated this persistence of cognitive deficits in several phases of the illness, but perhaps most striking is that the key cognitive deficits are present at the first psychotic episode and that performance in most cognitive domains typically changes to only a small degree over the initial years of the illness (Rund, 1998). One example of this tendency is from the study of first-episode schizophrenia patients by Hoff and colleagues (Hoff et al., 1999), which examined patients yearly for a 5-year period. The most prominent finding was that cognitive deficits in six domains were present at the first episode and at each of the yearly follow-ups. While there were small changes over time in some domains, the large deficit in each domain remained present.

While longitudinal studies that examine schizophrenia patients during clinical remission and during psychotic states are not as common, existing evidence suggests that several key cognitive deficits in schizophrenia do persist even during full clinical remission. For example, in a longitudinal study of recent-onset schizophrenia patients who could be examined a full clinical remission and a psychotic state, we found that early perceptual processing and sustained attention continued to be clearly abnormal during full clinical remission. Indeed, as shown in Fig. 1, sustained attention that demanded early perceptual processing showed a deficit with an effect size (Cohen's d) of 1.3–1.7 that did not even change significantly from the remitted to psychotic state (Nuechterlein et al., 1992). Thus, the cognitive deficits are not secondary to psychotic symptoms, but rather persist even in their absence.

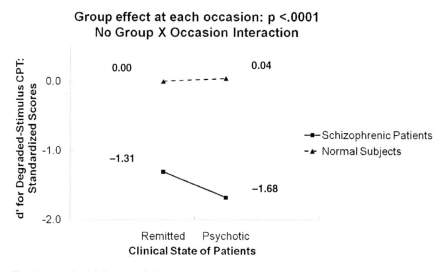

Fig. 1 Attention/vigilance deficits on the degraded-stimulus continuous performance test (CPT) are stable across remitted and psychotic states in recent-onset schizophrenia (adapted from Nuechterlein et al., 1992)

Presence Among First-Degree Relatives

A second key reason that cognitive deficits are believed to be core deficits in schizophrenia is that they are present in attenuated form among first-degree relatives of schizophrenia patients (Gur et al., 2007; Nuechterlein et al., 1998; Snitz, MacDonald, & Carter, 2006). Given that first-degree relatives have a 10-fold increased risk of schizophrenia compared to the general population and would often share some schizophrenia susceptibility genes with their ill family member, this pattern is consistent with the view that cognitive deficits may reflect core aspects of genetic vulnerability to develop this disorder. In Fig. 2, we summarize results of a recent meta-analysis by Snitz et al. (2006) using the comparison for studies that included demographically matched comparison samples. As shown there, first-degree relatives show a deficit on measures that represent several domains of cognition, including processing speed, sustained attention, working memory, verbal memory, visual memory, and reasoning and problem solving, with deficits in sustained attention being among the largest. Also noteworthy is that these cognitive deficits are approximately half the magnitude of those typically found among schizophrenia patients.

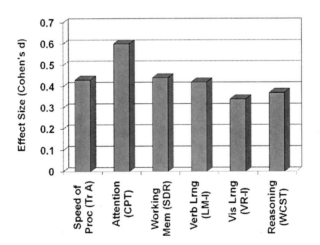

Fig. 2 Cognitive deficits in first degree relatives of schizophrenia probands compared to demographically matched comparison subjects (adapted from meta-analysis by Snitz et al., 2006)

Cognitive Deficits Predict Onset of Schizophrenia Spectrum Disorder

A third reason as to why cognitive deficits are viewed as core features of schizophrenia is that certain cognitive deficits precede and predict onset of schizophrenia spectrum disorder. While longitudinal studies that followed childhood high-risk samples into adulthood are not numerous, evidence from the New York High-Risk Study of children born to schizophrenic mothers indicates that immediate memory, gross motor skills, and attention from childhood assessments predict schizophrenia-related psychoses in early adulthood (Cornblatt, Obuchowski, Roberts, Pollack, & Erlenmeyer-Kimling, 1999; Erlenmeyer-Kimling et al., 2000). This relationship is readily evident in Fig. 3, which illustrates that the offspring of schizophrenic mothers who later developed schizophrenia spectrum disorders showed deficits in sustained attention starting at age 12 years (Cornblatt et al., 1999). The performance of these children of schizophrenic mothers who later developed schizophrenia spectrum disorder was distinguished not only from the typical performance of normal comparison children and children born to a parent with a major affective disorder but also from the remaining children born to schizophrenic mothers.

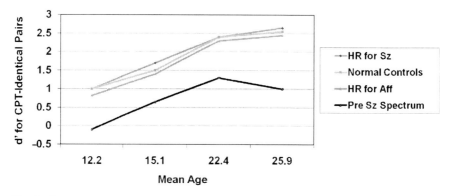

Fig. 3 Trait-like deficits in attention/vigilance (CPT-identical pairs version) occur before illness onset and predict schizophrenia spectrum disorder (reprinted from Cornblatt et al., 1999)

Cognitive Deficits Predict Functional Outcome in Schizophrenia

Finally, a fourth reason for considering cognitive deficits to be core features of schizophrenia is that they predict everyday work and social functioning and independent living after the onset of schizophrenia. The evidence for this conclusion has accumulated quickly in recent years and involves both cross-sectional and longitudinal analyses and several forms of functional outcome assessment (Green, 1996; Green, Kern, Braff, & Mintz, 2000; Green, Kern, & Heaton, 2004). Indeed, cognitive deficits have been considered to be a rate-limiting factor for everyday functioning in schizophrenia (Green, 1996). A meta-analysis by Green et al. (2000) examined the strength of the relationship between various cognitive domains and functional outcome. As shown in Table 1, a relationship to functional outcome was present for four major cognitive domains that had been sufficiently studied by 2000,

Table 1 Meta-analysis demonstrates that several neurocognitive domains predict functional outcome in schizophrenia (reprinted from Green et al., 2000)

Domain	Total sample size	Pooled estimater	Standard error	Effect size[1]	P value[2]
Immediate verbal memory	188	0.40	0.077	medium-large	<0.000001
Secondary verbal memory	727	0.29	0.039	medium	<0.000001
Card sorting	1002	0.23	0.033	small-medium	<0.000001
Attention/Vigilance	682	0.20	0.04	small-medium	<0.000001

[1] Estimates weighted by sample size
[2] Ratio of pooled estimate of r divided by its standard error referred to a normal distribution

with immediate verbal memory showing the strongest correlation with functional outcome and secondary verbal memory, card sorting (executive functioning), and attention/vigilance also being very clearly related to the level of everyday functioning. Composite cognitive measures that sum across several cognitive domains have in several studies shown even stronger relationships to functional outcome (Green, Kern et al., 2000; Green, Kern, & Heaton, 2004), probably because many situations in everyday life require a combination of specific cognitive skills to navigate successfully.

Issue 2: What Are the Key Separable Domains of Cognitive Functioning in Schizophrenia from an Empirical Perspective?

Given the evidence that cognitive deficits are core features of schizophrenia that endure over time and into clinical remission, apparently serving as a key limiting factor for everyday functioning, they have in recent years become a very prominent new target for treatment development (Hyman & Fenton, 2003). To develop new treatments for the core cognitive deficits in schizophrenia, we need to first identify the key cognitive targets. Identification of cognitive targets raises the question of separable cognitive dimensions or domains in schizophrenia.

One prominent recent approach to identifying the separable cognitive domains in schizophrenia is the one adopted by the initiative supported by the NIMH in the United States called Measurement and Treatment Approaches to Improve Cognition in Schizophrenia, or MATRICS. The MATRICS initiative was contracted to the University of California, Los Angeles (UCLA) to help the field overcome critical barriers to development of new treatments for the core cognitive deficits of schizophrenia (Green & Nuechterlein, 2004; Green, Nuechterlein et al., 2004). Among these barriers from the perspective of the NIMH and the US Food and Drug Administration (FDA) was the absence of a consensus among experts concerning the cognitive targets and the best current method for measuring them in clinical trials. The MATRICS Neurocognition Committee, headed by 2 of us and including 12 additional expert psychologists, psychiatrists, and statisticians representing academic, government, and patient advocate perspectives, was charged with finding ways to overcome these barriers. The MATRICS initiative integrated the existing data on cognitive performance in schizophrenia to determine how many separable cognitive domains are present in schizophrenia. It also brought together more than 130 experts in relevant fields to decide how to reliably and validly measure these cognitive domains.

A subgroup of the MATRICS Neurocognition Committee worked to identify the empirically separable cognitive domains in schizophrenia (Nuechterlein et al., 2004). We sought cognitive dimensions that were only weakly intercorrelated and were replicable across several studies. Because so many studies of cognition in schizophrenia focus intensively on only one cognitive domain and do not address the interrelationships among different domains, we viewed evidence from factor analytic studies of cognitive performance in schizophrenia across a number of measures as particularly relevant. We also examined the literature on cognitive dimensions in general community samples as an initial guide to the identification of cognitive domains in schizophrenia.

We identified 13 factor analytic studies of cognitive performance in schizophrenia, including both published analyses and as-yet unpublished results to enhance breadth of sampling (Nuechterlein et al., 2004). The results across studies were tallied, considering the cognitive processes in the measures studied, looking for replication of similar dimensions across studies. When past results were unclear, we completed additional factor analyses with existing data sets to shed light on the empirical separability of cognitive domains.

An example of the consistency of cognitive domains across studies is shown in the next table. In Table 2 we see that seven factor analytic studies of cognitive performance in schizophrenia revealed a dimension of attention/vigilance, which included various versions of the Continuous Performance Test (CPT) as well as some other measures emphasizing attention. Specific measures varied from study to study but the core content of the domain remained the same.

Table 2 Attention/vigilance Factors from factor analytic studies of cognition in schizophrenia (from Nuechterlein et al., 2004)

Study	Measures
Gold et al.	CPT-IP 2-, 3-, & 4-digit conditions
Goldberg et al.	Gordon CPT, 1-back, WCST persev. errors
Green et al.	DS-CPT, Span, Spatial Memory
Hobart et al.	Gordon CPT vigilance & distractibility
Kremen et al.	Auditory CPT, Dichotic Listening
Mirsky et al.	Visual CPT, Auditory CPT accuracy
Nuechterlein et al.	DS-CPT, 3-7 CPT, Backward Masking

Through this procedure, the MATRICS Neurocognition Committee concluded that there were six replicable domains of cognitive performance in schizophrenia that were sufficiently separable and potentially modifiable to deserve representation in a consensus cognitive battery designed for clinical trials (Nuechterlein et al., 2004). These cognitive domains are (1) Speed of Processing, (2) Attention/Vigilance, (3) Working Memory, (4) Verbal Learning and Memory, (5) Visual Learning and Memory, and (6) Reasoning and Problem Solving. At the initial MATRICS consensus conference, the assembled experts urged that Social Cognition be added as a seventh domain because its measures were too new in the schizophrenia literature to have been included in the factor analytic studies, yet it appeared to serve as a possible bridge between the traditional nonsocial aspects of cognition and everyday functioning (Green Nuechterlein et al., 2004; Nuechterlein et al., 2004; Sergi, Rassovsky, Nuechterlein, & Green, 2006). Following this recommendation, the MATRICS Neurocognition Committee concluded that the consensus cognitive battery for clinical trials should be structured to include reliable and valid measurement of the seven cognitive domains (Green Nuechterlein et al., 2004; Kern, Green, Nuechterlein, & Deng, 2004; Nuechterlein et al., 2004).

In addition, after hearing expert presentations on the critical features for measures for clinical trials, the MATRICS Neurocognition Committee concluded that the consensus cognitive battery should emphasize measures that (1) had high test–retest reliability, (2) high utility as repeated measures, (3) demonstrated relationships to functional outcome, and (4) demonstrated tolerability for patients and practicality for test administration and scoring (Green Nuechterlein et al., 2004). It was recommended that the entire battery be no longer than 90 min (Kern et al., 2004).

As described in a 2008 article in the *American Journal of Psychiatry* (Nuechterlein et al., 2008), the MATRICS Neurocognition Committee solicited over 90 nominations of tests for these seven cognitive domains from the group of more than 130 scientists at the first MATRICS consensus meeting and then systematically evaluated the available evidence based on the 4 criteria noted above to determine which 20 tests were the most promising. A direct comparison of these 20 cognitive tests in a new sample of 176 schizophrenia patients was then used to select the best 10 tests for the final MATRICS Consensus Cognitive Battery. The MATRICS Consensus Cognitive Battery was then normed on a community sample from five sites in the United States (Kern et al., 2008). The selected tests are shown in Table 3 and are now available in a convenient kit (www.matricsinc.org). The MATRICS Consensus Cognitive Battery was recommended by NIMH and accepted by the FDA in the

Table 3 Tests in the MATRICS consensus cognitive battery (from Nuechterlein et al., 2008)

Speed of Processing	**Verbal Learning**
• Category Fluency	• Hopkins Verbal Learning Test-R
• BACS Symbol Coding	**Visual Learning**
• Trial Making A	• Brief Visuospatial Memory Test-R
Attention / Vigilance	**Reasoning and Problem Solving**
• Continuous Performance Test	• NAB Mazes
–Identical Pairs version	**Social Cognition**
Working Memory	• MSCEIT Managing Emotions
• Letter Number Span	
• WMS-III Spatial Span	

United States as the standard cognitive battery for clinical trials of potential cognitive enhancers for schizophrenia. Translations of this battery into Spanish (for Spain and also South and Central America), German, Hindi, Russian, and Chinese have been completed and other translations are under way.

Issue 3: What Partitioning of Cognitive Processes Might Bring Us Closer to Neural Underpinnings?

While the MATRICS Consensus Cognitive Battery has now been established as the gold standard for clinical trials of cognition-enhancing interventionsin schizophrenia, research continues to seek a further parsing of cognitive processes, one that would be more tightly tied to underlying neural processes. Instead of emphasizing empirically separable processes through factor analysis and similar statistical techniques, this approach to identifying cognitive intervention targets draws heavily on cognitive psychology and cognitive neuroscience. This approach encourages the translation of the more differentiated constructs and paradigms of cognitive psychology and cognitive neuroscience into clinical research. Direct collaborations between basic and clinical investigators can greatly aid this process (Gold, Fuller, Robinson, Braun, & Luck, 2007; Luck & Gold, 2008; Nuechterlein, Pashler, & Subotnik, 2006).

One major initiative that is a follow-up to MATRICS and has emphasized this approach is called Cognitive Neuroscience to Improve Cognition in Schizophrenia (CNTRICS), led by Deanna Barch and Cameron Carter and an executive committee that includes the two of us (Barch, Carter et al., 2009; Carter et al., 2008). Although the cognitive domains identified by the MATRICS initiative are empirically separable based on cognitive research in schizophrenia, each domain includes several elementary cognitive subprocesses. The CNTRICS approach seeks to isolate more specific cognitive abnormalities in schizophrenia by examining these elementary cognitive processes. By drawing on developments in cognitive neuroscience, cognitive constructs and paradigms that have relevance to schizophrenia with close ties to neural substrates may be identified (Barch, Carter et al., 2009). Paradigms that measure these constructs can then be developed further in order to make them suitable at a future date for use in clinical trials of cognitive interventions.

An initial CNTRICS consensus meeting between experts in basic cognitive neuroscience, clinical research on cognition in schizophrenia, and animal psychopharmacology focused on the identification of cognitive constructs that have particular promise for future investigations attempting to link cognitive deficits to specific neural circuits. This discussion emphasized the clarity of the cognitive mechanisms involved, the ability to distinguish the construct through functional neuroimaging research, and evidence of links to neural circuits in normal humans or animals (Carter et al., 2008).

This discussion led to a list of cognitive constructs that the CNTRICS group believes are most ready for translation to schizophrenia research at this time (Carter

Table 4 CNTRICS list of cognitive constructs selected as most ready for translation to schizophrenia research (from Carter et al., 2008)

Perception	**Executive Control**
• Gain control	• Rule generation and selection
• Integration	• Dynamic adjustments of control
Working Memory	**Long Term Memory**
• Goal maintenance	• Relational encoding and retrieval
• Interference control	• Item encoding and retrieval
Attention	• Reinforcement learning
• Control of attention	**Social/Emotional Processing**
	• Affective recognition and evaluation

et al., 2008), as shown in Table 4. It is noteworthy that most of the broad cognitive domains are similar to those identified by the MATRICS initiative, although some domains are added (i.e., Perception) and others are combined (i.e., MATRICS' Verbal Learning and Visual Learning domains are merged into a Long-Term Memory domain in the CNTRICS list). In addition, however, certain subprocesses within cognitive domains are distinguished.

To illustrate the direction of the CNTRICS partitioning of cognitive constructs, let us use the Working Memory domain. The CNTRICS group distinguished two constructs within this domain that are believed to have promise for further translational development for schizophrenia research. The first one, goal maintenance, is defined as "the processes involved in activating task related goals or rules based on endogenous or exogenous cues, actively representing them in a highly accessible form, and maintaining this information over an interval during which that information is needed to bias and constrain attention and response selection" (Carter et al., 2008). The second construct, interference control, is defined as "the processes involved in protecting the contents of working memory from interference from either other competing representations or external stimuli" (Carter et al., 2008).

After identifying these cognitive constructs, the CNTRICS group selected individual measures of these constructs that have promise for further development into future measures for clinical trials. The issues of test–retest reliability, utility as repeated measures, relationship to functional outcome, tolerability, and practicality that were emphasized in the MATRICS selection process were not considered essential for selection at this point. Rather the emphasis was on the potential to differentiate more elementary component processes that can be studied through functional neuroimaging and other techniques to strengthen ties to neural substrates.

An example of a task selected by the CNTRICS group for its promise for further development is the Expectancy AX-CPT, which is a measure of the goal maintenance construct within working memory (Barch, Berman et al., 2009). This task involves visual presentations of a series of individual letters, with the instructions to press a button each time an "A" is followed by an "X". In a high proportion of the trials, the A is followed by an X. Goal maintenance in working memory is measured by examining the frequency of a particular form of error (pressing to a "B" followed by an "X"), which indicates that the task goal of using the preceding "A" to cue the response to the "X" is not being maintained. Initial support for the utility of this Expectancy AX-CPT to relate to biological systems includes evidence that amphetamine, an indirect D1 agonist, improves goal maintenance in healthy subjects, consistent with the D1 work of Goldman-Rakic (Barch & Braver, 2005). In addition, COMT val/val homozygotes have been shown to have selective goal maintenance deficits on a version of this task (MacDonald, Carter, Flory, Ferrell, & Manuck, 2007).

The approach to schizophrenia cognitive research illustrated by the CNTRICS cognitive constructs and measures has several strengths. A careful delineation of cognition processes that draws on basic cognitive psychology and cognitive neuro- science has excellent potential for isolating cognitive mechanisms in schizophrenia that can be examined through functional neuroimaging and neuropharmacological studies. These paradigms include control conditions that are well suited to finer separation of basic cognitive processes. These approaches may yield very useful measures for clinical trials of cognitive interventions in the future that have stronger links to individual neural circuits.

At this point, however, these paradigms typically have not been optimized for detection of individual differences and cognitive change. Thus, often very lim- ited data are available on the psychometrics of these measures, including test– retest reliability and utility as repeated measures, and many of the measures are too long and difficult to implement to use in large-scale clinical trials. It is also not clear whether these more finely differentiated cognitive measures will show the same substantial link to functional outcome that characterizes more global measures of cognitive domains. Future research will also need to evalu- ate whether the component processes identified by this approach are highly inter- correlated in schizophrenia or allow separation of several dimensions of cognitive deficit.

Issue 4: In Developing Treatments for Cognitive Deficits in Schizophrenia, Should We Focus on Separable Cognitive Processes or the Generalized Cognitive Deficit?

While most investigators have emphasized cognitive domains or their component processes in recent work on cognition in schizophrenia, some have argued that the global or generalized cognitive deficit in schizophrenia should be given more con- sideration (Dickinson & Harvey, 2009; Keefe et al., 2006). Empirical support comes from evidence that a substantial portion of the variance in the cognitive deficit in schizophrenia is due to the overall level of performance and that a smaller portion is accounted for by the pattern across cognitive domains (Dickinson, Iannone, Wilk, & Gold, 2004; Dickinson, Ragland, Calkins, Gold, & Gur, 2006).

Dickinson and Harvey (2009) have recently provided several thought-provoking examples of biological processes in schizophrenia that might lead to global cognitive deficits. A first one is the relatively broadly distributed gray matter reduction in schizophrenia. This gray matter reduction may reflect less arborization and connectivity in distal dendritic processes and thereby contribute to cognitive dysmetria (Andreasen, Paradiso, & O'Leary, 1998) or disconnection. White matter abnormalities in schizophrenia, which are receiving increased research attention (Bartzokis et al., 2003), are a second suggested possible source of generalized cognitive deficits. Reduced fiber tract coherence and myelin integrity would contribute to slowed processing across cognitive domains. A third possible biological source of global cognitive deficits is failure of integration in neural networks. Research has revealed abnormalities in beta and gamma bands in cortical oscillatory systems in schizophrenia that would be expected to contribute to reduced communication across neural assemblies, thereby affecting many cognitive processes. Finally, Dickinson and Harvey (2009) suggest that schizophrenia may be characterized by energy metabolism abnormalities and inflammatory processes that, similar to the insulin resistance and low-grade inflammation in diabetes, produce a broad range of cognitive deficits.

The suggestion that we should give additional thought to the generalized cognitive deficit in schizophrenia is an intriguing one, given that many investigators have viewed the global cognitive deficit as a nuisance factor that produces psychometric artifacts and obscures more specific deficits in schizophrenia (Chapman & Chapman, 1978; Strauss & Summerfelt, 2003). Considering possible biological sources of global cognitive deficits helps one to conceptualize ways in which a general deficit could be a reasonable outcome of disease processes. It is noteworthy, however, that neuropharmacologists tend to focus on particular cognitive domains as treatment targets, rather than the global cognitive deficit, and also identify domain-specific drug effects.

During the MATRICS initiative, a survey of neuropsychopharmacological experts was completed as part of a consensus meeting on promising molecular targets and mechanisms of action for cognition-enhancing drugs (Geyer & Tamminga, 2004). This survey, coordinated by Robert Kern, Ph.D., of UCLA, included questions that requested nominations for pharmacological mechanisms that were viewed as most likely to succeed in treatment of various cognitive disturbances. The results indicated that the most highly favored molecular target and pharmacological mechanism tended to differ from one cognitive domain to the next. Table 5 illustrates this for the cognitive domains of Attention/Vigilance and of Reasoning and Problem Solving. Neuropharmacological experts clearly viewed alpha-7 nicotinic receptor agonists as the most nominated processingdrugs for improving Attention/Vigilance disturbances, with glutamatergic agents being less often nominated. For Reasoning and Problem Solving, dopamine D1 receptor agonists and glutamatergic receptor agonists were viewed as most likely to succeed.

Similarly, when the neuropharmacological experts were asked about the likelihood that treatments targeted to affect specific neural circuits or brain regions would

Table 5 Favorite pharmacological targets for specific cognitive domains (MATRICS June 2003 Survey of Neuropharmacology Experts)

What molecular/pharmacological target has the greatest likelihood of success for treatment of disturbances in these cognitive domains?	
Target	Number of nominations
Attention/Vigilance	
Alpha-7 nicotinic receptor agonists	28
Dopamine D1 receptor agonists	13
Alpha-2 adrenergic receptor agonists	11
AMPA glutamatergic receptor agonists	8
NMDA glutamatergic receptor agonists	6
M1 muscarinic receptor agonists	6
Metabotropic glutamate receptors	5
Reasoning and Problem-Solving	
Dopamine D1 receptor agonists	13
AMPA glutamatergic receptor agonists	8
NMDA glutamatergic receptor agonists	6
Alpha-7 nicotinic receptor agonists	5
Alpha-2 adrenergic receptor agonists	5
Metabotropic glutamate receptors	4
Glycine reuptake inhibitors	3

If specific cognitive deficits are to be treated, what is the likelihood of success for treatments that are targeted to affect specific neurotransmitter receptors/systems?

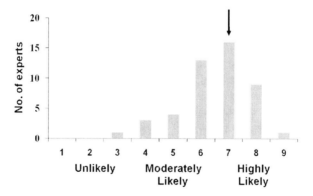

Fig. 4 MATRICS June 2003 survey of neuropharmacology experts: Likelihood of successful treatments for specific cognitive domains

successfully improve specific domains of cognitive functioning versus global cognitive deficits, they were more optimistic about improvements in specific cognitive domains. Their distributions of responses can be seen in Figs. 4 and 5.

If global cognitive deficits are to be treated, what is the likelihood of success for treatments that are targeted to affect specific neural circuits or brain regions?

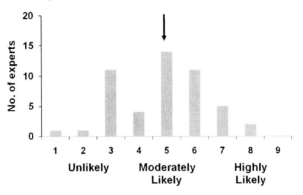

Fig. 5 MATRICS June 2003 survey of neuropharmacology experts: Likelihood of successful treatments for global cognitive deficits

Summary and Implications

Cognitive deficits are now widely recognized as a core feature of schizophrenia due to their persistence across time and clinical states, presence among first-degree relatives, predictive validity for illness onset, and relationship to functional outcome. This increasing recognition of the core nature of cognitive deficits and their relative resistance to change with traditional treatments has resulted in their emergence as a major target for new treatment development.

The MATRICS initiative identified seven separable cognitive domains in schizophrenia by emphasizing factor analytic methods for identifying cognitive dimensions. The most promising measures in each of these domains for reliable and valid measurement of cognitive change in a relatively brief assessment were selected by a panel of experts and directly compared within schizophrenia patients. The resulting MATRICS Consensus Cognitive Battery to allow standardized measurement of these deficits has been accepted by the US NIMH and FDA for use in clinical trials of potential new cognition-enhancing treatments.

The CNTRICS initiative is an ongoing attempt to develop measures of fine-grained cognitive processes with close ties to neural systems. This approach has excellent promise for developing future measures that will be very helpful in treatment development, but these measures require additional research and development to be appropriate for typical clinical trials.

While most investigators are emphasizing separable cognitive domains or even more fine-grained cognitive distinctions among deficits in schizophrenia, some have argued that the global or generalized deficit should be the major intervention target. Pharmacological and cognitive remediation approaches to schizophrenia have not yet resolved whether targeting the global cognitive deficit or differentiated cognitive processes will yield more effective interventions. Neuropharmacological experts tend to think that treatments for specific cognitive domains are more likely to be successful.

Given the rapid developments that are currently occurring in this area of schizophrenia research, the next few years should be an exciting period for addressing additional issues concerning cognitive deficits in schizophrenia and hopefully for developing cognitive interventions that truly improve everyday functioning in schizophrenia.

References

Andreasen, N. C., Paradiso, S., & O'Leary, D. S. (1998). Cognitive dysmetria as an integrative theory of schizophrenia: A dysfunction in cortical-subcortical-cerebellar circuitry. *Schizophrenia Bulletin, 24*, 203–218.

Barch, D. M., Berman, M. G., Engle, R., Jones, J. H., Jonides, J., Macdonald, A., 3rd, et al. (2009). CNTRICS final task selection: Working memory. *Schizophrenia Bulletin, 35*(1), 136–152.

Barch, D. M., & Braver, T. S. (2005). Cognitive control in schizophrenia: Psychological and neural mechanisms. In R. W. Engle, G. Sedek, U. von Hecker & A. M. McIntosh (Eds.), *Cognitive limitations in aging and psychopathology*. New York: Cambridge University Press.

Barch, D. M., Carter, C. S., Arnsten, A., Buchanan, R. W., Cohen, J. D., Geyer, M., et al. (2009). Selecting paradigms from cognitive neuroscience for translation into use in clinical trials: Proceedings of the third CNTRICS meeting. *Schizophrenia Bulletin, 35*(1), 109–114.

Bartzokis, G., Nuechterlein, K. H., Lu, P. H., Gitlin, M., Rogers, S., & Mintz, J. (2003). Dysregulated brain development in adult men with schizophrenia: A magnetic resonance imaging study. *Biological Psychiatry, 53*(5), 412–421.

Carter, C. S., Barch, D. M., Buchanan, R. W., Bullmore, E., Krystal, J. H., Cohen, J., et al. (2008). Identifying cognitive mechanisms targeted for treatment development in schizophrenia: An overview of the first meeting of the Cognitive Neuroscience Treatment Research to Improve Cognition in Schizophrenia Initiative. *Biological Psychiatry, 64*(1), 4–10.

Chapman, L. J., & Chapman, J. P. (1978). The measurement of differential deficit. *Journal of Psychiatric Research, 14*, 303–311.

Cornblatt, B., Obuchowski, M., Roberts, S., Pollack, S., & Erlenmeyer-Kimling, L. (1999). Cognitive and behavioral precursors of schizophrenia. *Development and Psychopathology, 11*, 487–508.

Dickinson, D., & Harvey, P. D. (2009). Systemic hypotheses for generalized cognitive deficits in schizophrenia: A new take on an old problem. *Schizophrenia Bulletin, 35*(2), 403–414.

Dickinson, D., Iannone, V. N., Wilk, C. M., & Gold, J. M. (2004). General and specific cognitive deficits in schizophrenia. *Biological Psychiatry, 55*(8), 826–833.

Dickinson, D., Ragland, J. D., Calkins, M. E., Gold, J. M., & Gur, R. C. (2006). A comparison of cognitive structure in schizophrenia patients and healthy controls using confirmatory factor analysis. *Schizophrenia Research, 85*(1–3), 20–29.

Erlenmeyer-Kimling, L., Rock, D., Roberts, S. A., Janal, M., Kestenbaum, C., Cornblatt, B., et al. (2000). Attention, memory, and motor skills as childhood predictors of schizophrenia-related psychosis: The New York High-Risk Project. *American Journal of Psychiatry, 157* (9), 1416–1422.

Geyer, M. A., & Tamminga, C. A. (2004). Measurement and treatment research to improve cognition in schizophrenia: Neuropharmacological aspects. *Psychopharmacology, 174*, 1–2.

Gold, J. M. (2004). Cognitive deficits as treatment targets in schizophrenia. *Schizophrenia Research, 72*(1), 21–28.

Gold, J. M., Fuller, R. L., Robinson, B. M., Braun, E. L., & Luck, S. J. (2007). Impaired top-down control of visual search in schizophrenia. *Schizophrenia Research, 94*(1–3), 148–155.

Gold, J. M., & Green, M. F. (2005). Neurocognition in Schizophrenia. In B. J. Sadock & V. A. Sadock (Eds.), *Kaplan & Sadock's comprehensive textbook of psychiatry* (Vol. 8th, pp. 1436–1448). Baltimore: Lippincott, Williams & Wilkins.

Green, M. F. (1996). What are the functional consequences of neurocognitive deficits in schizophrenia? *American Journal of Psychiatry, 153*(3), 321–330.

Green, M. F., Kern, R. S., Braff, D. L., & Mintz, J. (2000). Neurocognitive deficits and functional outcome in schizophrenia: Are we measuring the "right stuff"? *Schizophrenia Bulletin, 26*(1), 119–136.

Green, M. F., Kern, R. S., & Heaton, R. K. (2004). Longitudinal studies of cognition and functional outcome in schizophrenia: Implications for MATRICS. *Schizophrenia Research, 72*(1), 41–51.

Green, M. F., & Nuechterlein, K. H. (1999). Should schizophrenia be treated as a neurocognitive disorder? *Schizophrenia Bulletin, 25*, 309–319.

Green, M. F., & Nuechterlein, K. H. (2004). The MATRICS initiative: Developing a consensus cognitive battery for clinical trials. *Schizophrenia Research, 72*(1), 1–3.

Green, M. F., Nuechterlein, K. H., Gold, J. M., Barch, D. M., Cohen, J., Essock, S., et al. (2004). Approaching a consensus cognitive battery for clinical trials in schizophrenia: The NIMH-MATRICS conference to select cognitive domains and test criteria. *Biological Psychiatry, 56*(5), 301–307.

Gur, R. E., Calkins, M. E., Gur, R. C., Horan, W. P., Nuechterlein, K. H., Seidman, L. J., et al. (2007). The consortium on the genetics of schizophrenia: Neurocognitive endophenotypes. *Schizophrenia Bulletin, 33*(1), 49–68.

Hoff, A. L., Sakuma, M., Wieneke, M., Horon, R., Kushner, M., & DeLisi, L. E. (1999). Longitudinal neuropsychological follow-up study of patients with first-episode schizophrenia. *American Journal of Psychiatry, 156*(9), 1336–1341.

Hyman, S., & Fenton, W. (2003). What are the right targets for psychopharmacology? *299*, 350–351.

Keefe, R. S., Bilder, R. M., Harvey, P. D., Davis, S. M., Palmer, B. W., Gold, J. M., et al. (2006). Baseline Neurocognitive Deficits in the CATIE Schizophrenia Trial. *Neuropsychopharmacology, 31*(9), 2033–2046.

Kern, R. S., Green, M. F., Nuechterlein, K. H., & Deng, B. H. (2004). NIMH-MATRICS survey on assessment of neurocognition in schizophrenia. *Schizophrenia Research, 72*(1), 11–19.

Kern, R. S., Nuechterlein, K. H., Green, M. F., Baade, L. E., Fenton, W. S., Gold, J. M., et al. (2008). The MATRICS Consensus Cognitive Battery, part 2: Co-norming and standardization. *American Journal of Psychiatry, 165*(2), 214–220.

Luck, S. J., & Gold, J. M. (2008). The translation of cognitive paradigms for patient research. *Schizophrenia Bulletin, 34*, 629–644.

MacDonald, A. W., 3rd, Carter, C. S., Flory, J. D., Ferrell, R. E., & Manuck, S. B. (2007). COMT val158Met and executive control: A test of the benefit of specific deficits to translational research. *Journal of Abnormal Psychology, 116*(2), 306–312.

Nuechterlein, K. H., Asarnow, R. F., Subotnik, K. L., Fogelson, D. L., Ventura, J., Torquato, R., et al. (1998). Neurocognitive vulnerability factors for schizophrenia: Convergence across genetic risk studies and longitudinal trait/state studies. In M. F. Lenzenweger & R. H. Dworkin (Eds.), *Origins and Development of Schizophrenia: Advances in Experimental Psychopathology* (pp. 299–327). Washington, DC: American Psychological Association.

Nuechterlein, K. H., Barch, D. M., Gold, J. M., Goldberg, T. E., Green, M. F., & Heaton, R. K. (2004). Identification of separable cognitive factors in schizophrenia. *Schizophrenia Research, 72*(1), 29–39.

Nuechterlein, K. H., Dawson, M. E., Gitlin, M. J., Ventura, J., Goldstein, M. J., Snyder, K. S., et al. (1992). Developmental processes in schizophrenic disorders: Longitudinal studies of vulnerability and stress. *Schizophrenia Bulletin, 18*(3), 387–425.

Nuechterlein, K. H., Green, M. F., Kern, R. S., Baade, L. E., Barch, D. M., Cohen, J. D., et al. (2008). The MATRICS Consensus Cognitive Battery, part 1: Test selection, reliability, and validity. *American Journal of Psychiatry, 165*(2), 203–213.

Nuechterlein, K. H., Pashler, H. E., & Subotnik, K. L. (2006). Translating basic attentional paradigms to schizophrenia research: Reconsidering the nature of the deficits. *Development and Psychopathology, 18*(3), 831–851.

Rund, B. R. (1998). A review of longitudinal studies of cognitive functions in schizophrenia patients. *Schizophrenia Bulletin, 24*(3), 425–435.

Sergi, M. J., Rassovsky, Y., Nuechterlein, K. H., & Green, M. F. (2006). Social perception as a mediator of the influence of early visual processing on functional status in schizophrenia. *American Journal of Psychiatry, 163*(3), 448–454.

Snitz, B. E., MacDonald, A. W., 3rd, & Carter, C. S. (2006). Cognitive deficits in unaffected first-degree relatives of schizophrenia patients: A meta-analytic review of putative endophenotypes. *Schizophrenia Bulletin, 32*(1), 179–194.

Strauss, M. E., & Summerfelt, A. (2003). The neuropsychological study of schizophrenia: A methodological perspective. In M. F. Lenzenweger & J. M. Hooley (Eds.), *Principles of experimental psychopathology: Essays in honor of Brendan A. Maher* (pp. 119–134). Washington DC: American Psychological Association.

Cognitive and Social Processes in Psychosis: Recent Developments

Daniel Freeman

In general I'm paranoid about almost everything. Every nice compliment or comment I get given I take it as sarcasm, or I think the person will go away and laugh at me behind my back. Or sometimes if I walk over to people and they snigger or jerk a bit, I get worried they're plotting against me. I get worried about going to the shop, being followed. When I walk past people, I always get the feeling they're watching my back. Or they will throw something at me.

Ryan

I feel as if people that are close to me are trying to poison me, and every time I go to dinner they are giving me more of the poison and soon it will kill me. I know they wouldn't do it but the feeling is so strong that I feel as if they are. I even feel dizzy whilst eating the food and thinking of the poison. I can't be at home on my own as I feel scared that a ghost, an object or a person is going to kill me. I feel as if someone is going to break into my place and stab me. I feel a horrible feeling in my back where I am going to be stabbed, I hear voices telling me I ain't worth nothing, they tell me people are going to die.

Katherine

Introduction

These two personal accounts contain key aspects of paranoia: the individuals are making judgements about other people; the decision-making is influenced by fear, worry, and unusual 'feelings'; and danger is anticipated. This is consistent with an emerging body of psychological research that implicates – in the context of the social world – reasoning processes, negative affect, and anomalous internal

D. Freeman (✉)
Department of Psychology, Institute of Psychiatry, King's College London, Denmark Hill, London, SE5 8AF, UK
e-mail: d.freeman@iop.kcl.ac.uk

W.F. Gattaz, G. Busatto (eds.), *Advances in Schizophrenia Research 2009*,
DOI 10.1007/978-1-4419-0913-8_15, © Springer Science+Business Media, LLC 2010

experiences in the occurrence of delusions. In this chapter the advances in the cognitive and social understanding of psychosis will be illustrated with reference to the clinically important experience of persecutory delusions, where arguably the progress has been most rapid. The initial application of this theoretical knowledge to clinical practice via an interventionist causal model approach will be described.

The Cognitive Approach

A hallmark of the best cognitive studies is a clear focus on the phenomenon to be explained. Experiences such as delusions and hallucinations have drawn most attention recently, rather than diagnosis. Often these experiences are looked at individually (sometimes called 'the single-symptom approach'). There is recognition that there may be overlap in causal mechanisms, but, nonetheless, even statistical analyses with patient groups – where there is a bias to see co-occurrence of symptoms (Maric et al., 2004) – indicate a degree of independence for single psychotic experiences (Peralta & Cuesta, 1998; Vázquez-Barquero, Lastra, Nuñez, Castanedo, & Dunn, 1996). Delusions and hallucinations, for example, simply are different subjective experiences. Putting the experiences centre stage has helped to highlight two issues of conceptualisation with important implications for research: psychotic experiences are multi-dimensional and on a continuum of severity in the general population.

Debates on defining delusions (e.g. Strauss, 1969; Garety, 1985; Oltmanns, 1988), factor-analytic studies of patients' experiences (e.g. Kendler, Glazer, & Morgenstern, 1983; Harrow, Rattenbury, & Stoll, 1988; Garety, Everitt, & Hemsley, 1988), and evidence concerning treatment response (e.g. Mizrahi et al., 2006; Trower et al., 2004) all point to one conclusion: delusions are complex multi-dimensional experiences. For instance, assessing the presence of a delusion may best be accomplished by considering a list of characteristics or dimensions, none of which is necessary or sufficient, that with increasing endorsement produces greater agreement on the presence of a delusion (Oltmanns, 1988). The more a belief is implausible, unfounded, strongly held, not shared by others, distressing, and preoccupying, the more likely it is to be considered a delusion. So it is not simply the content of a delusion that needs to be explained but also the other elements that make up the experience, each of which is dimensional. The important implication for research is that multiple questions need to be asked about paranoid experience: what causes a thought of unfounded paranoid content, what causes the thought to become held as a belief, why does resistance to change occur, how does the thought become distressing, and why does it impact on day-to-day life? It is plausible that different factors are involved in the different dimensions of delusional experience. For example, the factors that lead a person to have a particular thought may be different from those that lead to strong belief conviction, which may in turn differ from the factors that make the thought preoccupying and distressing. The recent cognitive approaches to persecutory delusions make plausible connections to the experiences reported by patients. The explanations often have face validity. For example, that a cognitive style of seeking few data before reaching a decision ('jumping to conclusions') will lead to rapid acceptance of unlikely ideas (Garety et al., 2005). This is an important step before empirical testing.

Increasingly accepted is the view that psychotic symptoms are on a continuum with normal experience (e.g. Strauss, 1969; Chapman & Chapman, 1980; Claridge, 1997; van Os, Linscott, Myin-Germeys, Delespaul, & Krabbendam, in press). Delusions in psychosis would represent the severe end of a continuum, but such experiences would be present, often to a lesser degree, in the general population. Moreover, severe delusions would be related to milder, attenuated forms of the experience. For example, a clinical persecutory delusion about government attempts to kill the person would be considered related to non-clinical delusions about neighbours deliberately trying to distress the person that would in turn be considered as related to everyday suspicions and mistrust about the intentions of others. This view is based on three lines of empirical evidence showing the following: delusional ideation is not confined to psychotic groups (e.g. van Os, Hanssen, Bijl, & Ravelli, 2000; Freeman, Garety, Bebbington, Smith et al., 2005); non-clinical and clinical psychotic experiences have the same risk factors ('aetiological continuity'; Myin-Germeys, Krabbendam, & van Os, 2003); and the risk of clinical disorder is raised by the earlier presence of low-level symptoms (Poulton et al., 2000; Chapman, Chapman, Kwapil, Eckbald, & Zinser, 1994). Complete discontinuity between clinical and non-clinical experiences is therefore unlikely, although the exact nature of a paranoia spectrum remains to be established. The important implication for researchers is that studying non-clinical delusional ideation can inform the understanding of clinical phenomena, just as studying anxious or depressive states can inform the understanding of emotional disorders.

Cognitive Studies of Persecutory Ideation Using Virtual Reality

The recent virtual reality studies have the advantage of addressing a little-discussed spectre that accompanies the study of paranoia: justified suspicions. Paranoia is unfounded (or exaggerated) fear but it can be difficult to rule out perceived threats that are grounded in reality (Freeman, 2008a). Although never researched, the accuracy of questionnaire or interview methods will be related, to a degree, to the actual content of persecutory thoughts assessed. Physically impossible beliefs (e.g. there is a persecutor who has killed or removed the whole brain of the individual) are evidently less likely to be true than more plausible beliefs (e.g. the neighbours are trying to get the individual to move away). To confuse the issue further, paranoid thinking is, understandably, more likely following a real experience of victimisation (e.g. Johns et al., 2004; Gracie et al., 2007), and paranoid thinking may lead others into conspiratorial-type reactions, such as exclusion (Lemert, 1962). Justified suspicions are more likely to be a difficulty when studying non-clinical populations.

The personal accounts that head this chapter illustrate that paranoid fears concern perceived threats from others and misinterpretations of their behaviours. In essence, the social world is central to the experience. However, it is nearly impossible to give individuals exactly the same everyday experience in order to compare paranoid responses, or to be certain, within a given social situation, of the intentions of the putative persecutors. Moreover, people with paranoid thoughts often act differently with others (e.g. timidly) and thereby elicit different reactions. The solution developed was to exploit interactive computer-generated environments (virtual reality). Even though individuals in virtual reality know the environment is artificial, reactions similar to those in the real world are triggered (Sanchez-Vives & Slater, 2005; Freeman, 2008b). By presentation of exactly the same *neutral* social situation to individuals, any paranoid thinking that occurs will be known to be unfounded. No matter what a person does, the characters will remain neutral in their responses.

Recent virtual reality studies have confirmed that persecutory ideation is not confined to individuals diagnosed with severe mental illness, that it is understandable in terms of cognitive factors, and that the cognitive factors apply across the spectrum of paranoia severity (Freeman et al., 2003; Freeman, Garety, Bebbington, Slater et al., 2005; Freeman, Pugh, Antley et al., 2008; Freeman, Gittins et al., 2008; Freeman et al., submitted). In the first large-scale study, 200 members of the general population were recruited – screening out anybody who had a history of severe mental illness – for a study of 'reactions in virtual reality' (Freeman, Pugh, Antley et al., 2008). Each participant spent 5 min in a simulation of a London underground train ride (see Fig. 1). The train carriage was populated by about 15 neutral computer

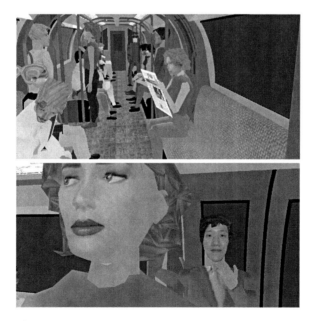

Fig. 1 Pictures of the tube train virtual environment

characters, which were animated using recordings of real people via the technique of optical motion capture. Even though all the participants were presented with the same virtual environment, there were striking differences in interpretation. Some people were very positive: 'It was nice – much nicer than a real experience – people aren't so forthcoming with their feelings in a real situation. Thought they were pretty friendly.' But others had more paranoid reactions: 'There was an aggressive person – intention was to intimidate me and make me feel uneasy. When he reacted like that I turned round and backed away.' The most common interpretation of the tube ride, as would be expected, was that it was neutral (e.g. 'No one had any particular feelings about me'). There were also a significant number of positive interpretations of the characters (e.g. 'I felt very safe in their company'). However, a significant minority had paranoid thoughts about the computer characters. The occurrence of persecutory thoughts was assessed using the State Social Paranoia Scale (Freeman et al., 2007). There was appreciable endorsement of the scale items such as 'Someone was hostile to me', 'Someone had it in for me', and 'Someone stared at me in order to upset me'. One in four of these non-clinical participants had significant endorsement of the scale items. Confirming the validity of the experimental procedure, individuals who had paranoid interpretations in virtual reality were significantly more likely to report having paranoid thoughts in day-to-day life.

The study also informed the theoretical understanding of paranoia. Before entering virtual reality, the participants completed a battery of tests based on a cognitive model of persecutory delusions (Freeman et al., 2002, 2006; Freeman & Freeman, 2008). In the model, it is explicitly acknowledged that there are multiple causes of paranoid thinking, but the following are identified as particularly important: *affective processes*, especially anxiety, worry, and interpersonal sensitivity; *anomalous experiences*, such as hallucinations and perceptual anomalies; *reasoning biases*, particularly jumping to conclusions and belief inflexibility; and *social factors*, such as adverse events and environments. In the virtual reality study, paranoid thinking was strongly predicted by higher levels of anxiety, depression, worry, everyday worries, catastrophic worry, interpersonal sensitivity, negative ideas about the self, negative ideas about others, cognitive inflexibility, perceptual anomalies, and loneliness associated with their family situation. The presence of perceptual anomalies distinguished the occurrence of paranoid thinking from social anxiety in VR (Freeman, Gittins et al., 2008). The results indicate a strong affective component to paranoid experience but also the importance of anomalies of experience and reasoning biases.

But do these findings with a non-clinical general population sample relate to clinical delusions seen in people diagnosed with psychosis? In order to examine this issue, three groups along the spectrum of paranoia were recruited: 30 individuals with persecutory delusions in the context of a nonaffective psychotic illness; 30 individuals with high levels of non-clinical paranoia; and 30 individuals with low levels of paranoia (Freeman et al., submitted). The levels of paranoia were validated by using the virtual reality train ride; the three groups significantly differed from each other in the expected directions. A number of factors from the psychological model were then examined across this paranoia spectrum. As levels of paranoia increased across the three groups, there were significant increases in anxiety, worry, interpersonal sensitivity, depression, anomalies of experience, and trauma history. This indicates a remarkable consistency in the occurrence of dose–response relationships for the model factors across the paranoia spectrum. The only exception was that the clinical group showed a strong bias in reasoning, while the two non-clinical groups did not differ, which is consistent with the evidence that reasoning difficulties specifically contribute to higher levels of belief conviction rather than simply the occurrence of paranoid thoughts (Garety et al., 2005; Freeman, Pugh, & Garety, 2008). This research clearly shows evidence of aetiological continuity across the paranoia spectrum and it is consistent with a series of studies that has examined single psychological variables across a hypothesised positive symptom continuum (Van Dael et al., 2006; Janssen et al., 2006; Vermissen et al., 2008).

The Cognitive Understanding of Persecutory Delusions

The findings of the virtual reality studies support an emerging research literature. At a cognitive level of explanation, persecutory delusions can broadly be considered as arising from an interaction of internal anomalous experience, negative affect, and reasoning. For a detailed review of the literature, see Freeman (2007).

Internal Anomalous Experience

The American psychologist Brendan Maher (1974) emphasises that delusional ideas spring from unusual internal experiences. He notes that 'the delusional belief is not being held "in the face of evidence normally sufficient to destroy it," but is being held because of evidence powerful enough to support it'. Delusions may be attempts by individuals to make sense of their experiences; odd experiences may lead to odd ideas. Supportive of this view, many people with psychosis have clearly anomalous experiences such as hallucinations, thought insertion, and replacement of will, and also a range of more subtle perceptual and attentional alterations in experience (e.g. McGhie & Chapman, 1961; Bunney et al., 1999) and, often, periods of arousal (e.g. Docherty, Van Kammen, Siris, & Marder, 1978; Hemsley, 1994). Non-clinical delusional ideation has been found to be associated with low-level perceptual anomalies such as changes in levels of sensory intensity, distorted sensory experience, and sensory flooding (e.g. Bell, Halligan, & Ellis, 2006; Freeman, Dunn et al., 2005). Kapur (2003) has highlighted the importance of aberrant feelings of salience in delusion formation, which is particularly of note since in this account the abnormal experience itself concerns processes of meaning ascription. A tradition in German psychiatry is to study anomalies of experience ('basic symptoms') for which 'delusions may provide new elaborative contexts to understand the dislocated or overly salient perceptual fragments' (Uhlhaas & Mishara, 2007). Explanations for the occurrence of anomalies of experience include dopamine dysregulation (e.g. Kapur, Mizrahi, & Li, 2005), core cognitive dysfunction (e.g. Hemsley, 1994), impairment in early-stage sensory processing (e.g. Butler & Javitt, 2005), illicit drug use (e.g. Henquet, Di Forti, Murray, & van Os, 2008), and hearing impairment (e.g. Thewissen et al., 2005).

Negative Affect

Anxiety and associated processes are likely to be central to understanding paranoia, as indicated in the virtual reality studies. Both persecutory and anxious thoughts concern the anticipation of threat; fears of physical, social, or psychological harm are apparent in anxious thoughts (e.g. Eysenck & van Berkum, 1992; Wells, 1994) and in persecutory thoughts (Freeman & Garety, 2000; Freeman et al., 2001). Anxiety, via threat anticipation, may lead to thoughts of a paranoid content. Anxiety has repeatedly been found to be associated with paranoid thoughts (e.g. Martin & Penn, 2001; Johns et al., 2004) and persecutory delusions (e.g. Freeman & Garety, 1999; Startup, Freeman, & Garety, 2007). Furthermore, anxiety is predictive of the occurrence of paranoid thoughts (e.g. Freeman et al., 2003; Freeman, Garety, Bebbington, Slater et al., 2005) and of the persistence of persecutory delusions (Startup et al., 2007; Harrow, Jobe, & Astrachan-Fletcher, 2008). Threat anticipation and paranoia have been found to be strongly associated (Bentall, Rowse et al., 2008; Bentall et al., in press). Several other anxiety-related processes have been linked to paranoia. For example, a worry cognitive style in individuals with persecutory delusions is associated with more catastrophic delusion content, higher levels of distress, and with paranoia persistence (Freeman & Garety, 1999; Morrison & Wells, 2007; Startup et al., 2007; Bassett, Sperlinger, & Freeman, in press).

Depression-related processes may also be important. Negative ideas about the self may be a first step in thinking about being a vulnerable target for others to mock, exploit, or harm. This may be especially likely when generally negative ideas about other people are also held, for example, that people are mostly bad, selfish, or devious. Fowler et al. (2006) found that in a non-clinical population of over 700 students, paranoia was associated with negative beliefs about the self, negative beliefs about others, and less positive beliefs about others. A related study of 100 patients with psychosis found that the severity, preoccupation, and distress of persecutory delusions were associated with negative beliefs about the self, negative beliefs about others, and low self-esteem (Smith et al., 2006). Richard Bentall and colleagues argue that self-esteem is central to understanding persecutory delusions (Bentall, Kinderman & Moutoussis, 2008; Thewissen, Bentall, Lecomte, van Os, & Myin-Germeys, 2008). The findings are consistent with repeated demonstrations that affective problems are associated with the positive symptoms of psychosis (e.g. Norman and Malla, 1994; Guillem, Pampoulova, Stip, Lalonde, & Todorov, 2005) and longitudinal evidence that low self-esteem predicts the development of the positive symptoms of psychosis (Krabbendam, Janssen, Bijl, Vollebergh, & van Os, 2002). The importance of affect in the development of paranoia is also highlighted by recent work on stress and psychosis. In particular, Myin-Germeys and colleagues provide evidence that increased emotional reactivity (increase in negative affect, decrease in positive affect) to stress underlies delusions and hallucinations (see reviews by Myin-Germeys & van Os, 2007; van Winkel, Stefanis, & Myin-Germeys, 2008).

Reasoning

If delusions are incorrect – or perhaps, more importantly, *uncorrected* – beliefs, then judgemental or reasoning processes are implicitly implicated in their cause. A number of researchers have tried to identify biases or deficits in reasoning in individuals with delusions. The most convincing empirical evidence is that a significant proportion of individuals with delusions are hasty in their data gathering (they 'jump to conclusions'), which is hypothesised to lead to the rapid acceptance of beliefs even if there is limited evidence to support them (e.g. Garety et al., 2005; van Dael et al., 2006; Moritz, Woodward, & Lambert, 2007; Broome et al., 2007). The bias has been found in studies that recruited individuals who all had persecutory delusions (Startup, Freeman, & Garety, 2008; Freeman et al., submitted). As expected, jumping to conclusions is specifically associated with degree of conviction in delusional ideas (Garety et al., 2005; Freeman, Pugh & Garety, 2008). It has also been plausibly suggested that individuals with persecutory delusions have a judgemental style of blaming other people for negative events (rather than the situation or themselves) (Bentall, Corcoran, Howard, Blackwood, & Kinderman, 2001). The research evidence here is more inconsistent (e.g. Lyon, Kaney, & Bentall, 1994; Martin & Penn, 2002; Langdon, Ward, & Coltheart, in press), which may be due to difficulties assessing the concept (e.g. Combs, Penn, Wicher, & Waldheter, 2007) or because the greater influence on attributional style is actually mood state. Finally, it should be noted that individuals with persecutory ideation are by definition misreading the intentions of other people and that theory of mind (ToM) dysfunction has been proposed as the cause (Frith, 1992, 2004). The empirical evidence indicates that ToM difficulties are apparent in people with a diagnosis of schizophrenia but that they may be most associated with negative symptoms and incoherent speech rather than paranoia (see reviews by Garety & Freeman, 1999; Brüne, 2004; Sarfati, Hardy-Baylé, Besche, & Widlöcher, 1997; Harrington, Siegert, & McClure, 2005; Freeman, 2007). The largest study of ToM in schizophrenia is by Greig, Bryson, and Bell (2004) and it best addresses the question of ToM and individual psychotic symptoms. A total of 128 out-patients with schizophrenia were assessed on the ability to understand hints. It was found that theory of mind performance was associated with thought disorder.

Combining the Factors

How do these factors combine to produce persecutory delusions? In essence, the anomalies of experience make the person feel *different* and in need of an explanation. Typically, individuals vulnerable to paranoid thinking try to make sense of internal unusual states by drawing in negative, discrepant, or ambiguous external information. For example, a person may go outside feeling in an unusual state and, rather than label this experience as such (e.g. 'I'm feeling somewhat odd and anxious today, probably because I've not been sleeping well'), the feelings are instead used as a source of evidence, together with the facial expressions of strangers in the street, that there is a threat (e.g. 'People don't like me and may harm me'). But why a suspicious interpretation of experiences? The internal and external events are interpreted in line with previous experiences, knowledge, memories, and emotional state, and therefore the origin of persecutory explanations lies in such factors (see Fig. 2). Emotion is key, especially anxiety. Suspicious thoughts often occur in the context of emotional distress, frequently triggered by stressful events (e.g. difficult interpersonal relationships, bullying, isolation). The theme of anxiety is the anticipation of danger and it is the origin of the threat content in persecutory ideation. Paranoid thoughts are often an anxious, ruminative extension of negative ideas about the self and others. Moreover, it is unsurprising that paranoid thoughts

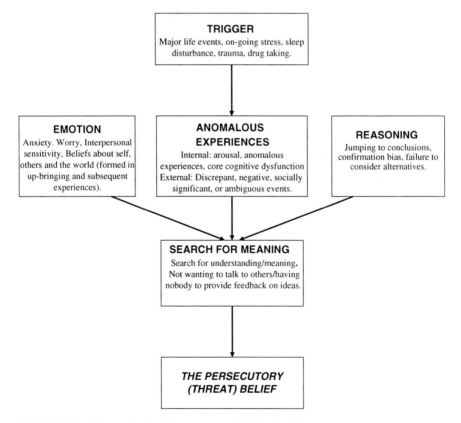

Fig. 2 Outline of factors involved in persecutory delusion development

pass through the mind, since the decision whether to trust or mistrust is at the heart of all social interactions. The persecutory ideas are most likely to reach delusional intensity when there are accompanying biases in reasoning such as reduced data gathering ('jumping to conclusions') (Garety & Freeman, 1999), a failure to consider alternative explanations for experiences (Freeman et al., 2004), and a strong confirmatory reasoning bias (Freeman, Garety, McGuire & Kuipers, 2005). When reasoning biases are present, the suspicions are more likely to become near certainties; the threat beliefs become held with a conviction unwarranted by the evidence and may then be considered delusional.

The Impact of Social Factors

The cognitive perspective on persecutory delusions can help make sense of recent advances in the epidemiological understanding of psychosis. Two illustrative examples are taken here: victimisation and urbanisation.

A number of studies link trauma and psychosis (see Larkin & Morrison, 2006). For instance, Janssen and colleagues (2004) in a longitudinal survey of 4,000 adults in the general population found that a history of childhood abuse increased the risk of subsequent development of psychotic symptoms by over 10 times. In a cross-sectional study, victimisation events were associated with a twofold increase in the likelihood of paranoid thoughts (Johns et al., 2004). In a survey of over 10,000 Australians, all types of trauma, but especially rape, were associated with delusional ideation, and a dose–response relationship was found (i.e. those who had been exposed to a greater number of different types of trauma were more likely to report delusions) (Scott, Chant, Andrews, Martin, & McGrath, 2007). How might such trauma increase the likelihood of paranoia? There is evidence that the effect of victimisation events may be mediated by levels of anxiety, depression, negative ideas about the self and others, and stress sensitivity (Gracie et al., 2007; Freeman & Fowler, 2008; Glaser, van Os, Portegijs, & Myin-Germeys, 2006). In other words, it is by the affective route that victimisation has its (non-specific) impact on paranoia.

McGrath (2007) has highlighted 'the surprisingly rich contours of schizophrenia epidemiology'. An impressively consistent literature now shows that the occurrence of psychosis is increased in urban environments (e.g. van Os, 2004; Sundquist, Frank, & Sundquist, 2004; Marcelis, Navarro-Mateu, Murray, Selten, & van Os, 1998; Kirkbride et al., 2006). For example, in a longitudinal study of 4.4 million people in Sweden those people living in the most densely populated areas had 68–77% greater risk of developing psychosis than those in the least populated areas (Sundquist et al., 2004). The cognitive impact of a deprived urban environment on individuals with persecutory delusions was examined in the Camberwell Walk Study (Ellett, Freeman, & Garety, 2008). Thirty patients with persecutory delusions were randomised to a 10-min exposure to a deprived urban environment or to a brief mindfulness relaxation task. After exposure, assessments of symptoms, reasoning, and affective processes were taken. Spending time in an urban environment made the participants more anxious and more paranoid. Compared with relaxation, walking in the main shopping street of Camberwell made patients think more negatively in general about themselves and other people and increased the jumping to conclusions reasoning bias. Work examining the psychological impact of social factors related to psychosis is at a very early stage, but, intriguingly, urban environments may well affect several factors identified by cognitive research.

Developing Treatments: An Interventionist Causal Model Approach

Interventions that target single factors identified by the theoretical literature have two benefits: they test the causal role of the factor and they may show the efficacy of a new therapeutic technique. This research method has been termed an 'interventionist causal model approach' (Woodward, 2003; Kendler & Campbell, in press). It has rarely been applied to psychosis, although there are exceptions (e.g. Trower et al., 2004). It is timely to take this approach to the theoretical advances in understanding paranoia. An example draws upon the findings noted earlier of a connection between worry and paranoia (Freeman & Garety, 1999; Startup et al., 2007; Morrison & Wells, 2007; Freeman, Pugh, Antley et al., 2008; Bassett et al., in press). In a recent study, the worry cognitive style in people with persecutory delusions was targeted (Foster, Startup, Potts, & Freeman, submitted). Twenty-four individuals with persistent persecutory delusions and high levels of worry were randomly assigned to receive a four-session cognitive behavioural worry intervention or treatment as usual. The worry intervention, drawing upon the generalised anxiety disorder literature (e.g. Borkovec, Ray, & Stober, 1998; Dugas & Ladouceur, 1998), was specifically designed not to target the content of delusions. The main prediction was that the worry intervention would reduce both worry and paranoia distress compared with treatment as usual. In this open-label evaluation, assessments of worry and paranoia were conducted at baseline, at 1 month (end of treatment), and at 2 months. The worry intervention achieved a statistically significant reduction in worry, which was maintained at 2-month follow-up (effect size = 1.1). A significant reduction in delusional distress was also reported (effect size = 1.4). There was an indication that the worry intervention may reduce the frequency of paranoid thoughts (effect size = 0.6). Changes in levels of worry were associated with changes in levels of paranoia. A larger and more rigorous examination is needed, but the results support a causal role for worry in paranoia and show encouraging efficacy for a very brief intervention. In similar early-stage research, a 45-min reasoning intervention has been shown to increase data gathering with potential effects on levels of delusion conviction (Ross et al., in press), and the interventionist model is being applied to recent findings of an association between insomnia and paranoia (Freeman et al., in press). This work is part of a (substantial) process of developing a new multi-component cognitive-behavioural intervention that draws upon the marked progress over the last 5 years in the cognitive and social understanding of persecutory delusions.

Acknowledgment The author is supported by a Wellcome Trust Fellowship.

References

Bassett, M., Sperlinger, D., & Freeman, D. (2009). Fear of madness and persecutory delusions. *Psychosis, 1*, 39–50.

Bell, V., Halligan, P.W., & Ellis, H.D. (2006). The Cardiff Anomalous Perceptions Scale (CAPS). *Schizophrenia Bulletin, 32*, 366–377.

Bentall, R. P., Corcoran, R., Howard, R., Blackwood, N., & Kinderman, P. (2001). Persecutory delusions: A review and theoretical interpretation. *Clinical Psychology Review, 21*, 1143–1192.

Bentall, R. P., Kinderman, P., & Moutoussis, M. (2008). The role of self-esteem in paranoid delusions: the psychology, neurophysiology, and development of persecutory beliefs. In D. Freeman, R. Bentall & P. Garety (Eds.), *Persecutory delusions* (pp. 143–173). Oxford: Oxford University Press.

Bentall, R. P., Rowse, G., Kinderman, P., Blackwood, N., Howard, R., Moore, R., et al. (2008). Paranoid delusions in schizophrenia spectrum disorders and depression: the transdiagnostic role of expectations of negative events and negative self-esteem. *Journal of Nervous & Mental Disease, 196*, 375–383.

Bentall, R. P., Rowse, G., Shryane, N. M., Kinderman, P., Howard, R., Blackwood, N., Moore, R., Corcoran, R. (2009). The cognitive and affective structure of paranoid delusions: A transdiagnostic investigation of patients with schizophrenia spectrum disorders and depression. *Archives of General Psychiatry, 66*(3), 236–247.

Borkovec, T. D., Ray W. J., & Stober, J. (1998). Worry: a cognitive phenomenon intimately linked to affective, physiological, and interpersonal behavioural processes. *Cognitive Therapy and Research, 22*, 561–576.

Broome, M. R., Johns, L. C., Valli, I., Woolley, J. B., Tabraham, P., Brett, C., et al. (2007). Delusion formation and reasoning biases in those at clinical high risk for psychosis. *British Journal of Psychiatry, 191*, s38–s42.

Brüne, M. (2005). "Theory of Mind" in schizophrenia. *Schizophrenia Bulletin, 31*, 21–42.

Bunney, W. E., Hetrick, W. P., Bunney, B. G., Patterson, J. V., Jin, Y., Potkin, S. G., et al. (1999). Structured interview for assessing perceptual anomalies (SIAPA). *Schizophrenia Bulletin, 25*, 577–592.

Butler, P. D., & Javitt, D. C. (2005). Early-stage visual processing deficits in schizophrenia. *Current Opinion in Psychiatry, 18*, 151–157.

Chapman, L. J., & Chapman, J. P. (1980). Scales for rating psychotic and psychotic-like experiences as continua. *Schizophrenia Bulletin, 6*, 476–489.

Chapman, L. J., Chapman, J. P., Kwapil, T. R., Eckbald, M., & Zinser, M. C. (1994). Putatively psychosis-prone subjects 10 years later. *Journal of Abnormal Psychology, 103*, 171–183.

Claridge, G. (1997). Theoretical background and issues. In G. Claridge (Eds.), *Schizotypy: Implications for illness and health* (pp. 3–18). Oxford: Oxford University Press.

Combs, D. R., Penn, D. L., Wicher, M., & Waldheter, E. (2007). The Ambiguous Intentions Hostility Questionnaire (AIHQ): A new measure for evaluating attributional biases in paranoia. *Cognitive Neuropsychiatry, 12*, 128–143.

Docherty, J. P., Van Kammen, D. P., Siris, S. G., & Marder, S. R. (1978). Stages of onset of schizophrenic psychosis. *American Journal of Psychiatry, 135*, 420–426.

Dugas, M. J., & Ladouceur, R. (1998). Analysis and treatment of generalised anxiety disorder: A preliminary test of a conceptual model. *Behaviour Research and Therapy, 36*, 215–226.

Ellett, L., Freeman, D., & Garety, P. A. (2008). The psychological effect of an urban environment on individuals with persecutory delusions: The Camberwell walk study. *Schizophrenia Research, 99*, 77–84.

Eysenck, M. W., & Van Berkum, J. (1992). Trait anxiety, defensiveness, and the structure of worry. *Personality and Individual Differences, 13*, 1285–1290.

Foster, C., Startup, H., Potts, L., & Freeman, D. (2009). A randomised controlled trial of a worry intervention for individuals with persistent persecutory delusions. *Journal of Behavior Therapy and Experimental Psychiatry*, in press.

Fowler, D., Freeman, D., Smith, B., Kuipers, E., Bebbington, P., Bashforth, H., et al. (2006). The Brief Core Schema Scales (BCSS): Psychometric properties and associations with paranoia and grandiosity in non-clinical and psychosis samples. *Psychological Medicine, 36*, 749–759.

Freeman, D. (2008a). The assessment of persecutory ideation. In D. Freeman, R. Bentall, & P. Garety (Eds.), *Persecutory delusions* (pp 23–52). Oxford: Oxford University Press.

Freeman, D. (2008b). Studying and treating schizophrenia using virtual reality (vr): A new paradigm. *Schizophrenia Bulletin, 34*, 605–610.

Freeman, D. (2007). Suspicious minds: The psychology of persecutory delusions. *Clinical Psychology Review, 27*, 425–457.

Freeman, D., Dunn, G., Garety, P.A., Bebbington, P., Slater, M., Kuipers, E., et al. (2005). The psychology of persecutory ideation I: A questionnaire study. *Journal of Nervous and Mental Disease, 193*, 302–308.

Freeman, D., & Fowler, D. (2009). Routes to psychotic symptoms: Trauma, anxiety and psychosis-like experiences. *Psychiatry Research, 169*(2), 107–112.

Freeman, D., & Freeman, J. (2008). *Paranoia: The 21st century fear*. Oxford: Oxford University Press.

Freeman, D., Freeman, J., & Garety, P. (2006). *Overcoming paranoid and suspicious thoughts*. London: Robinson.

Freeman, D., & Garety, P.A. (1999). Worry, worry processes and dimensions of delusions: An exploratory investigation of a role for anxiety processes in the maintenance of delusional distress. *Behavioural & Cognitive Psychotherapy, 27*, 47–62.

Freeman, D., & Garety, P.A. (2000). Comments on the content of persecutory delusions: Does the definition need clarification? *British Journal of Clinical Psychology, 39*, 407–414.

Freeman, D., Garety, P. A., Bebbington, P., Slater, M., Kuipers, E., Fowler, D., et al. (2005). The psychology of persecutory ideation II: A virtual reality experimental study. *Journal of Nervous and Mental Disease, 193*, 309–315.

Freeman, D., Garety, P. A., Bebbington, P. E., Smith, B., Rollinson, R., Fowler, D., et al. (2005). Psychological investigation of the structure of paranoia in a non-clinical population. *British Journal of Psychiatry, 186*, 427–435.

Freeman, D., Garety, P. A., Fowler, D., Kuipers, E., Bebbington, P., Dunn, G. (2004). Why do people with delusions fail to choose more realistic explanations for their experiences? An empirical investigation. *Journal of Consulting and Clinical Psychology, 72*, 671–680.

Freeman, D., Garety, P. A., & Kuipers, E. (2001). Persecutory delusions: developing the understanding of belief maintenance and emotional distress. *Psychological Medicine, 31*, 1293–1306.

Freeman, D., Garety, P. A., Kuipers, E., Fowler, D., & Bebbington, P.E. (2002). A cognitive model of persecutory delusions. *British Journal of Clinical Psychology, 41*, 331–347.

Freeman, D., Garety, P. A., McGuire, P., & Kuipers, E., (2005). Developing a theoretical understanding of therapy techniques: reasoning, therapy and symptoms. *British Journal of Clinical Psychology, 44*, 241–254

Freeman, D., Gittins, M., Pugh, K., Antley, A., Slater, M., & Dunn, G. (2008). What makes one person paranoid and another person anxious? The differential prediction of social anxiety and persecutory ideation in an experimental situation. *Psychological Medicine, 38*, 1121–1132.

Freeman, D., Pugh, K., Antley, A., Slater, M., Bebbington, P., Gittins, M., et al. (2008). A virtual reality study of paranoid thinking in the general population. *British Journal of Psychiatry, 192*, 258–263.

Freeman, D., Pugh, K., & Garety, P. (2008). Jumping to conclusions and paranoid ideation in the general population. *Schizophrenia Research, 102*, 254–260.

Freeman, D., Pugh, K., Green, C., Valmaggia, L., Dunn, G., & Garety, P. (2007). A measure of state persecutory ideation for experimental studies. *Journal of Nervous and Mental Disease, 195*, 781–784.

Freeman, D., Pugh, K., Vorontsova, N., Antley, A., & Slater, M. (2009). Establishing the continuum of delusional beliefs. *Journal of Abnormal Psychology*, in press.

Freeman, D., Pugh, K., Vorontsova, N., & Southgate, L. (2009). Insomnia and paranoia. *Schizophrenia Research, 108*(1–3), 280–284.

Freeman, D., Slater, M., Bebbington, P.E., Garety, P.A., Kuipers, E., Fowler, D., et al. (2003). Can virtual reality be used to investigate persecutory ideation? *The Journal of Nervous and Mental Disease, 191,* 509–514.

Frith, C. D. (1992). *The cognitive neuropsychology of schizophrenia.* Hove: LEA.

Frith, C. D. (2004). Schizophrenia and theory of mind. *Psychological Medicine, 34,* 385–389.

Garety, P. A. (1985). Delusions: Problems in definition and measurement.*British Journal of Medical Psychology, 58,* 25–34.

Garety, P. A., Everitt, B. S., & Hemsley, D. R. (1988). The characteristics of delusions. *European Archives of Psychiatry and Neurological Sciences, 237,* 112–114.

Garety, P. A., & Freeman, D. (1999). Cognitive approaches to delusions: a critical review of theories and evidence. *British Journal of Clinical Psychology, 38,* 113–154.

Garety, P.A., Freeman, D., Jolley, S., Dunn, G., Bebbington, P.E., Fowler, D., et al. (2005). Reasoning, emotions and delusional conviction in psychosis. *Journal of Abnormal Psychology, 114,* 373–384.

Glaser, J. P., van Os, J., Portegijs, P. J. M., & Myin-Germeys, I. (2006). Childhood trauma and emotional reactivity to daily life stress in adult frequent attenders of the General Practitioner. *Journal of Psychosomatic Research, 61,* 229–236.

Gracie, A., Freeman, D., Green, S., Garety, P. A., Kuipers, E., Hardy, A., et al. (2007). The association between traumatic experience, paranoia and hallucinations: A test of the predictions of psychological models. *Acta Psychiatrica Scandinavica, 116,* 280–289.

Greig, T. C., Bryson, G. J., & Bell, M. D. (2004). Theory of mind performance in schizophrenia. *The Journal of Nervous and Mental Disease, 192,* 12–18.

Guillem, F., Pampoulova, T., Stip, E., Lalonde, P., & Todorov, C. (2005). The relationships between symptom dimensions and dysphoria in schizophrenia. *Schizophrenia Research, 75,* 83–96.

Harrington, L., Siegert, R. J., & McClure, J. (2005). Theory of mind in schizophrenia. *Cognitive Neuropsychiatry, 10,* 249–286.

Harrow, M., Jobe, T. M., & Astrachan-Fletcher, E. B. (2008). Prognosis of persecutory delusions in schizophrenia: a 20-year longitudinal study. In D. Freeman, R. Bentall, & P. Garety (Eds.), *Persecutory delusions* (pp. 73–90). Oxford: Oxford University Press.

Harrow, M., Rattenbury, F., & Stoll, F. (1988). Schizophrenic delusions: an analysis of their persistence, of related premorbid ideas, and of three major dimensions. In T. F. Oltmanns & B. A. Maher (Eds.), *Delusional beliefs* (pp. 184–211). New York: Wiley.

Henquet, C., Di Forti, M., Murray, R. M., & van Os, J. (2008). The role of cannabis in inducing paranoia and psychosis. In D. Freeman, R. Bentall, & P. Garety (Eds.), *Persecutory delusions* (pp. 267–280). Oxford: Oxford University Press.

Hemsley, D. R. (1994). Perceptual and cognitive abnormalities as the bases for schizophrenic symptoms. In A. S. David & J. C. Cutting (Eds.), *The neuropsychology of schizophrenia* (pp. 97–116). Hove: Erlbaum.

Janssen, I., Krabbendam, L., Bak, M., Hanssen, M., Vollebergh, W, de Graaf, R., et al. (2004). Childhood abuse as a risk factor for psychotic experiences. *Acta Psychiatrica Scandinavica, 109,* 38–45.

Janssen, I., Versmissen, D., a Campo, J., Myin-germeys, I., van Os, J., & Krabbendam, L. (2006). Attribution style and psychosis. *Psychological Medicine, 36,* 771–778.

Johns, L. C., Cannon, M., Singleton, N., Murray, R. M., Farrell, M., Brugha, T., et al. (2004). The prevalence and correlates of self-reported psychotic symptoms in the British population. *British Journal of Psychiatry, 185,* 298–305.

Kapur, S. (2003). Psychosis as a state of aberrant salience: A framework linking biology, phenomenology, and pharmacology. *American Journal of Psychiatry, 160,* 13–23.

Kapur, S., Mizrahi, R., & Li, M. (2005). From dopamine to salience to psychosis – linking biology, pharmacology and phenomenology of psychosis. *Schizophrenia Research, 79,* 59-68.

Kendler, K. S., Glazer, W. M., & Morgenstern, H. (1983). Dimensions of delusional experience. *American Journal of Psychiatry, 140*, 466–469.

Kendler, K. S., Campbell, J. (2009). Interventionist causal models in psychiatry: repositioning the mind-body problem. *Psychological Medicine, 39*(6), 881–887.

Kirkbride, J. B., Fearon, P., Morgan, C., Dazzan, P., Morgan, K., Tarrant, J., et al. (2006). Heterogeneity in incidence rates of schizophrenia and other psychotic syndromes. *Archives of General Psychiatry, 63*, 250–258.

Krabbendam, L., Janssen, I., Bijl, R. V., Vollebergh, W. A. M., & van Os, J. (2002). Neuroticism and low self-esteem as risk factors for psychosis. *Social Psychiatry and Psychiatric Epidemiology, 37*, 1–6.

Langdon, R., Ward, P. B., & Coltheart, M. (in press). Reasoning anomalies associated with delusions in schizophrenia. *Schizophrenia Bulletin*.

Larkin, W., & Morrison, A. (Eds.). (2006). *Trauma and psychosis*. Hove, East Sussex: Routledge.

Lemert, E. M. (1962). Paranoia and the dynamics of exclusion. *Sociometry, 25*, 2–20.

Lyon, H. M., Kaney, S., & Bentall, R. P. (1994). The defensive function of persecutory delusions: evidence from attribution tasks. *British Journal of Psychiatry, 164*, 637–646.

Maher, B. A. (1974). Delusional thinking and perceptual disorder. *Journal of Individual Psychology, 30*, 98–113.

Marcelis, M., Navarro-Mateu, F., Murray, R., Selten, J. P., & van Os, J. (1998). Urbanisation and psychosis. *Psychological Medicine, 28*, 871–879.

Maric, N., Myin-Germeys, I., Delespaul, P., de Graaf, R., Vollebergh, W., Van Os, J. (2004). Is our concept of schizophrenia influenced by Berkson's bias? *Social Psychiatry and Psychiatric Epidemiology, 39*(8), 600–605.

Martin, J. A., & Penn, D. L. (2001). Brief report: social cognition and subclinical paranoid ideation. *British Journal of Clinical Psychology, 40*, 261–265.

Martin, J. A., & Penn, D. L. (2002). Attributional style in schizophrenia. *Schizophrenia Bulletin, 28*, 131–141.

McGhie, A., & Chapman, J. (1961). Disorders of attention and perception in early schizophrenia. *British Journal of Medical Psychology, 34*, 103–116.

McGrath, J. J. (2007). The surprisingly rich contours of schizophrenia epidemiology. *Archives of General Psychiatry, 64*, 14–16.

Mizrahi, R., Kiang, M., Mamo, D. C., Arenovich, T., Bagby, R. M., Zipursky, R. B., et al. (2006). The selective effect of antipsychotics on the different dimensions of the experience of psychosis in schizophrenia spectrum disorders. *Schizophrenia Research, 88*, 111–118.

Moritz, S., Woodward, T., & Lambert, M. (2007). Under what circumstances do patients with schizophrenia jump to conclusions? A liberal acceptance account. *British Journal of Clinical Psychology, 46*, 12–13.

Morrison, A. P., & Wells, A. (2007). Relationships between worry, psychotic experiences and emotional distress in patients with schizophrenia spectrum diagnoses and comparisons with anxious and non-patient groups. *Behaviour Research and Therapy, 45*, 1593–1600.

Myin-Germeys, I., Krabbendam, L., & van Os, J. (2003). Continuity of psychotic symptoms in the community. *Current Opinion in Psychiatry, 16*, 443–449.

Myin-Germeys, I., & van Os, J. (2007). Stress-reactivity in psychosis: evidence for an affective pathway to psychosis. *Clinical Psychology Review, 27*, 409–424.

Norman, R. M., & Malla, A. K. (1994). Correlations over time between dysphoric mood and symptomatology in schizophrenia. *Comprehensive Psychiatry, 35*, 34–38.

Oltmanns, T. F. (1988). Approaches to the definition and study of delusions. In T. F. Oltmanns & B. A. Maher (Eds.), *Delusional beliefs* (pp. 3–12). New York: Wiley.

Peralta, V., & Cuesta, M.J. (1998). Factor structure and clinical validity of competing models of positive symptoms in schizophrenia. *Biological Psychiatry, 44*, 107–114.

Poulton, R., Caspi, A., Moffitt, T. E., Cannon, M., Murray, R., & Harrington, H. (2000). Children's self-reported psychotic symptoms and adult schizophreniform disorder. *Archives of General Psychiatry, 57*, 1053–1058.

Sanchez-Vives, M. V., & Slater, M. (2005). From presence to consciousness through Virtual Reality. *Nature Reviews Neuroscience, 6*, 332–339.

Sarfati, Y., Hardy-Baylé, M., Besche, C., & Widlöcher, D. (1997). Attribution of intentions to others in people with schizophrenia. *Schizophrenia Research, 25*, 199–209.

Scott, J., Chant, D., Andrews, G., Martin, G., & McGrath, J. (2007). Association between trauma exposure and delusional experiences in a large community-based sample. *British Journal of Psychiatry, 190*, 339–343.

Smith, B., Fowler, D., Freeman, D., Bebbington, P., Bashforth, H., Garety, P., et al. (2006). Emotion and psychosis: direct links between schematic beliefs, emotion and delusions and hallucinations. *Schizophrenia Research, 86*, 181–188.

Startup, H., Freeman, D., & Garety, P. A. (2007). Persecutory delusions and catastrophic worry in psychosis: developing the understanding of delusion distress and persistence. *Behaviour Research and Therapy, 45*, 523–537.

Startup, H., Freeman, D., & Garety, P. (2008). Jumping to conclusions and persecutory delusions. *European Psychiatry, 23*, 457–459.

Strauss, J. S. (1969). Hallucinations and delusions as points on continua function. *Archives of General Psychiatry, 20*, 581–586.

Sundquist, K., Frank, G., & Sundquist, J. (2004). Follow-up study of 4.4 million women and men in Sweden. *British Journal of Psychiatry, 184*, 293–298.

Thewissen, V., Bentall, R. P., Lecomte, T., van Os, J., & Myin-Germeys, I. (2008). Fluctuations in self-esteem and paranoia in the context of daily life. *Journal of Abnormal Psychology, 117*, 143–153.

Thewissen, V., Myin-Germeys, I., Bentall, R., de Graaf, R., Vollebergh, W., & van Os, J. (2005). Hearing impairment and psychosis revisited. *Schizophrenia Research, 76*, 99–103.

Trower, P., Birchwood, M., Meaden, A., Byrne, S., Nelson, A., & Ross, K. (2004). Cognitive therapy for command hallucinations. *British Journal of Psychiatry, 184*, 312-320.

Uhlhaas, P. J., & Mishara, A. L. (2007). Perceptual anomalies in schizophrenia. *Schizophrenia Bulletin, 33*, 142–156.

Van Dael, F., Versmissen, D., Janssen, I., Myin-Germeys, I., van Os, J., & Krabbendam, L. (2006). Data gathering: biased in psychosis? *Schizophrenia Bulletin, 32*, 341–351.

Van Os, J. (2004). Does the urban environment cause psychosis? *British Journal of Psychiatry, 184*, 287–288.

Van Os, J., Hanssen, M., Bijl, R. V., & Ravelli, A. (2000). Strauss (1969) revisited: A psychosis continuum in the general population. *Schizophrenia Research, 45*, 11-20.

Van Os, J., Linscott, R. J., Myin-Germeys, I., Delespaul, P., & Krabbendam, L. (2009). A systematic review and meta-analysis of the psychosis continuum: evidence for a psychosis proneness–persistence–impairment model of psychotic disorder. *Psychological Medicine, 39*(2), 179–195.

Van Winkel, R., Stefanis, N. C., & Myin-Germeys, I. (2008). Psychosocial stress and psychosis. A review of the neurobiological mechanisms and the evidence for gene-stress interaction. *Schizophrenia Bulletin, 34*, 1095–1105.

Vázquez-Barquero, J. L., Lastra, I., Nuñez, M. J. C., Castanedo, S. H., & Dunn, G. (1996). Patterns of positive and negative symptoms in first episode schizophrenia. *British Journal of Psychiatry, 168*, 693–701.

Vermissen, D., Janssen, I., Myin-Germeys, I., Mengelers, R., à Campo, J., van Os, J., et al. (2008). Evidence for a relationship between mentalising deficits and paranoia over the psychosis continuum. *Schizophrenia Research, 99*, 103–110.

Wells, A. (1994). A multi-dimensional measure of worry: development and preliminary validation of the anxious thoughts inventory. *Anxiety, Stress and Coping, 6*, 289–299.

Woodward, J. (2003). *Making things happen: A theory of causal explanation*. New York: Oxford University Press.

The Impact of Early Intervention
in Schizophrenia

Alison R. Yung, Eoin J. Killackey, Barnaby Nelson, and Patrick D. McGorry

Introduction

Schizophrenia and other psychotic disorders are serious and potentially fatal illnesses that typically emerge during the sensitive developmental period of adolescence and emerging adulthood. For over 100 years, these disorders have been
viewed pessimistically, characterized by high levels of stigma and neglect. However, the last two decades have seen the rise of "the early intervention movement"
that advocates rapid access to care and comprehensive treatment in the initial stages
of disorder. The basis of this strategy is that the first few years of illness represent
a "critical period" (Birchwood et al. 1989, 1998), during which treatment will be
most effective and may prevent future deterioration and secondary morbidity. This
chapter examines the impact of and evidence related to early intervention.

What Is "Early Intervention"?

Schizophrenia usually begins with a prodromal phase, characterized by non-specific
symptoms at first, followed by the gradual acquisition of positive psychotic-like
experiences and often negative symptoms and deterioration in functioning, before
the development of a full-blown first psychotic episode. Unfortunately, there often
follows a period of time between the onset of the first psychotic episode and engagement in effective mental health care. This is referred to as the duration of untreated
psychosis (DUP) (McGlashan 1999; Norman and Malla 2001). The length of the
DUP depends on help-seeking patterns and service systems and can be prolonged,
for example, up to 52 weeks (Loebel et al. 1992). Upon reaching a treatment service,
acute management can begin, with an important aim of reducing distress and positive psychotic symptoms. This acute phase is then followed by the recovery phase,
in which broader issues such as re-engagement with family, peers, vocation and

A.R. Yung (✉)
Orygen Youth Research Centre, University of Melbourne, Australia
e-mail: aryung@unimelb.edu.au

W.F. Gattaz, G. Busatto (eds.), *Advances in Schizophrenia Research 2009*,
DOI 10.1007/978-1-4419-0913-8_16, © Springer Science+Business Media, LLC 2010

education can be addressed, as well as attention to treatment maintenance and relapse prevention. This brief (and simplistic) summary of the onset phases of schizophrenia underlines that there are three key foci for potential intervention. These are as follows:

1. the prodromal stage;
2. the period of untreated psychosis; and
3. the first episode of psychosis and the recovery phase.

"Early intervention" refers to early detection and intervention in any of these stages.

The aim of early intervention is to provide timely treatment, thus decreasing the disruption to the young person's life and preventing the development of chronic disabilities. Because symptoms and disability have already begun, early intervention in schizophrenia means early secondary prevention using the traditional primary, secondary and tertiary preventive framework. However, intervention in the prodromal phase can also be seen as indicated prevention, using the universal, selective and indicated prevention developed by the World Health Organization in 1994 (Mrazek and Haggerty 1994). The definition of indicated prevention is interventions targeted at individuals manifesting precursor signs and symptoms who have not yet met full criteria for diagnosis. As Mrazek and Haggerty (1994) note,

> The identification of individuals at this early stage, coupled with the introduction of pharmacological and psychosocial interventions, may prevent the development of the full-blown disorder.

Impact of Early Intervention

Focus 1: The Prodromal Phase

Detection of "The Prodrome"

In psychotic disorders, an early prepsychotic stage is known to exist, one in which much of the collateral psychosocial damage is known to occur (Yung and McGorry 1996). This earliest stage could, in retrospect, be termed the "prodrome", i.e., the precursor of the psychotic stage. However, since we can only apply the term "prodrome" with certainty if the definitive psychotic stage does indeed develop, terms such as the "ultra-high risk" (McGorry et al. 2003) or "clinical high risk" (Cornblatt et al. 2002) stage have been developed to indicate that psychosis is not inevitable and that false-positive cases also occur. This symptomatic yet prepsychotic stage is the earliest point at which preventive interventions for psychosis can currently be conceived (Mrazek and Haggerty 1994). Intervening during this prodromal phase may ameliorate, delay or even prevent onset of fully fledged disorder.

The challenge in detecting such a stage prospectively is first to define the clinical frontier for earliest intervention and "need for care", which represents the boundary between normal human experience and pathology. Second, a set of clinical and other predictors need to be defined, which identify a subgroup at imminent risk for psychotic disorder. This is a complex task and the main issues involved have been covered in many recent publications (Yung et al. 1996, 2003, 2004b; Cornblatt et al. 2001; Warner 2005; Haroun et al. 2006; Olsen and Rosenbaum 2006). A practical operational definition of a prepsychotic "at-risk" or "ultra-high risk" (UHR) mental state, which could be shown to confer a substantially high risk of full-blown psychotic disorder within a 12-month period, was then developed and tested in the early 1990s (Yung et al. 1996, 2003). This has captured the attention of the field and has been the focus of much subsequent research, focusing on prediction, treatment and neurobiological aspects.

The initial study of the predictive validity of the UHR criteria found that they identified a group at high risk of transition to psychotic disorder (Yung et al. 2003), with a transition rate of over 40%. Subsequently other research centres have used similar criteria and found transition rates of 9–54% (Olsen and Rosenbaum 2006) with an average of 36.7% within 1 year (Ruhrmann et al. 2003). The largest sample to date ($n = 291$) of UHR or "prodromal" individuals has recently been published (Cannon et al. 2008). This study found a transition rate of 35% over two and a half years, with an estimated relative risk of 40% compared to the incident rate of psychotic disorders in the general population.

Intervention in the UHR Stage

People have problems before they have diagnoses (Macmillan and Shiers 2000).

UHR individuals are clearly symptomatic and in need of some kind of help. They usually report sustained subjective and behavioral change, such as distress, social withdrawal and difficulties in relationships and educational and vocational performance, over many weeks, months or years. A point to emphasize is that the need for clinical care in these young people precedes, often by a long period, the capacity to diagnose a clear-cut DSM IV psychotic disorder.

Following advances in identification of the UHR or prodromal group, researchers began to investigate the possibility of intervening in these individuals. The aims of this "prodromal" intervention were first to prevent or delay transition to psychosis and second to treat current problems, such as comorbid depressive or anxiety symptoms or syndromes. A further aim was to ensure that should transition to schizophrenia or another psychotic disorder occur the individual is already well engaged with treatment and DUP is therefore minimized. In addition, non-traumatic entry into an early intervention programme could be facilitated, possibly avoiding the need for in-patient treatment (Yung et al. 2004a).

Psychotherapy and pharmacotherapy have been the main forms of intervention in UHR/prodromal clinics. Psychotherapy (usually cognitive in orientation (Morrison et al. 2004; Yung et al. 2004a)) can be targeted specifically at positive symptoms, or at comorbid syndromes or symptoms such as depression or anxiety. Similarly, pharmacotherapy can be targeted at mood or anxiety disorders, which frequently are present in people presenting to pre-onset clinics (Svirskis et al. 2005; Rosen et al. 2006), or specifically at subthreshold psychotic symptoms, and could include the use of low-dose antipsychotic medication (McGorry et al. 2002).

To date, three treatments trials have been published. These indicate that specific intervention, both psychological and pharmacological, may benefit individuals in terms of reducing the risk of transition from UHR state to full-threshold psychotic disorder or at least delaying or attenuating onset. The first randomized trial, conducted in Melbourne, Australia, at the PACE (Personal Assessment and Crisis Evaluation) Clinic between 1996 and 1999, aimed to determine whether a combination of up to 2 mg risperidone plus cognitive therapy (CT) ($n = 31$) was more effective than supportive counselling alone ($n = 28$) in preventing or delaying the onset of psychosis (McGorry et al. 2002). Significantly more people in the supportive counselling group developed a psychotic illness by the end of the 6-month treatment period (36 vs. 9.7%, $p = 0.03$). However, this difference was no longer significant at the end of the 6-month no-treatment follow-up (36 vs. 19.4%, $p = 0.24$), although individuals in the combined treatment group who were fully compliant with antipsychotic medication during the treatment phase were significantly less likely to develop psychosis over the follow-up period than the supportive counselling group. Members of both groups reported symptom improvement at the end of the 6-month follow-up phase and this was maintained when they were followed up 3–4 years later (Phillips et al. 2007). A number of limitations of this study have been noted (McGorry et al. 2002), including small sample size and lack of blind randomization to treatment group. In particular it was felt that treatment was not provided for long enough.

The PRIME (Prevention through Risk Identification Management & Education) North America study compared 12-month treatment with an antipsychotic (olanzapine, 5–15 mg daily, $n = 31$) with 12 months of placebo treatment ($n = 29$) (McGlashan 2003; McGlashan et al. 2006). At the end of the treatment phase, 16% of the olanzapine group developed a psychotic episode compared to 38% of the placebo group, a trend level difference ($p = 0.08$), and the olanzapine group reported greater improvement in level of positive psychotic symptoms than the placebo group. After a second 12-month period during which neither group received treatment, the difference in the transition rate remained. However, the participants who took olanzapine reported significantly greater weight gain over the treatment phase than the placebo group (mean = 8.79 kg, SD = 9.05 compared to mean = 0.30 kg, SD = 4.24). McGlashan and colleagues (2006) admit that recruitment was slower than anticipated and the study did not have sufficient power to fully assess the efficacy of the active treatment in preventing transition to psychosis or impact on symptom severity.

Finally, a trial conducted at Early Detection and Intervention Evaluation (EDIE) in Manchester, United Kingdom, reported that only 6% of UHR participants who received cognitive therapy ($n = 37$) for 6 months developed a psychotic disorder compared to 22% of individuals who did not receive any active psychological or medical treatment ($n = 23$) (Morrison et al. 2004). A logistic regression analysis indicated that CT was associated with significantly lower likelihood of developing psychotic disorder than no treatment ($p = 0.028$). This difference remained significant after another 6 months when no treatment was provided, suggesting that CT significantly reduced the likelihood of developing psychosis over a reasonably short follow-up period. Over a 3-year period, CT was associated with a significantly lower rate of transition to psychosis (when baseline cognitive factors were controlled for) and significantly reduced the likelihood of being prescribed antipsychotic medication (Morrison et al. 2007).

In a further development, a study has recently been completed, which examined the effect of eicosapentoic acid (EPA) (fish oil) in the UHR group. This randomized control trial compared fish oil with placebo. At 3-month follow-up, 1 (2.6%) of 38 individuals in the EPA group and 8 (21.1%) of 38 in the placebo group developed psychotic disorder (chi-square exact $p = 0.028$). At 6-month follow-up, 11 (28.9%) of 38 individuals developed psychotic disorder in the placebo group, while no further transitions occurred in the EPA group (chi-square exact $p = 0.002$) (Amminger et al. 2007).

One of the criticisms of intervention in the UHR phase is that people will be mislabelled, potentially stigmatized and exposed to treatments that they did not need because they were not going to develop psychosis ("false positives") (Bentall and Morrison 2002; Warner 2005). This is particularly a criticism targeted at interventions using antipsychotic medication. Morrison et al. (2004) specifically address this criticism in their choice of using only a psychological intervention, which they argue is less likely to lead to deleterious side effects than pharmacotherapy. While criteria for identification of those at risk of psychosis continue to detect large numbers of false positives, even the leading proponents of UHR/prodromal intervention advocate cautious use of medication, as do guidelines for treatment in this phase (Yung et al. 2004a, 2007b; International Early Psychosis Association et al. 2005; McGlashan et al. 2007).

Future research needs to focus on the continued improvement of the accuracy of predictive tools reducing the false-positive rate as much as possible and the development of knowledge about which interventions are required at what stage so as to reduce the exposure of people to unnecessary iatrogenic damage.

Focus 2: Reducing Duration of Untreated Psychosis

The controversy surrounding the importance of treatment delay in relation to poor outcome in schizophrenia seems to have been largely resolved following the publication of some key systematic reviews (Marshall et al. 2005; Perkins et al. 2005) and recent longitudinal research (Melle et al. 2004; Emsley et al. 2007). These studies have now established that longer DUP is both a marker and independent risk factor for poor outcome. The Early Treatment and Identification of Psychosis (TIPS) study in Scandinavia (Johannessen et al. 2005) examined the effect of early intervention – and a corresponding reduction in DUP – amongst two samples of patients with first-episode psychosis who were recruited from the same healthcare district in Norway but at different time periods. A historical control sample ($n = 43$) was assessed during the period 1993–1994, before the establishment of a community awareness programme and a system for early detection of psychosis, while an experimental first-episode sample ($n = 118$) was assessed during 1997–2000, after the interventions (community awareness programme and early detection system). The authors compared the 1-year clinical outcomes and course of illness variables between the groups (Larsen et al. 2007).

At first assessment, the mean DUP for the early detection group was significantly lower than in the historical control group (28.2 weeks compared to 114.2 weeks), showing that a community awareness campaign about psychosis coupled with an early psychosis outreach team could reduce DUP (Johannessen et al. 2005). The study found that reducing DUP led to early benefits in reducing suicidal risk and severity of illness at initial treatment. At 1-year follow-up, there were no significant differences between the groups, however, in terms of the clinical course of illness (e.g., proportion in remission, relapse or continuously psychotic) or positive symptoms. However, there was evidence of sustained benefits in terms of negative symptoms, even after adjusting for age and premorbid functioning (Larsen et al. 2007). The rate of suicide plans or attempts was significantly lower in patients in the early detection programme compared to those with standard treatment even after adjusting for known predictors of suicidality (Melle et al. 2004). The TIPS investigators acknowledged that their findings could be due to a lead time bias and that a longer period of follow-up would be necessary to exclude or confirm this possibility (Larsen et al. 2007). However even if this were the case, the change in the introduction into psychiatric services, which for many FEP patients is a highly traumatic experience, is still an important clinical finding. The reduction in DUP in the early detection group meant that these patients had milder symptoms at the time of first treatment and therefore could be significantly more often treated as outpatients rather than having to be admitted.

Another study that examined the impact of education about psychotic disorders coupled with an early detection programme was the Lambeth Early Onset Crisis Assessment Team (LEO CAT) study (Power et al. 2007a,b). This study evaluated the effectiveness of a brief general practitioner (GP) education programme (approximately 25 min duration) combined with the introduction of an early detection assessment team (LEO CAT) compared with no GP education programme and standard local mental health services (no access to LEO CAT) in reducing delays to access treatment. A total of 46 clusters of GP practices in the London borough of Lambeth were randomized, with 23 in the intervention group and 23 in the control group.

The study found that significantly more GP practices exposed to the early detection intervention referred their patients directly to mental health services compared with control GP practices (86.1 vs. 65.7%). Furthermore, fewer patients in the intervention practices experienced long delays (over 6 weeks) between first contact with the GP and being assessed by mental health services (13.9 vs. 37.1%). However, the overall mean DUP between the intervention and control groups did not differ significantly. Notably, this lack of difference in total DUP was due to the majority of DUP occurring before the patients reached the GPs. An important point from this study is that a brief, one-off GP education campaign plus the introduction of an accessible early detection team can reduce the delay between initial GP assessment and referral to specialist mental health services. In contrast, the long DUP before reaching GPs was still a problem. It may be that an intensive, targeted public education campaign, such as developed by the TIPS programme, is required to decrease this initial delay in help seeking.

Another finding apparent from the TIPS study was that although DUP is a malleable risk factor, it accounts for a relatively modest amount of outcome variance. This underlines the importance of not only treatment access in the first episode of psychosis but also the need for high-quality treatment during the early years of illness.

Focus 3: The First Episode of Psychosis and the Recovery Phase

The principles of early intervention continue after an individual has accessed treatment for a first episode of psychosis. That is, a preventive focus needs to be taken to reduce the trauma of initial presentation, enhance the therapeutic alliance and to vigorously treat the acute phase. In the recovery phase, the prevention or reduction of secondary morbidity is a focus, as well as attention to family, peer and vocational issues.

Acute Phase

Currently there are highly effective, if still imperfect, treatments to reduce symptoms and promote recovery of the first psychotic episode, and the probability of acute symptomatic recovery is high (70–90% depending on sampling and definition of response) (Lieberman et al. 1993; Robinson et al. 1999; Emsley et al. 2007). The International Clinical Practice Guidelines in Early Psychosis (International Early Psychosis Association et al. 2005) recommend the use of atypical antipsychotics as first-line therapy, because of better tolerability (a crucial issue in drug-naive first-episode patients) and reduced risk for tardive dyskinesia. The large multicentre European First Episode Schizophrenia Trial (EUFEST) (Kahn et al. 2008) supported this recommendation. This study found that while most patients responded well to both typical and atypical medications, with no significant efficacy differences, discontinuation rates and tolerability were clearly superior for atypical agents. This was true even when contrasted with very low-dose haloperidol. However, some atypicals have a particularly high risk of weight gain and metabolic problems and these risks need to be carefully managed and prevented wherever possible. A recent paper (Perez-Iglesias et al. 2008), however, suggests that weight gain is a problem in the first year of therapy for first-episode patients on both typicals and atypicals, with the key difference being the rate at which it develops.

Although the acute positive symptoms of a first episode of psychosis tend to respond well to antipsychotic medication, there is a risk of relapse, especially if individuals disengage with care or are non-adherent to medication (Tauscher-Wisniewski and Zipursky 2002; Emsley et al. 2007). Thus, services need to include out-reach components, which can recognize young people at risk of dropping out (Schley et al. 2008). There have been two trials that have used a randomized design to access the effectiveness of outcomes of intensive specialized first-episode services. The OPUS trial in Denmark randomly assigned 547 patients to either an integrated treatment in which they were provided with 2 years of service or a standard treatment (Thorup et al. 2005). The integrated treatment provided was intense and assertive and covered a wide range of domains including family therapy and social skills training. Caseload was 1:10. The control condition was treatment at a standard service in which caseloads were higher (1:25). The results from the study indicated that the integrated treatment had beneficial effects on symptomatic and functional outcome at 1 and 2 years (Petersen et al. 2005; Thorup et al. 2005) as well as a perceived reduction in family burden (Jeppesen et al. 2005). The more assertive nature of the early intervention model is reflected in the finding that patients receiving integrated treatment had an average of 77 contacts over the 2 years compared to 27 in the standard treatment group (Petersen et al. 2005; Thorup et al. 2005).

The second trial was the Lambeth Early Onset (LEO) trial (Craig et al. 2004). The LEO trial randomized people in Lambeth (South East London, England) presenting for a first-episode psychosis (or a second episode where there had been failure to engage previously) to either receive treatment from standard services or from a new early intervention service. It was found that there was a beneficial effect of the early intervention on re-admissions, relapses and drop-outs. However, when adjustments were made the relapse rate became non-significant. Further analysis of this study showed that the intervention group was more compliant with medication, spent more time engaged in educational or vocational pursuits, and established or re-established relationships better than the control group (Garety et al. 2006). The LEO trial shows that early intervention can achieve gains in both clinical and functional aspects of early psychosis.

Recovery Phase

The prevention or reduction of secondary problems requires the recognition of possible comorbidities and of the social impact of the onset of psychosis. Comorbidities include substance use disorders, smoking, forensic problems, social anxiety, depression and suicide. The social impact includes peer relationships, which tend to be crucial but fragile during this phase of life, the family network, educational and vocational trajectories and the evolution of the self and social identity. Early intervention in all these areas may increase the chances of a more complete functional recovery in the wake of symptom resolution. Clinical resources and skill are required to tackle these psychosocial challenges. Merely treating the psychotic symptoms during the acute phase leaves most of the therapeutic work undone, yet this is what often occurs if inadequate tenure of care is provided during this phase (McGorry and Yung 2003), which Birchwood et al. (1998) has referred to as "the critical period" – up to 5 years after the first treated episode. Such band-aid treatment of the acute phase with minimal specialist aftercare misses this key preventive opportunity.

Two psychosocial strands of management that have been investigated are that of family and vocational interventions.

Family Interventions

Since most first-episode patients live with their families (Edwards et al. 1994; Davis and Schultz 1998), it is important that family members are involved in management. Furthermore, family members of individuals with psychotic disorders, including those with first-episode psychosis, often report distress, including feelings of anxiety, depression and economic strain (Addington et al. 2003). Thus family interventions in early psychosis have two aims: to improve the management of the patient with the disorder and to reduce stress on the family members. Involving parents in the management plan, especially within programmes that offer family psychoeducation and support, has been found to reduce relapse rates (Falloon et al. 1984; McFarlane and Cunningham 1996; Cassidy et al. 2001; Dyck et al. 2002; McFarlane 2002), decrease length of hospital stay (Cassidy et al. 2001) and increase medication compliance (Lehman and Steinwachs 1998; Pitschel-Walz et al. 2001; Robinson et al. 2002). Indeed, the efficacy of family interventions in reducing relapse is now considered an evidence-based intervention (Lehman and Steinwachs 1998; Addington et al. 2005). There is also evidence that family interventions can reduce distress in family members of first-episode patients (Addington et al. 2005). The OPUS early intervention trial found that relatives of patients in the integrated treatment group (which included a family psychoeducation component) felt less burdened and were significantly more satisfied with treatment than relatives in standard treatment (Jeppesen et al. 2005).

Vocational Interventions

Rates of unemployment are high in first-episode psychosis, averaging between 40 and 50% (Killackey et al. 2006). For those who develop schizophrenia, unemployment rates are in excess of 75% (Marwaha and Johnson 2004). This is despite gaining competitive employment being the number one aim of people with serious mental illness (Secker et al. 2001). To date, there have been two reported studies of evidence-based employment interventions in first-episode psychosis. Rinaldi et al. (2004) conducted a non-randomized trial of individual placement and support (IPS) in London. They found that this intervention led to unemployment decreasing from 55 to 5%. Killackey et al. (2008) conducted the first RCT of IPS in first-episode psychosis in Melbourne, Australia. They found that in the group that received IPS, 85% had a positive vocational outcome – defined as getting a job, enroling in a course, or both – compared to 23% in the control condition. Furthermore, there was a significant reduction in the IPS group in the use of welfare benefits as opposed to no reduction in the control group. Another trial of IPS from North America is due to report soon (Nuechterlein, personal communication). The evidence to date strongly supports IPS as a form of vocational intervention in FEP. Vocational recovery is important as it leads to social and economic inclusion in a way that very few other interventions can. Consequently, the consensus statement of the International First Episode Vocational Recovery (iFEVR) group supports the use of IPS in FEP (iFEVR Group 2008).

Further Issues

Within the early intervention movement, there are two further questions that need addressing: how long should treatment in specialized early intervention services continue and how cost-effective are early intervention services?

In relation to tenure of treatment, although early psychosis programmes have been shown to improve outcome in the short term (OPUS, LEO), there is evidence that gains may not be sustained over the longer term if specialized services are withdrawn. The 5-year outcome data from the OPUS study have recently been published. After 2 years of access to an early intervention service, patients received standard care for the next 3 years. The outcome data showed that many of the gains in outcome evident at 2 years had been eroded by 5 years (Bertelsen et al. 2007). These findings, coupled with the high rate of relapse in young people with psychosis (Emsley et al. 2007), have led some to suggest that a longer continuity of care within first-episode programmes is warranted. Clearly, the tenure of treatment required in optimal early psychosis services warrants further investigation. It could be that if a longer period of more specialized care were provided, then the favourable difference in outcome that was established between early intervention and treatment as usual, as seen in the OPUS trial over the first years, could be maintained (McGorry et al. 2008).

Regarding the question of cost-effectiveness, some preliminary data addressing this issue are now available. The Parachute project (Cullberg et al. 2006) compared an early intervention model of service with both an historical control and a prospective control. Although there were no differences in patient cost between the programmes in the second and third years of the project, in the first year the total costs of the early intervention condition were significantly lower than the prospective control condition ($11,614 vs. $23,192 $p<0.05$). This was mainly due to lower in-patient costs as the early intervention model was more focused on treatment in the community. This was also found earlier by an early psychosis programme in Melbourne (Mihalopoulos et al. 1999, 2007). A recent report by an independent economics firm in Australia found that the potential savings to the health system in Australia if early intervention was routinely available would be AUD$210,000,000 per year (Access Economics 2008). This saving does not include the saving that would also accrue if some of the newer interventions that show great promise such as vocational intervention (Killackey et al. 2008) were also included. Clearly, more studies are needed to draw firm conclusions about cost-effectiveness of early psychosis services, but these preliminary data are promising.

Future Directions – Clinical Staging

With the advent of UHR (prodromal) detection and treatment, we have seen the frontier of early intervention pushed further distal from the end state of schizophrenia. Can intervention occur even earlier?

Currently there is no aetiopathological basis for diagnosing psychotic disorders. They can therefore only be diagnosed by the presence of characteristic symptoms or combinations of symptoms. In addition, we have no known risk factors that predict onset of psychotic disorder with any specificity. Thus, primary prevention is presently out of our reach. But can we detect the prodrome even earlier than our present system of relying mainly on attenuated psychotic symptoms? German researchers attempted to do this through their concept of "basic symptoms" – subtle subjectively noted changes in experience and behaviour (Gross 1989; Huber and Gross 1989; Klosterkotter 1992). These basic symptoms are theorized to be more closely related to the underlying schizophrenic-disease process than positive psychotic symptoms and are thought to form the psychopathological base from which Schneiderian first-rank symptoms develop (Yung et al. 2007a; Schultze-Lutter et al. in press). They are therefore seen as occurring earlier than attenuated psychotic symptoms. The Cologne Early Recognition (CER) study (Klosterkotter et al. 2001) sought to investigate the validity of these basic symptoms for the prediction of schizophrenia. In this study, 385 patients who were thought to be in the prodromal phase of schizophrenia were prospectively followed up after an average 9.6 (±7.6) years. Nearly half (49.4%) of the sample of 160 who were contacted at follow-up had developed schizophrenia. Only two patients who subsequently developed schizophrenia had not reported any basic symptom at baseline. Thus the presence/absence of any basic symptom predicted later presence/absence of conversion to schizophrenia in 78.1% correctly. Hence the basic symptoms concept and methodology may represent a strategy for diagnosing and intervening even earlier in psychotic disorders. Surprisingly, until recently the basic symptoms have had limited impact in Anglophone psychiatry. However, since the growth of the UHR/prodromal field, they are beginning to have some influence and are now being more widely researched through the EPOS study (Klosterkotter et al. 2005), are included in the CAARMS instrument (Yung et al. 2005), a specialized tool for assessing the UHR group and are now more readily assessable through a specific instrument (Schultze-Lutter et al. 2004).

An alternative to the basic symptoms approach to earlier detection and intervention would be to attempt to identify the prodrome of psychotic disorder through the earliest signs of change from premorbid mental state and functioning. The earliest clinical stages of psychotic disorder are non-specific and overlap phenotypically with the initial stages of other disorders. For example, it has been shown that the prodromal phase of schizophrenia is indistinguishable from that of major depression (Hafner et al. 2005). Yet individuals do seek help for these symptoms and syndromes, even though a DSMIV diagnosis may not be possible at this early stage and considerable disability may already be present (Angold et al. 1999; Cosgrave et al. 2007). The idea would be to detect such help-seeking young people and offer them appropriate non-stigmatizing health care, without the expectation of a high rate of transition to psychotic disorder. That is, the aim would not be to expect a high degree of specificity but to detect individuals in need of treatment, some of whom may be at risk of psychotic disorder, some of whom may be at risk of a non-psychotic disorder and some of whom would spontaneously recover. Interventions would need to be benign and targeted at non-specific symptoms and could include, for example, supportive therapy, neuroprotective agents such as fish oil or exercise. This approach is consistent with the clinical staging model (McGorry 2007; McGorry et al. 2007). Clinical staging differs from conventional diagnostic practice in that it defines the extent of progression of disease at a particular point in time, and where a person lies currently along the continuum of the course of illness. The differentiation of early and milder clinical phenomena from those that accompany illness extension, progression and chronicity lies at the heart of the concept. It enables the clinician to select treatments relevant to earlier stages and assumes that such early interventions will be both more effective and less harmful than treatments delivered later in the course. Using this model to treat help-seeking individuals before onset of frank disorders would solve many of the second-order issues raised by the early psychosis reform process, such as diagnostic uncertainty despite a clear-cut need for care.

The aim of developing a system for detecting a range of mental problems in young people and treating them would be to provide cheap and non-toxic interventions to prevent worsening of problems. At the same time, young people who are identified through such systems could be assessed regarding potential markers of schizophrenia or other disorders. A clinical staging model, which allows the relationship of biological markers to stage of illness to be mapped, may help to validate the boundaries of current or newly defined clinical entities, distinguish core biological processes from epiphenomena and sequelae, and enable existing knowledge to be better represented and understood.

Conclusion

The growth of the early intervention movement has seen the advent of preventive thinking in relation to psychotic disorders. This has required a shift in the way schizophrenia and other psychotic disorders are viewed. Rather than seeing them as having inevitably poor prognoses with deterioration in social and functional outcome as the norm, more recent concepts and strategies, backed up by evidence, view the course of these disorders as much more fluid and malleable. As the International Early Psychosis Association states,

> Comprehensive programmes for the detection of early psychosis and in supporting the needs of young people with early psychosis carry the important function of promoting recovery, independence, equity and self-sufficiency and of facilitating the uptake of social, educational and employment opportunities (International Early Psychosis Association et al. 2005).

It is hoped that continued optimism can be backed by further evidence and translation of evidence into practice. There are now hundreds of early intervention programmes worldwide, of varying intensity and duration, which focus on the special needs of young people and their families. International clinical practice guidelines and a consensus statement have been published (Edwards and McGorry 2003) and clinical practice guidelines for the treatment of schizophrenia now typically have a major section on early psychosis (National Institute of Clinical Excellence 2003; Royal Australian and New Zealand College of Psychiatrists Clinical Practice Guidelines Team for the Treatment of Schizophrenia and Related Disorders 2005). The International Early Psychosis Association (www.iepa.org.au), an international organization which seeks to improve knowledge, clinical care and service reform in early psychosis, has been in existence for over 10 years. This association has over 3,000 members from over 60 different countries and has held 6 international conferences, stimulating and capturing a large volume of research and experience. In 2008, responding to the widespread international momentum, the US National Institute of Mental Health announced a new funding initiative to study and promote the development of better services for patients with first-episode psychosis (www.nimh.nih.gov). However, while this large international investment in early intervention is promising, many countries have made no progress at all and others have achieved only sparse coverage (McGorry et al. 2008). Governments worldwide need to recognize the public health importance of untreated and poorly treated mental disorders.

References

Access Economics. 2008. Cost Effectiveness of Early Intervention for Psychosis. Orygen Youth Health Research Centre, Melbourne.

Addington, J., E. Coldham, B. Jones, T. Ko, and D. Addington. 2003. The first episode of psychosis: The experience of relatives. Acta Psychiatr Scand 108:285–289.

Addington, J., A. McCleery, and D. Addington. 2005. Three year outcome of family work in an early psychosis program. Schizophr Res 79:107–116.

Amminger, G. P., M. R. Schaefer, K. Papageorgiou, J. Becker, N. Mossaheb, S. M. Harrigan, P. D. McGorry, and G. E. Berger. 2007. Omega-3 fatty acids reduce the risk of early transition to psychosis in ultra-high risk individuals: A double-blind randomized, placebo-controlled treatment study. Schizophr Bull 33:418–419.

Angold, A., E. J. Costello, E. Farmer, B. J. Burns, and A. Erkanli. 1999. Impaired but undiagnosed. J Am Acad Child Adolescent Psychiatry 38:129–137.

Bentall, R. P., and A. P. Morrison. 2002. More harm than good: The case against using antipsychotic drugs to prevent severe mental illness. Journal of Mental Health 11:351–356.

Bertelsen, M., P. Jeppesen, L. Petersen, and et al. 2007. Suicidal behaviour and mortality in first-episode psychosis: The OPUS trial. Br J Psychiatry 191(Suppl. 51):s140–s146.

Birchwood, M., J. Smith, F. Macmillan, B. Hogg, R. Prasad, C. Harvey, and S. Bering. 1989. Predicting relapse in schizophrenia: The development and implementation of an early signs monitoring system using patients and families as observers, a preliminary investigation. Psychol Med 19:649–656.

Birchwood, M., P. Todd, and C. Jackson. 1998. Early intervention in psychosis: The critical period hypothesis. Br J Psychiatry 172 (Suppl. 33):53–59.

Cannon, T. D., K. Cadenhead, B. Cornblatt, S. W. Woods, J. Addington, E. Walker, L. J. Seidman, D. Perkins, M. Tsuang, T. McGlashan, and R. Heinssen. 2008. Prediction of psychosis in youth at high clinical risk: A multisite longitudinal study in North America. Arch Gen Psychiatry 65:28–37.

Cassidy, E., S. Hill, and E. O'Callaghan. 2001. Efficacy of a psychoeducational intervention in improving relatives' knowledge about schizophrenia and reducing rehospitalisation. Eur Psychiatry 16:446–450.

Cornblatt, B., T. Lencz, C. Correll, A. Author, and C. Smith. 2002. Treating the prodrome: Naturalistic findings from the RAP program. Acta Psychiatr Scand 106:44.

Cornblatt, B. A., T. Lencz, and J. M. Kane. 2001. Treatment of the schizoporenia prodome: It is presently ethical? Schizophr Res 51:31–38.

Cosgrave, E. M., A. R. Yung, E. J. Killackey, J. A. Buckby, K. A. Godfrey, C. A. Stanford, and P. D. McGorry. 2008. Met and unmet need in youth mental health. J Mental Health, 17(6):618–628.

Craig, T. K. J., P. A. Garety, P. Power, N. Rahaman, S. Colbert, M. Fornells-Ambrojo, and G. Dunn. 2004. The Lambeth Early Onset (LEO) Team: Randomised controlled trial of the effectiveness of specialised care for early psychosis. Br Med J 329:1067.

Cullberg, J., M. Mattsson, S. Levander, R. Holmqvist, L. Tomsmark, C. Elingfors, and I. M. Wieselgren. 2006. Treatment costs and clinical outcome for first episode schizophrenia patients: A 3-year follow-up of the Swedish 'Parachute Project' and two comparison groups. Acta Psychiatr Scand 114:274–281.

Davis, D. J., and C. L. Schultz. 1998. Grief, parenting and schizophrenia. Soc Sci Med 46: 369–379.

Dyck, D. G., M. S. Hendryx, R. A. Short, W. D. Voss, and W. R. McFarlane. 2002 Service use among patients with schizophrenia in psychoeducational multiple family groups. Psychiatric Services 53:749–754.

Edwards, J., S. M. Francey, P. D. McGorry, and H. J. Jackson. 1994. Early psychosis prevention and intervention: Evolution of a comprehensive community-based specialised service. Behav Change 11:223–233.

Edwards, J., and P. D. McGorry. 2003. Implementing early intervention in psychosis: A guide to establishing early psychosis services. Aust NZ J Psychiatry 37.

Emsley, R., J. Rabinowitz, R. Medori, and Early Psychosis Global Working Group. 2007. Remission in early psychosis: Rates, prediction, and clinical and functional correlates. Schizophr Res 89:129–139.

Falloon, I., J. Boyd, and C. McGill. 1984. Family Care of Schizophrenia: A Problem Solving Approach to the Treatment of Mental Illness. Guilford Press, New York.

Garety, P. A., T. K. Craig, G. Dunn, M. Fornells-Ambrojo, S. Colbert, N. Rahaman, J. Read, and P. Power. 2006. Specialised care for early psychosis: Symptoms, social functioning and patient satisfaction: Randomised controlled trial. Br J Psychiatry 188:37–45.

Gross, G. 1989. The "basic" symptoms of schizophrenia. Br J Psychiatry 155(Suppl. 7):21–25.

Hafner, H., K. Maurer, G. Trendler, W. a. d. Heiden, M. Schmidt, and R. Konnecke. 2005. Schizophrenia and depression: Challenging the paradigm of two separate diseases – A controlled study of schizophrenia, depression and healthy controls. Schizophr Res 77: 11–24.

Haroun, N., L. Dunn, A. Haroun, and K. Cadenhead. 2006. Risk and protection in prodromal schizophrenia: Ethical implications for clinical practice and future research. Schizophr Bull 32:166–178.

Huber, G., and G. Gross. 1989 The concept of basic symptoms in schizophrenic and schizoaffective psychoses. Recenti Prog Med 80:646–652.

iFEVR Group. 2008. Meaningful Lives: Supporting Young People with Psychosis in Education, Training and Employment. International First Episode Vocational Recovery Group; 2008.www.iris-initiative.org.uk), Melbourne.

International Early Psychosis Association J. Addington, G. P. Amminger, A. Barbato, S. Catts, E. Chen, S. Chhim, S. A. Chong, J. Cullberg, J. Edwards, L. Grosso, M. Louza, M. Hambrecht, M. Keshavan, J. O. Johannessen, D. L. Johnson, S. Lewis, J. Lieberman, W. MacEwan, A. Malla, R. May, T. H. McGlashan, P. McGorry, M. G. Merlo, M. Nordentoft, S. Nightingale, D. Perkins, R. Thara, K. Yamamoto, and A. Yung. 2005. International clinical practice guidelines for early psychosis. Br J Psychiatry 187:120–124.

Jeppesen, P., L. Petersen, A. Thorup, et al. 2005. Integrated treatment of first-episode psychosis: Effect of treatment on family burden: OPUS trial. Br J Psychiatry 187(Suppl. 48): s85–s90.

Johannessen, J. O., T. K. Larsen, and I. Joa. 2005. Pathways to care for first-episode psychosis in an early detection healthcare sector: Part of the Scandinavian TIPS study. Br J Psychiatry 187(Suppl. 48):s24–s28.

Kahn, R. S., W. W. Fleischhacker, H. Boter, et. al. 2008. Effectiveness of antipsychotic drugs in first-episode schizophrenia and schizophreniform disorder: An open randomised clinical trial. Lancet 371:1085–1097.

Killackey, E. J., H. J. Jackson, J. Gleeson, I. B. Hickie, and P. D. McGorry. 2006. Exciting career opportunity beckons! early intervention and vocational rehabilitation in first episode psychosis: Employing cautious optimism. Aust NZ J Psychiatry 40:951–962.

Killackey, E., H. J. Jackson, and P. D. McGorry. 2008. Vocational intervention in first-episode psychosis: A randomised controlled trial of individual placement and support versus treatment as usual. Br J Psychiatry 193:114–120.

Klosterkotter, J. 1992. The meaning of basic symptoms for the development of schizophrenic psychoses. Neurology, Psychiatry and Brain Res 1:30–41.

Klosterkotter, J., M. Birchwood, D. Linszen, R. Salokangas, S. Ruhrmann, G. Juckel, A. Morrison, S. Lewis, and H. Graf von Reventlow. 2005. Overview on the recruitment, sample characteristics, and distribution of inclusion criteria of the European Prediction of Psychosis Study (EPOS). Eur Psychiatry 20:48.

Klosterkotter, J., M. Hellmich, E. M. Steinmeyer, and F. Schultze-Lutter. 2001. Diagnosing schizophrenia in the initial prodromal phase. Arch Gen Psychiatry 58:158–164.

Larsen, T. K., I. Melle, S. Friis, I. Joa, J. O. Johannessen, S. Opjordsmoen, E. Simonsen, P. Vaglum, and T. H. McGlashan. 2007. One-year effect of changing duration of untreated psychosis in a single catchment area. Br J Psychiatry 51:s128–s132.

Lehman, A. F., and D. M. Steinwachs. 1998. Patterns of usual care for schizophrenia: Initial results from the schizophrenia patient outcomes research team (PORT) client survey. Schizophr Bull 24:11–20.

Lieberman, J., D. Jody, S. Geisler, J. Alvir, A. Loebel, S. Szymanski, M. Woerner, and M. Borenstein. 1993. Time course and biologic correlates of treatment response in first-episode schizophrenia. Arch Gen Psychiatry 50:369–376.

Loebel, A. D., J. A. Lieberman, J. M. Alvir, D. I. Mayerhoff, S. H. Geisler, and S. R. Szymanski. 1992. Duration of psychosis and outcome in first-episode schizophrenia. Am J Psychiatry 149:1183–1188.

Macmillan, F., and D. Shiers. 2000. The IRIS programme. In M. Birchwood, D. Fowler, and C. Jackson (eds.) Early Intervention in Psychosis: A Guide to Concepts, Evidence and Interventions, pp. 315–326. Wiley, Chichester.

Marshall, M., S. Lewis, A. Lockwood, R. Drake, P. Jones, and T. Croudace. 2005. Association between duration of untreated psychosis and outcome in cohorts of first-episode patients. Arch Gen Psychiatry 62:975–983.

Marwaha, S., and S. Johnson. 2004. Schizophrenia and employment: A review. Soc Psychiatry Psychiatr Epidemiol 39:337–349.

McFarlane, W. R. 2002. Multifamily Groups in the Treatment of Severe Psychiatric Disorders. Guilford Press, New York, USA.

McFarlane, W. R., and K. Cunningham. 1996. Multiple-family groups and psychoeducation: Creating therapeutic social networks. J.V. Vaccaro and G.H. Clark Jr. (eds.) Practicing Psychiatry in the Community: A Manual, pp. 387–406, xxii, 510 pp.

McGlashan, T. H. 1999. Duration of untreated psychosis in first episode schizophrenia: Marker or determinant of course. Biol Psychiatry 46:729–739.

McGlashan, T. H., J. Addington, T. Cannon, M. Heinimaa, P. McGorry, M. O'Brien, D. Penn, D. Perkins, R. K. R. Salokangas, B. Walsh, S. W. Woods, and A. Yung. 2007. Recruitment and treatment practices for help-seeking "prodromal" patients. Schizophr Bull 33:715–726.

McGlashan, T. H., R. B. Zipursky, D. Perkins, J. Addington, T. J. Miller, S. W. Woods, K. A. Hawkins, R. Hoffman, S. Lindborg, M. Tohen, and A. Breier. 2003. The PRIME North America randomized double-blind clinical trial of olanzapine versus placebo in patients at risk of being prodromally symnptomatic for psychosis: I. Study rationale and design. Schizophr Res 61:7–18.

McGlashan, T. H., R. B. Zipursky, D. Perkins, J. Addington, T. Miller, S. W. Woods, K. A. Hawkins, R. E. Hoffman, A. Preda, I. Epstein, D. Addington, S. Lindborg, Q. Trzaskoma, M. Tohen, and A. Breier. 2006. Randomized, double-blind trial of olanzapine versus placebo in patients prodromally symptomatic for psychosis. Am J Psychiatry 163:790–799.

McGorry, P. D. 2007. Issues for DSM-V: Clinical staging: A heuristic pathway to valid nosology and safer, more effective treatment in psychiatry. Am J Psychiatry 164:859–860.

McGorry, P. D., E. Killackey, and A. R. Yung. 2008. Early intervention in psychosis: Concepts, evidence and future directions. World Psychiatry 7:148–156.

McGorry, P. D., R. Purcell, I. Hickie, A. R. Yung, C. Pantelis, and H. J. Jackson. 2007. Clinical staging: A heuristic model for psychiatry and youth mental health. Med J Aust 187:40–42.

McGorry, P. D., and A. R. Yung. 2003. Early intervention in psychosis: An overdue reform. Aust NZ J Psychiatry 37:393–398.

McGorry, P. D., A. R. Yung, and L. J. Phillips. 2003. The 'close-in' or ultra high risk model: A safe and effective strategy for research and clinical intervention in prepsycxhotic mental disorder. Schizophr Bull 29:771–790.

McGorry, P. D., A. R. Yung, L. J. Phillips, H. P. Yuen, S. Francey, E. M. Cosgrave, J. Bravin, S. Adlard, T. MacDonald, A. Blair, and H. Jackson. 2002. Randomized controlled trial of interventions designed to reduce the risk of progression to first episode psychosis in a clinical sample with subthreshold symptoms. Arch Gen Psychiatry 59:921–928.

Melle, I., T. K. Larsen, U. Haahr, S. Friis, J. O. Johannessen, S. Opjordsmoen, E. Simonsen, B. R. Rund, P. Vaglum, and T. McGlashan. 2004. Reducing the duration of untreated first-episode psychosis: Effects on clinical presentation. Arch Gen Psychiatry 61:143–150.

Mihalopoulos, C., M. Harris, and L. Henry, et al. 2007. Are the short-term cost savings and benefits of an early psychosis program maintained at 8-year follow-up? Schizophr Bull 33:487.

Mihalopoulos, C., P. D. McGorry, and R. C. Carter. 1999. Is phase-specific, community oriented treatment of early psychosis an economically viable method of improving outcome? Acta Psychiatr Scand 100:47–55.

Morrison, A. P., P. French, S. Parker, M. Roberts, H. Stevens, R. P. Bentall, and S. W. Lewis. 2007. Three-year follow-up of a randomized controlled trial of cognitive therapy for the prevention of psychosis in people at ultra high risk. Schizophr Bull 33:682–687.

Morrison, A. P., P. French, L. Walford, S. W. Lewis, A. Kilcommons, J. Green, S. Parker, and R. P. Bentall. 2004. Cognitive therapy for the prevention of psychosis in people at ultra-high risk: Randomised controlled trial. Br J Psychiatry 185:291–297.

Mrazek, P. J., and R. J. Haggerty, eds. 1994. Reducing Risks for Mental Disorders: Frontiers for Preventive Intervention Research. National Academy Press, Washington DC.

National Institute of Clinical Excellence. 2003. Schizophrenia: Full National Clinical Guideline on Core Interventions in Primary and Secondary Care. Gaskell and the British Psychological Society, London.

Norman, R. M. G., and A. K. Malla. 2001. Duration of untreated psychosis: A critical examination of the concept and its importance. Psychol Med 31:381–400.

Olsen, K. A., and B. Rosenbaum. 2006. Prospective investigations of the prodromal state of schizophrenia: Review of studies. Acta Psychiatr Scand 113:247–272.

Perez-Iglesias, R., B. Crespo-Facorro, and O. Martinez-Garcia. 2008. Weight gain induced by haloperidol, risperidone and olanzapine after 1 year: Findings of a randomized clinical trial in a drug-naive population. Schizophr Res 99:13–22.

Perkins, D. O., H. Gu, and K. Boteva. 2005. Relationship between duration of untreated psychosis and outcome in first-episode schizophrenia: A critical review and meta-analysis. Am J Psychiatry 162:1785–1804.

Petersen, L., M. Nordentoft, P. Jeppesen, et al. 2005. Improving 1-year outcome in first-episode psychosis: OPUS trial. Br J Psychiatry 187(Suppl. 48):s98–s103.

Phillips, L. J., P. D. McGorry, H. P. Yuen, J. Ward, K. Donovan, D. Kelly, S. M. Francey, and A. R. Yung. 2007. Medium term follow-up of a randomized controlled trial of interventions for young people at Ultra High Risk of psychosis. Schizophr Res 96:25–33.

Pitschel-Walz, G., S. Leucht, J. Bauml, W. Kissling, and R. R. Engel. 2001. The effect of family interventions on relapse and rehospitalization in schizophrenia – a meta-analysis. Schizophr Bull 27:73–92.

Power, P., E. Iacoponi, N. Reynolds, H. Fisher, M. Russell, P. Garety, P. K. McGuire, and T. Craig. 2007a. The Lambeth Early Onset Crisis Assessment Team Study: General practitioner education and access to an early detection team in first-episode psychosis. . Br J Psychiatry 51: s133–s139.

Power, P., P. McGuire, E. Iacoponi, P. Garety, E. Morris, L. Valmaggia, D. Grafton, and T. Craig. 2007b. Lambeth early onset (LEO) and outreach & support in south London (OASIS) service. Early Intervention in Psychiatry 1:97–103.

Rinaldi, M., K. McNeil, M. Firn, M. Koletsi, R. Perkins, and S. P. Singh. 2004. What are the benefits of evidence-based supported employment for patients with first-episode psychosis? Psychiatric Bull 28:281–284.

Robinson, D., M. G. Woerner, J. M. Alvir, R. M. Bilder, G. Hinrichsen, and J. A. Lieberman. 2002. Predictors of medication discontinuation by patients with first episode schizophrenia and schizoaffective disorder. Schizophr Res 57:209–219.

Robinson, D., M. G. Woerner, J. M. Alvir, S. Geisler, A. Koreen, B. B. Sheitman, M. Chakos, D. Mayerhoff, R. M. Bilder, R. Goldman, and J. A. Lieberman. 1999. Predictors of treatment response from a first episode of schizophrenia or schizoaffective disorder. Am J Psychiatry 156:544–549.

Rosen, J. L., T. J. Miller, J. T. D'Andrea, T. H. McGlashan, and S. W. Woods. 2006. Comorbid diagnoses in patients meeting criteria for the schizophrenia prodrome. Schizophr Res 85(1–3) Jul 2006, 124–131.

Royal Australian and New Zealand College of Psychiatrists Clinical Practice Guidelines Team for the Treatment of Schizophrenia and Related Disorders. 2005. Royal Australian and New Zealand College of Psychiatrists clinical practice guidelines for the treatment of schizophrenia and related disorders. Aust NZ J Psychiatry 39:1–30.

Ruhrmann, S., F. Schultze-Lutter, and J. Klosterkotter. 2003. Early detection and intervention in the initial prodromal phase of schizophrenia. Pharmacopsychiatry 36:S162–S167.

Schley, C., V. Ryall, L. Crothers, S. Radovini, K. Fletcher, K. Marriage, S. Nudds, C. Groufsky, and H. P. Yuen. 2008. Early intervention with difficult to engage, 'high-risk' youth: Evaluating an intensive outreach approach in youth mental health. Early Intervention in Psychiatry 2: 195–200.

Schultze-Lutter, F., E. M. Steinmeyer, and J. Klosterkotter. in press. Early detection of schizophrenia. Schizophr Res.

Schultze-Lutter, F., A. Wieneke, H. Picker, Y. Rolff, E. M. Steinmeyer, S. Ruhrmann, and J. Klosterkoetter. 2004. The Schizophrenia Prediction Instrument, Adult Version (SPI-A). Schizophr Res 70/1S:76–77.

Secker, J., B. Grove, and P. Seebohm. 2001. Challenging barriers to employment, training and education for mental health service users: The service user's perspective. J Mental Health 10:395–404.

Svirskis, T., J. Korkeila, M. Heinimaa, J. Huttunen, T. Ilonen, T. Ristkari, T. McGlashan, and R. K. Salokangas. 2005. Axis-I disorders and vulnerability to psychosis. Schizophr Res 75(2–3) Jun 2005:439–446.

Tauscher-Wisniewski, S., and R. Zipursky. 2002. The role of maintenance pharmacotherapy in achieving recovery from a first episode of schizophrenia. Int Rev Psychiatry 14:284–292.

Thorup, A., L. Petersen, P. Jeppesen, J. Ohlenschlaeger, T. Christensen, G. Krarup, P. Jorgensen, and M. Nordentoft. 2005. Integrated treatment ameliorates negative symptoms in first episode psychosis – results from the danish OPUS trial. Schizophr Res 79:95–105.

Warner, R. 2005. Problems with early and very early intervention in psychosis. Br J Psychiatry 48:s104–s107.

Yung, A. R., E. Killackey, S. Hetrick, A. G. Parker, F. Schultze-Lutter, J. Klosterkoetter, R. Purcell, and P. D. McGorry. 2007a. The prevention of schizophrenia. Int Rev Psychiatry 19:1–14.

Yung, A. R., and P. D. McGorry. 1996. The prodromal phase of first episode psychosis: Past and current conceptualisations. Schizophrenia Bull 22:353–370.

Yung, A. R., P. D. McGorry, S. M. Francey, B. Nelson, K. Baker, L. J. Phillips, G. Berger, and G. P. Amminger. 2007b. PACE- A specialised service for young people at risk of psychotic disorders. Med J Aust 187:43–47.

Yung, A. R., P. D. McGorry, C. A. McFarlane, H. J. Jackson, G. C. Patton, and A. Rakkar. 1996. Monitoring and care of young people at incipient risk of psychosis. Schizophr Bull 22:283–303.

Yung, A. R., L. J. Phillips, and P. D. McGorry. 2004a. Treating Schizophrenia in the Prodromal Phase. Taylor and Francis, London.

Yung, A. R., L. J. Phillips, H. P. Yuen, S. M. Francey, C. A. McFarlane, M. Hallgren, and P. D. McGorry. 2003. Psychosis prediction: 12-month follow up of a high-risk ("prodromal") group. Schizophr Res 60:21–32.

Yung, A. R., L. J. Phillips, H. P. Yuen, and P. D. McGorry. 2004b. Risk factors for psychosis in an ultra high-risk group: Psychopathology and clinical features. Schizophr Res 67:131–142.

Yung, A. R., H. P. Yuen, P. D. McGorry, L. Phillips, D. Kelly, M. Dell'Olio, S. Francey, E. Cosgrave, E. Killackey, C. Stanford, K. Godfrey, and J. Buckby. 2005. Mapping the onset of psychosis – the Comprehensive Assessment of At Risk Mental States (CAARMS). Aust NZ J Psychiatry 39:964–971.

The Cross-Sectional and Longitudinal Architecture of Schizophrenia: Significance for Diagnosis and Intervention?

Wolfgang Gaebel, Wolfgang Wölwer, Mathias Riesbeck, and Jürgen Zielasek

Introduction

In the course of revising the current psychiatric classification systems, one of the major questions relates to the classification of schizophrenia. While cross-sectional issues of the pathogenesis of schizophrenia are duly reviewed in other chapters of this book, recent discussions have put aspects of the longitudinal time course of schizophrenia into their focus. Considering the onset of schizophrenia, initial prodromal symptoms have been characterized but yet yield a low sensitivity and specificity with progression rates to full-blown schizophrenia or "psychosis" in general (including affective disorders) ranging from approximately 15 to 40% in different studies. Thus, the question arises whether such findings warrant the inclusion of a novel "prodromal state" into the mental disorders chapter of the *International Classification of Diseases* (11th revision, hence ICD-11) or the *Diagnostic and Statistical Manual* issued by the American Psychiatric Association (5th revision, hence DSM-V). What may be the new diagnostic and therapeutic strategies to be employed in the obviously prognostically very important early stages of schizophrenia? Once schizophrenia has fully developed, cognitive dysfunctions like reduced attention and impairments of working memory play a major role in the determination of the further disease course in particular considering functional disabilities. This suggests these factors to be prime targets for novel therapeutic approaches. But can schizophrenia be regarded as a cognitive disorder and may the pathophysiological processes be regarded as exerting their pathogenetic actions on predefined and functionally discernible brain modules? Finally, social cognition has turned out to be a central determinant of functions of daily living including such important aspects as vocational functioning and integration into society. All these aspects were covered in the presentations of the session on "Psychopathology, cognition, outcome" at the 6th Symposium on the Search for the Causes of Schizophrenia in Sao Paulo, Brazil,

W. Gaebel (✉)
Department of Psychiatry and Psychotherapy, Heinrich-Heine-University Duesseldorf, Clinics of the Rhineland Regional Council, Bergische Landstraße 2, D-40629 Düsseldorf, Germany
e-mail: wolfgang.gaebel@uni-duesseldorf.de

W.F. Gattaz, G. Busatto (eds.), *Advances in Schizophrenia Research 2009*, DOI 10.1007/978-1-4419-0913-8_17, © Springer Science+Business Media, LLC 2010 in February 2009. This chapter will review the central ideas of the contributions in this session and will emphasize aspects of the time course of schizophrenia starting with the (potential) prodromal syndrome, followed by a discussion of the role of cognitive dysfunctions with an emphasis on social cognition in schizophrenia and novel preventive and therapeutic approaches based on such findings.

Diagnosis and Classification: From Description to Function, to Brain Modules – and Beyond?

Already Emil Kraepelin in 1920 claimed that the "patterns of mental disorders" were the "natural response of the human machinery," which could be traced back to the "interplay of preformed mechanisms of our organism" due to the disturbance of "identical areas" (Kraepelin 1920). Today, in the course of revising ICD-10 and DSM-IV, similar ideas are being proposed, which take the shape of "disorder clusters" as a novel means of structuring the classification of mental disorders. For instance, Andrews and coworkers (unpublished) suggested defining a neurocognitive cluster (including such disorders as delirium, dementias, amnestic and other cognitive disorders), a developmental cluster (mental retardation, learning, motor skill and communication disorders, pervasive developmental disorders), a psychosis cluster (including schizophrenia, bipolar disorders, and schizotypal personality disorder), an emotional cluster (encompassing depression, anxiety disorders, post-traumatic stress disorder, and dissociative and somatoform disorders), and an "externalizing cluster" (with substance use disorders and impulse control disorders among others). The underlying guiding principle is that mental disorders – which are of a complex nature – may be decomposed into different symptom complexes that may have different neural substrates and etiological factors. A disorder like "schizophrenia" may then be decomposed into a cluster of "positive symptoms," "negative symptoms," "cognitive symptoms," and "mood symptoms" (Hyman and Ivleva 2008). Many non-affected relatives may have minor symptoms or correlated structural and functional deficits, giving the clusters a dimensional characteristic. The current task is to define such clusters and validate them in field trials. For the cognitive symptoms, several initiatives are underway to define the most relevant cognitive domains, identify the clinical tests available for their assessment, and investigate the neural basis of these functions. The definition of neural circuits for disorder domains is still in its infancy, but several basic cognitive functions can be assigned to specific interconnected brain areas, like the amygdalae and their connections for the recognition of fearful facial expressions, or the hippocampus with its connections to the anterior cingulate and the dorsolateral prefrontal cortex for memory functions (Tamminga 2008). Viewing such functionally specified "modules" of the brain, a modular concept of psychiatric classification may be constructed in which these basic functional brain units become the targets of pathophysiological effects of genetic or environmental factors (Murphy and Stich 2000; Zielasek and Gaebel 2008). Recent applications of functional network analyses have shown disturbed hierarchical organizations of brain networks in schizophrenia and the assessment of modularity has become one of the parameters of such network analyses (cf. Bullmore and Spoons 2009, and references therein). While Kraepelin's idea was focused on anatomically localizable, functionally specified brain areas, today's neuroscience informs us that the localization of functionally specified brain areas is possible, but that their connectivity with other brain areas is of similar importance and that such networks are dynamical in nature.

Regarding the application of such principles to schizophrenia, it appears that schizophrenia is composed of a psychotic core found in all patients supplemented with varying additional symptom clusters like negative symptoms, cognitive impairments, reality distortion, disorganization, and affective symptoms. These may, however, become the leading factors for social disintegration in the course of the disorder. Several different ways are theoretically possible to "deconstruct" psychotic disorders (recently reviewed by Gaebel and Zielasek 2008), and the main issue here will be to define selection criteria and design field trials to validate such "clusters."

The cross-sectional architecture of schizophrenia in such a modular approach would necessitate the assessment of all relevant modular dysfunctions leading to a profile of disturbances of functional brain circuits (here termed "modules"). These different modules would be affected in different degrees and each clinical syndrome or "cluster" may be composed of a different set of disturbances. Figure 1 gives an example of such a profile in the case of severe delusions of persecution and auditory hallucinations. Obviously, the pattern would be quite different in a hebephrenic patient with a "deficit syndrome," in which motor, social cognitive, or affective modules would be preferentially affected (cf. arrows in Fig. 1). Most importantly, such a cross-sectional architecture would not be stable over time, due to either the natural disease course or the effects of therapeutic measures. This may also influence

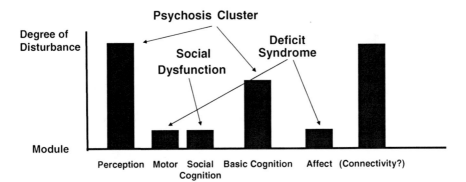

Fig. 1 Cross-sectional architecture of "schizophrenia" in a modular approach. An example of the cross-sectional architecture of a psychotic syndrome with severe delusions of persecution and auditory hallucinations, with the height of each bar denoting the degree of disturbance of the respective module. A putative "psychosis cluster" would mainly involve elements of basic cognition and perception. Alternatively, in a severe hebephrenic syndrome, modules comprising the deficit syndrome including social dysfunctions would be more severely affected

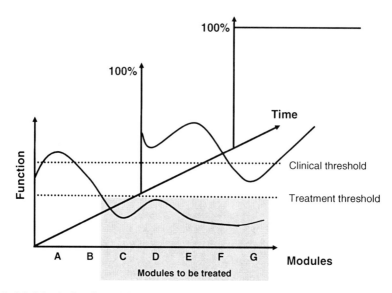

Fig. 2 Modular dysfunction, clinical diagnosis, and treatment decisions. Mental disorders are conceived of as a pattern of dysfunctions of functionally defined neural networks ("modules"). The y-axis gives the degree of functioning, with "100%" denoting normal function. In the first graph, the function of module A is slightly impaired (i.e., not 100% functional), but this does not lead to clinically detectable signs or symptoms (the clinical threshold is denoted by the upper dotted line). Module B is more severely impaired and its dysfunction may be clinically detected, but its dysfunction does not yet reach a degree to warrant therapy (note the lower dotted line, which indicates the treatment threshold). Modules C–G are most markedly dysfunctional and have fallen below the treatment threshold. With time (z-axis), the pattern of affected modules may change (second graph in time) and successful treatment or the natural course of the disorder may lead to full functional recovery (top line indicating that all modules have regained full functionality)

the continuous reassessment of treatment decisions, which may change over time given that the pattern of affected modules varies with time. Also, there may be a significant difference between a clinical threshold (i.e., the degree of disturbance of a module that makes its dysfunction clinically detectable) and a treatment threshold (i.e., the degree of disturbance of a module that makes treatment necessary). Thus, both the pattern of affected modules and the points where treatment decision have to be made are of a dynamic nature and need to be reassessed continuously during the disease course (Fig. 2).

Cognitive Function as a Criterion for Diagnosis, Course, and Prognosis?

The importance of cognitive functions as major determinants of functional outcomes in schizophrenia was addressed by Nuechterlein in this conference and may be summarized as follows: Cognitive impairments in schizophrenia are stable across different stages of the disorder including periods of remissions; they can even be detected in non-affected first-degree relatives. Cognitive impairments are good predictors of the functional outcome in schizophrenia and they may also be suitable to predict the clinical course both before (e.g., Brewer et al. 2005, Lencz et al. 2005, Keefe et al. 2006, Whyte et al. 2006) and after the onset of schizophrenia (e.g., Wölwer et al. 2008). However, the neuropsychological tests usually used are not sensitive and specific enough to warrant their use for individual predictions. Several separable cognitive domains of functional importance have been identified by the MATRICS initiative (Nuechterlein et al. 2008). By drawing from developments in cognitive neuroscience, the CNTRICS initiative is currently in the process of selecting elementary cognitive paradigms with close ties to neural substrates as putative additional treatment targets in schizophrenia (Carter et al. 2008). Not surprisingly, the latter include domains of visual perception, working memory, attention, executive control, long-term memory, and social/emotional processing. In contrast to this deconstructionist approach, Dickinson and Harvey (2008) have suggested focusing on the generalized or more global cognitive deficit in schizophrenia. Neural network integration, reduced arborization and connectivity in distal dendritic processes, reduced fiber tract coherence, and myelin abnormalities may all be determinants of such generalized cognitive impairments.

An important question is how cognition and functional outcome are linked. Social cognitive processes appear to be of central importance concerning this relationship. Recent studies have shown that a two-factor model using both social cognition and basic cognition (often termed "neurocognition") better explains observational data than a one-factor model of "general cognition" (Sergi et al., 2007), and that social cognition qualifies as a separable factor in addition to factors representing basic cognition (Allen et al. 2007). A recent workshop organized by the National Institutes of Mental Health has defined relevant terms in this area and identified suggestions for future research (Green et al. 2008). Despite social and basic cognition seeming to be separable factors, they are not independent of each other. Schmidt et al. (2008) reported a shared variance of about 50% between basic cognitive and social cognitive impairments. There is accumulating evidence that social cognitive processes mediate the impact of basic cognition on functional outcome, e.g., Schmidt and coworkers found that social cognition explains approximately 17% of the functional outcome impairment in schizophrenia, whereas the direct impact of basic cognition on functional outcome explained only about 9% (see also Addington et al. 2006, Sergi et al. 2006). In a similar type of analysis, Bowie and coworkers (2006, 2008) developed models predicting real-world behavior with data from specific neuropsychological and functional capacity measures in schizophrenia. Neuropsychological functioning showed a high degree of correlation with functional capacity, which in turn showed a high degree of correlation with work skill performance, community activities and interpersonal activities. More specifically, certain outcome measures were best correlated with some specific cognitive domains, for example, only processing speed and measures of attention/working memory predicted social competence, and the latter domain was directly related to work skill performance. Symptoms were directly related to outcomes, with fewer relationships with competences. Thus, it appears feasible to identify the relative contributions of symptoms and specific cognitive domains to predefined functionally relevant outcome measures. This information will be very useful to identify those cognitive domains that may be prime targets to achieve improvements in "real-world behavior."

Given the before-mentioned importance of cognitive functions for fulfilling one's everyday role in family and community life, an important question is how far schizophrenia may be conceptualized as a cognitive disorder, with the acute delusional or hallucinatory delusions being consequences of such cognitive dysfunctions. But how specific are cognitive dysfunctions for schizophrenia as compared to affective disorders? Recent reviews by Buchanan et al. (2005) and Keefe and Fenton (2007) indicate that the patterns of cognitive dysfunctions in schizophrenia and affective disorders are not so much different regarding the areas of cognition that are affected, but rather the severity of dysfunction is more pronounced and more stable in the course of schizophrenia than in major depressive disorders or in euthymic bipolar disorder. Thus, due to their importance for functional outcome, cognitive factors were proposed to be included in the future definition of schizophrenia (Keefe and Fenton 2007; Keefe 2008, and discussion therein).

A second question addresses the issue whether the appearance of cognitive dysfunctions may serve as a predictor for future illness manifestation, and may qualify as a determinant of future illness progression. Keefe and coworkers (2006) showed that the total cognitive capacity is most impaired in patients with first-episode schizophrenia, followed by those at a high risk of developing schizophrenia who later develop schizophrenia, as compared to those not progressing to frank schizophrenia. Likewise, other studies have shown that the degree of impairments in memory functions in high-risk individuals may predict the subsequent transition to manifest psychosis (Brewer et al. 2005, Lencz et al. 2005, Whyte et al. 2006). But how may the link between functional outcome and cognitive function be constructed? Obviously, normal psychophysiological function depends on a physiological balance of neurotransmitters and neuroanatomic integrity. This sustains normal basic cognitive functions like attention, memory, and other types of information processing, which are the building blocks of integrative complex cognitive functions like abstract mental representations, volition, or social cognition. Several models have been proposed to explain psychotic symptoms with disturbed cognitive functions, like cognitive neuropsychiatric models of persecutory delusions (Blackwood et al. 2001; Freeman 2007) or Kapur et al.'s (2003) model of aberrant salience. Couture and coworkers (2006) extended these approaches to formulate a conceptual model of social cognition and functional outcome. Freeman and coworkers (this conference) investigated the cognitive and social processes underlying psychotic phenomenology focusing on persecutory delusions. Virtual reality studies provide novel experimental evidence that individual factors play a very important role in determining the "meaning" of social situations and that internal anomalous experiences, negative affects like anxiety, and reasoning biases (for example, jumping to conclusions or failure to consider alternatives) may all be involved in a complex and inter-individually variable combination. Social factors like traumatic experiences or an urban development add to these cognitive factors. Thus, a range of triggers like major (critical?) life events may lead to anomalous experiences. These, combined with reasoning biases and emotional dysfunctions like increased worry, may misguide a (physiological!) search for meaning into a pathologic persecutory (threat) belief. Most importantly, interventions that target such contributing factors are being developed and initial evidence indicates that, for example, a "worry intervention" may reduce distress in psychotic individuals. These approaches may lead to the development of a multi-component behavioral intervention in the future.

Considering the potential for treating separable cognitive domains in schizophrenia, recent meta-analyses showed a significant reduction in positive symptoms after cognitive-behavioral interventions in schizophrenia (Zimmermann et al. 2005), but only mild improvements in cognitive functions following the administration of antipsychotic medication (Woodward et al. 2005). Cognitive remediation programs produce modest improvements in cognitive performance and – when combined with psychiatric rehabilitation – also improve functional outcome (McGurk et al. 2007). Such cognitive remediation programs differ with regard to the scope of cognitive domains addressed, i.e., whether the program focuses on only one cognitive domain like affect recognition or whether several subcomponents are addressed in parallel. Considering social cognition, impairments in the recognition of facial affect have been shown to be remediable by domain-specific, "focused" programs (e.g. Training of Affect Recognition, TAR, Wölwer et al. 2005) as well as by "broader" social cognitive skills training (SCST, Horan et al. 2009) addressing affect perception, social perception, attributional style, and Theory of Mind. The fact that the SCST improves affect recognition independently both of changes in basic cognitive functions and of other social cognitive functions may indicate that facial affect recognition is a separable cognitive domain (Horan et al. 2009). Importantly, practice effects in training programs must be considered in the analysis of putative domain-specific therapeutic (in particular drug-related) effects (Goldberg et al. 2007), which poses an additional challenge to trial designers. The more the knowledge gained about the neural networks underlying the relatively basic but still complex cognitive functions such as affect recognition or memory, the more likely it becomes that novel targets not only for training programs but also for pharmacological interventions will be identified. A recent review by Gray and Roth (2007) listed several neurotransmitters, their receptors and metabolic pathways including dopamine, nicotine, serotonine, and gamma-aminobutyric acid (GABA) among the most promising candidates. Some clinical studies lend reason to cautious optimism that novel domain-specific cognitive therapies will be developed in the near future and may lead to clinically meaningful improvements for patients with schizophrenia. Still, several conceptual questions as discussed by Keith Nuechterlein in this conference are currently open and need to be clarified in carefully designed clinical studies:

1. Will it be preferable to target specific cognitive functions or rather a generalized cognitive deficit in schizophrenia trials?
2. What are the therapeutically most relevant cognitive functions and what is the biological basis of their dysfunction in schizophrenia?

3. Can we develop therapies that specifically target social cognition or other cognitive functions based on their neurobiological underpinnings?

Time for Early Diagnosis, Early Intervention – and Prevention?

Given this progress on the role of cognitive dysfunctions in the pathogenesis of schizophrenia, a critical analysis is warranted of the question whether it is time to consider early diagnosis and early prevention for those who are at an increased risk of developing schizophrenia. The early illness course of schizophrenia is characterized by a premorbid and a prodromal phase, characterized by unspecific (e.g., impairments in concentration, sleep disturbances, restlessness, depressed mood) or more specific symptoms (e.g., ideas of reference, impression of being controlled, perceptual disturbances). Such pre-psychotic symptoms may be elements of a dynamic process in which symptoms come and go, in which coping strategies may limit the clinical effects of such symptoms and in which the threshold of clinical detection may be passed in both directions several times over time. In a modular approach to mental disorders, this may be depicted as in Fig. 3. But what is the meaning of a "prodromal syndrome" considering schizophrenia? It may be a subthreshold illness variant with certain determinants for a progressive disease course, which may be amenable to treatment. Alternatively, it may be a comorbid disorder independent of the genuine schizophrenia disease process (this is suggested by the frequent affective symptoms in the prodromal phase, which may be part of an

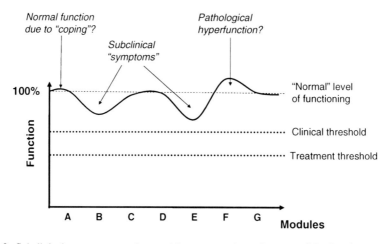

Fig. 3 Subclinical symptoms, prodrome, risk status – a dynamic process? During the prodromal illness state, the function of one or several modules may be impaired without reaching the threshold of clinical signs or symptoms, but may be detectable by specific clinical tests. Also, coping strategies may successfully limit the development of impairment of modules leading even back to normal function. Also, the pathological hyperfunction of modules may play a role, like acoustic perception modules with spontaneous activity leading to acoustic hallucinations

underlying comorbid affective disorder). Prodromal symptoms may also be mere indicators of vulnerability, and may be completely unrelated to the disease process. They may also be part of a physiological stress reaction that occurs due to the separate underlying schizophrenia process leading to cognitive disturbances like persecutory misinterpretations of environmental signals. Together with epidemiological studies, the identification of the elements of a prodromal state may also lead to the definition of an "early" and a "late" prodromal state (Bechdolf et al. 2005; Ruhrmann et al. 2007). Both psychological and pharmacological interventions appear to be moderately effective in preventing progression to manifest schizophrenia in these early stages of the disorder. However, while previous studies had shown rather high spontaneous conversion rates in the range 30–40% (Cannon et al. 2008; Klosterkötter et al. 2008), a recent study from Australia showed a conversion rate of only 16% even in "ultra-high risk" individuals (Yung et al. 2008, and this conference). Given these epidemiological discrepancies, the factors governing the progression need to be identified and may encompass genetic factors, psychological factors, social factors, and a history of substance abuse. As an example, cognitive disease course predictors in high-risk persons were identified including memory functions and sustained attention (Brewer et al. 2005; Lencz et al. 2006; Keefe et al. 2006; Whyte et al. 2006), but it remains to be determined whether therapeutically addressing these dysfunctions is of any functional efficacy. Generally, one of the central questions is whether future studies should focus on a reduction in functional disability in prodromal states rather than on a reduction of the progression rate to schizophrenia and whether biological measures can increase sensitivity and specificity of the prediction (Cannon 2008). Recently published Italian guidelines for early intervention in schizophrenia clearly state that due to scarce evidence, recommendations for interventions targeting prodromal (non-psychotic) persons cannot be given, but that early intervention programs are highly recommended for the early psychotic phase. Needs-orientation of these services and independence of the traditional mental health services were recommended (DeMasi et al. 2008; Gaebel and Riesbeck 2008).

How can the predictive sensitivity and specificity of prognostic features in prodromal schizophrenia be increased in order to reliably identify those individuals who are at risk of developing the full clinical picture? In this context, it is interesting that some genetic factors seem to indicate a rather high conversion rate, but larger field trials are necessary to show whether such information is already sensitive enough on a population level to warrant inclusion in preventive trials (Hall et al. 2006; Keri et al. 2009). While the neuregulin 1 gene apparently is a risk factor for an extended or intermediate phenotype, current research is focusing also on the COMTval158met polymorphism and its predictive validity including its effects in neuroimaging studies ("imaging genetics"; Lawrie et al. 2008). Neuroimaging is also considered as a means to improve the prediction of disease progression. Cortical volume loss – most pronounced in the right prefrontal area – was found to be associated with psychosis onset (Sun et al. 2009), and white matter volume changes were shown in people developing psychosis (Walterfang et al. 2008). Furthermore, once the disorder has progressed to the first manifest episode of schizophrenia, cortical volume loss was found to be positively associated with a poorer clinical course (Wobrock et al., in press). Further studies are needed to verify that such changes are also detectable on the individual and not just a group comparison level, and are sufficiently sensitive and specific to be useful for individual counseling in high-risk persons. In a positron emission tomography study, Howes et al. (2009) recently showed that elevated striatal dopamine function is associated with prodromal signs of schizophrenia and neuropsychological impairment. This novel approach may yield important new links in the intricate chain of events between morphology, function, and outcome in the early stages of schizophrenia, but currently only in the framework of clinical studies.

Given the many open questions regarding the optimal definition of the prodromal state, it appears unlikely that "prodromal schizophrenia" is already sufficiently characterized on a diagnostic level to warrant inclusion as a novel diagnostic category in the incipient revised psychiatric classification systems. The most relevant problems preventing inclusion so far are the heterogeneity of disorders prodromal states may transit to and the high number of false-positive classifications occurring on the basis of the current definition criteria. Beyond the theoretical and methodological implications of these two major problems, a premature inclusion of prodromal states as a new diagnostic category would also face the problem of stigmatizing people who never may transit to a mental disorder. Thus, the ethical issue arises as to how to avoid stigmatizing healthy high-risk individuals with a "prodrome label" on the one hand, but on the other hand also to provide counseling and clinical follow-up visits for those prodromal individuals without a psychiatric diagnosis but in high distress.

More research is warranted to quickly resolve such open scientific questions in this important area. In the meantime, McGorry and coworkers suggested including prodromal states into clinical staging for psychotic disorders by defining disease stages, corresponding target populations, and potential interventions. The proposed prodromal stages range from a genetic risk in first-degree relatives, when information and skills training may be most important, to ultra-high-risk individuals in which more specific therapeutic interventions may be warranted (McGorry et al. 2008, and this conference). Following such a staging scheme may hopefully lead to earlier, safer, and more effective interventions.

Conclusions

Currently, discussions about the reclassification of schizophrenia in DSM-V and ICD-11 focus on the role of the prodromal syndrome and its putative inclusion as a new diagnostic category, and the importance of cognitive dysfunctions for functional outcome and how to assess them. The inclusion of the prodromal states as novel diagnostic entities, however, appears to be premature given the high number of false-positive classifications (resulting in insufficient positive predictive values of the current diagnostic criteria), the heterogeneity of transitions from the same prodromal states into different mental disorders, and the problem of early stigmatization.

Much more research is needed to demonstrate which modules of brain functions are affected in schizophrenia, how this pattern changes over time, how therapeutic interventions alter the disease course, and which prognostic factors are best for predicting disease progression. The importance of cognitive dysfunctions for the functional outcome is becoming increasingly realized and it therefore appears likely that cognitive domains will be included into the definition of schizophrenia. Other clusters or dimensions of symptoms like affective disturbances may also become included.

Considering the exploitation of these novel findings for an improvement of our therapeutic armamentarium in schizophrenia, several options in the fields of both pharmacotherapy and psychotherapy appear. Studies are needed to clarify whether targeting specific cognitive domains (tailored to individual impairments) or general cognitive and/or functional impairments will be more efficacious and cost-effective. Functional outcome assessments will probably play a more important role in the future supplementing classical outcome measures like the severity of psychotic symptoms or relapse/remission rates. Thus, the diagnosis and therapy of schizophrenia will become increasingly sophisticated for the better of our patients with schizophrenia and those at risk for developing schizophrenia.

References

Addington, J., Saeedi, H., & Addington D. Facial affect recognition: a mediator between cognitive and social functioning in psychosis? Schizophrenia Research 85: 142–150, 2006

Allen, D.N., Strauss, G.P., Donohue, B., & Vankammen, D.P. Factor analytic support for social cognition as a separable cognitive domain in schizophrenia. Schizophrenia Research 93: 325–333, 2007

Bechdolf, A., Veith, V., Schwarzer, D., Schormann, M., Stamm, E., Janssen, B., Berning, J., Wagner, M., & Klosterkötter, J. Cognitive-behavioral therapy in the pre-psychotic phase: an exploratory study. Psychiatry Research 136: 251–255, 2005

Blackwood, N.J., Howard, R.J., Bentall, R.P., & Murray, R.M. Cognitive neuropsychiatric models of persecutory delusions. American Journal of Psychiatry 158: 527–539, 2001

Bowie, C.R., Reichenberg, A., Patterson, T.L., Heaton, R.K., & Harvey, P.D. Determinants of real-world functional performance in schizophrenia subjects: correlations with cognition, functional capacity, and symptoms. American Journal of Psychiatry 163: 418–425, 2006

Bowie, C.R., Leung, W.W., Reichenberg, A., McClure, M.M., Patterson, T.L., Heaton, R.K., & Harvey, P.D. Predicting schizophrenia patients' real-world behavior with specific neuropsychological and functional capacity measures. Biological Psychiatry 63: 505–511, 2008

Brewer, W.J., Francey, S.M., Wood, S.J., Jackson, H.J., Pantelis, C., Phillips, L.J., Yung, A.R., Anderson, V.A., & McGorry, P.D. Memory impairments identified in people at ultra-high risk for psychosis who later develop first-episode psychosis. American Journal of Psychiatry 162(Suppl. 1): 71–78, 2005

Buchanan, R.W, Davis, M., Goff, D., Green, M.F., Keefe, R.S.E., Leon, A.C., Nuechterlein, K.H., Laughren, T., Levin, R., Stover, E., Fenton, W., & Marder, S.R. A summary of the FDA-NIMH-MATRICS workshop on clinical trial design for neurocognitive drugs for schizophrenia. Schizophrenia Bulletin 33: 5–19, 2005

Bullmore, E., & Spoons, O. Complex brain networks: graph theoretical analysis of structural and functional systems. Nature Reviews Neuroscience 10: 186–198, 2009

Cannon, T.D. Neurodevelopment and the transition from schizophrenia prodrome to schizophrenia: Research imperatives. Biological Psychiatry 64: 737–738, 2008

Cannon, T.D., Cadenhead, K., Cornblatt, B., Woods, S.W., Addington, J., Walker, E., Seidman, L.J., Perkins, D., Tsuang, M., McGlashan, T., & Heinssen, R. Prediction of psychosis in youth at high clinical risk: A multisite longitudinal study in North America. Archives of General Psychiatry 65: 28–37, 2008

Carter, C.S., Barch, D.M., Buchanan, R.W., Bullmore, E., Krystal, J.H., Cohen, J., Geyer, M., Green, M., Nuechterlein, K.H., Robbins, T., Silverstein, S., Smith, E.E., Strauss, M., Wykes, T., & Heinssen, R. Identifying cognitive mechanisms for treatment development in schizophrenia: An overview of the first meeting of the Cognitive Neuroscience Treatment Research Initiative in Schizophrenia Initiative. Biological Psychiatry 64: 4–10, 2008

Couture, S.M., Penn, D.L., & Roberts, D.L. The functional significance of social cognition in schizophrenia: A review. Schizophrenia Bulletin 32(Suppl. 1): 44–63, 2006

Dickinson, D., & Harvey, P.D. Systemic hypotheses for generalized cognitive deficits in schizophrenia: A new take on an old problem. Schizophrenia Bulletin 2008 Aug 9. [Epub ahead of print] PMID: 18689868

Demasi, S., Sampaolo, L., Mele, L., Morciano, C., Cappello, S., Meneghelli, A., & Degirolamo, G. The Italian guidelines for early intervention in schizophrenia: development and conclusions. Early Intervention in Psychiatry 2: 291–302, 2008

Freeman, D. Suspicious minds: the psychology of persecutory delusions. Clinical Psychology Reviews 27(4): 425–57, 2007

Gaebel, W., & Riesbeck, M. Evidence-based treatment guidelines for the early illness phase in schizophrenia. Comment on DeMasi et al.'s 'The Italian guidelines for early intervention in schizophrenia: development and recommendations'. Early Intervention in Psychiatry 2: 303–306, 2008

Gaebel, W., & Zielasek, J. The DSM-V initiative 'Deconstructing Psychosis' in the context of Kraepelin's concept on nosology. European Archives of Psychiatry and Clinical Neuroscience 258(Suppl. 2): 41–47, 2008

Goldberg, T.E., Goldman, R.S., Burdick, K.E., Malhotra, A.K., Lencz, T., Patel, R.C., Woerner, M.G., Schooler, N.R., Kane, J.M., & Robinson, D.G. Cognitive improvement after treatment with second-generation antipsychotic medications in first-episode schizophrenia. Is it a practice effect? Archives of General Psychiatry 64: 1115–1122, 2007

Gray, J.A., & Roth, B.L. Molecular targets for treating cognitive dysfunction in schizophrenia. Schizophrenia Bulletin 33: 1100–1119, 2007

Green, M.F., Penn, D.L., Bentall, R., Carpenter, W.T., Gaebel, W., Gur, R.C., Kring, A.M., Park, S., Silerstein, S.M., & Heinssen, R. Social cognition in schizophrenia: An NIMH Workshop on definitions, assessment, and research opportunities. Schizophrenia Bulletin 34: 1211–1220, 2008

Hall, J., Whalley, H.J., Job, D.E., Baig, B.J., Mcintosh, A. M., Evans, K.I., Thomson, P.A., Porteou, D. J., Cunningham-Owens, D.G., Johnstone, E.C., & Lawrie, S.M. A neuregulin 1 variant associated with abnormal cortical function and psychotic symptoms. Nature Neuroscience 9: 1477–1478, 2006

Horan, W.P., Kern, R.S., Shokat-Fadai, K., Sergi, M.J., Wynn, J.K., & Green, M.F. Social cognitive skills training in schizophrenia: An initial efficacy study of stabilized outpatients. Schizophrenia Research 107: 47–54, 2009

Howes, O.D., Montgomery, A.J., Asselin, M.-C., Murray, R.M., Valli, I., Tabraham, P., Bramon-Bosh, E., Valmaggia, L., Johns, L., Broome, M., Mcguire, P.K., & Grasby, P.M. Elevated striatal dopamine function linked to prodromal signs of schizophrenia. Archives of General Psychiatry 66(Suppl. 1): 13–20, 2009

Hyman, S., & Ivleva, E. Cognition in schizophrenia. American Journal of Psychiatry 165: 312, 2008

Kapur, S. Psychosis as a state of aberrant salience: A framework linking biology, phenomenology, and pharmacology in schizophrenia. American Journal of Psychiatry 160: 13–23, 2003

Keefe, R.S.E. Should cognitive impairment be included in the diagnostic criteria for schizophrenia? World Psychiatry 7: 22–28, 2008

Keefe, R.S.E., & Fenton, W.S. How should DSM-V criteria for schizophrenia include cognitive impairment? Schizophrenia Bulletin 33: 912–920, 2007

Keefe, R.S.E., Perkins, D.O., Gu, H., Zipursky, R.B., Christensen, B.K., & Lieberman, J.A. A longitudinal study of neurocognitive function in individuals at-risk for psychosis. Schizophrenia Research 88: 26–35, 2006

Keri, S., Kiss, I., & Kelemen, O. Effects of neuregulin 1 variant on conversion to schizophrenia and schizophreniform disorder in people a high risk for psychosis. Molecular Psychiatry 14: 118–122, 2009

Klosterkötter, J., Schultze-Lutter, F., & Ruhrmann, S. Kraepelin and psychotic prodromal conditions. European Archives of Psychiatry and Clinical Neuroscience 258(Suppl. 2): 74–84, 2008

Kraepelin, E. Die Erscheinungsformen des Irreseins. Zeitschrift für die gesamte Neurologie und Psychiatrie 62: 1–29, 1920

Lawrie, S.M., Mcintosh, A.M., Cunningham-Owens, D.G., & Johnstone, E.C. Neuroimaging and molecular genetics of schizophrenia: pathophysiological advances and therapeutic potential. British Journal of Pharmacology 153: 120–124, 2008

Lencz, T., Smith, C.W., McLaughlin, D., Auther, A., Nakayama, E., Hovey, L., & Cornblatt, B.A. Generalized and specific neurocognitive deficits in prodromal schizophrenia. Biological Psychiatry 59: 863–871, 2005

Lencz, T., Smith, C.W., McLaughlin, D. Generalized and specific neurocognitive deficits in prodromal schizophrenia. Biological Psychiatry 59: 863-871, 2006

McGorry, P.D., Killackey, E., & Yung, A. Early intervention in psychosis: concepts, evidence and future directions. World Psychiatry 7: 148–156, 2008

McGurk, S.R., Twamley, E.W., Sitzer, D.I., McHugo, G.J., & Mueser, K.T. A meta-analysis of cognitive remediation in schizophrenia. American Journal of Psychiatry 164: 1791–1802, 2007

Murphy, D. & Stich, S. Darwin in the Madhouse. Evolutionary Psychology and the Classification of Mental Disorders. In: Carruthers, P. & Chamberlain, A. (eds.) Evolution and the Human Mind. Modularity, Language, and Meta-Cognition, Cambridge University Press, Cambridge, MA, pp. 62–92, 2000

Nuechterlein, K.H., Green, M.F., Kern, R.S., Baade, L.E., Barch, D.M., Cohen, J.D., Essock, S., Fenton, W.S., Freese III, F.J., Gold, J.M., Goldberg, T., Heaton, R.K., Keefe, R.S., Kraemer, H., Mesholam-Gately, R., Seidman, L.J., Stover, E., Weinberger, D.R., Young, A.S., Zalcman, S., & Marder, S.R. The MATRICS consensus cognitive battery, part 1: test selection, reliability, and validity. American Journal of Psychiatry 165: 203–213, 2008

Ruhrmann, S., Bechdolf, A., Kühn, K.U., Wagner, M., Schultze-Lutter, F., Janssen, B., Maurer, K., Häfner, H., Gaebel, W., Möller, H.J., Maier, W., & Klosterkötter, J. LIPS study group. Acute effects of treatment for prodromal symptoms for people putatively in a late initial prodromal state of psychosis. British Journal of Psychiatry 51: 88–95, 2007

Schmidt, S., Müller, D.S., Reinecker, H., & Roder, V. Soziale Kognition als Mediatorvariable zwischen Neurokognition und psychosozialem Funktionsniveau bei schizophren Erkrankten? Erste empirische Ergebnisse einer Anwendung von Strukturgleichungsmodellen. Presentation at the annual congress of the German Psychiatric Society, Berlin, Abstract in Nervenarzt (Suppl. 4): 181, 2008

Sergi, M.J., Rassovsky, Y., Nuechterlein, K.H., & Green, M.F. Social perception as a mediator of the influence of early visual processing on functional status in schizophrenia. American Journal of Psychiatry 163: 448–454, 2006

Sergi, M.J., Rassovsky, Y., Widmark, C., Reist, C., Erhart, S. Braff, D.L., Marder, S.R., & Green, M.F. Social cognition in schizophrenia: relationships with neurocognition and negative symptoms. Schizophrenia Research 90: 316–324, 2007

Sun, D., Phillips, L.J., Velakoulis, D., Yung, A., McGorry, P.D., Wood, S.J., Vanerp, T.G.M., Thompson, P.M., Toga, A.W., Cannon, T.D., & Pantelis, C. Progressive brain structural changes mapped as psychosis develops in 'at risk' individuals. Schizophrenia Research 108: 85–92, 2009

Tamminga, C. Neuropsychiatric aspects of schizophrenia. In: Yudofsky, S.C. & Hales, R.E., (eds.) Neuropsychiatry and Behavioral Neurosciences, American Psychiatric Association Publications, Washington, DC, pp. 969–1001, 2008

Walterfang, M., McGuire, PK, Yung, A.R., Phillips, L.J., Velakoulis, D., Wood, S.J., Suckling, J., Bullmore, E., Brewer, W., Soulsby, B., Desmond, P., McGorry, P.D., & Pantelis, C. White matter volume changes in people who develop psychosis. British Journal of Psychiatry 193: 210–215, 2008

Whyte, M.-C., Brett, C., Harrison, L.K., Byrne, M., Miller, P., Lawrie, S.M., & Johnstone, E.C. Neuropsychological performance over time in people at high risk of developing schizophrenia and controls. Biological Psychiatry 59: 730–739, 2006

Wobrock, T., Gruber, O., Schneider-Axmann, T., Wölwer, W., Gaebel, W., Riesbeck, M., Maier, W., Klosterkötter, J., Schneider, F., Buchkremer, G., Möller, H.J., Schmitt, A., Bender, S., Schloesser, R., & Falkai, P. Internal capsule size associated with outcome in first-episode schizophrenia. European Archives of Psychiatry and Clinical Neuroscience, 259: 278–283, 2009

Woodward, N.D., Purdon, S.E., Meltzer, H.Y., & Zald, D.H. A meta-analysis of neuropsychological change to clozapine, olanzapine, quetiapine, and risperidone in schizophrenia. The International Journal of Neuropsychopharmacology 8(Suppl. 3): 457–472, 2005

Wölwer, W., Frommann, N., Halfmann, S., Piaszek, A., Streit, M., & Gaebel, W. Remediation of impairments in facial affect recognition in schizophrenia: Efficacy and specificity of a new training program. Schizophrenia Research 80: 295–303, 2005

Wölwer, W., Brinkmeyer, J., Riesbeck, M., Freimüller, L., Klimke, A., Wagner, M., Möller, H.J., Klingberg, S., & Gaebel, W., for the German Study Group on First Episode Schizophrenia. Neuropsychological impairments predict the clinical course in schizophrenia. European Archives of Psychiatry and Clinical Neuroscience 258(Suppl. 5): 28–34, 2008

Yung, A.R., Nelson, B., Stanford, C., Simmons, M.B., Cosgrave, E.M., Killackey, E., Phillips, L.J., Bechdolf, A., Buckby, J., & McGorry, P.D. Validation of "prodromal" criteria to detect individuals at ultra-high risk of psychosis: 2 year follow-up. Schizophrenia Research 105: 10–17, 2008

Zielasek, J., & Gaebel, W. Modern modularity and the road towards a modular psychiatry. European Archives of Psychiatry and Clinical Neuroscience 258(Suppl. 5): 60–65, 2008

Zimmermann, G., Favrod, J., Trieu, V.H., & Pomini, V. The effect of cognitive-behavioral treatment on the positive symptoms of schizophrenia spectrum disorders: A meta-analysis. Schizophrenia Research 77: 1–9, 2005

Part V
Schizophrenia and Other Psychotic Disorders: Boundaries and Similarities

Continua or Classes? Vexed Questions on the Latent Structure of Schizophrenia

Richard J. Linscott, Mark F. Lenzenweger, and Jim van Os

Introduction

Continuum and its various forms, synonyms, and antonyms frequently appear in the literature on schizophrenia, typically with two main referents. One concerns the nature of the signs or symptoms of the disorder and their relationships to normal psychological experience. For example, some speak of the phenotypic psychosis continuum comprising culturally normal experiential phenomena, subclinical experience, and clinically significant psychosis. Certainly, it seems that there is a phenomenological continuum of psychotic experience (van Os et al., 2008). The second concerns the latent structure[1] of the population: A population has a continuous structure if its members comprise one group, and a class structure if its members comprise two, three, or more commingled types. Our focus here is on this latter sense of *continuum*

Anecdotally, the prevailing view seems to be that the latent structure of schizophrenia is continuous. That is, if we take a view of schizophrenia that is broader than the construct the World Health Organization (2004) or the American Psychiatric Association (2000) describes and that encapsulates liability, the prodrome, and benign outcomes, there is no qualitative difference distinguishing individuals who are and are not affected by schizophrenia. A narrower version of this same view is that there is no latent boundary between affective and nonaffective psychosis, or dividing different psychosis phenotypes

There is a small cohort of studies from the 1970s and 1980s that is often cited in support of this viewpoint, as a basis for rejecting the notion of a class boundary between affective and nonaffective psychosis (e.g., Kendell and Gourlay, 1970; Brockington et al., 1979; Kendell and Brockington, 1980). However, the

---

R.J. Linscott (✉)
Department of Psychology, University of Otago, Dunedin, New Zealand
e-mail: linscott@psy.otago.ac.nz

[1] By *latent* we mean the underlying structure, unobserved and unobservable, but inferred. Latent contrasts with *manifest*, which is the directly observed phenotype or endophenotype variable. See also Meehl (2004).

W.F. Gattaz, G. Busatto (eds.), *Advances in Schizophrenia Research 2009*,
DOI 10.1007/978-1-4419-0913-8_18, © Springer Science+Business Media, LLC 2010

influence of these studies appears to outweigh their merit. In the first of these studies (Kendell and Gourlay, 1970), discriminant function scores were computed from clinical ratings obtained from a mixed sample of patients with affective psychosis or schizophrenia. The scores generated a trimodal distribution that was interpreted as inconsistent with a class distinction between schizophrenia and affective psychosis. A replication study in the same paper yielded the same conclusion.

The principal difficulty with this and similar papers is that the analysis approach that was used—seeking evidence of bimodality—is not suited to address the question of the latent structure of a population. First, when the latent structure is discontinuous, bimodality will not necessarily result (Murphy, 1964; Maxwell, 1971). Second, bimodality can arise in situations in which the latent structure is continuous, such as where logistic functions underlie the probability of phenotype expression (Grayson, 1987).

This early cohort of studies also gives rise to a broader implication: Statistical methods that are used to arrive at interpretations about latent structure subsequently may be found not to be suitable for addressing such questions. This has certainly been the case for the bimodal criterion. It is also the case for cluster analytic methods (Golden and Meehl, 1980; Cleland et al., 2000; Beauchaine and Beauchaine, 2002; Ruscio and Ruscio, 2004). Moreover, it may turn out to be the case for contemporary methods that, at this point in time, appear to work quite well. With this proviso in mind, we recently suggested there are two statistical approaches that may serve to model or test, respectively, hypotheses about the latent structure of schizophrenia (Linscott et al., 2009): factor mixture modeling (FMM; also called *item-response mixture modeling*) and coherent cut kinetic (CCK) methods (Meehl, 1973; Muthén and Asparouhov, 2006).

Briefly, FMM may be conceived of as the combination of two modeling methods: factor analysis and latent class analysis (Fig. 1). In factor analysis, latent continuous variables, or factors, account for observed variance among items. In latent class analysis, latent categorical variables representing classes account for observed variance among people. When combined in FMM, analyses can shed light on whether variance in data is best described in terms of latent classes, latent factors, or both (Muthén and Asparouhov, 2006).

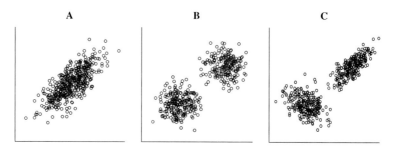

Fig. 1 Idealized depictions of (**A**) a latent factor structure identified by factor analysis, (**B**) a latent class or mixture structure with zero within-class covariance, and (**C**) a hybrid involving latent classes, each with distinct within-class factors

In contrast, CCK methods involve scrutinizing observed data for anomalies that are inconsistent with a latent continuous structure. For example, one of the most frequently used CCK methods, maximum covariance analysis, is based on a statistical theorem that covariance between two variables measured on a sample comprising two subsamples is a function of the covariances within the respective subsamples and the sizes and degree of separations of the subsamples. In practice, this means that latent structure can be evidenced by predictable patterns of covariance across subsamples in an ordered series. Conformity with a flat pattern favors a dimensional interpretation; conformity with a peaked pattern favors a class interpretation (Meehl, 1995; Waller and Meehl, 1998).

FMM and CCK methods are quite distinct in their mechanics. An important commonality is that these can each be used to contrast competing hypotheses about latent structure, especially dimensional vs. categorical hypotheses. Importantly, both approaches are constrained by their sensitivity to design and psychometric limitations. CCK methods are limited in that a single analysis cannot distinguish latent structures with more than two groups; the indicators (whether clinical ratings, self-report, or objective performance measures) must be monotonically related; and the primary results are graphical, requiring subjective judgments of shape. FMM is limited in that distinguishing among competing latent models is achieved by examining the fit of distributions that are composed using hypothetical latent structures, rather than by observing phenomena in the data that are indicative of latent structure (Linscott et al., 2009); alternative models can be indistinguishable in fit; the primary statistical results, although numeric, also require subjective appraisal; and they present a complex interpretive challenge, similar to that faced in factor analysis (Meehl, 1979). Given these limitations, CCK and FMM are complementary methods.

The primary reason we regard CCK and FMM methods as providing pertinent evidence is that these methods are unbiased, contrasting continuous and class hypotheses such that the resulting evidence can favor either of these alternatives (Meehl, 2004; Muthén and Asparouhov, 2006). In contrast, there are many studies of clinical features of schizophrenia in which latent class (Linscott et al., 2009) or factor (Peralta and Cuesta, 2001) analyses have been used to test ideas about the heterogeneity of schizophrenia. Those using factor analysis are, in essence, seeking to resolve heterogeneity through the identification of latent continua and those using latent class analysis, through the identification of latent classes. However, used in isolation, factor analysis cannot serve to discount a latent class structure, and latent class analysis cannot serve to discount a latent continuous structure. In short, factor analysis can (and always will) only find dimensions in data and latent class analysis, including cluster analysis, can (and always will) only find evidence for latent classes in data.

Review Aims and Method

Our objective is to determine whether there is a body of evidence that is inconsistent with the prevailing view that the latent structure of schizophrenia—broadly defined so as not to exclude liability—is continuous. We sought four sets of CCK- or FMM-derived evidence. First, we sought evidence from analyses of clinical features of schizophrenia that make up Criterion A in *DSM-IV*. Second, we sought evidence from analyses of biological liability and, third, psychometric liability for schizophrenia. Fourth, we sought evidence from analyses of putative endophenotypes of schizophrenia, such as eye movement dysfunction.

In order to obtain an unbiased sample of research, we searched MEDLINE (1950 to December 2008) content for papers that contained any reference to schizophrenia spectrum disorders or schizotypy (search terms: *schizophren$*, *schizaffect$*, *psychosis*, *psychotic*, and *schizotyp$*, where term truncation is indicated by the $ suffix), and reference to *class* or a synonym of *class* (search terms: *class, kind, category, type, subtype, taxa, taxon, taxanomic, taxonomic, categorical, categorial, continu$, discontinu$, discrete*, or *mixture*), and reference to *latent* or one of its synonyms (search terms: *latent, underlying, structure, structural, hidden*, or *unobserv$*). This search yielded 1,222 papers, and 863 papers when limited to non-review human research. The latter were systematically reviewed, first by reading the titles and then, as necessary, the abstracts, to identify pertinent original research. Citations in pertinent original research were also searched for reference to other potentially relevant papers, which were appraised in the same manner as outlined above.

In reviewing this research, we have divided the papers into four subsets: those concerned with criterion symptoms of schizophrenia, those concerned with biological risk, those concerned with psychometric risk, and those concerned with putative endophenotypes of schizophrenia.

Discontinuity in Clinical Features of Schizophrenia

Whereas the first CCK methods were described and implemented in the mid- to late 1960s (Meehl, 1973), FMM has emerged only recently, within the last 10 years. Not surprisingly, then, nearly all the research we identified as pertinent involved the application of CCK methods. From what we can determine, the first study to approximate a contrast of continuum and class latent models using measures of clinical features of schizophrenia was reported by Kendell and Brockington (1980). It is not clear whether Kendell and Brockington were aware of the similarity between their statistical approach and CCK methods, and their approach was more rudimentary than that which Meehl described in 1973. Nevertheless, the Kendell and Brockington paper provides a useful orientation to the logic of CCK methods and so we review this in somewhat more detail than other studies.

Kendell and Brockington (1980) proposed that latent discontinuity between schizophrenia and affective psychosis would be evidenced by a nonlinear relationship between continuous measures of symptoms and measures of outcome. To test for nonlinearity, they divided a mixed psychosis sample ($n = 127$) into 10 subgroups ordered on a continuous symptom index. Then, outcome indices, including measures of clinical outcome and social and occupational functioning, were plotted against subgroup position. They reasoned that nonlinear variation in outcome across the ordered subgroups—more specifically, a sigmoid relationship—would constitute evidence of a latent class boundary. In contrast, if the latent structure were continuous, there would be a linear relationship between symptom ratios and outcome.

Figure 2 shows two hypothetical simulations illustrating these alternatives. The first simulation has a discontinuous structure, with 42% belonging to a schizophrenia class and a group effect size in the order of $d = 2.0$. Here, the mean correlation between symptom and outcomes in the mixed sample was $r = 0.50$. In the second, a correlated dimensional data set was simulated. The second simulation has correlated indicators (mean $r = 0.55$) but a continuous structure. Analyses of both simulations proceeded as Kendell and Brockington (1980) specified, by dividing the respective samples into 10 ordered subgroups (ordered on a symptom scores, with low scores indicating affective psychosis and high scores indicating schizophrenic psychosis) and plotting mean outcome against each group (Fig. 2).

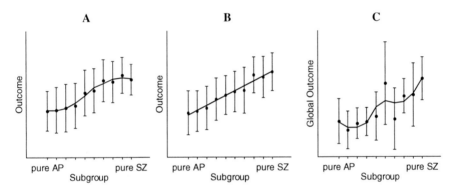

Fig. 2 Kendell and Brockington's (1980) kinetic cut method using ordered symptom subgroups. (**A**) Discontinuous simulation ($n = 130$, with 42% falling in the schizophrenia class): there is a nonlinear relationship between symptoms and outcome as subsample composition shifts from being pure affective psychosis (AP) to pure schizophrenia (SZ). (**B**) Continuous simulation ($n = 130$): there is a linear relationship between symptoms and outcome. (**C**) Observed global outcomes reported by Kendell and Brockington (1980, $n = 127$). Each plot shows mean outcomes for ordered subgroups. Error bars are standard deviations. The line in B is a least squares regression line and the curves in A and C are Lowess-smoothed averages

One of Kendell and Brockington's (1980) results is shown in Fig. 2. On this basis, Kendell and Brockington concluded that the evidence did not demonstrate discontinuity, that there was no significant departure from linearity among the relationships between the outcome variables and the symptomatology index. However, although the logic was sound, the steps they took in their analysis were insufficient in two important respects. First, there was no consideration of the likely outcome of the procedure given the competing latent models. Kendell and Brockington did not simulate continuous and discontinuous data to determine the degree of departure from linearity associated with each model, nor did they consider the effects of the sample parameters on the analysis (e.g., effect of sample size, indicator validity, and taxa ratios). Second, the analysis ended somewhat prematurely, after only considering the distribution of means.

Kendell and Brockington's (1980) results are sufficient, given certain assumptions, to allow supplementary analysis of their data. In their results (Kendell and Brockington, 1980, p. 328), 6 plots are presented showing each of the 10 symptom subgroup means and errors on 6 outcome indices. If it is assumed that the symptom subgroups are of approximately equal size (about 13 people per group) and that the errors are standard deviation for each subgroup, two additional results can be considered, both of which are based on the same analysis logic and only use the results they reported.

First, the logic underlying Kendell and Brockington's analysis also underpins the CCK method, mean above minus below a cut (Meehl and Yonce, 1994). This procedure works in essentially the same way, except that the y-axis gives the mean outcome difference between those above and below the cut, and the sliding cut takes steps of $n = 1$. When the underlying structure is continuous, differences in outcomes across changing symptom ratios will tend to be flat or dish shaped (Fig. 3). In contrast, when the underlying structure is discontinuous, differences in outcomes will tend to be peaked, with the peak occurring at the point that best separates two latent classes. The observed curve for global outcome data reported by Kendell and Brockington (1980) has a clear peak: it is neither flat nor dish shaped (Fig. 3).

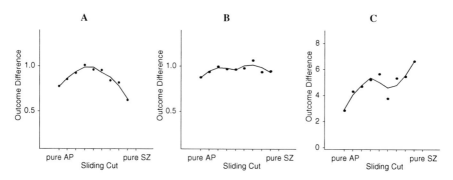

Fig. 3 MAMBAC curves for (**A**) discontinuous and (**B**) continuous simulations ($n = 130$) and for (**C**) global outcome data reported by Kendell and Brockington (1980). Curves are Lowess-smoothed averages. AP = affective psychosis; SZ = schizophrenia

The second supplementary result requires a small extension of Kendell and Brockington's logic: If the underlying structure is discontinuous and if within the latent classes outcome is not correlated with symptomatology, there will be a predictable pattern of variance across the ordered symptomatology subgroups. Specifically, variance will maximize as the ratio of the two latent classes approaches 1:1 and minimize at the extremes where the class composition is almost pure (0:1 or 1:0). An increase in variation should occur as symptom ratios approach 1:1 because between-class variance would make increasingly substantial contributions to the subgroup variance. If the latent structure is continuous, variance across the ordered subgroups should be constant. This logic approximates that which underlies the CCK method, maximum covariance analysis (Meehl, 1973). This second analysis

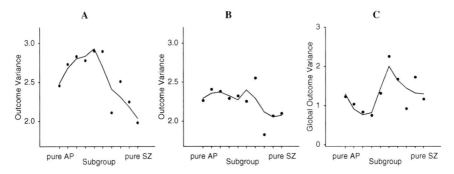

Fig. 4 Maximum variance curves (Lowess smoothed) for the (**A**) discontinuous and (**B**) continuous simulations, and for (**C**) the Kendell and Brockington (1980) data. AP = affective psychosis; SZ = schizophrenia

was performed on the simulated data and the observed data, which yield a peaked maximum covariance curve (Fig. 4).

Although results from both these supplementary CCK analyses yield evidence consistent with the presence of a latent class boundary, the evidence is not strong for two reasons: First, there are multiple analysis limitations in these supplementary results: the analyses are ad hoc; additional corroborating statistical analyses cannot be performed; and it is not clear whether selected ranges of the y-axes are appropriate. Second, the symptom scores are discriminant function scores based on the provision of a diagnostic gold standard. Consequently, the CCK results simply corroborate that the discriminant analysis was effective in identifying a discriminating score. Interpreting these supplementary data as evidence of a latent class boundary would require the assumption that the diagnostic gold standard was accurately aligned with a latent class boundary and constitute a critical logical error. A significant advantage of CCK and FMM methods is that these can be applied where no gold standard is available (Meehl, 1973). Moreover, in an exploratory context, it is critical that such gold standards can be set aside.

Other studies of clinical symptoms have appeared only recently. Blanchard et al. (2005) provided a comprehensive analysis of negative symptom ratings on patients with schizophrenia-spectrum disorders with a view to testing the theory that the deficit syndrome has a latent class structure with a prevalence of 30%. Evidence from two CCK methods (maximum covariance analysis and mean above minus below a cut) converged to support the predicted structure, with an observed prevalence between 28 and 36%. However, two sample characteristics complicate the interpretation of this finding.

As with any analysis method, CCK and FMM are not intelligent systems. These detect anomalies in observed variance or recreate variance patterns, respectively, regardless of the source of the observed variance. Consequently, any systematic error variance in the observed data could resemble a meaningful latent class boundary. In the Blanchard et al. (2005) study, participants were patients in a 24-month multisite treatment outcome study (Schooler et al., 1997) and the indicators were the average of negative symptom ratings obtained at baseline and 6 months into the intervention. Evidence indicates there were both significant site effects and treatment effects in the outcome data (Schooler et al., 1997). Although Blanchard et al. (2005) demonstrated the resulting latent class was not associated with any of the treatment *conditions* included in the original study, the observed latent class boundary may reflect variance introduced by site differences or by response vs. nonresponse to treatment. Unfortunately, it is not possible to disentangle these competing accounts of their findings.

Cuesta et al. (2007) conducted CCK analyses on reality distortion, disorganization, and negative factor scores obtained from SANS and SAPS ratings on 660 consecutively admitted patients who exhibited one or more psychotic symptoms at admission. In earlier research on the same sample, index psychosis and affective symptoms comprising more than a dozen indicators were subject to latent class analysis and yielded evidence for a five-class structure: a general schizophrenia class (prevalence = 42%) and classes characterized as psychotic with poor insight (19%), schizo-manic (17%), schizo-depressive (12%), and mixed psychotic-cycloid (10%) (Peralta and Cuesta, 2003). Unfortunately, the results from the CCK analyses were ambiguous, allowing neither a class nor a continuum interpretation (Cuesta et al., 2007). The primary cause of this ambiguity appears to have been the inclusion of, what Meehl refers to as, *parataxonic* indicators in the analyses, that is, indicators that were not monotonically related, thereby violating the assumptions of the CCK analysis methods they used (Meehl, 1999). In Cuesta et al. (2007), whereas disorganization and negative factor indices were positively correlated ($r = 0.31$), each of these was negatively correlated with reality distortion ($r = -0.07$ and -0.15, respectively). Given a two-group mixture (e.g., Fig. 1), it is readily understandable that indicators that are sensitive to a two-class mix will be monotonically related. Consequently, a better strategy in the case of this data set would have involved separating the CCK analysis of the items contributing to the reality distortion factor from the CCK analysis of items comprising the negative and disorganized factors. Alternatively, CCK methods could have been used to validate one or more of the class boundaries implied by the results of the earlier latent class analysis by focusing on those indicators found to have discriminated one of the five classes from the remaining four (Meehl, 1979; Linscott et al., 2009).

Disorganization features have been analysed in isolation in two reports. An abstract from Morris Bell (1997) described three studies of cognitive disorganization using 6 items from the PANSS and samples sizes of around 400. Maximum covariance analyses were reported to yield evidence of latent class structures in the three samples. However, as full reports were never published (personal communication, Jan 18, 2008), it is difficult to evaluate the quality of these studies. Also, Blanchard et al. (2005) conducted limited CCK analyses on BPRS disorganization ratings on the same patients described earlier. In contrast to the relatively clear results obtained on the negative symptom indicators, disorganization ratings yielded ambiguous results and were not fully reported.

We found no studies of Criterion A symptoms in which investigators employed FMM in an exploratory fashion. The study that came the closest to doing so involved reanalyses of hallucination and delusion ratings from two large epidemiological data sets, the National Comorbidity Survey and the Netherlands Mental Health Survey and Incidence Study (Shevlin et al., 2007a; see also Shevlin et al., 2007b). The critical limitation of these reanalyses was that the analysis model incorporated the assumption that any latent classes would be ordered along a single underlying dimension. That is, the analysis did not involve a contrast of continuum vs. class explanations. Consequently, it is no surprise that the classes they identified—four in all, labeled *psychosis-like, intermediate, low,* and *normative*—were consistent across the two samples and were interpreted as arising from a single underlying continuum.

Discontinuities in Biological Risk for Schizophrenia

Two reports described taxometric analyses of biological risk groups. The first of these involved analyses of data from the New York High-Risk Project, participants in which included offspring of schizophrenia ($n = 55$), major affective disorder ($n = 38$), and control ($n = 92$) parents (Erlenmeyer-Kimling et al., 1989). Indicators were performance measures of attention, motor control, visuomotor integration, and intelligence, and these were analyzed using a forerunner to maximum covariance analysis (Golden, 1982). The results from the analysis were consistent with a latent class structure with a class-of-interest prevalence of 0.26, of whom 61% were offspring of parents with schizophrenia. The class prevalence varied with parent diagnosis, with the highest prevalence being among offspring of parents with schizophrenia (0.55), followed by affective disorder (0.32) and control (0.08) group offspring. Equivalent data from a replication sample (with $n = 46$, $n = 39$, and $n = 65$, respectively), described in the same report, produced similar results, with an overall prevalence of 0.18.

The second study of biological risk followed an analysis of data from the Copenhagen High Risk Project (Tyrka et al., 1995). In this, social withdrawal, social anxiety, flat affect, passivity, poor prognosis, and peculiarity indices from 311 healthy offspring of normal mothers ($n = 104$) or mothers with schizophrenia ($n = 207$) were subject to the CCK method, maximum covariance analysis. The results suggested the combined sample had a latent class structure, with the clinically interesting latent class comprising approximately 49% of the sample, 81% of whom were offspring of mothers with schizophrenia; 58% of offspring of mothers with schizophrenia were in the latent class.

A continuum model of schizophrenia cannot readily explain these findings. This notwithstanding, there are significant problems with these studies that may compromise the validity of the results. First, the study samples both comprised participants drawn from two sources, the distinction between which might have engendered an artifactual latent class boundary. This is particularly the case in the Tyrka et al. (1995) sample. Whereas high-risk offspring had mothers with schizophrenia, the control offspring had no recorded family history of psychiatric disorder spanning two prior generations. This artificial gap in the gene–environment baggage carried by the respective subsamples might have given rise to the appearance of a latent class boundary in the mixed data set. Alternatively, a gap such as this might have distorted or obscured a genuine latent class boundary.

The second problem concerns Tyrka et al. (1995) only. Here, the primary variables, or *indicators*, used in the analysis were selected on the basis of their sensitivity to offspring heritage. Indicators that were not sensitive to heritage were excluded from the analysis. Whereas indicator validity is a critical issue in the design of taxometric (FMM and CCK) studies, it is reasonable to argue that indicator validity should not be determined on the basis of sensitivity to those subgroups that are to be included in the taxometric analysis. A better strategy might have been to determine indicator validity on the basis of sensitivity to offspring heritage but to conduct the CCK analysis only with offspring of the mothers with schizophrenia. Given that fewer than 60% of those in the biological risk group were classified as being in the class of interest and given evidence on the heritability of schizophrenia (Gottesman, 1991), it would be reasonable to predict a taxonic outcome in this situation also.

Discontinuities in Psychometric Risk for Schizophrenia

The majority of reports we identified concern psychometric risk for schizophrenia (Table 1). The earliest of these studies was the first published application of CCK methods to the problem of the liability for schizophrenia. Golden and Meehl (1979) examined the latent structure of select MMPI item ratings obtained from nonpsychotic male psychiatric in-patients. In separate analyses, the items were demonstrated to distinguish schizophrenia and healthy respondents. Two analyses using distinct indicators yielded convergent evidence of a latent class boundary and a class-of-interest prevalence of approximately 0.40. The authors' tentative assertion that the study provided evidence of a schizoid taxon has been strongly corroborated by a body of evidence comprising 12 subsequent published reports (Table 1) as well as several unpublished works or theses (Lowrie and Raulin, 1990; Brenner and Raulin, 1994; Brenner et al., 1995; Lowrie and Raulin, 1996; MacFarlane, 1996; Whitehead, 2005). Specific replication of Golden and Meehl (1979) was reported by Whitehead (2005) who obtained responses from an unselected sample of psychiatric patients on a direct (cf. criterion keyed) measure of psychometric risk. In contrast to Golden and Meehl (1979), Whitehead (2005) did not exclude patients with psychosis. Maximum covariance analysis yielded clear evidence of a latent class boundary with a prevalence of approximately 0.30.

The modal methodology in this body of research involved collecting self-report responses on a schizotypy questionnaire from a convenience sample of undergraduate participants. There is also relatively limited diversity in the assessment instruments that have been used, with 8 of 14 investigations in these 12 reports relying primarily on one or more of the Chapmans' scales (Chapman et al., 1976, 1978; Eckblad and Chapman, 1983; Mishlove and Chapman, 1985). Only one study used

Table 1 Summary of studies of psychometric risk for schizophrenia

First author (year)	Sample (n)	Measures (items)	Analysis (indicators)	Result
Golden and Meehl (1979)	Male in-patients, without psychosis (221)	MMPI Schizoidia Scale (7)	MAMBAC (7 items)	T, 0.37
Lenzenweger and Korfine (1992)	Undergraduates (1,093)	MMPI schizoid (113)	MAXCOV (3 factors)	T, 0.40
		Perceptual aberration (35)	MAXCOV (8 items)	T, 0.10
Korfine and Lenzenweger (1995)	Undergraduates (1,646)	Perceptual aberration (35)	MAXCOV (8 items)	T, 0.05
Lenzenweger (1999)	Undergraduates (429)	Perceptual aberration (35), magical ideation (30), referential thinking (34)	MAXCOV (3 scales)	T, 0.13
van Kampen (1999)	Primary health care patients (2,118)	4DPT pre-schizophrenic personality, insensitivity (16)	MAXCOV (7 items)	T, 0.24
		4DPT pre-schizophrenic personality, introversion (16)	MAXCOV (7 items)	T, 0.41
		4DPT pre-schizophrenic personality, neuroticism (16)	MAXCOV (7 items)	T, 0.40
Blanchard et al. (2000)	Undergraduates (1,526)	Social anhedonia (40)	MAXCOV (4 factors)	T, 0.08
			MAXEIG (4 factors)	T, NR
Meyer and Keller (2001)	Students and employees (809)	Perceptual aberration (35)	MAXCOV (6 items)	T, 0.11
		Magical ideation (30)	MAXCOV (8 items)	D
		Physical anhedonia (50)	MAXCOV (7 items)	T, 0.13

Table 1 (continued)

First author (year)	Sample (n)	Measures (items)	Analysis (indicators)	Result
Keller et al. (2001)	Undergraduates (1,103)	SPQ perceptual aberration (9)	MAXCOV, (7 items)	D
			Mixed Rasch and LCA (7 items)	D
		SPQ odd speech (9)	MAXCOV (7 items)	D
		SPQ social anxiety (8)	MAXCOV, (7 items)	T, 0.18
			Mixed Rasch and LCA (7 items)	2-class, 0.24
		SPQ constricted affect (8)	MAXCOV (7 items)	D
		SPQ positive schizotypy	MAXCOV (4 scales)	A, 0.17
		SPQ negative schizotypy	MAXCOV (3 scales)	T, 0.11
Horan et al. (2004)	Undergraduates (1,560)[a]	Social anhedonia (40)	MAXCOV (4 factors)	T, 0.08
			MAMBAC (4 factors)	T, 0.18
			MAXCOV (8 items)	T, 0.07
		Magical ideation (30)	MAMBAC (2 factors)	A, 0.25
			MAXCOV (8 items)	T, 0.22
		Social anhedonia, magical ideation (70)	MAXCOV (6 factors)	T, 0.12–0.21
			MAMBAC (2 scales)	D
	Undergraduates (2,574)	Social anhedonia (40)	MAXCOV (4 factors)	T, 0.11
			MAMBAC (4 factors)	T, 0.19
			MAXCOV (8 items)	T, 0.06
		Magical ideation (30)	MAMBAC (2 factors)	A, 0.31
			MAXCOV (8 items)	D
		Perceptual aberration (35)	MAXCOV (8 items)	T, 0.06
		Magical ideation, perceptual aberration (65)	MAMBAC (2 scales)	T, 0.29
		Social anhedonia, magical ideation, perceptual aberration (105)	MAXCOV (3 scales)	D
			MAMBAC (3 scales)	D

Table 1 (continued)

First author (year)	Sample (n)	Measures (items)	Analysis (indicators)	Result
Linscott et al. (2006)	High school children (387)	Magical thinking, hallucinatory tendency, self-reference, perceptual aberration (26)	MAXCOV (4 scales)	T, 0.13
			MAXEIG (4 scales)	T, 0.07
			L-MODE (4 scales)	T, 0.09
Fossati et al. (2007)[b]	High school children, without history of mental disorder (929)	SPQ, STA, and SS Schizophrenism (123)	MAXCOV (3 scales)	D
	Undergraduates, without history of mental disorder (803)	SPQ, STA, and SS Schizophrenism (123)	MAXCOV (3 scales)	T, 0.15
Linscott (2007)	Undergraduates (1,543)	TPSQ-positive schizotypy (66)	MAXCOV (6 scales)	T, 0.13
			MAXEIG (6 scales)	T, 0.12
		TPSQ hypohedonia (33)	MAXCOV (6 scales)	D
			MAXEIG (6 scales)	D

Table 1 (continued)

First author (year)	Sample (n)	Measures (items)	Analysis (indicators)	Result
Rawlings et al. (2008)[c]	Undergraduates, university staff, subject pool participants, and respondents to advertising (1,073)[c]	Perceptual aberration (35)	MAXEIG (4 scales)	D
			MAMBAC (4 scales)	A, 0.19
		Magical ideation (30)	MAXEIG (4 scales)	D
			MAMBAC (4 scales)	T, 0.34
		Social anhedonia (40)	MAXEIG (4 scales)	D
			MAMBAC (4 scales)	D
		Physical anhedonia (59)	MAXEIG (4 scales)	D
			MAMBAC (4 scales)	D

Note: 4DPT = Four-Dimensional Personality Test; A = ambiguous structure; D = dimensional (nontaxonic) structure; LCA = latent class analysis; L-MODE = latent modes analysis; MAMBAC = mean above minus below a cut; MAXCOV = maximum covariance analysis; MAXEIG = maximum eigenvalue analysis; MMPI = Minnesota Multiphasic Personality Inventory; SPQ = Schizotypal Personality Questionnaire (Raine, 1991); SS = Schizotypy Scale (Venables et al., 1990); STA = Schizotypal Personality Scale (Claridge and Broks, 1984); T = taxonic class structure; TPSQ = Thinking and Perceptual Style Questionnaire (Linscott and Knight, 2004).

[a] Of these, 845 participants (54.2%) came from the Blanchard et al. (2000) sample.

[b] High correlations among indicators suggests redundancy and violation of MAXCOV assumptions.

[c] Sampling methodology introduced significant systematic bias. Indicator construction method suggests redundancy and violation of MAXCOV assumptions.

both CCK- and FMM-type methods of analysis (Keller et al., 2001). The majority of these studies are free of major threats to their internal validity.

Two exceptions deserve brief mention. First, Fossati et al. (2007) examined the latent structure of total scores on three schizotypy measures in two samples, one comprising university students and the other adolescent school children, using maximum covariance analysis (Table 1). A significant limitation of this study was that the scale total scores were highly correlated (mean $r = 0.65$). Given their hypothesis there is a latent class structure with a prevalence of 0.10, and given class effect sizes on indicators that are in the order of $d = 2.0$, the expected correlation among indicators is just $r = 0.36$ (Meehl, 1992). Consequently, the assumption of conditional independence (or, zero nuisance covariance) was likely to have been substantially violated, undermining the result of the CCK method they used by elevating covariance across the sample. An alternative more conventional approach, involving the identification of moderately correlated subscale or item scores, might have provided a sounder test of the hypothesis.

Second, Rawlings et al. (2008) presented a reanalysis of data from four Chapman scales collected for the development of the Oxford-Liverpool Inventory of Feelings and Experiences (Claridge et al., 1996; Claridge, 1997). One vital problem with study was the introduction of systematic bias in the sampling method. Participants comprised a mix of undergraduates and professional staff at two universities, general public who were members of an experimental participant pool, and respondents to advertisements seeking people for a study of out-of-body experiences. Advertisement respondents constituted 38% of the sample. A second vital problem affected indicator selection, which consisted of random within-scale item pooling without any minimization of indicator redundancy. This strategy likely resulted in significant violation of conditional independence. Beauchaine et al. (2008) discuss other important problems with this study.

These two studies aside, results from undergraduate samples were remarkably consistent and substantially in favor of a latent class model of liability for schizophrenia (Table 1). This was the case for indicators of both positive and negative features of schizotypy (Fig. 5). Of 16 unambiguous findings based on positive indicators, 11 were interpreted as evidence of a latent class boundary, with a median prevalence of 0.105, and 5 as evidence of a latent continuum. Of 10 unambiguous findings from negative indicators, one was interpreted as evidence of a latent continuum, with the remainder evidence of a latent class with a median prevalence of 0.085.

These studies are not without limitations. Despite significant encouragement to use indicators that span multiple modes of assessment (e.g., Meehl, 1973), virtually all of these studies relied on a single mode, namely self-report. Similarly, many studies relied on just one analysis method, typically maximum covariance analysis. Often, studies focused on narrowly defined indicators, such as perceptual aberration, and few studies sought to validate any classes that were identified using independent measures.

One unresolved question arising from this research is whether positive and negative features of liability indicate the same latent class. Horan et al. (2004) attempted

Fig. 5 Class-of-interest prevalence estimates, and dimensional interpretations, from studies of psychometric risk in undergraduate and school children samples. (Estimates base on the mean-above-minus-below-a-cut CCK method are excluded as this procedure tends to over-estimate prevalence. Results from Fossati et al. (2007) and Rawlings et al. (2008) are excluded for reasons specified in the main text.) The horizontal marker indicates median estimates. A = ambiguous result, not included in calculation of median

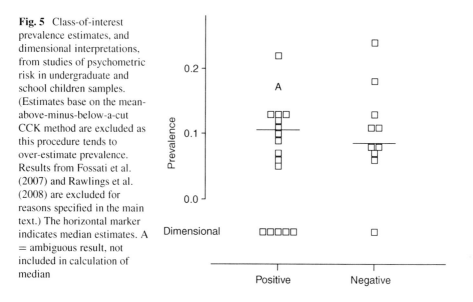

to address this question in two studies and their results provide some evidence that classes identified by positive and negative indicators are neither independent nor redundant, with an overlap that is somewhat greater than chance (Linscott, 2007). The parataxonic correlations Cuesta et al. (2007) observed among their three factors are consistent with the notion that positive and negative indicators tap distinct latent classes, as is evidence of similar nonmonotonic relationships among other self-report measures (Chapman et al., 1982; Linscott, 2007).

Discontinuities in Schizophrenia Endophenotypes

A notable body of research has examined the latent structure of a small number of putative schizophrenia endophenotypes, including ventricular enlargement (Harvey et al., 1990; Daniel et al., 1991), disturbances in eye movement (Gibbons et al., 1984; Sweeney et al., 1993; Pauler et al., 1996; Ross et al., 1996, 1997, 2002; Rubin and Wu, 1997), impaired memory (Lo et al., 2002), impaired attention (Erlenmeyer-Kimling et al., 1989), or a combination of these (Lenzenweger et al., 2007) in patients with schizophrenia, affective disorder, or other psychoses, in their biological relatives, or in general population samples. Unfortunately, only two of these studies have used CCK or FMM: Erlenmeyer-Kimling et al. (1989), which was described above, and Lenzenweger et al. (2007).

Lenzenweger et al. obtained data on sensitivity of attention, measured with a continuous performance test, and pursuit gain and catch-up saccades, measured with an eye-tracking task, from a self-selected general population sample ($n = 294$). Maximum covariance analysis and finite mixture modeling both supported a latent class model, with a class-of-interest prevalence of 0.27. Importantly, given the indicators, the liability status of this class was validated with two independent measures: self-reported features of schizotypal personality and family history of schizophrenia among first-degree relatives.

Discussion

The notion that schizophrenia, broadly construed, is on a continuum with normality affects research methodology, clinical practice, thinking about schizophrenia, and the direction of research. Our objective in this review was to seek evidence that might challenge this notion, purposively setting a standard of evidence that, if met, would cast doubt on the adequacy of a continuum model.

Evidence from studies of criterion symptoms of schizophrenia is, generally speaking, quite weak. Whereas this research could be interpreted as favoring a latent class viewpoint, serious methodological limitations suggest this research should be viewed with caution (Linscott et al., 2009). In contrast, studies of biological and psychometric risk and studies of putative endophenotypes provide a significant challenge to the continuum viewpoint. Several consistencies emerged. First, the majority of findings favor a latent class interpretation. Second, the estimates of the size of the latent class are high in studies of psychiatric patients and offspring of probands with schizophrenia and low in studies of general population and undergraduate samples. Third, evidence of taxonicity was not restricted to a particular measurement methodology. Finally, the level of replication of findings from studies of psychometric risk is very high (Beauchaine et al., 2008).

The evidence is consistent with a boundary that lies well beyond the clinical syndrome, presumably capturing related disorders, prodromal states, and trait liability. However, this interpretation comes with several important qualifications. First, although there are consistencies despite methodological variability, the methodological variability is not great and only the self-report-based evidence is well replicated. Moreover, the methodological variability only exists between studies. No studies have ventured to include indicators from a multilevel multimodal battery of measures (cf. Meehl, 1973). In the absence of within-study variability in measurement, doubts persist about the potential contribution of psychometric or measurement artifacts, on the one hand, and about the clinical relevance of the findings on the other (Linscott et al., 2009). That is, whereas a multilevel multimodal battery would simultaneously preempt concerns about measurement artifacts and clarify interpretation by linking clinical phenotypes, endophenotypes, exploratory measures, and latent structure, this approach has not yet been used despite early recommendations (Meehl, 1973).

Second, while the concept of a dichotomous class may be appealing and makes intuitive sense, it can be shown that common phenotypes are unlikely to be entirely dichotomous in nature if their origin is multifactorial. For example, diseases caused by a single dominant gene defect that is fully penetrant may exist as a truly dichotomous phenomenon. If nothing else influences the expression of the genetic defect, the disease in question will have the same distribution as the genetic defect itself. However, in the case of multifactorial traits, such as the behavioral phenotype of schizotypy, where multiple interacting causes contribute to the phenotypic distribution, it can be shown, using statistical simulations, that the most likely distribution is half-normal (van Os et al., 2009). It may be argued that it would still be possible that multiple interacting factors contribute to an underlying continuous abnormality that, when a certain threshold is reached, gives rise to a dichotomous behavioral phenotype. Although this may be possible, it is unlikely given the fact that the biological and cognitive abnormalities associated with (the genetics of) schizotypy and schizophrenia have all been demonstrated to behave as linear risk indicators without evidence of threshold effects (Jones et al., 1994a,b). Therefore, to the degree that etiology dictates that the schizotypy phenotype must be continuous, it cannot be excluded that CCK and related statistical methods pick up a class where the phenotype exists as a severely skewed but continuous phenotype.

Third, the consistency between findings from studies measuring negative and positive features of psychometric risk should not be mistaken as evidence that the latent classes are one and the same. It is equally the case—given the design limitations of the available literature—that the evidence is consistent with the existence of distinct positive and negative latent risk taxa (Horan et al., 2004; Linscott, 2007). Indeed, the common observation of nonmonotonic associations between positive and negative markers of risk (Chapman et al., 1982; Cuesta et al., 2007; Linscott, 2007) is consistent with a three-group latent structure, comprising two risk groups and a large normative group (Meehl, 1999).

Finally, there is relatively little evidence on the validity of the latent class (or classes) of interest. More importantly, prospective evidence on the outcomes associated with class membership is particularly weak. There is some evidence from prospective biological high-risk cohorts that class-of-interest membership is associated with high rates of schizophrenia-spectrum disorders (Tyrka et al., 1995) and need for care (Erlenmeyer-Kimling et al., 1989). However, there is no prospective data from taxometrically defined psychometric risk groups. This notwithstanding, there is evidence that quantitative measures of psychometric risk are associated with schizophrenia-spectrum outcomes (Chapman et al., 1994; Poulton et al., 2000).

Professor Doug Melton (personal communication, February 19, 2009) often comments that one of the key hurdles to the advancement of research into neurological disorders is the dependence of research on participants who can only be identified once symptoms emerge. If a disorder has an early-life developmental etiology, the benefits of research into the end stages of the disorder are clearly constrained. Biological high-risk studies and research into prodromal states provide important means of moving beyond this constraint in the context of schizophrenia. However, given only a small minority of patients with schizophrenia have a parent with schizophrenia (Gottesman, 1991), a substantial proportion of the disease burden falls outside risk groups defined by inheritance. Similarly, prodromal research requires symptomatic help seekers and so is also constrained. In this context, psychometric methods for identifying liability for schizophrenia offer an important window for research into the causes of schizophrenia. If it is the case that liability is continuously distributed in the general population, with no nonarbitrary boundary, venturing beyond the clinical syndrome carries the risk that research could become bogged down in personality variables and other individual differences (McGrath, this volume). In contrast, significant methodological efficiencies would be afforded if one or more natural boundaries exist.

Given the limitations of the available evidence, the growing recognition that *DSM* classes do not correspond to natural disease boundaries (e.g., Cannon, this volume), and the methodological significance of a nonarbitrary liability, it is time for more comprehensive analyses of continuum vs. class viewpoints. Three types of studies are required. Sound epidemiological general population studies are required to determine whether the latent class evidence obtained in psychometric risk studies can be corroborated using meaningful multilevel multimodal assessment batteries. Second, taxometric analyses of theoretically meaningful variables collected from unselected help seekers (i.e., samples unmodified by diagnosis- or symptom-related service parameters or inclusion and exclusion criteria) should be used to examine questions about the totality or unity of psychosis or about conceptual divisions between classes of schizophrenia (e.g., deficit vs. nondeficit). Third, where any evidence for latent class boundaries is found, prospective validation of the class of interest is essential.

Finally, in undertaking research in this area, design is critical. As mentioned, the statistical methods used in the literature we have reviewed are not intelligent systems, somehow only divining the latent structure of the theoretical notion the researcher is thinking about. In early studies, researchers devoted particularly careful attention to many—although not all—design issues beyond the technical application of the statistical procedures themselves: indicator selection, indicator validity, and the many issues involved in setting sample recruitment and composition protocols. It is concerning that this has not been the case generally, particularly in some of the more recent studies (e.g., Fossati et al., 2007; Rawlings et al., 2008). However, serious design-related oversights are not specific to CCK and FMM research. We recently suggested that similar serious design issues were so prevalent among research into Criterion A features of schizophrenia using latent class analyses that the body of literature itself provided no reasonable test of the latent structure of these features (Linscott et al., 2009).

References

American Psychiatric Association Diagnostic and Statistical Manual of Mental Disorders. Author, Washington, DC, 2000.

Beauchaine, T. P. & Beauchaine, R. J., III A comparison of maximum covariance and *k*-means cluster analysis in classifying cases into known taxon groups. Psychological Methods 7: 245–261, 2002.

Beauchaine, T. P., Lenzenweger, M. F. & Waller, N. G. Schizotypy, taxometrics, and disconfirming theories in soft science. Personality and Individual Differences 44: 1652–1662, 2008.

Bell, M. Cognitively disorganized schizophrenia: a taxometric analysis of PANSS ratings. Schizophrenia Research 24: 98, 1997.

Blanchard, J. J., Gangestad, S. W., Brown, S. A. & Horan, W. P. Hedonic capacity and schizotypy revisited: A taxometric analysis of social anhedonia. Journal of Abnormal Psychology 109: 87–95, 2000.

Blanchard, J. J., Horan, W. P. & Collins, L. M. Examining the latent structure of negative symptoms: Is there a distinct subtype of negative symptom schizophrenia? Schizophrenia Research 77: 151–165, 2005.

Brenner, V. & Raulin, M. L. Validation of the Schizotypal Taxon Using Graphical Taxometric Techniques. 102nd Annual American Psychological Convention, Los Angeles, CA, 1994.

Brenner, V., Raulin, M. L. & Young, B. L. Comparing the Sensitivity of Two Taxometric Techniques in Detecting the Schizotypal Taxonomy. Annual Convention of the Society for Research on Psychopathology, Iowa City, IA, 1995.

Brockington, I. F., Kendell, R. E., Wainwright, S., Hillier, V. F. & Walker, J. The distinction between the affective psychoses and schizophrenia. British Journal of Psychiatry 135: 243–248, 1979.

Chapman, L. J., Chapman, J. P., Kwapil, T. R., Eckblad, M. & Zinser, M. C. Putatively psychosis-prone subjects 10 years later. Journal of Abnormal Psychology 103: 171–183, 1994.

Chapman, L. J., Chapman, J. P. & Miller, E. N. Reliabilities and intercorrelations of eight measures of proneness to psychosis. Journal of Consulting and Clinical Psychology 85: 374–382, 1982.

Chapman, L. J., Chapman, J. P. & Raulin, M. L. Scales for physical and social anhedonia. Journal of Abnormal Psychology 85: 374–382, 1976.

Chapman, L. J., Chapman, J. P. & Raulin, M. L. Body-image aberration in schizophrenia. Journal of Abnormal Psychology 87: 399–407, 1978.

Claridge, G. Schizotypy: Implications for Illness and Health. Oxford University Press, New York, 1997.

Claridge, G. & Broks, P. Schizotypy and hemispheric function-I. Theoretical considerations and the measurement of schizotypy. Personality and Individual Differences 5: 633–648, 1984.

Claridge, G., et al. The factor structure of 'schizotypal' traits: A large replication study. British Journal of Clinical Psychology 35:103–115, 1996.

Cleland, C. M., Rothschild, L. & Haslam, N. Detecting latent taxa: Monte Carlo comparison of taxometric, mixture model, and clustering procedures. Psychological Reports 87: 37–47, 2000.

Cuesta, M. J., Ugarte, M. D., Goicoa, T., Eraso, S. & Peralta, V. A taxometric analysis of schizophrenia symptoms. Psychiatry Research 150: 245–253, 2007.

Daniel, D. G., Goldberg, T. E., Gibbons, R. D. & Weinberger, D. R. Lack of a bimodal distribution of ventricular size in schizophrenia: A Gaussian mixture analysis of 1056 cases and controls. Biological Psychiatry 30: 887–903, 1991.

Eckblad, M. L. & Chapman, L. J. Magical ideation as an indicator of schizotypy. Journal of Consulting and Clinical Psychology 51: 215–225, 1983.

Erlenmeyer-Kimling, L., Golden, R. R. & Cornblatt, B. A. A taxometric analysis of cognitive and neuromotor variables in children at risk for schizophrenia. Journal of Abnormal Psychology 98: 203–208, 1989.

Fossati, A., Raine, A., Borroni, S. & Maffei, C. Taxonic structure of schizotypal personality in nonclinical subjects: Issues of replicability and age consistency. Psychiatry Research 152: 103–112, 2007.

Gibbons, R. D., Dorus, E., Ostrow, D. G., Pandey, G. N., Davis, J. M. & Levy, D. L. Mixture distributions in psychiatric research. Biological Psychiatry 19: 935–961, 1984.

Golden, R. R. A taxometric model for the detection of a conjectured latent taxon. Multivariate Behavioral Research 17: 389–416, 1982.

Golden, R. R. & Meehl, P. E. Detection of the schizoid taxon with MMPI indicators. Journal of Abnormal Psychology 88: 217–233, 1979.

Golden, R. R. & Meehl, P. E. Detection of biological sex: An empirical test of cluster methods. Multivariate Behavioral Research 15: 475–496, 1980.

Gottesman, I. I. Schizophrenia Genesis: The Origins of Madness. Freeman, New York, 1991.

Grayson, D. A. Can categorical and dimensional views of psychiatric illness be distinguished? British Journal of Psychiatry 151: 355–361, 1987.

Harvey, I., Mcguffin, P., Williams, M. & Toone, B. K. The ventricle-brain ratio (VBR) in functional psychoses: An admixture analysis. Psychiatry Research: Neuroimaging 35: 61–69, 1990.

Horan, W. P., Blanchard, J. J., Gangestad, S. W. & Kwapil, T. R. The psychometric detection of schizotypy: Do putative schizotypy indicators identify the same latent class? Journal of Abnormal Psychology 113: 339–357, 2004.

Jones, P., Rodgers, B., Murray, R. & Marmot, M. Child development risk factors for adult schizophrenia in the British 1946 birth cohort. Lancet 344: 1398–1402, 1994a.

Jones, P. B., et al. Cerebral ventricle dimensions as risk factors for schizophrenia and affective psychosis: An epidemiological approach to analysis. Psychological Medicine 24: 995–1011, 1994b.

Keller, F., Jahn, T. & Klein, C. Anwendung von taxometrischen methoden und von mischverteilungsmodellen zur erfassung der schizotypie. In: Andresen, B. & Mas, R. (eds.) Schizotypie: Psychometrische entwicklungen und biopsychologische forschungsansätze, Hogrefe, Göttingen, Germany, pp. 391–412, 2001.

Kendell, R. E. & Brockington, I. F. The identification of disease entities and the relationship between schizophrenic and affective psychoses. British Journal of Psychiatry 137: 324–331, 1980.

Kendell, R. E. & Gourlay, J. The clinical distinction between the affective psychoses and schizophrenia. British Journal of Psychiatry 117: 261–266, 1970.

Korfine, L. & Lenzenweger, M. F. The taxonicity of schizotypy: A replication. Journal of Abnormal Psychology 104: 26–31, 1995.

Lenzenweger, M. F. Deeper into the schizotypy taxon: On the robust nature of maximum covariance analysis. Journal of Abnormal Psychology 108: 182–187, 1999.

Lenzenweger, M. F. & Korfine, L. Confirming the latent structure and base rate of schizotypy: A taxometric analysis. Journal of Abnormal Psychology 101: 567–571, 1992.

Lenzenweger, M. F., Mclachlan, G. & Rubin, D. B. Resolving the latent structure of schizophrenia endophenotypes using expectation-maximization-based finite mixture modeling. Journal of Abnormal Psychology 116: 16–29, 2007.

Linscott, R. J. The latent structure and coincidence of hypohedonia and schizotypy and their validity as indices of psychometric risk for schizophrenia. Journal of Personality Disorders 21: 225–242, 2007.

Linscott, R. J., Allardyce, J. & Van Os, J. Seeking verisimilitude in a class: A systematic review of evidence that the criterial clinical symptoms of schizophrenia are taxonic. Schizophrenia Bulletin in press: 1–19, 2009.

Linscott, R. J. & Knight, R. G. Potentiated automatic memory in schizotypy. Personality and Individual Differences 37: 1503–1517, 2004.

Linscott, R. J., Marie, D., Arnott, K. L. & Clark, B. L. Over-representation of Maori New Zealanders among adolescents in a schizotypy taxon. Schizophrenia Research 84: 289–296, 2006.

Lo, Y., Matthysse, S., Rubin, D. B. & Holzman, P. S. Permutation tests for detecting and estimating mixtures in task performance within groups. Statistics in Medicine 21: 1937–1953, 2002.

Lowrie, G. S. & Raulin, M. L. Search for Schizotypic and Nonschizotypic Taxonomies in a College Population. Sixty-First Annual Convention of the Eastern Psychological Association, Philadelphia, PA, 1990.

Lowrie, G. S. & Raulin, M. L. Testing the construct validity of Meehl's taxonic model of schizotypy: Taxometric search techniques applied to self-report measures of schizotypic signs. Unpublished manuscript, 1996.

Macfarlane, R. M. Taxometric analysis of schizotypy. Unpublished thesis, University of Iowa, 1996.

Maxwell, A. E. Multivariate statistical methods and classification problems. British Journal of Psychiatry 119: 121–127, 1971.

Meehl, P. E. Maxcov-Hitmax: A taxonomic search method for loose genetic syndromes. In: Meehl, P. E. (eds.) Psychodiagnosis: Selected papers, University of Minnesota Press, Minneapolis, pp. 200–224, 1973.

Meehl, P. E. A funny thing happened to us on the way to the latent entities. Journal of Personality Assessment 43: 564–581, 1979.

Meehl, P. E. Factors and taxa, traits and types, differences of degree and differences in kind. Journal of Personality 60: 117–174, 1992.

Meehl, P. E. Bootstraps taxometrics: Solving the classification problem in psychopathology. American Psychologist 50: 266–275, 1995.

Meehl, P. E. Clarifications about taxometric method. Applied and Preventive Psychology 8: 165–174, 1999.

Meehl, P. E. What's in a taxon? Journal of Abnormal Psychology 113: 39–43, 2004.

Meehl, P. E. & Yonce, L. J. Taxometric analysis: I. Detecting taxonicity with two quantitative indicators using means above and below a sliding cut (MAMBAC procedure). Psychological Reports 74: 1059–1274, 1994.

Meyer, T. D. & Keller, F. Exploring the latent structure of the perceptual aberration, magical ideation, and physical anhedonia scales in a German sample. Journal of Personality Disorders 15: 521–535, 2001.

Mishlove, M. & Chapman, L. J. Social anhedonia in the prediction of psychosis proneness. Journal of Abnormal Psychology 94: 384–396, 1985.

Murphy, E. A. One cause? Many causes? The argument from the bimodal distribution. Journal of Chronic Diseases 17: 301—324, 1964.

Muthén, B. & Asparouhov, T. Item response mixture modeling: Application to tobacco dependence criteria. Addictive Behaviors 31: 1050–1066, 2006.

Pauler, D. K., Escobar, M. D., Sweeney, J. A. & Greenhouse, J. Mixture models for eye-tracking data: A case study. Statistics in Medicine 15: 1365–1376, 1996.

Peralta, V. & Cuesta, M. J. How many and which are the psychopathological dimensions in schizophrenia? Issues influencing their ascertainment. Schizophrenia Research 49: 269–285, 2001.

Peralta, V. & Cuesta, M. J. The nosology of psychotic disorders: A comparison among competing classification systems. Schizophrenia Bulletin 29: 413–425, 2003.

Poulton, R., Caspi, A., Moffitt, T. E., Cannon, M., Murray, R. & Harrington, H. Children's self-reported psychotic symptoms and adult schizophreniform disorder: A 15-year longitudinal study. Archives of General Psychiatry 57: 1053–1058, 2000.

Raine, A. The SPQ: A scale for the assessment of schizotypal personality based on DSM-III-R criteria. Schizophrenia Bulletin 17: 555–564, 1991.

Rawlings, D., Williams, B., Haslam, N. & Claridge, G. Taxometric analysis supports a dimensional latent structure for schizotypy. Personality and Individual Differences 44: 1640–1651, 2008.

Ross, D. E., Ochs, A. L., Pandurangi, A. K., Thacker, L. R. & Kendler, K. S. Mixture analysis of smooth pursuit eye movements in schizophrenia. Psychophysiology 33: 390–397, 1996.

Ross, D. E., et al. Eye tracking disorder in schizophrenia is characterized by specific ocular motor defects and is associated with the deficit syndrome. Biological Psychiatry 42: 781–796, 1997.

Ross, R. G., et al. Admixture analysis of smooth pursuit eye movements in probands with schizophrenia and their relatives suggests gain and leading saccades are potential endophenotypes. Psychophysiology 39: 809–819, 2002.

Rubin, D. B. & Wu, Y. N. Modeling schizophrenic behavior using general mixture components. Biometrics 53: 243–261, 1997.

Ruscio, J. & Ruscio, A. M. Clarifying boundary issues in psychopathology: The role of taxometrics in a comprehensive program of structural research. Journal of Abnormal Psychology 113: 24–38, 2004.

Schooler, N. R., et al. Relapse and rehospitalization during maintenance treatment of schizophrenia. The effects of dose reduction and family treatment. Archives of General Psychiatry 54: 453–463, 1997.

Shevlin, M., Adamson, G., Vollebergh, W., De Graaf, R. & Van Os, J. An application of item response mixture modelling to psychosis indicators in two large community samples. Social Psychiatry and Psychiatric Epidemiology 42: 771–779, 2007a.

Shevlin, M., Murphy, J., Dorahy, M. J. & Adamson, G. The distribution of positive psychosis-like symptoms in the population: A latent class analysis of the National Comorbidity Survey. Schizophrenia Research 89: 101–109, 2007b.

Sweeney, J. A., Clementz, B. A., Escobar, M. D., Li, S., Pauler, D. K. & HAAS, G. L. Mixture analysis of pursuit eye-tracking dysfunction in schizophrenia. Biological Psychiatry 34: 331–340, 1993.

Tyrka, A. R., et al. The latent structure of schizotypy: I. Premorbid indicators of a taxon of individuals at risk for schizophrenia-spectrum disorders. Journal of Abnormal Psychology 104: 173–183, 1995.

Van Kampen, D. Genetic and environmental influences on pre-schizophrenic personality: MAXCOV-HITMAX and LISREL analyses. European Journal of Personality 13: 63–80, 1999.

Van Os, J., Linscott, R. J., Myin-Germeys, I., Delespaul, P. & Krabbendam, L. A systematic review and meta-analysis of the psychosis continuum: Evidence for a psychosis proneness-persistence-impairment model of psychotic disorder. Psychological Medicine 39(2):179–195, 2009.

Van Os, J., Linscott, R. J., Myin-Germeys, I., Delespaul, P. & Krabbendam, L. A systematic review and meta-analysis of the psychosis continuum: Evidence for a psychosis proneness-persistence-impairment model of psychotic disorder. Psychological Medicine 39: 179–195, 2009.

Venables, P. H., Wilkins, S., Mitchell, D. A., Raine, A. & Bailes, K. A scale for the measurement of schizotypy. Personality and Individual Differences 11: 481–495, 1990.

Waller, N. G. & Meehl, P. E. Multivariate Taxometric Procedures: Distinguishing Types from Continua. Sage, Thousand Oaks, CA, 1998.

Whitehead, K. V. Precursors for Schizophrenia: Are Schizotaxia and Schizotypy Related? Unpublished thesis, University of Otago, 2005.

World Health Organization. ICD-10: International Statistical Classification of Diseases and Related Health Problems (10th ed.). World Health Organization, Geneva, 2004.

Integrating the Epidemiology and Pathogenesis of Schizophrenia from the Street to the Striatum: Integrating the Epidemiology and Pathogenesis of Schizophrenia

Robin M. Murray, Marta Di Forti, and Oliver Howes

Research into schizophrenia has proceeded in a patchwork manner as if isolated portions of a giant jigsaw were being completed with little thought as to how these might contribute to the whole picture. For example, investigations into the two major pathogenic theories of schizophrenia, namely the dopamine hypothesis and the neurodevelopmental hypothesis, proceeded for many years in parallel with little crosstalk. Only recently have there been attempts to integrate the two theories, with our group concluding that dopamine dysregulation is the final step in a complex developmental cascade that starts early in life and ends with the onset of full-blown psychosis (Murray et al., 2008a).

The neurodevelopmental hypothesis originally supposed that variants of developmental genes interacted with early neurological insults to produce developmental deviance and ultimately schizophrenia. As a result of epidemiological studies this hypothesis has been modified to include the pathogenic effects of abuse of certain drugs and also of chronic social adversity; therefore, it is perhaps now more appropriately termed the developmental hypothesis (Howes et al., 2004).

Unfortunately, there has been no such productive interchange between epidemiologists and dopamine theorists. Given the central role that dopamine dysregulation appears to play in the proximal pathogenesis of psychosis (Howes and Kapur, 2009), one inevitably must consider the causes of this dysregulation. We have elsewhere briefly outlined some of the evidence that various established risk factors for schizophrenia impact on the dopamine system (Di Forti et al., 2007). A logical extension of such reasoning is to consider whether the epidemiology of schizophrenia may be explained on the basis of what we know about the pathophysiology of dopamine. This chapter will address this question. However, first we will briefly review the modern view of how dopamine dysregulation underlies psychotic symptoms.

R.M. Murray (✉)
Division of Psychological Medicine and Psychiatry, Institute of Psychiatry, King's College London, De Crespigny Park, London SE5 8AF, UK
e-mail: robin.murray@kcl.ac.uk3

W.F. Gattaz, G. Busatto (eds.), *Advances in Schizophrenia Research 2009*,
DOI 10.1007/978-1-4419-0913-8_19, © Springer Science+Business Media, LLC 2010

Striatal Dopamine as the 'Wind of Psychotic Fire'

The 'classical' dopamine hypothesis of schizophrenia was proposed over 30 years ago and states that schizophrenia is associated with an exaggerated dopaminergic function in the central nervous system (Snyder, 1976). We now know that this is a synaptic excess of dopamine: patients with schizophrenia show elevated baseline striatal availability of dopamine (Abi-Dargham, 2004; Howes et al., 2007) and increased release of dopamine in the striatum following amphetamine challenge (Laruelle et al., 1996; Breier et al., 1997; Abi-Dargham et al., 1998; Laruelle and Abi-Dargham, 1999a, b). Furthermore, the degree of dopamine release is directly related to the severity of symptoms, particularly psychotic symptoms (Laruelle et al., 1999).

Recently we have begun to understand how excessive release of dopamine facilitates the development of the classic positive symptoms of psychosis, hallucinations, and delusions. Building on the evidence that dopamine normally mediates the attachment of salience to ideas and objects, Kapur et al. (2005) proposed that heightened dopaminergic neurotransmission leads to aberrant assignment of salience to normal external and internal stimuli and that delusions arise from attempts to explain this. Until recently this remained only a theory. However, now Murray et al. (2008b) have shown that first-episode psychotic patients show less ability than controls to distinguish between motivationally salient stimuli as opposed to neutral stimuli, i.e., they showed rapid reactivity even to stimuli that predicted no reward. Furthermore, fMRI demonstrated that the patients showed smaller differences than controls in midbrain activation in response to stimuli that either predicted the possibility of reward or did not. Thus the patients showed both behavioral and physiological evidence of abnormality in dopamine-based reinforcement learning and provide empirical support for Kapur's theory.

When does this dopaminergic dysregulation develop? We know that it occurs before the onset of frank psychosis and that there is excess release of dopamine from the striatum in individuals who are at ultra high risk of psychosis, as well as those experiencing their first psychotic episode (Howes et al., 2009). This suggests that, somewhere around their late teens, patients develop an abnormality of the dopamine system such that there is an exaggerated release of dopamine to normal stimuli.

We will now proceed to discuss how what we know about the epidemiology of schizophrenia might be related to the pathophysiology of dopamine.

Age of Onset and Gender Distribution

The most striking epidemiological characteristics of schizophrenia are (a) its predominant onset between late adolescence and early 30s and (b) the fact that it is more common and more severe in men. This distribution is paralleled by that of minor psychotic symptoms in the general population. Verdoux and Van Os (2002) who studied this latter showed a predominance of delusional ideas in young people, especially males. Is it possible that young men are particularly vulnerable to development of psychotic symptoms both mild and severe because of the characteristics of their dopamine systems?

The age of onset distribution of schizophrenia fits well with what we know regarding the age-related activity of dopamine neurones. It is well established that there are significant reductions in pre- and post-synaptic markers during normal aging with losses in dopamine receptors and transporters (Reeves et al., 2002). The significance of this for the motor system is evident in the fact that Parkinson's disease is mainly a disorder of later life. However, until recently little attention had been paid to the effects on behavior. Now Dreher and colleagues (2008) have investigated the neurofunctional consequences of this age-related dopaminergic decline. Using FluroDOPA PET and event-related fMRI, they showed that normal aging induces functional changes in the dopamine-based reward system and, in particular, in the relationship between subcortical dopamine availability and pre-frontal activity in reward processing (Dreher et al., 2008).

Gender differences in schizophrenia were the cause of much speculation in the 1990s. Two main theories were proposed to explain the early onset in males and male preponderance and severity. The first noted that schizophrenia is at least in part a neurodevelopmental disorder and that all neurodevelopmental disorders are more common in men (Castle and Murray, 1991). The second proposed that young females were spared schizophrenia by the antidopaminergic effects of estrogen (Hafner et al., 1993). However neither of these theories is satisfactory.

A more immediately relevant notion arises from recent evidence that men have a more positive subjective responsive to the effects of amphetamine. Munro et al. (2006) confirmed this in the course of a PET study examining the magnitude of displacement of raclopride binding following an amphetamine challenge. Importantly men showed robustly greater dopamine release in the ventral striatum and indeed in three out of four other striatal regions. The primary conclusion of the authors was that this greater effect on reward might explain why men are more likely to abuse drugs. However, they did also note the earlier onset and greater severity of schizophrenia in men though they did not suggest any mechanism underlying this. If indeed psychotic symptoms arise out of a dopaminergic disturbance of the normal process of attribution of salience, then could it be that males with their more reactive striatal dopamine system might be more prone to both the onset of disturbance and of its persistence.

Abuse of Drugs

Abuse of some but not all drugs is associated with schizophrenia-like psychosis.

Stimulants: Amphetamine-induced psychosis was clearly described in the 1950s (Connell, 1958), and more recently the psychosis associated with methamphetamine use has been more fully examined in recent years by Chen et al. (2003). These investigators reported that methamphetamine users with psychosis presented a clinical picture that closely mimicked the positive symptoms of schizophrenia. How does abuse of amphetamine or methamphetamine lead to psychosis? Repeated use of stimulants has been shown to result in sensitization of the dopaminergic system in healthy volunteers (Boileau et al., 2006). Furthermore there is evidence for cross-sensitization (Boileau et al., 2007). For example, ketamine, a stimulant that induces psychotic-like symptoms, increases the dopamine release to levels seen in patients with schizophrenia when given with amphetamine but not when given alone (Kegeles et al., 2000, 2002). These findings are consistent with the idea that in individuals who have a 'sensitive striatal dopaminergic system,' arising from either genetic reasons or through early environmental damage, repeated use of stimulants may induce sensitization of the dopamine system, to a point that it becomes dysregulated and results in disordered salience and ultimately psychosis.

Cannabis: There are now a number of longitudinal prospective studies that indicate that the use of cannabis leads to an increased risk of schizophrenia-like psychosis or psychotic symptoms (Andréasson et al., 1987; Arseneault et al., 2002; Fergusson et al., 2005). Several reviews and meta-analyses have been carried out, reaching the conclusion that heavy use of cannabis is a contributory cause of schizophrenia in a dose-responsive manner (Arseneault et al., 2004; Henquet et al., 2005; Murray et al., 2007).

Does cannabis or its main psychoactive ingredient tetrahydrocannabinol (THC) affect striatal dopamine? As yet only one published study has examined this following a challenge dose of THC. Bossong et al. (2009), using the PET and raclopride displacement paradigm in seven healthy males, noted significant displacement of raclopride compatible with THC having provoked the release of endogeneous dopamine. These data suggesting that the psychotogenic effects of THC are mediated by dopamine are compatible with the findings of Caspi et al. (2005) who showed that those adolescent cannabis users who carry the val allele of the catechol-O-methyltransferase (COMT) gene are more likely to subsequently develop psychosis than those with the met allele; COMT, of course, is responsible for the breakdown of dopamine in the pre-frontal cortex.

Susceptibility Genes

Schizophrenia is highly heritable but identifying susceptible genes has proved far from easy. So far the evidence suggests the operation of many genes of small effect. Two particular types of susceptibility genes have recently been associated with schizophrenia. First are neurodevelopmental genes, such as neuregulin, dysbindin, and DISC 1 (Harrison and Owen, 2003; O'Donovan et al., 2008; Sullivan, 2008). Second, genes associated with dopamine regulation such as the COMT gene just mentioned and dopamine DRD3 have been reported as possibly implicated. Talkowski (2008) has suggested that possibly a number of small effects operating at different points in the dopamine system may act together to produce susceptibility.

Should this be the case then one might expect that the relatives of people with schizophrenia would share some of the dopaminergic abnormalities demonstrated by their affected kin. Indeed this seems to be the case. Finnish research has shown that the first-degree relatives of people with schizophrenia show an increased capacity to synthesize dopamine in the caudate and the putamen (Huttunen et al., 2007).

Obstetric Events

Many studies have also shown that early environmental 'insults,' especially obstetric complications, such as hypoxia, are more common in people with schizophrenia than in the general population (Cannon et al., 2002), and there is increasing evidence that an interaction between genetically predisposed individuals and obstetric events may occur (Schulze et al., 2003) and that those patients who have suffered obstetric events are particularly to have decreased volume of the hippocampus (Stefanis et al., 1999).

Such early environmental factors may impact on the development of the dopamine system. For example, hippocampal lesions made in neonatal rats result in increased striatal dopamine levels in post-pubertal rats (Alquicer et al., 2004).

Animal studies indicate that perinatal damage leads to a labile dopaminergic system vulnerable to sensitization. Moore et al. (1999) suggested that developmental disruption of the hippocampus cortex can result in dysregulation of the dopaminergic inputs to the striatum, increasing the response to novelty, mild stress, or psychotomimetics.

Social Adversity

There has been a resurgence of interest in the effects of social adversity on risk of schizophrenia.

Childhood: Childhood trauma such as physical or sexual abuse, or emotional neglect is reported to be associated with a significant, although relatively moderate, increase in risk of later developing schizophrenia (Morgan and Fisher, 2007). Animal studies indicate that environmental effects post-natally may modulate striatal dopaminergic systems and that this may depend on gene–environmental interactions. For example, isolation rearing elevates striatal dopaminergic turnover in mice and is associated with deficits in pre-pulse inhibition (Eells et al., 2006b). The effects of isolation rearing on pre-pulse inhibition can be reversed by depleting dopamine levels in the nucleus accumbens (Powell et al., 2003). Maternal separation has similar effects on young rats, leading to alterations in striatal dopaminergic function (Hall et al., 1999).

Later Effects: It is well known that the incidence of schizophrenia is increased among migrants and minority populations (Harrison, et al., 1988; Bhugra, 2000; Selten et al., 2001). The incidence of schizophrenia among people from non-white ethnic minorities has been investigated by comparing neighborhoods where they constituted a smaller or larger proportion of the total population (Boydell et al., 2001). The incidence ratio of schizophrenia increased significantly as the proportion of minorities in the local population fell, from 2.4 in areas where the

Developmental Cascade towards Schizophrenia

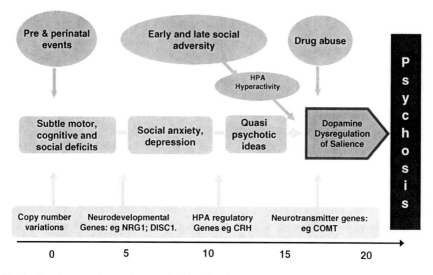

Fig. 1 Developmental cascade toward schizophrenia

minorities formed a larger proportion of the local population to 4.4 in the areas where they formed a smaller proportion. This suggests that social isolation and the lack of social support for people living in an alien environment may be factors contributing to schizophrenia. Such population-based data are supported by animal studies that show that social isolation, social stress, subordination, or defeat are also associated with changes in the dopaminergic system (Shively, 1998; Isovich et al., 2000, 2001). Hence, not only certain drugs of abuse but also certain types of social adversity could induce dopamine sensitization, disordered salience, and ultimately psychosis.

Of course such factors presumably operate particularly on those with a susceptible genotype. The nurr1 gene is required for terminal differentiation of dopamine neurons and abnormalities in it have been associated with schizophrenia (Castillo et al., 1998; Chen et al., 2001). Mice heterozygous for the Nurr-1 null genotype show additional effects of isolation rearing. Isolation disrupted pre-pulse inhibition and reduced markers of pre-frontal cortical dopamine in Nurr-1 null heterozygotes compared to wild-type isolation-reared mice, whereas the group raised with Nurr-1 null heterozygotes did not show alterations in pre-frontal dopamine markers (Eells et al., 2006a).

Conclusion

In most medical disorders what is known about epidemiology maps directly onto theories of pathogenesis. This has not been the case for schizophrenia. However, now that we know the main risk factors for schizophrenia and that dopamine-driven dysfunction of the process of attribution of salience underlies some of the positive symptoms of psychosis, the way is open to attempt to attempt to link the two, as outlined in Fig. 1.

Of course, it is likely that there are many steps in between risk factors and the dopamine system, involving, for example, GABA and glutamate systems. However, the evidence that we have briefly discussed suggests that there is merit in setting up hypotheses to test the relationship between identified risk factors and striatal dopamine regulation.

References

Abi-Dargham A, Gil R, Krystal J, Baldwin RM, Seibyl JP, Bowers M, van Dyck CH, Charney DS, Innis RB, Laruelle M (1998). Increased striatal dopamine transmission in schizophrenia: confirmation in a second cohort. American Journal of Psychiatry, 155(6), 761–767.

Abi-Dargham A (2004). Do we still believe in the dopamine hypothesis? New data bring new evidence. International Journal Neuropsychopharmacology, 7(Suppl 1), S1–S5.

Alquicer G, Silva-Gomez AB, Peralta F, Flores G (2004). Neonatal ventral hippocampus lesion alters the dopamine content in the limbic regions in postpubertal rats. International Journal of Developmental Neuroscience, 22, 103–111.

Andréasson S, Allebeck P, et al. (1987). Cannabis and schizophrenia. A longitudinal study of Swedish conscripts. Lancet 2(8574), 1483–1486.

Arseneault L, Cannon M, Poulton R, Murray R, Caspi A, Moffitt TE (2002). Cannabis use in adolescence and risk for adult psychosis: longitudinal prospective study. British Medical Journal, 325(7374), 1212–1213.

Arseneault L, Cannon M, Witton J, Murray R M (2004). Causal association between cannabis and psychosis: Examination of evidence. British Journal of Psychiatry 184, 110–117.

Bhugra D (2000). "Migration and schizophrenia." Acta Psychiatrica Scandinava Suppl 102(407), 68–73.

Boileau I, Dagher A, Leyton M, et al. (2006). Modeling sensitization to stimulants in humans: An [11C]raclopride/positron emission tomography study in healthy men. Archive of General Psychiatry, 63, 1386–1395.

Boileau I, Dagher A, Leyton M, et al. (2007). Conditioned dopamine release in humans: A positron emission tomography [11C]raclopride study with amphetamine. Journal of Neuroscience, 27, 3998–4003.

Bossong MG, Van Berckel BN, Boellaard R, Zuurman L, Schuit RC, Windhorst AD, Van Gerven JM, Ramsey NF, Lammertsma AA, Kahn RS (2009). Delta 9-tetrahydrocannabinol induces dopamine release in the human striatum. Neuropsychopharmacology 34, 759–766.

Boydell J, Van Os J, Mckenzie K, Allardyce J, Goel R, Mccreadie RG, Murray RM (2001). Incidence of schizophrenia in ethnic minorities in London: ecological study into interactions with environment. British Medical Journal 323(7325), 1336–1338.

Breier A, Su TP, Saunders R, et al. (1997). Schizophrenia is associated with elevated amphetamine-induced synaptic dopamine concentrations: Evidence from a novel positron emission tomography method. Proceedings of the National Academy of Science USA, 94, 2569–2574.

Cannon M, Jones PB, Murray RM (2002). Obstetric complications and schizophrenia: historical and meta-analytic review. American Journal of Psychiatry, 159, 1080–1092.

Caspi A, Moffitt TE, Cannon M, Mcclay J, Murray R, Harrington HL, Taylor A, Arsenault L, Williams B, Braithwaite A, Poulton R, Craig IW. (2005). Moderation of the effect of adolescent-onset cannabis use on adult psychosis by a functional polymorphism in the

Catechol-O-Methayltransferase Gene: Longitudinal evidence of a gene X environment interaction. Biological Psychiatry 57, 1117–1127.

Castillo SO, Baffi JS, Palkovits M, Goldstein DS, Kopin IJ, Witta J, Magnuson MA, Nikodem VM (1998). Dopamine biosynthesis is selectively abolished in substantia nigra/ventral tegmental area but not in hypothalamic neurons in mice with targeted disruption of the Nurr1 gene. Molecular Cell Neuroscience, 11, 36–46.

Castle DJ, Murray RM (1991). The neurodevelopmental basis of sex differences in schizophrenia. Psychological Medicine, 21, 565–575.

Chen C-K, Lin S-K, Sham P, Ball D, Loh E-W, Hsiao C-C, Chiang Y-L, Ree S-C, Lee C-H, Murray RM (2003). Pre-morbid characteristics and co-morbidity of methamphetamine users with and without psychosis. Psychological Medicine, 33, 1407–1414.

Chen YH, Tsai MT, Shaw CK, Chen CH (2001). Mutation analysis of the human NR4A2 gene, an essential gene for midbrain dopaminergic neurogenesis, in schizophrenic patients. American Journal of Medical Genetics, 105, 753–762.

Connell PH (1958). Amphetamine Psychosis Maudsley Monograph No. 5, Chapman and Hall, London.

Di Forti M, Lappin JM, Murray RM (2007). Risk factors for schizophrenia – all roads lead to dopamine. European Neuropsychopharmacology, 17, S101–S107.

Dreher JC, Meyer-Lindenberg A, Kohn P, Berman KF (2008). Age-related changes in midbrain dopaminergic regulation of the human reward system. Proceedings of the National Academy of Science USA, 105, 15106–15111.

Eells JB, Misler JA, Nikodem VM (2006a). Early postnatal isolation reduces dopamine levels, elevates dopamine turnover and specifically disrupts prepulse inhibition in Nurr1-null heterozygous mice. Neuroscience, 140, 1117–1126.

Eells JB, Misler JA, Nikodem VM (2006b). Early postnatal isolation reduces dopamine levels, elevates dopamine turnover and specifically disrupts prepulse inhibition in Nurr1-null heterozygous mice. Neuroscience, 140, 1117–1126.

Fergusson DM, Horwood LJ, Ridder EM (2005). Tests of causal linkages between cannabis use and psychotic symptoms. Addiction, 100(3), 354–366.

Hafner H, Reicher-Rossler A, Hambrecht M, Maurer K, et al. (1993). The influence of age and sex on the onset and early course of schizophrenia. British Journal of Psychiatry, 162, 80–86.

Hall FS, Wilkinson LS, Humby T, et al. (1999). Maternal deprivation of neonatal rats produces enduring changes in dopamine function. Synapse, 32, 37–43.

Harrison PJ, Owen MJ (2003). Genes for schizophrenia? Recent findings and their pathophysiological implications. Lancet, 361(9355), 417–419.

Harrison G, Owens D, et al. (1988). A prospective study of severe mental disorder in Afro-Caribbean patients. Psychological Medicine, 18(3), 643–657.

Henquet C, Krabbendam L, Spauwen J, Kaplan C, Lieb R, Wittchen HU (2005). Prospective cohort study of cannabis use, predisposition for psychosis, and psychotic symptoms in young people. British Medical Journal, 330(7481), 11.

Howes OD, Mcdonald CM, Cannon M, Arsenault L, Boydell J, Murray RM (2004). Pathways to schizophrenia: The impact of environmental factors. International Journal of Neuropsychopharmacology, 7(Suppl. S1), 7–13.

Howes OD, Kapur S (2009). The dopamine hypothesis of schizophrenia: Version III – The final common pathway. Schizophrenia Bulletin. March Online advanced publication: doi:10.1093/schbul/sbp006.

Howes OD, Montgomery AJ, Asselin MC, et al. (2007). Molecular imaging studies of the striatal dopaminergic system in psychosis and predictions for the prodromal phase of psychosis. British Journal of Psychiatry, Suppl. 51, s13–s18.

Howes OD, Montgomery AJ, Asselin MC, et al. (2009). Elevated striatal dopamine function linked to prodromal signs of schizophrenia. Archive of General Psychiatry, 66, 13–20.

Huttunen J, Heinimaa M, Svirskis T, Nyman M, Kajander J, Forsback S, Solin O, Ilonen T, Korkeila J, Ristkari T, Mcglashan T, Salokangas RK, Hietala J (2007). Striatal dopamine synthesis in first-degree relatives of patients with schizophrenia. Biological Psychiatry, 63, 114–117.

Isovich E, Engelmann M, Landgraf R, et al. (2001). Social isolation after a single defeat reduces striatal dopamine transporter binding in rats. European Journal of Neuroscience, 13, 1254–1256.

Isovich E, Mijnster MJ, Flugge G, et al. (2000). Chronic psychosocial stress reduces the density of dopamine transporters. European Journal of Neuroscience, 12, 1071–1078.

Kapur S, Mizrahia R, Lia M (2005). From dopamine to salience to psychosis – linking biology, pharmacology and phenomenology of psychosis. Schizophrenia Research 79, 59–68.

Kegeles LS, Abi-Dargham A, Zea-Ponce Y, et al. (2000). Modulation of amphetamine-induced striatal dopamine release by ketamine in humans: Implications for schizophrenia. Biological Psychiatry, 48, 627–640.

Kegeles LS, Martinez D, Kochan LD, et al. (2002). NMDA antagonist effects on striatal dopamine release: positron emission tomography studies in humans. Synapse, 43, 19–29.

Laruelle M, Abi-Dargham A (1999b). Dopamine as the wind of the psychotic fire: new evidence from brain imaging studies. Journal of Psychopharmacology, 13, 358–371.

Laruelle M, Abi-Dargham A, Gil R, et al. (1999). Increased dopamine transmission in schizophrenia: Relationship to illness phases. Biological Psychiatry, 46, 56–72.

Laruelle M, Abi-Dargham A, Van Dyck CH, et al. (1996). Single photon emission computerized tomography imaging of amphetamine-induced dopamine release in drug-free schizophrenic subjects. Proceedings of the National Academy of Science USA, 93, 9235–9240.

Laruelle M, Abi-Dargham A (1999a). Dopamine as the wind of the psychotic fire: New evidence from brain imaging studies. Journal of Psychopharmacology, 13, 358–371.

Moore H, West AR, et al. (1999). The regulation of forebrain dopamine transmission: Relevance to the pathophysiology and psychopathology of schizophrenia. Biological Psychiatry, 46(1), 40–55.

Morgan C, Fisher H (2007). Environment and schizophrenia: environmental factors in schizophrenia: Childhood trauma – a critical review. Schizophrenia Bulletin, 33, 3–10.

Munro CA, Mccaul ME, Wong DF, Oswald LM, Zhou Y, Brasic J, Kuwabara H, Kumar A, Alexander M, Ye W, Wand GS (2006). Sex differences in striatal dopamine release in healthy adults. Biological Psychiatry, 59(10), 966–974.

Murray GK, Corlett PR, Clark L, Pessiglione M, Blackwell AD, Honey G, Jones PB, Bullmore ET, Robbins TW, Fletcher PC (2008b). Substantia nigra/ventral tegmental reward prediction error disruption in psychosis. Molecular Psychiatry 13, 267–276.

Murray R, Diforti M, Henquet C, Morrison P (2007). Cannabis, mind and society: The hash reality. Nature Reviews Neuroscience, 8(11), 885–895.

Murray, RM, Lappin, J, Di Forti M (2008a). Schizophrenia: From developmental deviance to dopamine dysregulation. European Neuropsychopharmacology, 18, S129–S134.

O'Donovan MC, Craddock N, Owen M (2008). Schizophrenia: Complex genetics, not fairy tales. A commentary on "the emperors of the schizophrenia polygene have no clothes by T. Crow, 2008". Psychological Medicine, 38, 1687–1691.

Powell SB, Geyer MA, Preece MA, Pitcher LK, Reynolds GP, Swerdlow NR (2003). Dopamine depletion of the nucleus accumbens reverses isolation-induced deficits in prepulse inhibition in rats. Neuroscience, 119, 233–240.

Reeves S, Bench C, Howard R (2002). Ageing and the nigrostriatal dopaminergic system. International Journal of Geriatric Psychiatry, 17, 359–370.

Schulze K, McDonald C, Frangou S, Sham P, Grech A, Toulopoulou T, Walshe M, Sharma T, Sigmundsson T, Taylor M, Murray RM (2003). Hippocampal volume in familial and non-familial chizophrenic probands and their unaffected relatives. Biological Psychiatry, 53(7), 562–570.

Selten JP, Veen N, Feller W, Blom JD, Schols D, Camoenie W, Oolders J, Van Der Velden M, Hoek HW, Rivero VM, Van Der Graaf Y, Kahn R (2001). Incidence of psychotic disorders in immigrant groups to The Netherlands. British Journal of Psychiatry, 178, 367–372.

Shively CA (1998). Social subordination stress, behavior, and central monoaminergic function in female cynomolgus monkeys. Biological Psychiatry, 44, 882–891.

Snyder SH (1976). The dopamine hypothesis of schizophrenia: Focus on the dopamine receptor. American Journal of Psychiatry, 133, 197–202.

Stefanis N, Frangou S, Yakeley J, Sharma T, O'connell P, Morgan K, Sigmundsson T, Taylor M, Murray RM (1999). Hippocampal volume reduction in schizophrenia: effects of genetic risk and pregnancy and birth complications. Biological Psychiatry, 46, 697–702.

Sullivan PF (2008). The dice are rolling for schizophrenia genetics. A commentary on "The Emperors of the schizophrenia polygene have no clothes by T. Crow, 2008". Psychological Medicine, 38(12), 1693–1696.

Talkowski ME, Kirov G, Bamne M, Georgieva L, Torres H, Mansour G, Chowdari KV, Milanova V, Wood J, McClain L (2008). A network of dopaminergic gene variations implicated as risk factors for schizophrenia. Human Molecular Genetics, 17(5), 747–758.

Verdoux H, Van Os J (2002). Psychotic symptoms in non-clinical populations and the continuum of psychosis. Schizophrenia Research 54, 59–65.

Cannabis: A Clue or a Distraction in the Search for 'Causes' of Psychosis?

John McGrath and Louisa Degenhardt

Introduction

Has cannabis been a distraction for the process of finding causes for schizophrenia or has it been a useful clue along the path to discovery? Good science is all about looking for clues, going down various pathways and then backing out if we come to a dead end. Sometimes we realize we have taken a wrong path in time to change directions quickly. Often it takes decades before we learn of our mistakes. However, it is important to note that regardless of what future researchers think about cannabis as a risk factor for psychosis, setting up and rejecting hypotheses is a defining feature of the scientific process. Rejecting a hypothesis is not an occasion for derision or hubristic scorn.

Cannabis rated only two brief mentions in the index of the proceedings of the 4th Search for the Cause of Schizophrenia meeting (Gattaz and Hafner 1999). At the meeting 5 years later, it was accorded an entire chapter (Witton et al. 2004). Over the past 4 years, studies that examine cannabis use as a potential cause of schizophrenia have continued to accumulate. It has remained a focus of research and a trigger for intense public debate. It could be argued that it has been a distraction for some – in particular politicians and social commentators. Politicians have eagerly examined the evidence linking cannabis and adverse mental health outcomes in order to justify changes to (or the maintenance of) the legal status of cannabis. However, it is doubtful whether changing the legal status of the drug would affect levels of cannabis use (Hall and Degenhardt 2003, 2006). Some might regard this distraction in a negative sense – as a futile waste of time. One man's clue is another man's distraction.

J. McGrath (✉)
Queensland Centre for Mental Health Research, The Park Centre for Mental Health, Wacol, QLD 4076, Australia
e-mail: john_mcgrath@qcmhr.uq.edu.au

W.F. Gattaz, G. Busatto (eds.), *Advances in Schizophrenia Research 2009*,
DOI 10.1007/978-1-4419-0913-8_20, © Springer Science+Business Media, LLC 2010

A Glut of Narrative and Systematic Reviews

In recent years the field has been well served by narrative or systematic reviews of the association between cannabis use and risk of schizophrenia (Hall et al. 2004; Macleod et al. 2004; Fergusson et al. 2005; Degenhardt and Hall 2006; Murray et al. 2007b; Hall and Degenhardt 2008). Several papers have integrated the data using meta-analytic techniques (Henquet et al. 2005a; Semple et al. 2005; Moore et al. 2007). The conclusions of these reviews have been consistent: on balance, the best available epidemiological evidence suggests that the regular use of cannabis is associated with an increased risk of later schizophrenia and related disorders. As part of the revision of the Global Burden of Disease, the Expert Group on Mental Disorders and Illicit Drug Use once again reviewed the evidence linking cannabis as a risk factor for psychosis and, in particular, reviewed the multiple reviews conducted in recent years (Degenhardt et al. 2008). The summary table from this most recent review is shown in Table 1.

Table 1 Global Burden of Disease revision: summary of two systematic reviews investigating cannabis use as a risk factor for psychosis (Degenhardt et al. 2008)

Study	Study type	Adjusted pooled estimate (95% CI)
Moore et al. (2007)	Searched Medline, Embase, CINAHL, PsycINFO, ISI Web of Knowledge, ISI Proceedings, ZETOC, BIOSIS, LILACS and MEDCARIB from their inception to September 2006, searched reference lists of studies selected for inclusion, and contacted experts Studies were included if longitudinal and population based Seven studies were included (some multiple papers) (Andreasson et al. 1987; Tien and Anthony 1990; Arseneault et al. 2002; van Os et al. 2002; Zammit et al. 2002; Fergusson et al. 2003, 2005; Caspi et al. 2005; Henquet et al. 2005b; Wiles et al. 2006). Data extraction and quality assessment were done independently and in duplicate	Ever used pooled AOR 1·41 (CI 1·20–1·65) 'heavy' use pooled AOR 2·09 (1·54–2·84)
Arsenault et al. (2002)	The research strategies used were computerized Medline and PsycLIT searches; cross-referencing of original studies; and contact with other researchers in the field Studies (Arseneault et al. 2002; van Os et al. 2002; Zammit et al. 2002; Fergusson et al. 2003) that included a well-defined sample drawn from population-based registers or cohorts and used prospective measures of cannabis use and adult psychosis	Pooled AOR 2.34 (1.69–2.95)

Note: AOR: pooled adjusted odds ratio; CI: confidence interval; HR: hazard ratio.

Multiple attempts have been made to explore the potential role of issues such as residual confounding, reverse causality, and a range of other methodological biases. For some, constant regurgitation of the primary data has not been sufficient to convince them that the association between cannabis is a causal agent of psychosis. Some of these concerns have been outlined in commentaries or letters to the editor that have followed target articles (Anthony and Degenhardt 2007; Macleod et al. 2007; Perkonigg et al. 2008). This leads us to ask: What further evidence do we need to consider the evidence sufficient and how do we define a cause?

What Is a Cause?

Mervyn Susser (1991) wrote an influential paper 18 years ago titled 'What is a cause and how do we know one? A grammar for pragmatic epidemiology'. In this article, the criteria made popular by Hill (1965) were refreshed and pragmatic definitions were provided to guide researchers. Many of the commentators on the topic of cannabis and psychosis have allocated the evidence to these headings (Witton et al. 2004; Degenhardt and Hall 2006). Apart from the epidemiological evidence, there is an ever-growing body of neurobiological evidence implicating cannabis in neurobiological pathways associated with schizophrenia (Murray et al. 2007b).

Commentators acknowledge that the application of causal criteria to evidence is not a straightforward process (Rothman and Greenland 2005) and belief systems related to competing epidemiological theories can cloud the debate. These issues have contributed to a debate around the interpretation of the association between cannabis and psychosis. Because observational data are prone to important errors, some commentators with a more cautious temperament do not interpret the cannabis evidence as 'sufficient' to warrant giving it the label of a 'risk factor' or a 'component cause' of schizophrenia.

A recent review process has brought these issues into sharp relief. As part of the revision of the Global Burden of Disease (Murray and Lopez 1996; Murray et al. 2007a), estimates of the prevalence of cannabis use and dependence have been compiled from around the world (Calabria et al. 2008), which will progressively be made available in reports and peer-reviewed publications. Material related to this exercise can also be found at the following website: www.gbd.unsw.edu.au. As part of this process, Comparative Risk Assessments (CRA) are being undertaken exploring the potential to avert disability by reducing or eliminating various risk factors associated with the outcome of interest (Degenhardt et al. 2008). Such exercises have been particularly valuable in modelling the potential impact of tobacco and alcohol use on morbidity and mortality, but no such global estimates have ever been made for cannabis use. Considerable discussion has occurred about whether there is sufficient evidence to justify undertaking a CRA for cannabis as risk factor for psychosis (Degenhardt et al. under review).

Why Might Cannabis Use Be Associated with Schizophrenia?

It is useful to define the ways in which cannabis use could be a 'cause' of psychosis (Degenhardt 2003; Arseneault et al. 2004). The strongest form of causal link is that heavy cannabis use causes a psychosis that would not otherwise have occurred, that is, that cannabis use increases the incidence of psychosis.

A second hypothesis is that cannabis use is a contributory cause: it might precipitate psychosis in vulnerable individuals and is one factor among many (including genetic predisposition and other unknown causes) that act together to cause psychotic disorders. The evidence suggests that it is more likely that cannabis use precipitates psychosis in vulnerable persons. This is consistent with other lines of evidence suggesting that there is a complex constellation of factors leading to the development of psychosis (i.e., the stress–diathesis model of schizophrenia) and with studies suggesting that gene–environment interactions may provide some explanation of the association (Degenhardt 2003; Arseneault et al. 2004).

Does Cannabis Use Influence the Prevalence of Psychotic Symptoms?

Leaving aside the issue of whether or not cannabis use leads to an increased incidence of the clinical diagnosis of schizophrenia, let us rephrase the question from a different perspective. Does cannabis use cause isolated psychotic symptoms (e.g., delusions and hallucinations)? Several large population-based studies have reported an unexpectedly high prevalence of psychotic-like experiences among cannabis users (Eaton et al. 1991; van Os et al. 2000; Krabbendam et al. 2004; Hanssen et al. 2005; Scott et al. 2007b). A recent systematic review of population-based prevalence studies of subclinical psychotic experiences found a median prevalence rate of around 5% (van Os et al. 2008). This same study undertook a meta-analysis of risk factors and reported that cannabis use was associated with a twofold risk of endorsing psychotic-like experiences.

Does Cannabis Use Influence Remission from Psychosis?

For those with established schizophrenia, there is robust evidence that cannabis use is associated with reduced remission (and thus, persistent psychotic symptoms) (Linszen et al. 1994; Ferdinand et al. 2005; Henquet et al. 2005b; Degenhardt et al. 2007; Zammit et al. 2008). Thus, from the perspective of active psychosis in the community, increased cannabis use could increase the point prevalence of psychosis via two mechanisms. It could lead to an increased incidence of symptoms (subclinical or clinical) and it could also decrease remission of people with established psychotic disorders. As a consequence, the higher prevalence of psychotic symptoms and disorders translates into a greater disease burden, as measured by personal suffering, disability adjusted life years (DALYs), and demands on services (Saha et al. 2008).

Different Levels of Proof Are Required for Different Scenarios

Within any developing science, hypotheses flux in and out of fashion. Sometimes the literature reflects more the opinion of influential researchers rather than the objective data (McGrath 2005). History tells us that data can be wrong, and as new data accumulate we must remain vigilant to revise cherished hypotheses. It is entirely feasible that cannabis per se *does not* contribute to the risk of developing schizophrenia.

The uncertainty around the quality of data derived from observational epidemiology is cause of some angst within our field at the moment. Put bluntly, observational epidemiology can get it wrong – very wrong on occasions (Davey Smith and Ebrahim 2001; Smith 2001). With respect to cannabis, the findings from prospective longitudinal studies may still be vulnerable to residual confounding. The best way to deal with both known and unknown confounding is to use randomized controlled trials to explore the impact of an exposure on the health outcome of interest. Clearly, this strategy cannot be used to explore the association between cannabis and psychosis. Thus, we must have realistic expectations for this field. The evidence will never reach the 'beyond reasonable proof' level required in many criminal procedures. In the absence of this level of evidence we have no choice but to fall back on more relaxed evidential criteria, such as the thresholds used in civil courts. At this level, evidence is judged on 'balance of probability' or 'preponderance of evidence' criteria. Reassuringly, similar criteria have been recommended for the interpretation of the evidence for susceptibility genes for schizophrenia (Sullivan 2008).

Few, if any, commentators in the field believe that the evidence linking cannabis as a cause of schizophrenia is proven beyond reasonable doubt. Most, but not all, commentators would rank the current aggregation of epidemiological and biological evidence as somewhere between 'moderate' and 'strong'. Within this level of proof, what actions should we take?

Regardless of how governments deal with cannabis use, there is widespread agreement that the research community needs to monitor cannabis use and related mental health outcomes closely in the years to come. For example, in sites with rising or falling prevalence of cannabis use, can we monitor changes in the incidence and prevalence of psychosis? Are there 'natural experiments' that could be used to examine changes in the frequency or dose of cannabis exposure? What would we expect to find if cannabis use increases in the years to come? Modelling exercises are now available that allow us to explore these questions (Anthony and Degenhardt 2007; Hickman et al. 2007; Saha et al. 2008).

The research community should also use genetic epidemiology to explore biologically plausible gene by environment interactions (Smith and Ebrahim 2004). Studies that have examined the interaction between cannabis and polymorphisms in genes such as COMT have been particularly interesting (Caspi et al. 2005; Henquet et al. 2006; van Winkel et al. 2007). One can safely assume that currently we are only scratching the surface with respect to understanding the genetic factors that may influence or moderate the associations between cannabis and psychosis.

Cannabis-Induced Apathy: What Are the Risks of Doing Nothing?

Regardless of the arcane and Jesuitical disputes amongst epidemiologists about whether the evidence is sufficient to accept cannabis as a cause of psychosis, there may be other criteria upon which to judge the debate. From a public health perspective, there is an argument that some interventions should be implemented in the absence of complete and definitive proof. For example, if the health outcomes are severe and there is lack of effective treatments, then it can be argued that relatively safe and cheap interventions could be trialled based on incomplete evidence. For example, observational epidemiology identified an association between infant sleeping positions and risk of sudden infant death syndrome ('cot death') (Moon et al. 2007). While there is still much work to be done in further reducing the incidence of this particular disorder and unravelling the biological correlates underpinning the condition, the simple public health advice about placing infants on their back to sleep has been a public health success story.

The aim in this instance would primarily be the reduction or prevention of cannabis use among young people, particularly those at risk of developing psychotic symptoms or disorder (Hall and Degenhardt 2006). Some might argue that an association with adverse effects of cannabis provides sufficient justification for maintaining or strengthening prohibition of cannabis use, but as has been argued in some length (Hall and Degenhardt 2003), this logic is flawed: prohibition has clearly failed to prevent many young people from using cannabis. Drugs such as alcohol and tobacco have been shown to have many serious adverse effects, yet remain legal. Finally, there is a need to balance the potential benefits of prohibition against the costs that society might bear due to aggressive implementation of such a scheme (Hall and Degenhardt 2003).

Educating young people about the risks of cannabis use is relatively cheap, safe and could avert adverse health outcomes if some choose not to use the drug. Such education needs to be carefully given, however, in ways that do not overly exaggerate the risks (Hall and Degenhardt 2006). Because it seems unlikely that the evidence base will ever be beyond reasonable doubt, maybe we should act sooner rather than later?

The Fertile Intersection Between Schizophrenia Epidemiology and Neurobiology

Apart from research that translates the epidemiological clues linking cannabis and psychosis into the arena of public health, the research community also benefits from translating these clues into the field of neurobiology. While the epidemiological data base has grown slowly over the past few decades, the pace of discovery has recently quickened as groups have used animal models to explore the impact of THC and related compounds on brain function (Gorriti et al. 1999; Boucher et al. 2007;

Murray et al. 2007b; Vigano et al. 2008). In the absence of a stimulus from schizophrenia epidemiology, it is feasible that these cannabinoid-related pathways would have remained poorly understood and under-appreciated.

Cannabis remains an important clue for the neuroscience community. Various animal models can help explore the neurobiological correlates of intermediate phenotypes of interest to our field (e.g., differential sensitivity to glutaminergic or dopaminergic agents). Invertebrate systems such as Drosophila or zebra fish can also provide powerful and efficient research platforms to explore research questions related to how cannabinoid-related mechanisms interact with brain functioning (Swinderen 2005; Scott et al. 2007a; van Swinderen 2007).

Conclusions

From all perspectives, the pace of discovery related to cannabis and psychosis has quickened in recent years. There is a general consistency in the epidemiological evidence base – cannabis use is associated with an increased risk of psychosis. Entwined with this evidence, there is a balanced appreciation that the evidence base needs to be interpreted with caution. Molecular, cellular and behavioural neuroscience has been energized by the clues linking cannabis to psychosis (Murray et al. 2007b).

Schizophrenia remains a poorly understood group of disorders. Even our best treatments are suboptimal (Andrews et al. 2003, 2004). In the absence of better treatments, the most effective way to reduce the disability associated with schizophrenia is to prevent the disorder (Saha et al. 2008). When considering potential risk factors for schizophrenia, we argue that candidates that offer the opportunity for public health interventions should be accorded more attention. Such research attention should be focused at the clinical and the population health level. Even if cannabis use is found to be a relatively small contributor to disease burden, such a finding nonetheless carries importance. Rather than a futile distraction, we argue that the links between cannabis use and schizophrenia remain a fertile and productive focus for investigation.

References

Andreasson S, Allebeck P, Engstrom A, Rydberg U. 1987. Cannabis and schizophrenia. A longitudinal study of Swedish conscripts. Lancet 2(8574): 1483–6.

Andrews G, Sanderson K, Corry J, Issakidis C, Lapsley H. 2003. Cost-effectiveness of current and optimal treatment for schizophrenia. Br J Psychiatry 183: 427–35; discussion 436.

Andrews G, Issakidis C, Sanderson K, Corry J, Lapsley H. 2004. Utilising survey data to inform public policy: comparison of the cost-effectiveness of treatment of ten mental disorders. Br J Psychiatry 184: 526–33.

Anthony JC, Degenhardt L. 2007. Projecting the impact of changes in cannabis use upon schizophrenia in England and Wales: the role of assumptions and balance in framing an evidence-based cannabis policy. Addiction 102(4): 515–6; discussion 516–8.

Arseneault L, Cannon M, Poulton R, Murray R, Caspi A, Moffitt TE. 2002. Cannabis use in adolescence and risk for adult psychosis: longitudinal prospective study. BMJ 325(7374): 1212–3.

Arseneault L, Cannon M, Witton J, Murray RM. 2004. Causal association between cannabis and psychosis: examination of the evidence. Br J Psychiatry 184. 110–7.

Boucher AA, Arnold JC, Duffy L, Schofield PR, Micheau J, Karl T. 2007. Heterozygous neuregulin 1 mice are more sensitive to the behavioural effects of Delta9-tetrahydrocannabinol. Psychopharmacology (Berl) 192(3): 325–36.

Calabria B, Degenhardt L, Mclaren J, Nelson P, Roberts A, Sigmundsdottir L, Callaghan B, Baxter A, Whiteford HA. 2008. Summary of data collected and decision rules used in making regional and global estimates of cannabis dependence (available at http://www.med.unsw.edu.au/gbdweb.nsf).

Caspi A, Moffitt TE, Cannon M, Mcclay J, Murray R, Harrington H, Taylor A, Arseneault L, Williams B, Braithwaite A and others. 2005. Moderation of the effect of adolescent-onset cannabis use on adult psychosis by a functional polymorphism in the catechol-O-methyltransferase gene: longitudinal evidence of a gene × environment interaction. Biol Psychiatry 57(10): 1117–27.

Davey Smith G, Ebrahim S. 2001. Epidemiology – is it time to call it a day? Int J Epidemiol 30(1): 1–11.

Degenhardt L. 2003. The link between cannabis use and psychosis: furthering the debate. Psychol Med 33(1): 3–6.

Degenhardt L, Hall W. 2006. Is cannabis use a contributory cause of psychosis? Can J Psychiatry 51(9): 556–65.

Degenhardt L, Hall W, Lynskey M, Mclaren J, Calabria B. 2008. Cannabis use as a risk factor for mental disorders. Global Burden of Disease Mental Disorders and Illicit Drug Use Expert group, Illicit drugs discussion paper No. 2.

Degenhardt L, Tennant C, Gilmour S, Schofield D, Nash L, Hall W, Mckay D. 2007. The temporal dynamics of relationships between cannabis, psychosis and depression among young adults with psychotic disorders: findings from a 10-month prospective study. Psychol Med 37(7): 927–34.

Eaton WW, Romanoski A, Anthony JC, Nestadt G. 1991. Screening for psychosis in the general population with a self-report interview. J Nerv Ment Dis 179(11): 689–93.

Ferdinand RF, Sondeijker F, Van Der Ende J, Selten JP, Huizink A, Verhulst FC. 2005. Cannabis use predicts future psychotic symptoms, and vice versa. Addiction 100(5): 612–18.

Fergusson DM, Horwood LJ, Swain-Campbell NR. 2003. Cannabis dependence and psychotic symptoms in young people. Psychol Med 33(1): 15–21.

Fergusson DM, Horwood LJ, Ridder EM. 2005. Tests of causal linkages between cannabis use and psychotic symptoms. Addiction 100(3): 354–66.

Gattaz WF, Hafner H. ed. 1999. Search for the Causes of Schizophrenia, Volume 4: Balance of the Century. Darmstadt, Springer-Verlag.

Gorriti MA, Rodriguez DE Fonseca F, Navarro M, Palomo T. 1999. Chronic (-)-delta9-tetrahydrocannabinol treatment induces sensitization to the psychomotor effects of amphetamine in rats. Eur J Pharmacol 365(2–3): 133–42.

Hall W, Degenhardt L. 2003. Medical marijuana initiatives: are they justified? How successful are they likely to be? CNS Drugs 17(10): 689–97.

Hall W, Degenhardt L. 2006. What are the policy implications of the evidence on cannabis and psychosis? Can J Psychiatry 51(9): 566–74.

Hall W, Degenhardt L. 2008. Cannabis use and the risk of developing a psychotic disorder. World Psychiatry 7(2): 68–71.

Hall W, Degenhardt L, Teesson M. 2004. Cannabis use and psychotic disorders: an update. Drug Alcohol Rev 23(4): 433–43.

Hanssen M, Bak M, Bijl R, Vollebergh W, Van Os J. 2005. The incidence and outcome of subclinical psychotic experiences in the general population. Br J Clin Psychol 44(Pt 2): 181–91.

Henquet C, Murray R, Linszen D, Van Os J. 2005a. The environment and schizophrenia: the role of cannabis use. Schizophr Bull 31(3): 608–12.

Henquet C, Krabbendam L, Spauwen J, Kaplan C, Lieb R, Wittchen HU, Van Os J. 2005b. Prospective cohort study of cannabis use, predisposition for psychosis, and psychotic symptoms in young people. BMJ 330(7481): 11.

Henquet C, Rosa A, Krabbendam L, Papiol S, Fananas L, Drukker M, Ramaekers JG, Van Os J. 2006. An experimental study of catechol-o-methyltransferase Val158Met moderation of delta-9-tetrahydrocannabinol-induced effects on psychosis and cognition. Neuropsychopharmacology 31(12): 2748–57.

Hickman M, Vickerman P, Macleod J, Kirkbride J, Jones PB. 2007. Cannabis and schizophrenia: model projections of the impact of the rise in cannabis use on historical and future trends in schizophrenia in England and Wales. Addiction 102(4): 597–606.

Hill AB. 1965. The environment and disease: association or causation? Proc R Soc Med 58: 295–300.

Krabbendam L, Myin-Germeys I, De Graaf R, Vollebergh W, Nolen WA, Iedema J, Van Os J. 2004. Dimensions of depression, mania and psychosis in the general population. Psychol Med 34(7): 1177–86.

Linszen DH, Dingemans PM, Lenior ME. 1994. Cannabis abuse and the course of recent-onset schizophrenic disorders. Arch Gen Psychiatry 51(4): 273–9.

Macleod J, Oakes R, Copello A, Crome I, Egger M, Hickman M, Oppenkowski T, Stokes-Lampard H, Davey Smith G. 2004. Psychological and social sequelae of cannabis and other illicit drug use by young people: a systematic review of longitudinal, general population studies. Lancet 363(9421): 1579–88.

Macleod J, Davey Smith G, Hickman M, Egger M. 2007. Cannabis and psychosis. Lancet 370(9598): 1539; author reply 1539–40.

McGrath JJ. 2005. Myths and plain truths about schizophrenia epidemiology – the NAPE lecture 2004. Acta Psychiatr Scand 111(1): 4–11.

Moon RY, Horne RS, Hauck FR. 2007. Sudden infant death syndrome. Lancet 370(9598): 1578–87.

Moore TH, Zammit S, Lingford-Hughes A, Barnes TR, Jones PB, Burke M, Lewis G. 2007. Cannabis use and risk of psychotic or affective mental health outcomes: a systematic review. Lancet 370(9584): 319–28.

Murray CJ, Lopez AD. 1996. The Global Burden of Disease. Boston, Harvard School of Public Health.

Murray CJ, Lopez AD, Black R, Mathers CD, Shibuya K, Ezzati M, Salomon JA, Michaud CM, Walker N, Vos T. 2007a. Global burden of disease 2005: call for collaborators. Lancet 370(9582): 109–10.

Murray RM, Morrison PD, Henquet C, Di Forti M. 2007b. Cannabis, the mind and society: the hash realities. Nat Rev Neurosci 8(11): 885–95.

Perkonigg A, Goodwin RD, Behrendt S, Beesdo K, Lieb R, Wittchen HU. 2008. Cannabis use – do we have solutions? A reply to Macleod. Addiction 103(9): 1575.

Rothman KJ, Greenland S. 2005. Causation and causal inference in epidemiology. Am J Public Health 95(Suppl 1): S144–50.

Saha S, Barendregt JJ, Vos T, Whiteford H, McGrath J. 2008. Modelling disease frequency measures in schizophrenia epidemiology. Schizophr Res 104(1–3): 246–54.

Scott EK, Mason L, Arrenberg AB, Ziv L, Gosse NJ, Xiao T, CHI NC, Asakawa K, Kawakami K, Baier H. 2007a. Targeting neural circuitry in zebrafish using GAL4 enhancer trapping. Nat Methods 4(4): 323–6.

Scott J, Chant D, Andrews G, Martin G, McGrath J. 2007b. Association between trauma exposure and delusional experiences in a large community-based sample. Br J Psychiatry 190: 339–43.

Semple DM, Mcintosh AM, Lawrie SM. 2005. Cannabis as a risk factor for psychosis: systematic review. J Psychopharmacol 19(2): 187–94.

Smith GD. 2001. Reflections on the limitations to epidemiology. J Clin Epidemiol 54(4): 325–31.

Smith GD, Ebrahim S. 2004. Mendelian randomization: prospects, potentials, and limitations. Int J Epidemiol 33(1): 30–42.

Sullivan PF. 2008. The dice are rolling for schizophrenia genetics. Psychol Med: 1–4.

Susser M. 1991. What is a cause and how do we know one? A grammar for pragmatic epidemiology. Am J Epidemiol 133(7): 635–48.

Swinderen B. 2005. The remote roots of consciousness in fruit-fly selective attention? Bioessays 27(3): 321–30.

Tien AY, Anthony JC. 1990. Epidemiological analysis of alcohol and drug use as risk factors for psychotic experiences. J Nerv Ment Dis 178(8): 473–80.

Van Os J, Hanssen M, Bijl RV, Ravelli A. 2000. Strauss (1969) revisited: a psychosis continuum in the general population? Schizophr Res 45(1–2): 11–20.

Van Os J, Bak M, Hanssen M, Bijl RV, De Graaf R, Verdoux H. 2002. Cannabis use and psychosis: a longitudinal population-based study. Am J Epidemiol 156(4): 319–27.

Van Os J, Linscott RJ, Myin-Germeys I, Delespaul P, Krabbendam L. 2008. A systematic review and meta-analysis of the psychosis continuum: evidence for a psychosis proneness-persistence-impairment model of psychotic disorder. Psychol Med: 1–17.

Van Swinderen B. 2007. Attention-like processes in Drosophila require short-term memory genes. Science 315(5818): 1590–3.

van Winkel R, Henquet C, Rosa A, Papiol S, Fananás L, De Hert M, Peuskens J, van Os J, Myin-Germeys I. 2008. Evidence that the COMT(Val158Met) polymorphism moderates sensitivity to stress in psychosis: an experience-sampling study. American Journal of Medical Genetics Part B: Neuropsychiatric Genetics, 147B(1): 10–17.

Vigano D, Guidali C, Petrosino S, Realini N, Rubino T, Di Marzo V, Parolaro D. 2008. Involvement of the endocannabinoid system in phencyclidine-induced cognitive deficits modelling schizophrenia. Int J Neuropsychopharmacol: 1–16.

Wiles NJ, Zammit S, Bebbington P, Singleton N, Meltzer H, Lewis G. 2006. Self-reported psychotic symptoms in the general population: results from the longitudinal study of the British National Psychiatric Morbidity Survey. Br J Psychiatry 188: 519–26.

Witton J, Arseneault L, Cannon M, Murray R. 2004. Cannabis as a causal factor for psychosis – a review of the evidence. In: Gattaz WF, Hafner H (ed.) Search for the Causes of Schizophrenia. Darmstadt, Steinkopff-Verlag, pp. 133–49.

Zammit S, Allebeck P, Andreasson S, Lundberg I, Lewis G. 2002. Self reported cannabis use as a risk factor for schizophrenia in Swedish conscripts of 1969: historical cohort study. BMJ 325(7374): 1199.

Zammit S, Moore TH, Lingford-Hughes A, Barnes TR, Jones PB, Burke M, Lewis G. 2008. Effects of cannabis use on outcomes of psychotic disorders: systematic review. Br J Psychiatry 193(5): 357–63.

The 'Totality' of Psychosis: Epidemiology and Developmental Pathobiology

Olabisi Owoeye, Tara Kingston, Robin J. Hennessy, Patrizia A. Baldwin, David Browne, Paul J. Scully, Anthony Kinsella, Vincent Russell, Eadbhard O'Callaghan, and John L. Waddington

Introduction

Among numerous impediments to further advancement between the fifth and sixth symposia on Search for the Causes of Schizophrenia, several uncertainties endure: (i) What are the boundaries of psychotic illness? (ii) Where do we position what we currently conceptualise and diagnose as schizophrenia within the much broader reality of psychotic disorder among those with serious mental illness and, indeed, of psychotic phenomena among the general population? (iii) To what extent are those components of psychotic illness that we resolve into separate diagnostic categories actually distinct in any fundamental way in terms of their epidemiological, clinical and pathobiological 'signature'?

These challenges achieve their greatest currency via contemporary re-evaluation of the Kraepelinian dichotomy between schizophrenia and bipolar disorder in terms of phenomenology, epidemiology, pathobiology, course and treatment (Jablensky 1999; Maier et al. 2006; Ivleva et al. 2008), but in fact extend to the full breadth of psychotic disorder that places such demands on individuals, families, society and health-care provision. As we wrestle with such long-standing but still unresolved issues regarding the validity and meaning of conventional diagnostic categories, it is salutary to reflect anew on whether the use of such diagnoses facilitates or confounds our 'search for the causes of schizophrenia'. A radical approach to this debate would be to study the 'totality' of psychotic illness naturalistically in the absence of a priori diagnostic restriction; subsequent post hoc imposition of contemporary diagnostic criteria would then allow the epidemiological, clinical and pathobiological characteristics of those categories to be compared systematically.

In contemplating a study of the 'totality' of psychotic illness, additional challenges are evident. There is now a wealth of evidence that factors such as urban birth (March et al. 2008) and migration status (Selten et al. 2007) can exert marked

J.L. Waddington (✉)
Molecular & Cellular Therapeutics, Royal College of Surgeons in Ireland,
St Stephen's Green, Dublin 2, Ireland
e-mail: jwadding@rcsi.ie

W.F. Gattaz, G. Busatto (eds.), *Advances in Schizophrenia Research 2009*,
DOI 10.1007/978-1-4419-0913-8_21, © Springer Science+Business Media, LLC 2010

influences on risk for psychosis, as usually assessed in terms of schizophrenia. While such epidemiological findings surely contain important clues to causality, inevitable diversity in such factors confounds comparison between studies and obscures the fundamental nature of psychotic illness; this can only be clarified in the absence of such factors. Here we present an update on preliminary findings from the Cavan–Monaghan First-Episode Study, specifically designed to incept the 'totality' of psychosis in an unusually favourable social/demographic setting for such a purpose, together with initial findings relating to the developmental pathobiology of psychosis beyond schizophrenia.

The Cavan–Monaghan First-Episode Study

In 1995 we initiated a study of first-episode psychosis in Cavan and Monaghan, two rural border counties in the Republic of Ireland having an ethnically homogeneous population totalling 109,139. The basic methods of this study have been described previously (Scully et al. 2002; Baldwin et al. 2005).

In outline, the study involves the following ascertainment procedures: mental health care provided via strict catchment areas, involving home-base treatment with minimal recourse to in-patient care (Russell et al. 2003; McCauley et al. 2003); cases identified from (a) all treatment teams in the catchment areas, including services for the elderly, (b) cases from the catchment areas who present privately to St. Patrick's Hospital or St. John of God Hospital, Dublin, which together account for >90% of all national private psychiatric admissions, and (c) cases from the catchment areas having forensic admission to the Central Mental Hospital, Dublin; primary entry criterion of a first lifetime episode of any psychotic illness, to include a first manic episode; no exclusion criteria other than a previously treated episode of psychosis/mania or psychosis occurring with a prior, overriding diagnosis of gross neurodegenerative disease (e.g., Alzheimer's disease, Huntington's disease or Parkinson's disease); presentation at age 16 or above, with no upper age cut-off or loss of cases to services for the elderly; DSM-IV diagnosis intrinsic to (rather than an entry/exclusion criterion for) study at inception, together with psychopathological and cognitive assessments, and repeat DSM-IV diagnosis at 6 months; Research Ethics Committee approvals for all procedures, to include obtaining diagnostic/demographic information from case notes/treating teams for those declining formal assessment.

The Challenge of the 'Totality' of Psychosis

Over the period 1995–2008 we have to date identified 372 cases of first-episode psychosis, to include a first manic episode [mean age 38.4 years (SD 19.5, range 16–92); 216 males, age 35.7 years (18.5); 156 females, age 42.3 years (20.3)]. The incidence of psychosis was 33.5 (95% CI 30.1–37.0)/100,000 of population age

>15 years [males, 38.9 (33.9–44.5); females, 28.0 (23.8–32.8)]; risk for psychosis in males exceeded that in females [relative risk (RR) = 1.39 (95% CI 1.13–1.71, $P < 0.01$].

Among these 372 cases of first-episode psychosis, DSM-IV diagnoses at 6 months following inception were as follows: schizophrenia, $N = 71$; schizophreniform disorder, $N = 21$; schizoaffective disorder, $N = 20$; delusional disorder, $N = 22$; brief psychotic disorder, $N = 21$; bipolar disorder, $N = 73$; major depressive disorder with psychotic features, $N = 77$; substance-induced psychosis, $N = 21$; substance-induced mood disorder (selective serotonin reuptake inhibitor-induced mania), $N = 6$; psychosis due to a general medical condition, $N = 11$; mood disorder (mania) due to a general medical condition, $N = 4$; psychosis not otherwise specified, $N = 23$; and 'simple deteriorative disorder' (a DSM-IV – Appendix B exploratory entity relating to all the hallmarks of schizophrenia in terms of negative symptoms and functional decline but without sufficiently prominent positive symptoms to satisfy criteria for schizophrenia), $N = 2$. There were three cases of completed suicide over the first 6 months following inception, with the 'last observation' diagnosis prior to demise being carried forward.

Major Post Hoc Diagnostic Nodes: Demographics and Psychopathology

Among this 'totality' of psychosis, the three largest diagnostic nodes were as follows: schizophrenia [$N = 71$, age 31.3 years (14.7, range 16–79), incidence 6.4 (5.0–8.1); 53 males, age 29.2 years (13.5), incidence 9.6 (7.2–12.5); 18 females, age 37.5 years (16.7), incidence 3.2 (1.9–5.1)]; bipolar disorder [$N = 73$, age 32.6 years (15.7, range 16–80), incidence 6.6 (5.2–8.3); 38 males, age 31.2 years (13.3), incidence 6.9 (4.5–9.0); 35 females, age 34.1 years (14.7), incidence 6.3 (4.4–8.7)]; and major depressive disorder with psychotic features [$N = 77$, age 50.8 years (22.4, range 16–87), incidence 6.6 (5.2–8.3); 36 males, age 48.9 years (23.7), incidence 6.5 (3.7–9.1); 41 females, age 52.6 years (21.4), incidence 7.4 (5.3–10.0)]. For schizophrenia, risk in males exceeded that in females [RR = 2.95 (1.73–5.04), P < 0.001]; conversely, risk for bipolar disorder and major depressive disorder with psychotic features was indistinguishable between males and females.

In relation to psychopathology, total scores for the seven positive symptom items on the Positive and Negative Syndrome Scale (PANSS) were similar for cases of schizophrenia [17.0 (6.0), $N = 51$], bipolar disorder [16.2 (8.1), $N = 46$] and major depressive disorder with psychotic features [14.6 (6.5), $N = 37$]; total scores for the seven negative symptom items on the PANSS were only marginally higher for cases of schizophrenia than those of major depressive disorder with psychotic features, while total scores were considerably lower for bipolar disorder.

For cases of bipolar disorder categorised by DSM-IV as 'with psychotic features', total scores for the seven positive symptom items on the PANSS [17.3 (8.7), $N = 31$] were only slightly higher than those for all other cases of bipolar disorder [14.0 (6.4), $N = 15$]; total scores for the seven negative symptom items on the PANSS were low and indistinguishable between these two groups of bipolar patients.

It will be necessary to clarify whether similar total subscale scores reflect similar individual scale items, altered distribution in item scores and/or confounding between domains of psychopathology such as negative vs. depressive symptoms.

Major Post Hoc Diagnostic Nodes: Long-Term Follow-Up

To clarify the stability of these diagnostic nodes and whether other diagnoses converge on these nodes, we conducted a long-term follow-up of those cases incepted over the first 8 years of the Cavan–Monaghan First-Episode Study ($N = 202$), to include DSM-IV diagnosis with multiple psychopathological and functional assessments. In an interim analysis of the first 178 of these cases (88%), followed up at a mean of 6.4 (SD 2.3) years post inception, diagnostic stability was as follows: schizophrenia/schizoaffective disorder, $N = 34$: 100% at 6 months, 85% at 6 years; bipolar disorder, $N = 31$: 97% at 6 months, 84% at 6 years; major depressive disorder with psychotic features, $N = 35$: 94% at 6 months, 74% at 6 years.

Among other diagnoses, schizophreniform disorder ($N = 21$), delusional disorder ($N = 11$) and psychosis not otherwise specified ($N = 14$) evolved primarily to schizophrenia or schizoaffective disorder from 6 months to 6 years. However, while 11 cases of brief psychotic disorder at inception resolved readily over subsequent weeks, by 6 years all had evolved to show serious mental illness: schizophrenia, $N = 3$; schizoaffective disorder, $N = 1$; delusional disorder, $N = 1$; bipolar disorder, $N = 5$; and major depressive disorder with psychotic features, $N = 1$.

Major Post Hoc Diagnostic Nodes: Developmental Pathobiology

While much theorising indicates an important role for early disturbance in brain development in the origins of psychotic illness (Waddington et al. 1999; McGrath et al. 2003; Rapoport et al. 2005), there is little understanding of the nature of this process and the extent to which it might generalise from schizophrenia to bipolar disorder (Dutta et al. 2007). Facial dysmorphologies in disorders of early brain development reflect the embryological intimacy with which the anterior brain and face evolve over early foetal life (Diewert et al. 1993; Waddington et al. 1999; Marcucio et al. 2005). Though anthropometric studies (Lane et al. 1997; McGrath et al. 2002; Hennessy et al. 2004) have indicated subtle facial dysmorphology in schizophrenia, this has yet to be studied systematically in bipolar disorder.

Using the 3D digitisation technology of laser surface imaging and geometric morphometric analysis of resultant 3D facial surfaces (Hennessy et al. 2002, 2005), we have recently identified a characteristic topography of frontonasal and associated dysmorphologies in schizophrenia (Hennessy et al. 2007). Identical methods have now been applied to 13 male [age 45.0 years (SD 14.3)] and 14 female [age 44.7 years (SD 16.3)] patients with bipolar disorder, who include participants in the Cavan–Monaghan First-Episode study together with additionally recruited prevalent cases (Scully et al. 2004), in comparison with 61 male [age 40.7 years (SD 10.7)] and 75 female [age 38.0 years (SD 9.7)] control subjects from the Cavan–Monaghan community.

On application of Procrustes ANOVA to facial landmark-based data and regression analysis of those principal components of facial landmark-based and facial surface-based data that statistically distinguish patients from controls, both male and female bipolar patients evidenced significant [$P < 0.05$] dysmorphology: common to male and female patients were overall facial widening, increased width of nose, narrowing of mouth and upward displacement of the chin; dysmorphology differed between male and female patients for nose length, lip thickness and tragion height. The same analytical approaches indicated few morphological differences between patients with bipolar disorder and those in our previous study in schizophrenia (Hennessy et al. 2007).

Epidemiology of the 'Totality' of Psychosis

In the Cavan–Monaghan First-Episode Study we have sought, since 1995, the continuing inception of *all* incident cases of psychosis, to include a first manic episode, among a rural region of socioeconomic homogeneity that minimises the confounds of urbanicity and ethnic migration. To the extent that these aspirations are realised, the findings may be highly representative and so define the baseline epidemiology of psychotic illness on which urbanicity and ethnic migration act. Our 'sister' study, based in urban areas in and around Dublin city and using very similar methods (Browne et al. 2000; Clarke et al. 2006), will allow us to examine systematically and prospectively several issues related to urbanicity and, as the demographics of Irish society continue their secular evolution, to ethnic migration.

Results from the study to date indicate the striking diversity of the 'totality' of psychosis. On post hoc application of DSM-IV criteria to *all* cases of psychosis incepted in the absence of a priori diagnostic restriction, it was confirmed, as expected, that schizophrenia and bipolar disorder would constitute major diagnostic groupings. Yet these diagnoses each accounted for less than one-fifth of cases; furthermore, extension to 'schizophrenia spectrum' diagnoses (schizophrenia, schizophreniform disorder and schizoaffective disorder) increased the proportion only to less than one-third of cases. One contributory factor was the unexpectedly high incidence of a third major diagnostic grouping, i.e. a first psychotic episode on a background of major depressive disorder.

Risk for schizophrenia was threefold greater in men than in women, while risk for bipolar disorder and for major depressive disorder was essentially identical across the sexes; inception of cases without any arbitrary upper age cut-off yielded: (a) for schizophrenia a mean age at inception in the early 1930s, somewhat older for women than for men, with a median below the mean indicating emergence primarily in the early phases of adulthood but extending upwards throughout the lifespan; (b) for bipolar disorder a mean age at inception in the early 1930s, at similar ages for men and women, with a median below the mean indicating emergence primarily in the early phases of adulthood but extending upwards throughout the lifespan; and (c) for major depressive disorder with psychotic features a mean age at inception in the early 1950s, with a median above the mean indicating emergence primarily in the later phases of adulthood but extending downwards throughout the lifespan.

Yet these varying epidemiological 'signatures' must be juxtaposed with substantive homogeneity in terms of indistinguishable overall incidence, presentation throughout the lifespan, indistinguishable total scores for the seven positive symptom items on the PANSS and substantial stability for up to 6 years of follow-up. Similarly, dichotomisation of bipolar disorder into two subgroups on the basis of the DSM-IV qualifier 'with psychotic features' revealed only minimal difference in terms of total scores for the seven positive symptom items on the PANSS; psychosis in bipolar disorder appears to be a generic characteristic, most likely evident along a continuum, rather than any basis for arbitrary subtyping of the disorder. Additional analyses will be necessary to examine (i) the factor structure of psychopathology for similarities vs. differences between and within these diagnostic *nodes* and (ii) whether any of their quantitative characteristics evidence unimodal vs. bimodal or higher order distributions to further address the issue of subgroups therein.

On long-term follow-up, schizophrenia, bipolar disorder and major depressive disorder with psychotic features were generally stable diagnostic categories, while schizophreniform disorder, delusional disorder and psychosis not otherwise specified evolved primarily to schizophrenia or schizoaffective disorder from 6 months to 6 years. A diagnosis of brief psychotic disorder appeared superficially benign, with psychosis invariably resolving over the weeks immediately following emergence and little evidence of recrudescence over 6 months. However, by 6 years all cases had relapsed to a more portentious diagnosis, most notably schizophrenia/schizoaffective disorder and particularly bipolar disorder. Brief psychotic disorder appears to be a deceptive entity that can be the harbinger of long-term evolution to serious psychotic illness and may repay more vigorous, sustained intervention.

Developmental Pathobiology of the 'Totality' of Psychosis

3D laser surface imaging and geometric morphometrics were applied to identify any domains of facial shape that distinguish bipolar patients from controls and bipolar patients from those with schizophrenia. Both male and female bipolar patients evidenced significant facial dysmorphology as a putative index of brain dysmorphogenesis. Furthermore, that dysmorphology of the frontonasal prominences and related facial regions in bipolar disorder is more similar to, than different from, that found in schizophrenia suggests some shared dysmorphogenic process.

This appears to involve disruption to the primarily midline process of normal growth of the anterior face and brain, narrowing of the anterior mid-facial region, primary palate formation, dissociation of cranial base width from anterior facial and cerebral changes, and more rapid forward growth of the face than of the brain; frontonasal and adjacent facial areas are related embryologically to the forebrain and anterior midline cerebral regions and function as a single developmental unit in terms of 3D gene expression domains (Waddington et al. 1999; Schneider et al. 2001; Marcucio et al. 2005; Hennessy et al. 2007). On the basis of current knowledge as to the timing of these processes, the dysmorphologies characterising bipolar disorder and schizophrenia implicate dysmorphogenesis over a time frame that has limits of gestational weeks 6–19 but suggest a common denominator of weeks 9/10–14/15 of gestation (Waddington et al. 1999; Hennessy et al. 2007). Bipolar disorder and schizophrenia may reflect similar disturbances(s) acting over slightly differing time frames or slightly differing disturbances(s) acting over a similar time frame. Aspects of underlying developmental pathobiology may be tractable using mice that are mutant for genes associated with risk for schizophrenia, some of which are intimately involved in essential aspects of cerebral-craniofacial development (Waddington et al. 2007).

Synthesis

Focus on the 'totality' of first-episode psychosis, rather than on one or more a priori diagnostic categories, presents several challenges: (i) schizophrenia constitutes only a limited component of psychotic illness that presents to our health services for care; (ii) the three major diagnostic *nodes* of schizophrenia, bipolar disorder and major depressive disorder with psychotic features evidence some homogeneity for overall incidence, presentation throughout the lifespan and indistinguishable total scores for positive symptoms, and are substantially stable over several years of follow-up; (iii) brief psychotic disorder appears to be deceptive in its 'transience', as it can be the harbinger of long-term evolution to serious psychotic illness that may warrant more vigorous, sustained intervention; (iv) psychosis in bipolar disorder appears to be a generic characteristic, most likely evident along a continuum, rather than any basis for arbitrary subtyping; (iv); dysmorphology joins molecular genetics, structural brain pathology and cognitive dysfunction in indicating some shared pathobiology between schizophrenia and bipolar disorder and implicating some common process of dysmorphogenesis. The extent to which these concepts generalise to other components of the 'totality' of psychosis remains to be determined, yet they may inform importantly on how we structure health-care provision for the practical reality of psychotic illness and its disrespect for what are increasingly recognised to be arbitrary diagnostic impositions.

Acknowledgments The Cavan–Monaghan First-Episode Study was supported initially by the Stanley Medical Research Institute and, subsequently, by Cavan–Monaghan Mental Health Service. Studies on the developmental pathobiology of psychosis are supported by Science Foundation Ireland. We thank the clinical teams and associated staff of Cavan–Monaghan Mental Health

Service for their important contributions and Dr. Ronan Conroy, Department of Epidemiology, for assistance with incidence analyses.

References

Baldwin PA, Scully PJ, Quinn JF, Morgan MG, Kinsella A, Owens JM, O'Callaghan E, Waddington JL (2005) Schizophrenia Bulletin 31:624–638, 2005

Browne S, Clarke M, Gervin M, Waddington JL, Larkin C, O'Callaghan E (2000) Determinants of quality of life at first presentation with schizophrenia. British Journal of Psychiatry 176: 173–176

Clarke M, Whitty P, Browne S, McTigue O, Kamali M, Gervin M, Kinsella A, Waddington JL, Larkin C, O'Callaghan, E (2006) Untreated illness and outcome of psychosis. British Journal of Psychiatry 189:235–240

Diewert VM, Lozanoff S, Choy, V (1993) Computer reconstructions of human embryonic craniofacial morphology showing changes in relations between the face and brain during primary palate formation. Journal of Craniofacial Genetics and Developmental Biology 13:193–201

Dutta R, Greene T, Addington J, McKenzie K, Phillips M, Murray RM (2007) Biological, life course, and cross-cultural studies all point toward the value of dimensional and developmental ratings in the classification of psychosis. Schizophrenia Bulletin 33:868–876

Hennessy RJ, Kinsella A, Waddington JL (2002) 3D laser surface scanning and geometric morphometric analysis of craniofacial shape as an index of cerebro-craniofacial morphogenesis: initial application to sexual dimorphism. Biological Psychiatry 51:507–514

Hennessy RJ, Lane A, Kinsella A, Larkin C, O'Callaghan E, Waddington JL (2004) 3D morphometrics of craniofacial dysmorphology reveals sex-specific asymmetries in schizophrenia. Schizophrenia Research 67:261–268

Hennessy RJ, McLearie S, Kinsella A, Waddington JL (2005) Facial surface analysis by 3D laser scanning and geometric morphometrics in relation to sexual dimorphism in cerbral-craniofacial morphogenesis and cognitive function. Journal of Anatomy 207:283–296

Hennessy RJ, Baldwin PA, Browne DJ, Kinsella A, Waddington JL (2007) Three-dimensional laser surface imaging and geometric morphometrics resolve frontonasal dysmorphology in schizophrenia. Biological Psychiatry 61:1187–1194

Ivleva E, Thaker G, Tamminga CA (2008) Comparing genes and phenomenology in the major psychoses: schizophrenia and bipolar 1 disorder. Schizophrenia Bulletin 34:734–742

Jablensky A (1999) The conflict of the nosologists: views on schizophrenia and manic-depressive illness in the early part of the 20th century. Schizophrenia Research 39:95–100

Lane A, Kinsella A, Murphy P, Byrne M, Keenan J, Colgan K, Cassidy B, Sheppard N, Horgan R, Waddington JL, Larkin C, O'Callaghan E (1997) The anthropometric assessment of dysmorphic features in schizophrenia as an index of its developmental origins. Psychological Medicine 27:1155–1164, 1997

Maier W, Zobel A, Wagner M (2006) Schizophrenia and bipolar disorder: differences and overlap. Current Opinion in Psychiatry 19:165–170

Marcucio RS, Cordero DR, Hu D, Helms JA (2005) Molecular interactions coordinating the development of the forebrain and face. Developmental Biology 284:48–61

McCauley M, Rooney S, Clarke C, Carey T, Owens J (2003) Home-based treatment in Monaghan: the first two years. Irish Journal of Psychological Medicine 20:11–14

McGrath JC, El-Saadi O, Grim V, Cardy S, Chapple B, Chant D, Lieberman D, Mowry B (2002) Minor physical anomalies and quantitative measures of the head and face in psychosis. Archives of General Psychiatry 59:458–464

McGrath JJ, Féron FP, Burne TH, Mackay-Sim A, Eyles DW (2003) The neurodevelopmental hypothesis of schizophrenia: a review of recent developments. Annals of Medicine 35(2):86–93

Rapoport JL, Addington AM, Frangou S (2005) The neurodevelopmental model of schizophrenia: update 2005. Molecular Psychiatry 10:434–449

Russell V, McCauley M, McMahon J, Casey S, McCullagh H, Begley J (2003) Liaison psychiatry in rural general practice. Irish Journal of Psychological Medicine 20:65–68

Schneider RA, Hu D, Rubenstein JLR, Maden M, Helms JA (2001) Local retinoid signaling coordinates forebrain and facial morphogenesis by maintaining FGF8 and SHH- Development 128:2755–2767

Scully PJ, Quinn JF, Morgan MG, Kinsella A, O'Callaghan E, Owens JM, Waddington JL (2002) First episode schizophrenia, bipolar disorder and other psychoses in a rural Irish catchment area: incidence and gender in the Cavan–Monaghan study at 5 years. British Journal of Psychiatry 181 (Suppl. 43):s3–s9

Scully PJ, Owens JM, Kinsella A, Waddington JL (2004) Schizophrenia, schizoaffective and bipolar disorder within an epidemiologically complete, homogeneous population in rural Ireland: small area variation in rate. Schizophrenia Research 67:143–155

Selten JP, Cantor-Graae E, Kahn RS (2007) Migration and schizophrenia. Current Opinion in Psychiatry 20:111–115

Waddington JL, Lane A, Larkin C, O'Callaghan E (1999) The neurodevelopmental basis of schizophrenia: clinical clues from cerebro-craniofacial dysmorphogenesis, and the roots of a lifetime trajectory of disease. Biological Psychiatry 46:31–39

Waddington JL, Corvin AP, Donohue G, O'Tuathaigh CMP, Mitchell KJ, Gill M (2007) Functional genomics and schizophrenia: endophenotypes and mutant models. Psychiatric Clinics of North America 30:365–399

Part VI
Treatment

Comparative Efficacy and Safety of First- and Second-Generation Antipsychotics in the Treatment of Schizophrenia: Facts and Fiction

Rajiv Tandon, and Babu Rankapalli

Introduction

The introduction of chlorpromazine into clinical practice a half-century ago revolutionized the pharmacological treatment of schizophrenia (Nasrallah and Tandon, 2009). Fifty typical or first-generation antipsychotics (FGAs) have since become available around the world (Table 1). These agents are extremely effective in reducing the positive symptoms of schizophrenia (delusions, hallucinations, disorganized thinking, and paranoia) and allowed deinstitutionalization of persons with schizophrenia. These agents are found to be minimally effective, however, against negative and cognitive symptoms that contribute to much of the disability associated with schizophrenic illness. Additionally, they do not substantially diminish the suicidality and social dysfunction associated with the illness. Furthermore, these medications cause a range of adverse effects including acute extrapyramidal symptoms and tardive dyskinesia. To a considerable extent because of their poor tolerability, patients often do not take these medications as prescribed and this, in turn, leads to psychotic relapses and poor outcome.

Clozapine, the first so-called atypical or second-generation antipsychotic (SGA), was introduced into clinical practice in the late 1960s. It did not cause EPS or tardive dyskinesia. Its other significant adverse effects, however, substantially limited its utilization and agranulocytosis kept it out of most parts of the world until the 1990s. The fact that it was more effective than FGAs in treatment-refractory patients (Kane et al., 1988), specifically reduced suicidality (Meltzer et al., 2003), and was devoid of significant short- and long-term motor side effects led to optimism that better antipsychotic treatments for schizophrenia were possible. Substantial efforts to develop "a better clozapine" have led to the introduction of 10 additional SGAs (Table 1) into clinical practice. Believed to be more effective and safer than the 50 first-generation neuroleptics, these 11 "atypical" or second-generation antipsychotics (in order of introduction, clozapine, amisulpride, zotepine, risperidone,

R. Tandon (✉)
University of Florida Medical School, Gainesville, Florida, USA
e-mail: tandon@ufl.edu

Table 1 List of first- and second-generation antipsychotics

First-generation antipsychotics (N = 50)
  I. *PHENOTHIAZINES*
      (A) *Aliphatic side chain* (low–medium potency agents)
           Chlorpromazine, chlorproethazine, cyamemazine, levomepromazine,
           promazine, triflupromazine
      (B) *Piperidine side chain* (low–medium potency agents)
           Mesoridazine, piperacetazine, pipoptiazine, propericiazine, sulforidazine,
           thioridazine
      (C) *Piperazine side chain* (medium–high potency agents)
           Fluphenazine, acetophenazine, butaperazine, dixyrazine, perazine,
           perphenazine, prochlorperazine, thiopropazate, thioproperazine, trifluoperazine
  II. *BUTYROPHENONES* (high-potency agents)
      Haloperidol, benperidol, bromperidol, droperidol, fluanisone, melperone,
      moperone, pipamperone, timiperone, trifluperidol.
 III. *THIOXANTHENES* (medium–high potency agents)
      Thiothixene, chlorprothixene, clopenthixol, flupenthixol, zuclopenthixol
  IV. *DIHYDROINDOLONES* (low–medium potency agents)
      Molindone, oxypertine
  V. *DIBENZOEPINES* (low–medium potency agents)
      Loxapine, clotiapine
  VI. *DIPHENYLBUTYLPIPERIDINES* (high-potency agents)
      Pimozide, fluspirilene, penfluridol
 VII. *BENZAMIDES* (low-potency agents)
      Sulpiride, nemonapride, sultopride, tiapride
VIII. *IMINODIBENZYL* (medium-potency agents)
      Clocapramine, mosapramine

Second-generation antipsychotics (N = 11)
  I. *BENZO (DIAZE- or THIAZE-) PINES* (low and medium–high potency agents)
      Clozapine, olanzapine, quetiapine
  II. *INDOLONES and DIONES* (low–medium and high-potency agents)
      Aripiprazole, paliperidone, perospirone, risperidone, sertindole, ziprasidone
 III. *BENZAMIDE* (low-potency agents)
      Amisulpride
  IV. *AMINES* (low–medium potency agents)
      Zotepine

olanzapine, quetiapine, sertindole, ziprasidone, aripiprazole, perospirone, and paliperidone) have rapidly displaced the older agents in the treatment of schizophrenia (Jibson and Tandon, 1998; Kapur and Remington, 2001; Kane et al., 2003; Miller et al., 2004) and have become the standard of care.

Varying definitions of what it means to be an "atypical" antipsychotic (Fig. 1) have been utilized based on differential efficacy ("atypicals" considered more effective than "typicals" in neuroleptic-refractory patients; "atypicals" more effective than "typicals" with regard to negative, cognitive, and mood symptoms), differential safety (lower liability of "atypicals" to cause acute and long-term motor side effects), and distinctive pharmacology (e.g., "atypicals" being serotonin–dopamine antagonists as opposed to "typicals," which are merely dopamine antagonists)

Fig. 1 What is atypicality?

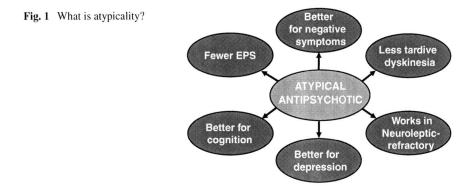

(Moller, 2000).Even though none of these definitions strictly dichotomized the existing 61 antipsychotic agents into "atypical" and "typical" categories, the idea that the 11 so-called "atypical" agents were fundamentally different from the other 50 antipsychotic agents prevailed. Because a range of different clinical and pharmacological definitions were utilized to characterize atypicality, however, it was suggested that these 11 agents might be better named "second-generation antipsychotics" (SGAs) to distinguish them from the supposedly less-effective and more risky "first-generation" agents (FGAs) even as attempts to clarify the nature of atypicality continued.

Clinicians and patients were excited about the possibilities for better outcome afforded by these newer agents and this considerable enthusiasm led to SGAs completely supplanting FGAs in the treatment of schizophrenia. Since SGAs cost about 10–30 times more than FGAs and much of the data indicating the substantial superiority of SGAs over FGAs were derived from industry-sponsored clinical trials (Montgomery et al., 2004; Heres et al., 2006), payors were somewhat dubious about these claims, leading to the conduct of two major government-supported trials of comparative FGA versus SGA effectiveness in schizophrenia in the United States (CATIE, Lieberman et al., 2005) and England (CUtLASS, Lewis et al., 2006). The results of these trials have been published over the past several years and appear to indicate that SGAs are no more effective than FGAs and are not associated with better cognitive or social outcomes (Lieberman et al., 2005; Jones et al., 2006; Lewis et al., 2006; McEvoy et al., 2006; Rosenheck et al., 2006; Stroup et al., 2006; Davies et al., 2007; Keefe et al., 2007; Swartz et al., 2007).

Amidst controversy about the implications and interpretation of these significant results (Moller, 2005; Meltzer and Bobo, 2006; Lewis and Lieberman, 2008; Tandon et al., 2008), the currently available 61 antipsychotic medications continue to be classified into FGA and SGA classes. In this chapter, the appropriateness of this classification is explored with particular reference to the following questions:

1. Do first- and second-generation antipsychotic agents constitute distinctive classes with reference to their efficacy?

2. Do first- and second-generation antipsychotic agents constitute distinctive classes with regard to their safety and tolerability?
3. Should we continue with the current dichotomization of existing antipsychotic agents into "first-generation" and "second-generation" agents?
4. Is "atypicality" still a relevant construct and, if so, what does it really mean?
5. What are the implications for best clinical practice?

Do First- and Second-Generation Antipsychotics Differ in Efficacy?

We separately examine the assumptions about the greater efficacy of second-generation over first-generation agents with regard to overall efficacy, efficacy in otherwise "neuroleptic-refractory" patients, and their presumed broader spectrum of efficacy.

Comparing FGAs and SGAs in Overall Efficacy

Meta-analyses comparing the efficacy of various SGAs to FGAs have found SGAs to constitute a heterogeneous class in this regard with only some SGAs being found to be more effective than both haloperidol and low-potency FGAs (Davis et al., 2003; Leucht et al., 2009). Results from the most recent and comprehensive meta-analytic comparison (Leucht et al., 2009) in this regard are graphically depicted in Fig. 2. Although methodological constraints hinder efficacy comparisons between different SGAs (Tandon and Fleischhacker, 2005), they confirm the absence of any categorical distinction between SGAs and FGAs in terms of overall efficacy. Results of both CATIE (Lieberman et al., 2005) and CUtLASS band-1 (Jones et al., 2006) support the absence of any categorical difference between SGAs and FGAs in overall efficacy. Even among first-episode and early-onset schizophrenia patients, no categorical difference in overall efficacy between SGAs and FGAs has been found (Sikich et al., 2008).

Comparing FGAs and SGAs in Neuroleptic-Refractory Patients

Among patients with treatment-refractory schizophrenia, clozapine has the largest body of evidence supporting its greater efficacy (Kane et al., 1988; Chakos et al., 2001). The extent to which other SGAs share this property is unclear (Tuunainen et al., 2002). In band 2 of CUtLASS (Lewis et al., 2006), 136 patients exhibiting a poor response to ≥ 2 antipsychotic agents were randomized to receive either clozapine or a non-clozapine SGA and their quality of life compared over 1 year. Clozapine was found to be significantly superior to non-clozapine SGAs with reference to symptoms ($p = 0.01$) and exhibited a trend towards superiority with regard to quality

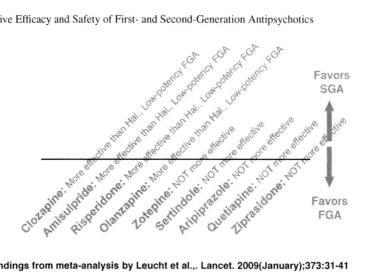

Findings from meta-analysis by Leucht et al.,. Lancet. 2009(January);373:31-41

Fig. 2 Nine second-generation antipsychotics compared to haloperidol and low-potency FGAs

of life ($p = 0.08$) in this group of patients. Results from the efficacy arm of phase-2 in CATIE (McEvoy et al., 2006) also support the greater efficacy of clozapine in poorly responsive schizophrenia patients. These data suggest that clozapine may be unique among the SGAs with regard to superior efficacy in schizophrenia patients who do not respond to FGA treatment. The similar efficacy of aripiprazole and per-phenazine among patients unresponsive to 4–6 weeks of treatment with risperidone or olanzapine (two SGAs) (Kane et al., 2007) supports the view that non-clozapine SGAs and FGAs may not differ in efficacy among schizophrenia patients refractory to treatment with two or more antipsychotic agents.

Do FGAs and SGAs Differ in Spectrum of Efficacy: Cognitive, Negative, and Mood Symptoms?

The preponderance of clinical trial data prior to CATIE and CUtLASS indicated that SGAs provide a broader spectrum of efficacy than FGAs (equivalent efficacy in positive symptoms and greater efficacy in negative, mood, and cognitive symptoms) (Kane et al., 2003; Meltzer, 2004). Much of these data were derived from industry-supported clinical trials (Heres et al., 2006), however, and studies of SGAs compared to high doses of haloperidol utilized as the FGA comparator (Geddes et al., 2000; Hugenholtz et al., 2006). CATIE and CUtLASS did not find any clear difference between SGAs and FGAs with regard to efficacy in any of these symptom domains. Furthermore, the most recent meta-analytic comparison (Leucht et al., 2009) also did not find any categorical difference between SGAs and FGAs in this regard. Again, although methodological constraints hinder efficacy comparisons between different SGAs (Tandon and Nasrallah, 2006; Johnsen et al., 2008), they confirm the absence of any categorical distinction between SGAs and FGAs in terms of spectrum of efficacy.

Making Sense of It All: What Might Explain Contradictory Findings About Differential Efficacy Between SGAs and FGAs?

Understanding the original basis of differentiating SGAs from FGAs might help to resolve the confusion. "Atypicality" of an antipsychotic agent originally referred to the ability to produce a robust antipsychotic effect without causing extrapyramidal side effects (EPS) (Jibson and Tandon, 1998; Meltzer, 2004). The principal distinction between so-called SGAs and FGAs is the ability of the former to provide an equivalent antipsychotic effect with a lower liability to cause EPS, although there is substantial variation within each class in this regard. In clinical trials comparing SGAs to FGAs, heightening the EPS differential (using high-dose haloperidol as the FGA comparator, for example) leads to observations of a broader spectrum of efficacy of SGAs versus FGAs (Hugenholtz et al., 2006; Tandon et al., 2008). On the other hand, minimizing this EPS differential (by using low-dose and low-potency FGAs as the comparator or the study of low-EPS risk samples as in CATIE) is associated with findings of no SGA–FGA difference. In CATIE, for example, the inclusion–exclusion criteria for the study led to a sample that was at very risk for developing EPS with any agent – this resulted in very low overall EPS rates in this 18-month study and there were no differences in EPS rates between SGA and FGA treatment arms (Miller et al., 2008).

These apparent discrepancies reveal a crucial clinical lesson – the apparently broader spectrum of efficacy of SGAs than FGAs is substantially related to their generally lower propensity to cause motor side effects. By eliminating differences in EPS between FGAs and SGAs, one can also eliminate differential efficacy between them in terms of negative, cognitive, and depressive symptoms. Essentially, the purported benefits of SGAs are related to their greater ability to be "atypical" (Fig. 3), i.e., the greater ease and consistency with which they can provide a robust antipsychotic effect without EPS (Tandon et al., 2007). As will be discussed in the next section, this distinction between the various SGAs and FGAs is relative and not categorical.

Do First- and Second-Generation Antipsychotics Differ in Adverse Effects?

Substantial differences in the adverse effect profiles of the 61 currently available antipsychotic medications are very well documented. Generally, SGAs have a lower propensity to induce EPS than FGAs, although there are substantial differences among both groups of agents with regard to the ease and consistency with which an adequate antipsychotic effect can be achieved without EPS (Weiden, 2007; Leucht

Fig. 3 Why is avoidance of
EPS so important?

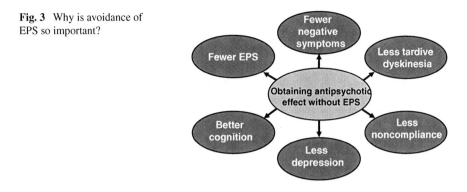

et al., 2009). Dichotomizing antipsychotic agents into SGAs and FGAs based on EPS liability obscures the significant heterogeneity within both these groups in this regard and suggests a categorical distinction that does *not* exist.

Metabolic side effects that increase the risk of ischemic heart disease (weight gain, dyslipidemia, diabetes mellitus) have recently received particular attention (Newcomer, 2005; Franciosi et al., 2005; Fleischhacker et al., 2008). In view of their likely contribution to the increased mortality of persons with schizophrenia, they warrant close attention (Meyer and Nasrallah, 2009). Although SGAs are *generally* associated with metabolic adverse effects to a greater extent than FGAs, there are variations among both SGAs and FGAs with regard to their liability to cause these side effects. CATIE, for example, found olanzapine to cause more weight gain and related metabolic side effects than perphenazine, risperidone, and quetiapine to cause equivalent weight gain to perphenazine, while ziprasidone caused fewer metabolic problems than perphenazine. Again, SGAs and FGAs do *not* categorically discriminate with regard to the risk of metabolic side effects (Leucht et al., 2009).

Other adverse effects differ *among* FGAs and SGAs as well (Tandon et al., 2006; Leucht et al., 2009); these groups *do not categorically differ* with regard to risks of sedation, hypotension, prolactin elevation, or other adverse effects.

Is the Categorization of Antipsychotics into FGAs and SGAs then Meaningful?

Based on the absence of absolute categorical differences between SGAs and FGAs in either efficacy or safety/tolerability, there is little justification to preserve this dichotomous classification. FGAs and SGAs both constitute very heterogeneous classes of antipsychotic medications. The principal *loose* distinction between SGAs and FGAs is the ability of the former to provide an equivalent antipsychotic effect with a lower liability to cause EPS, although there is substantial variation within each class in this regard. Clinical trial data that indicate that SGAs may demonstrate a broader spectrum of efficacy than FGAs (equivalent efficacy in positive symptoms and variably greater efficacy in negative, mood, and cognitive symptoms) also indicate that these benefits are substantially related to their lower propensity to cause motor side effects. Thus the effect of atypicality (a robust antipsychotic effect without EPS) is an important attribute, but this depends on the interaction between agent (greater or lesser degree of ease in providing a robust antipsychotic effect without EPS), patient (high or lower degree of vulnerability to develop EPS), and therapeutic strategy (dosing, rate of titration).

Thus both FGA and SGA classes exhibit substantial heterogeneity across a range of clinical and pharmacological attributes and no single property can consistently distinguish the existing 61 antipsychotic agents into these two subgroups. In addition to the above anomalies, the dichotomy of first-generation versus secondary-generation antipsychotics results in some obvious misclassifications. For example, the so-called second-generation agent clozapine was developed before several so-called first-generation agents such as molindone.

Therefore the dichotomy between SGAs and FGAs should be abandoned (Table 2).

Table 2 Abandon dichotomy between first- and second-generation antipsychotics

---

1. There are no consistent differences in efficacy across agents (except for clozapine in some populations!)
2. The efficacy advantage of clozapine in this population appears independent of its EPS and TD benefit
3. On average, so-called second-generation antipsychotics cause less EPS and more metabolic side-effects than first-generation agents
4. *But there are varying degrees of risk of EPS, metabolic side effects, and other adverse effects WITHIN both classes*

Abandon dichotomy between first- and second-generation antipsychotics as it is not useful and, in fact, misinforms

---

Atypicality Is Relevant but SGA/FGA Dichotomization Is Not

Recent findings reinforce the importance of achieving an antipsychotic effect without EPS. The inconsistently observed greater spectrum of efficacy of SGAs over FGAs is substantially explained by their *generally* reduced propensity to cause EPS, and when EPS differences between these antipsychotic agents are eliminated, efficacy spectrum differences disappear as well. Thus using any antipsychotic agent as an "atypical" (*a robust antipsychotic effect without EPS and without using an anticholinergic agent*) is of importance – this leads to modestly greater effects on negative, cognitive, and depressive symptoms. Clozapine is more effective than other antipsychotic agents in treatment-refractory schizophrenia patients (specifically antipsychotic-refractory positive symptoms), ameliorating symptoms in about one-third of such patients. Reduced EPS liability does not explain this greater efficacy of clozapine.

Indirect comparisons of efficacy across studies and direct comparisons in the relatively few randomized, controlled head-to-head studies between other SGAs suggest that they are essentially similar with regard to overall efficacy and efficacy in treating positive and negative symptoms; if differences exist, these are small (Tandon et al., 2008). The occasional observation of the superior efficacy of some SGAs over others (Leucht et al., 2009) may be explained by the fact that optimal dose ranges for olanzapine, risperidone, and amisulpride are somewhat better defined than those for quetiapine, ziprasidone, and aripiprazole and other methodological differences (Tandon et al., 2008).

The concept of atypicality as originally conceived is still meaningful – the ability to obtain a robust antipsychotic effect without EPS. This "atypical effect" is associated with a perceived broader spectrum of efficacy (advantages with reference to negative, cognitive, and mood symptoms) and a lower risk of tardive dyskinesia. Disagreement about the basic definition of atypicality and efforts to define its pharmacological basis led to the replacement of "atypical antipsychotic" by the term "second-generation antipsychotic." While the dichotomous classification of existing antipsychotic agents into these two subgroups is not valid or useful, the property of atypicality is still relevant. Efforts to elucidate its pharmacological substrate is still of great importance. The term second-generation antipsychotic should be abandoned as it is both uninformative and misleading.

Implications for Clinical Practice

Existing antipsychotic agents are broadly similar in terms of overall efficacy with the exception of clozapine's greater efficacy in those with neuroleptic-refractory schizophrenia. If there are differences in efficacy between agents, these differences are likely to be small. In view of the significant individual variability in drug pharmacokinetics and treatment responsivity, however, it should be emphasized that equivalent overall efficacy across patient groups does not translate into equal efficacy in each individual patient. Furthermore, different antipsychotic agents present different challenges with regard to the speed and possibility of achieving the most efficacious dose of that agent across patients. Some agents have to be titrated more slowly than others because of the potential for uncomfortable side effects (e.g., akathisia and other EPS; sedation) or for potentially risky adverse effects (e.g., hypotension). Since tolerance to these side effects develops to a certain extent, it is possible to titrate agents causing these adverse effects up to their optimal dose, but this has to be done slowly.

Individual patients differ in their response to different antipsychotic agents and in their vulnerability to different adverse effects. Some patients may not be able to tolerate the maximally efficacious dose of particular agents because of adverse effects. There is no best agent or a best dose of any agent for all patients. It is not currently possible to prospectively predict which antipsychotic medication might be optimal for a given patient. Decisions about antipsychotic therapy consequently entail a trial and error process with careful monitoring of clinical response and adverse effects and an ongoing risk-benefit assessment. A minimum protocol for monitoring adverse effects should be implemented and this needs to be customized to the patient's specific vulnerabilities/needs and the agent selected (Marder et al., 2004; Constantine et al., 2006; Tandon et al., 2008).

Treatment targets should be explicitly defined and the impact of treatment on the individual carefully monitored. Adjustments in treatment should be made based on response. Data related to reliable measures of symptomatology, side effects, risk factors for metabolic and other diseases, appropriate laboratory tests, measurement of mild EPS, and other relevant individualized risk-benefit data should be obtained in a timely manner and utilized to assist decision making. Pharmacological treatment decisions made by the psychiatrist in conjunction with the individual receiving treatment for schizophrenia include initial choice of antipsychotic, dosing strategy of chosen agent, determination of specific treatment target and assessment of response, and choosing between available options (e.g., allowing more time, changing the dose, adding another medication, switching antipsychotics) in the event of an unsatisfactory response.

The most proximate objective of antipsychotic treatment of schizophrenia is to achieve an "atypical antipsychotic effect" – maximum reduction of positive symptoms while avoiding EPS or using anticholinergic medications. Although it is possible to achieve this goal with suitably dosed FGA treatment in a fair number of individuals, SGA treatment *on average* may provide a better likelihood of more predictably accomplishing this objective. But this distinction is *not* categorical and hence the dichotomy should be abolished.

If the initially selected treatment does not accomplish this goal, appropriate treatment adjustments need to be made. Other objectives include optimizing reduction of other symptom domains while minimizing adverse effects considering individual patient vulnerabilities and preferences.

Conclusion

The terms first-generation antipsychotic and second-generation antipsychotic should be abandoned. They are neither useful nor valid. The concept of "atypicality" as originally conceived is still meaningful – it refers to the ability to obtain a robust antipsychotic effect without any extrapyramidal side effect. Although so-called SGAs are *on average* better able than so-called FGAs to be *atypical*, there is no dichotomy with overlaps across these supposed groups and substantial heterogeneity within both of them.

Some other assertions that can be made about antipsychotic treatment of schizophrenia include

(i)   achieving a robust antipsychotic effect without any EPS is of enormous clinical importance because a broader spectrum of efficacy and a lower risk of tardive dyskinesia accompany this "atypical antipsychotic effect";

(ii) different challenges exist in balancing efficacy and tolerability with different agents;

(iii) given enormous individual variability in drug handling, responsivity, and susceptibility to and tolerance of different adverse effects, no single approach works for all patients; and

(iv) clozapine is still the gold standard in the treatment of otherwise unresponsive schizophrenia.

There is no question that we need better treatments for schizophrenia and that existing treatments are neither completely effective nor devoid of significant side effects. But they do meaningfully help. Just as it is important not to exaggerate what existing treatments for schizophrenia can offer, it is equally important not to discount what they can do. Even as we strive to develop more effective treatments for the future, we can do better in utilizing existing treatments to optimize individual outcomes and reduce the considerable morbidity and mortality associated with schizophrenia. To be able to do so, we need a realistic understanding of what available treatments can and cannot do, how they compare, and how this information can be translated to optimize individualized treatment for each person with schizophrenia (Tandon et al., 2006). Antipsychotic treatment needs to be individually tailored and this requires careful monitoring and ongoing joint decision making by the clinician–patient team about choice of antipsychotic agent, dosing, continuation/switching, and augmentation. Although existing antipsychotic treatments for schizophrenia are not completely satisfactory, they can meaningfully reduce the devastating effects of the illness. Even as we try to develop better treatments, we need to better characterize and compare existing treatments. A balanced understanding of our extensive data repository on treatments for schizophrenia is essential and effective mechanisms for fair dissemination of this information are necessary. A meticulous application of this understanding can reduce the significant gap between what we know and how we provide antipsychotic pharmacotherapy for persons with schizophrenia. Collectively, we can do much to better utilize existing treatments to optimize individual outcomes and reduce the considerable morbidity and mortality associated with the illness.

References

Chakos M, Lieberman J, Hoffman E, Bradford D, Sheitman B. Effectiveness of second-generation antipsychotics in patients with treatment-resistant schizophrenia: a review and meta-analysis of randomized trials. *Am J Psychiatry*, 2001; 158:518–526.

Constantine RJ, Richard SM, Surles RC, et al. Optimizing pharmacotherapy of schizophrenia: tools for the psychiatrist. *Curr Psychosis Ther Rep*, 2006; 4:5–11.

Davies LM, Lewis S, Jones PB, et al. Cost-effectiveness of first- v. second-generation antipsychotic drugs: results from a randomized controlled trial in schizophrenia responding poorly to previous therapy. *Br J Psychiatry*, 2007; 191:14–22.

Davis JM, Chen N, Glick ID. A meta-analysis of the efficacy of second-generation antipsychotics. *Arch Gen Psychiatry*, 2003; 60:553–564.

Fleischhacker WW, Cetkovich-Bakmas M, De Hert M, Hennekens CH, Lambert M, Leucht S, Maj M, McIntyre RS, Naber D, Newcomer JW, Olfson M, Osby U, Sartorius N, Lieberman JA. Comorbrid somatic illnesses in patients with severe mental disorders: clinical, policy, and research challenges. *Journal of Clinical Psychiatry*, 2008; 69(4): 514–519.

Franciosi LP, Kasper S, Garber AJ, et al. Advancing the treatment of people with mental illness: A call to action in the management of metabolic issues. *J Clin Psychiatry*, 2005; 66:790–798.

Geddes J, Freemantle N, Harrison P, Bebbington P. Atypical antipsychotics in the treatment of schizophrenia: systematic overview and meta-regression analysis. *British Medical Journal*, 2000; 321(7273): 1371–1376.

Heres S, Davis J, Maino K, et al. Why olanzapine beats risperidone, risperidone beats quetiapine, and quetiapine beats olanzapine: an exploratory analysis of head-to-head comparison studies of second-generation antipsychotics. *Am J Psychiatry*, 2006; 163:185–194.

Hugenholtz GW, Heerdink ER, Stolker JJ, et al. Haloperidol dose when used as active comparator in randomized controlled trials with atypical antipsychotics in schizophrenia: comparison with officially recommended doses. *J Clin Psychiatry*, 2006; 67:897–903.

Jibson MD, Tandon R. New atypical antipsychotic medications. *J Psychiatr Res*, 1998; 32: 215–228.

Johnsen E, Jørgensen HA. Effectiveness of second generation antipyschotics: a systematic review of randomized trials. *BMC Psychiatry*, 2008; 8:31.

Jones PB, Davies L, Barnes TR, et al. Randomized controlled trial of effect on quality of life of second-generation versus first generation antipsychotic drugs in schizophrenia. *Arch Gen Psychiatry*, 2006; 63:1079–1087.

Kane JM, Honigfeld G, Singer J, Meltzer HY. Clozapine for the treatment-resistant schizophrenic: A double-blind comparison with chlorpromazine. *Arch Gen Psychiatry*, 1988; 45: 789–796.

Kane JM, Leucht S, Carpenter D, et al. Expert consensus guideline series: optimizing pharmacologic treatment of psychotic disorders. *J Clin Psychiatry*, 2003; 64(Suppl. 12):1–100.

Kane JM, Meltzer HY, Carson WH, et al. Aripiprazole for treatment-resistant schizophrenia: results of a multi-center, randomized, double-blind, comparison study versus perphenazine. *J Clin Psychiatry*, 2007; 68:213–223.

Kapur S, Remington G. Atypical antipsychotics: New directions and new challenges in the treatment of schizophrenia. *Annu Rev Med*, 2001; 52:503–517.

Keefe RSE, Bilder RM, Davis SM, et al. Neurocognitive effects of antipsychotic medications in patients with chronic schizophrenia in the CATIE trial. *Arch Gen Psychiatry*, 2007; 64: 633–647.

Leucht S, Corves C, Arbter D, et al. second-generation versus first-generation antipsychotic drugs for schizophrenia: a meta-analysis. *Lancet*, 2009; 373:31–41.

Lewis S, Lieberman J. CATIE and CUtLASS: can we handle the truth? *Br J Psychiatry*, 2008; 192:161–163.

Lewis SW, Barnes TR, Davies L, et al. Randomized controlled trial of effect of prescription of clozapine versus other second-generation antipsychotic drugs in resistant schizophrenia. *Schizophr Bull*, 2006; 32:715–723.

Lieberman JA, Stroup ST, McEvoy JP, et al. Effectiveness of antipsychotic drugs in patients with chronic schizophrenia. *N Engl J Med*, 2005; 353:1209–1223.

Marder SR, Essock SM, Miller AM, et al. Physical health monitoring of patients with schizophrenia. *Am J Psychiatry*, 2004; 161:1334–1349.

McEvoy JP, Lieberman JA, Stroup TS, et al. Effectiveness of clozapine versus olanzapine, quetiapine, and risperidone in patients with chronic schizophrenia who did not respond to prior antipsychotic treatment. *Am J Psychiatry*, 2006; 163:600–610.

Meltzer HY. What's atypical about atypical antipsychotic drugs? *Curr Opin Pharmacol*, 2004; 4:53–57.

Meltzer HY, Alphs L, Green AI, et al. Clozapine treatment for suicidality in schizophrenia: International Suicide Prevention Trial (InterSePT). *Arch Gen Psychiatry*, 2003; 60:82–91.

Meltzer HY, Bobo WV. Interpreting the efficacy findings in the CATIE study: what the clinician should know. *CNS Spectrums*, 2006; 11(Suppl. 7):14–24.

Miller AL, Hall CS, Buchanan RW, et al. The Texas Medication Algorithm Project antipsychotic algorithm for schizophrenia: 2003 update. *J Clin Psychiatry*, 2004; 65:500–508.

Miller DD, Caroff SN, Davis SM, et al. Extrapyramidal side-effects of antipsychotics in a randomized trial. *Br J Psychiatry*, 2008; 193:279–288.

Moller H-J. Definition, psychopharmacological basis and clinical evaluation of novel/atypical neuroleptics: methodological issues and clinical consequences. *World J Biol Psychiatry*, 2000; 1:75–91.

Moller H-J. Are the new antipsychotics no better than the classical neuroleptics? The problematic answer from the CATIE study. *Eur Arch Psychiatry Clin Neurosci*, 2005; 255:371–372

Montgomery JH, Byerly M, Carmody T, et al. An analysis of the effect of funding source in randomized clinical trials of second-generation antipsychotics for the treatment of schizophrenia. *Control Clin Trials*, 2004; 25:598–612.

Nasrallah HA, Tandon R: Conventional antipsychotics. In Nemeroff C, Schatzberg A (eds) American Psychiatric Press Textbook of Psychopharmacology, 4th Edition, American Psychiatric Press, Washington DC, 2009.

Newcomer JW. Second-generation (atypical) antipsychotics and metabolic effects: a comprehensive literature review. *CNS Drugs*, 2005; 19(Suppl. 1):1–93.

Rosenheck RA, Leslie DL, Sindelar J, et al. Cost-effectiveness of second-generation antipsychotics and perphenazine in a randomized trial of treatment for chronic schizophrenia. *Am J Psychiatry*, 2006; 163:2080–2089.

Sikich L, Frazier JA, McClellan J, et al. Double-blind comparison of first- and second- generation antipsychotics in early-onset schizophrenia and schizoaffective disorder: Findings from the treatment of early-onset schizophrenia study (TEOSS). *Am J Psychiatry*, 2008; 165:1420–1431.

Stroup TS, Lieberman JA, McEvoy JP, et al. Effectiveness of olanzapine, quetiapine, risperidone, and ziprasidone in patients with chronic schizophrenia following discontinuation of a previous atypical antipsychotic. *Am J Psychiatry*, 2006; 163:611–622.

Swartz MS, Perkins DO, Stroup ST, et al. Effects of antipsychotic medications on psychosocial functioning in patients with chronic schizophrenia: findings from the NIMH CATIE study. *Am J Psychiatry*, 2007; 164:428–436.

Tandon R, Belmaker RH, Gattaz WF, et al. World Psychiatric Association Pharmacopsychiatry Section statement on comparative effectiveness of antipsychotics in the treatment of schizophrenia. *Schizophr Res*, 2008; 100:20–38.

Tandon R, Carpenter WT, Davis JM. First- and second-generation antipsychotics: Learning from CUtLASS and CATIE. *Arch Gen Psychiatry*, 2007; 64:977–978.

Tandon R, Fleischhacker WW. Comparative efficacy of antipsychotics in the treatment of schizophrenia: A critical assessment. *Schizophr Res*, 2005; 79:145–155.

Tandon R, Nasrallah HA. Subjecting meta-analyses to closer scrutiny: little support for differential efficacy among second-generation antipsychotics. The authors reply. *Arch Gen Psychiatry*, 2006; 63:935–939.

Tandon R, Targum SD, Nasrallah HA, Ross R. Strategies for maximizing clinical effectiveness in the treatment of schizophrenia. *J Psychiatr Pract*; 2006 12:348–363.

Tuunainen A, Wahlbeck K, Gilbody SM. Newer atypical antipsychotic medication in comparison to clozapine: a systematic review of randomized trials. *Schizophr Res*, 2002; 56:1–10.

Weiden PJ. EPS profiles: the atypical antipsychotics are not all the same. *Journal of Psychiatric Practice*, 2007; 13(1): 13–24.

Long-Acting Antipsychotic Medication and the Outcome of Schizophrenia

Anthony S. David, Ayana Gibbs, and Maxine X. Patel

History

Long-acting injectable antipsychotic medication or depots are an important element in the treatment of schizophrenia. Before assessing the pros and cons of such treatment and determining whether it has a significant impact on outcome over and above oral medication, it may be useful to consider where the idea of depot injections came from. There is surely a history behind this idea though it appears that a full account of this has yet to be written.

In his brief history of 'depot neuroleptics' George Simpson wrote in 1984 that the pharmaceutical company Squibb were first to consider adapting their phenothiazine drug fluphenazine, developed in 1957, into an agent with relatively long activity. The chemical compound had an alcohol group on a side chain and Simpson noted that scientists at Squibb who had developed long-acting preparations of hormones such as testosterone experimented with attaching a variety of long-chain fatty acids to the alcohol group, thus delaying the availability of the free drug. This created an ester and required that the long-chain fatty acid be hydrolysed before the fluphenazine, in this case, could be released. Further experimentation with vehicles such as sesame oil followed and thus the first depot neuroleptic was born. This was fluphenazine enanthate, which was followed by fluphenazine decanoate.

The ability to give these drugs, which at that time had been shown by study after study to be effective in treatment of schizophrenia, as an injection every 2, 3 or 4 weeks was, according to Simpson, 'hailed as a great advance'. However, looking back on the earliest publications in the field and attempts to summarise them, one is struck by two recurrent themes. First, the notion that benefits of long-acting injections are quite simply obvious and self-evident while at the same time a notion emerges that they are in some sense under-utilised. One contemporary advocate of depots has estimated that 50% of patients are not treated prophylactically at all or only for inadequate duration (Kissling, 1994, 1997), the implication being that

A.S. David (✉)
Section of Cognitive Neuropsychiatry, Institute of Psychiatry, KCL, London SE5 8AF, UK
e-mail: anthony.david@iop.kcl.ac.uk

W.F. Gattaz, G. Busatto (eds.), *Advances in Schizophrenia Research 2009*,
DOI 10.1007/978-1-4419-0913-8_23, © Springer Science+Business Media, LLC 2010

depots may solve at least part of this problem, a view widely echoed (Glazer and Kane, 1992; Gerlach, 1995; Kane et al., 1998).

David Healey (2000), in the third of his published interviews with psychophar-macologists, discusses the early days of depots with Pierre Lambert, a senior French pharmacologist and psychiatrist. He noted how the first drugs manufactured by Squibb were quickly followed by those from Specia and then Lundbeck. The pos-sible application in forensic populations was an early suggestion according to Lam-bert. However, he noted, "it is all too easy to give a depot neuroleptic to patients and then to forget about them for a fortnight or three weeks". He recalled that this led to adverse affects and might even have contributed to some suicides in the early usage of the drugs. Again this remark during the interview echoes another theme in the literature on depots that somehow this form of treatment alters the way physicians practice and perhaps alters too the doctor–patient relationship.

Early Use and Utilisation

Perhaps the first clinical report of the use and effectiveness of a long-acting antipsy-chotic injection was by Kinross-Wright and colleagues in 1963 as a 'clinical note' in the *American Journal of Psychiatry*. The brief report describes the first use of fluphenazine enanthate in a double-blind, presumably placebo-controlled, study of 147 patients, all but one suffering from schizophrenia. Injections mostly of 25 re given every 2 weeks for a duration that ranged between 2 weeks and 6 months. The authors reported that 17 (12%) were unimproved or worse, 40 (27%) showed relief of some symptoms, 68 (46%) showed relief of many symptoms and made 'a good adaptation to the hospital situation' and 22 (15%) 'achieved remission' and were discharged. Extra-pyramidal side effects were noted as were dizziness, insomnia, etc. The authors note also that "lack of insight or co-operation on the part of the patient or his family more often than not leads to rejection of medi-cation" and they go on, ". . . a slow release preparation of an effective phenoth-iazine . . . would solve much of the problem". This support was followed by studies on the deaconate form in the following years in the United States and around the world. Early initial trials in the United Kingdom led to fairly heated correspon-dence in the *British Medical Journal* late in 1966 with a report by Hicks and Oven-stone initially recording a high level of dystonic reactions although this was fol-lowed by numerous other reports essentially of open-label trials that were far more positive, although the need to prescribe additional anticholinergic medication was emphasised. The first full study from Britain was published in the *British Journal of Psychiatry* in 1968 by Haider working in Edinburgh, which contrasted the oral and injectable forms of fluphenazine in a double-blind cross-over design. Interest-ingly there were few marked differences between the two formulations noted at that time.

There are great regional and international variations in the use and uptake of long-acting injectable antipsychotics, which again may be explained through a complex sociology and history. Prescribing practices for depot antipsychotics have been found to differ significantly between countries, with higher rates of depot prescribing in Denmark, Sweden and the United Kingdom, and lower rates in France and the United States (Dencker and Axelsson, 1996). Such factors as the manufacturing base of pharmaceutical company and its national prominence in the case of Lundbeck and the Scandinavian countries may be relevant. Also apposite is the relative deference that patients give to doctors in certain cultures and perhaps most importantly and in our view most relevant to the current situation, the ease with which the long-acting injection treatment paradigm fitted into the organisation of health care for people with chronic and enduring mental illness such as in the UK National Health Service with its strong primary care ethos and community-orientated outlook. Prescribing habits can also vary greatly within a region and between regions (Taylor et al., 1999). The prescribing practice of an individual psychiatrist is subject to a multitude of influencing factors including psychiatrists' beliefs about adverse side effects, patients' acceptance of depots, stigma, nursing-staff involvement, external forces in health-care systems, prescribing knowledge and experience (Patel and David, 2005).

One element inherent in the use of long-acting injections is the allied notion of maintenance therapy. Here, the idea is that it is not simply the treatment of acute symptoms that is important but the maintenance of the person in health and prevention of relapse. The term 'maintenance therapy' becomes embedded in the psychiatric literature around the early 1970s as exemplified by the study by Leff and Wing (1971), which compared in what would now be described a pragmatic fashion, treatment of 'recovered' patients with schizophrenia with either oral trifluoperazine or chlorpromazine on the one hand versus placebo on the other. The results showed that 12 out of 15 (80%) relapsed on placebo compared to 7 out of 20 (35%) on oral medication at 1 year. This seemed to pave the way for an influential and prestigious study by Hirsch et al. (1973) again published in the *British Medical Journal* and funded by the Medical Research Council of Great Britain. This was a double-blind placebo-controlled trial with long-acting fluphenazine and it was found that at 9 months, 25 out of 38 patients (66%) relapsed whilst on placebo, while only 3 out of 36 (8%) relapsed on depot medication. The authors concluded that fluphenazine had a powerful effect in preventing and ameliorating both symptoms and deterioration but they also highlighted the need for adequate community services to make the most of this treatment. It should also be emphasised that the comparator here was placebo and not the oral version of the drug.

Depots in Current Practice

We can now fast-forward 20 years to a landmark article by Davis and colleagues in 1994, which provided a scholarly and comprehensive overview of the then relevant literature. This was not confined to randomised controlled trials as in the *Cochrane Reviews* (see below). It included the so-called 'mirror image' studies, which are essentially cohort studies in which a period prior to the introduction of the new agent is compared to the period post introduction. These studies tended to show positive benefits, particularly in terms of reduced number of days spent in hospital. However, it must be borne in mind that the studies tended not to be randomised and often led to the introduction of a new treatment at the point in the patient's clinical history when they were perhaps at their worst so that some improvement was very likely. Also the studies carried out in the 1970s and the 1980s could not control for general 'period' effects, that is the general reduction in lengths of hospital stay and admissions as part of 'de-institutionalisation' and the development of community care. Some years later, a series of systematic reviews and meta-analyses conducted under the auspices of the *Cochrane* collaboration (Adams et al., 2001) was published, which attempted to evaluate the efficacy of depot antipsychotic drugs as a group. It was also possible to review at that stage other non-clinical trial data that considered attitudes of both professionals and patients towards this treatment.

Those randomised controlled trials meeting the exacting standards of the Cochrane collaboration were less persuasive. Demonstrating superiority of depots in relation to placebo was confirmed but hardly surprising. What the clinician should be interested in is whether the depot formulation of the drug is superior to the oral formulation, in other words strict pharmacological factors are controlled while the effect of formulation is the variable under test. A number of studies have been carried out which use this sort of comparison, for example, fluphenazine in its oral and depot forms and haloperidol in the two forms, although most of the studies were short term. In the meta-review published by Adams and colleagues (2001) relapse rates overall were remarkably similar in groups randomised to oral or depot preparations, the rates being between 30 and 40%. Relapse rates are chosen here as it is surely a clear-cut outcome that one would hope would show a benefit for long-acting maintenance treatment. Relapse rates in a comparison of high- or standard-dose depot versus low-dose depot encompassing well over 600 patients, again mostly from short-term studies, showed a clear benefit of the high/standard-dose regime with only 19% showing relapse compared to 46% in the low-dose group, a relative risk of 2.5 (95% confidence intervals 1.07–5.89). The only other outcome that differentiated the depot from the oral treatment forms was a measure of global outcome that favoured depot. It should also be noted that adverse effects including abnormal movements were not any worse in the depot versus oral groups.

Finally on the subject of relapse it is worth highlighting the study by Hogarty et al. (1979), which is a rare example of a study that considered the outcome of relapse over 24 months. The design was complex and examined the interaction between psychosocial input, depot and oral fluphenazine. However, when a contrast is made simply between the two formulations it is clear that at the 12-month point there is little to distinguish the two while at the 24-month point there is an advantage in terms of patients remaining in the community in the depot fluphenazine group. This study more than any other makes the case that if one is to see a true benefit of long-acting injections, the study has to be of a duration sufficient to capture relapsed rates over a realistic time frame.

Attitudes

In terms of acceptance of long-acting injections, work in the United Kingdom by Patel et al. (2003a, b) has shown that experienced psychiatrists in general claim to be very positive towards depot antipsychotics, that they see them as solving problems of non-compliance and deny that they need necessarily be stigmatising. A coercive element to depot administration is however noted. It is also shown that psychiatric nurses hold similar views and attitudes to physicians (Patel et al., 2005) that are, if anything, more positive about their effectiveness in certain patient groups although somewhat more alert to the side effects of injections. In Germany, depot rates are approximately 20%, and in one study (Heres et al., 2006), only 36% of patients with schizophrenia or schizoaffective disorder treated by psychiatrists had ever been offered a depot. The authors also found that for 80% of the psychiatrists, presumed sufficient compliance with oral antipsychotics was an important factor in resisting depot prescription. It seems therefore that depots are not favourably perceived by significant numbers of psychiatrists.

In terms of patient acceptance a number of studies have shown that if patients on depot medication are asked whether they favour this form of treatment they tend to answer in the affirmative. Walburn et al. (2001) conducted a systematic review of satisfaction with depot antipsychotic medication. In total, 12 main studies were considered: in 10, a positive opinion towards depot antipsychotics was expressed, in 1 a neutral opinion and in 1 a negative opinion. Five out of six studies that compared depots with oral antipsychotics showed patient preference for depots, although again, patients tended to state a preference for the formulation that they were taking at the time. This is clearly a finding subject to bias. More recently, Heres et al. (2007) sampled in-patients shortly before discharge from hospital. Acceptance of depots was highest for those currently on depot (73%), less for those with previous depot experience (45%) and least for those who were depot naïve (23%) ($p<0.001$).

Thus if all patients, including those who have been exposed to depots but have subsequently stayed on oral medication, are included in the surveys their attitudes to the prospect of depots is strikingly negative (Patel et al., 2009). This is important research for two reasons. First, it tells us that once the 'barrier' to accepting a depot has been overcome in the minds of the patient, they can appreciate the benefits of this form of treatment in terms of its convenience and effectiveness. However, leaping over that barrier is a formidable test. Patel et al. (2008) have explored the possible reasons behind this and the one that seems to emerge most powerfully was experience of coercion. Even patients who are being treated voluntarily with long-acting injections tend to perceive the treatment as coercive and entailing less choice in comparison to patients similar in their social and demographic profile who are treated with oral medication (Patel et al., 2007). Enabling the use of long-acting injectable antipsychotics while avoiding the taint of coercion is a challenge for mental health-care professionals. That said, it is also noteworthy that in the study by Heres et al. (2007), approximately a quarter of depot-naïve patients think a depot is an acceptable formulation for treatment.

Forensic Psychiatry

There is incontrovertible evidence that violent offending is an adverse outcome associated with serious mental illness, including schizophrenia (Arseneault et al., 2000; Hodgins 1992; Swanson et al., 2006; Walsh et al., 2002; Schanda et al., 2004). Although the most serious violence (homicide) is still rare, it has tragic consequences for both patients and victims. Less serious, but often more frequent, violent acts also have significant clinical and social consequences. The relationship between violent offending and active psychotic symptoms is more ambiguous (Appelbaum et al., 2000; Arseneault et al., 2000; Swanson et al., 2006). Yet there is a growing body of evidence indicating that positive symptoms, particularly certain types of delusional beliefs, are linked to violent offending in some patients (Hodgins et al., 2003; Link et al., 1998; Swanson et al., 2006; Teasdale et al., 2006; Junginger et al., 1998). Also relevant is the emerging evidence linking poor insight to increased risk of violence although it is unclear whether this is independent of severity of positive symptoms (Arango et al., 1999; Buckley et al., 2004).

Research in this area has therefore turned naturally to consider the impact of antipsychotic treatment on violence reduction. Early studies conducted in in-patients demonstrated an anti-aggressive effect of both first- and second-generation drugs that was reported to be independent of sedation or general antipsychotic effects (Volavka 1999; Buckley et al., 1995, 1997; Steinert et al., 2000). A number of recent community-based studies have focused on the anti-aggressive effect of second-generation relative to first-generation antipsychotics, the rationale being that the former should be more efficacious due to improved medication adherence as a result of reduction in side effects. This approach made use of the increasingly apparent link between non-adherence and violence (Swartz et al., 1998a, b). The first such report was a naturalistic study of patients with schizophrenia in the community, which demonstrated a significant reduction in risk of violent behaviour associated with second-, but not first-, generation antipsychotics (Swanson et al., 2006).

This was supported by another large naturalistic study demonstrating that depot perphenazine performed similarly to olanzapine and clozapine in reducing discontinuation of medication and rehospitalisation, relative to haloperidol (Tiihonen et al., 2006). Yet in contrast, two large recent double-blind studies (CATIE and CUtLASS) have failed to demonstrate any difference between first- and second-generation antipsychotic medications on a number of outcome measures including adherence, although neither of these reports examined violence as a primary outcome measure (Lieberman et al., 2005; Jones et al., 2006). Further analysis of the former study, including violent behaviour as a treatment outcome, also found no difference between medication groups. Although notably, medication adherence emerged as a significant factor associated with reduced violence in patients without a history of personality disorder (Swanson et al., 2008). This suggests that enhancing medication adherence in certain patients with schizophrenia may be critical to the reduction of violence risk.

The evidence supporting the use of second-generation antipsychotics to enhance adherence remains weak. An alternative approach is the use of depot preparations in preference to oral, irrespective of class of drug. To date there has only been one longitudinal randomised, controlled trial specifically examining the effect of oral versus depot medication on violence. This relatively small study compared oral and depot preparations of a single first-generation antipsychotic (zuclopenthixol) over a 1-year period. The authors found a lower frequency of violent acts in the depot group and again demonstrated that treatment non-adherence was the best predictor of violence (Arango et al., 2006). This may be of particular relevance in jurisdictions where such treatment can be enforced in the community (Swartz et al., 2001). However, the evidence to support this remains limited.

Future Prospects

Since the review by Adams et al. there are now two licensed long-acting injectable second-generation or atypical antipsychotics. The first was risperidone long-acting injection and began to be used in the early years of the new millennium. The long-acting injection is based on microsphere technology rather than the traditional depot. This puts certain constraints on its use, most notably the lack of clinical effects before at least 2–3 cycles of 2 weekly injections have been completed. This formulation again was able to show obvious superiority in comparison to placebo in short-term trials (Kane et al., 2003) and several long-term non-randomised studies have supported its effectiveness (e.g. Fleischhaker et al., 2003; review by Hosalli and Davis, 2003). A relatively short-term trial of the oral versus the long-acting injectable forms by Chue and colleagues (2005) was aimed at showing equivalence or at least non-superiority of the oral agent, and this study was successful. Both groups tended to improve over the course of the 12-week trial but there was no real difference between the oral and long-acting injectable form. This somewhat echoes experience in traditional depot randomised controlled trials as noted earlier. Most recent of all is the introduction of olanzapine pamoate, which again is a novel twist on the long-acting injectable technology field. The compound becomes soluble when in contact with blood and it is available in up to 4 weekly injectable forms. An initial placebo-controlled study showed its clear effectiveness (Lauriello et al., 2008) and longer term comparative trials are awaited with interest.

Demonstration of Effect

Depots

So why is it so difficult to demonstrate the presumed benefits of long-acting injections given that the problem of non-adherence with medication as noted by early practitioners in the field who championed depots remains as deeply problematic as it always was? A clue comes from work by Ioannidis et al. (2001).

This author contrasted controlled trials and observational studies across many branches of medicine and found that their results generally correlated extremely highly, suggesting that in some ways the additional effort needed to carry out a randomised control trial was an unnecessary waste. However, when one looks more deeply, what this work showed was that there are particular instances where the controlled trial tends to strongly favour the experimental treatment and other instances where the observational study strongly favours the experimental treatment. This leads one to consider what factors might influence the ability of a randomised controlled trial to show a theoretically true benefit of an experimental treatment.

For example, consider a population of patients recruited to a randomised controlled clinical trial, particularly one that was commercially sponsored and aimed at licensing a new agent. It is likely that the trial will be rather onerous in terms of numbers of assessments and would entail safety as well as efficacy measures including biological samples. It is also likely that inclusion criteria would aim to enrol restricted, relatively pure diagnostic groups. Exclusions would be patients with comorbidities and possibly those with various forms of treatment resistance and certainly those likely to be non-adherent to treatment regimes. Contrast this with a slightly idealised view of population and observational or pragmatic study. In these, patients may be somewhat less adherent, may have a range of diagnoses in the schizophrenia spectrum in this case and may show higher rates of psychopathology in general as well as comorbid psychopathology. Considering these two groups it is quite possible that one or the other might respond well to a particular treatment. A treatment that had general 'broad-spectrum' therapeutic effects would likely produce significant benefits in the less-selected group.

However, if there was a treatment that was highly specific for schizophrenia (if such a treatment ever were to be discovered) then by definition its benefits would only appear, or would appear more strongly, in the highly selected group. However, considering any treatment aimed at counteracting non-adherence such as a long-acting formulation or a psychosocial intervention, it becomes obvious that a group selected in part because of superior adherence and compliance, such as that needed to consent for a randomised controlled trial, will always show relatively little benefit from the compliance-enhancing intervention. This might be one of the few examples where the randomised controlled trial is not the ideal method of choice for demonstrating the true benefit of an experimental treatment.

Finally, quantifying adherence to depot treatments in observational or experimental studies is not trivial. In fact we know of three studies that have investigated adherence in patients who have remained on depots for 12 months. Heysue et al. (1998) reported an overall 'adherence proportion' of 0.96 (whereby the adherence proportion is the ratio of kept appointments to scheduled appointments for depot administration). In a later study, 26% were reported to have poor adherence, based on the duration of missed injections (Tattan and Creed, 2001). Most recently, Shi et al. (2007) calculated the mean medication possession ratio (cumulative number of days covered by depot divided by 365 days) to be 91% for patients on typical depots.

Psychosocial Interventions

Reviewing such adherence-related interventions in schizophrenia, Zygmunt and colleagues (2002) showed that only one-third reported significant treatment effects, but that interventions based on the principles of motivational interviewing were 'promising' as exemplified by the Maudsley study by Kemp et al. (1996, 1998). A later subsequent meta-analysis concluded that clinical interventions for reducing patient non-adherence can be effective but the benefit is more evident in the short term (Nose et al., 2003). However, an attempt to replicate the Kemp et al. study (O'Donnell et al., 2003) found no clear advantage at 1 year in a relatively small sample. This prompted a large European-wide study that recruited over 400 community patients with a research diagnosis of schizophrenia with evidence of clinical instability in the previous year. Patients were randomised to receive eight sessions of adherence therapy or health education. Adherence therapy turned out to be no more effective than health education in improving antipsychotic medication adherence, psychiatric symptoms or quality of life (all of which tended to improve over the 1-year follow-up; Gray et al., 2006). One possible explanation for this inconsistency is that the sample in the Kemp et al. study, based on acute in-patients with psychosis, was less selected and hence as a group had more 'room for improvement' in terms of adherence in response to a simple but structured intervention.

Conclusions

In summary, long-acting injections were developed with the explicit aim of countering non-adherence in patients with schizophrenia and related disorders. They appeared to emerge once the technology was available rather than following motivated development and this may in part have prevented a more rational and programmatic search for their true potential benefit. In so far as non-compliance is covert, long-acting injections do offer a solution as it is immediately obvious to the clinician when the patient has not been given their injection. However, we do not of course solve the problem of stated and overt treatment refusal as not all patients are willing to accept a depot (Glazer and Kane, 1992; Barnes and Curson, 1994; Gerlach, 1995). In such cases, the clinical team can respond appropriately to reduce the risk of relapse by actively trying to re-engage the patient (Weiden and Glazer, 1997). This clearly requires other kinds of intervention such as psychologically orientated compliance therapies or, when all else fails, legal controls. This in itself probably contributes to the inherently coercive perception patients seem to have of long-acting injections.

If a patient discontinues depot treatment their risk of relapse increases, but if a patient relapses despite regular depot injections then non-adherence can be safely excluded as the cause (Barnes and Curson, 1994). Depot antipsychotics are unable to prevent relapse completely; even in clinical trials there is an irreducible 20–25% of patients who relapse, despite receiving depots (Adams et al., 2001).

Newer agents, regardless of any real or claimed superiority in terms of efficacy and side effect profile, will have to overcome these same barriers that have afflicted all depot treatments from their inception. Given the clear relationship between treatment discontinuation and relapse in schizophrenia (Robinson et al., 1999; Valenstein et al., 2002), efforts to ensure consistent maintenance treatment are fully justified.

References

Adams, C.E., Fenton, M.K.P., Quraishi, S., & David, A.S. (2001) Systemic meta-review of depot antipsychotic drugs for people with schizophrenia. British Journal of Psychiatry 179: 290–299

Appelbaum, P.S., Robbins, P.C., & Monahan, J. (2000). Violence and delusions: data from the MacArthur violence risk assessment study. American Journal of Psychiatry 157: 566–572

Arango, C., Barba, A.C., Gonzalez-Salvador, T., & Ordonez, A.C. (1999). Violence in inpatients with schizophrenia: a prospective study. Schizophrenia Bulletin 25: 493–503

Arango, C., Bombin, I., Gonzalez-Salvador, T., Garcia-Cabeza, I., & Bobes, J. (2006). Randomised clinical trial comparing oral versus depot formulations of zuclopenthixol in patients with schizophrenia and previous violence. European Psychiatry 21: 34–40

Arseneault, L., Moffitt, T.E., Caspi, A., Taylor, P.J., & Silva, P.A. (2000). Mental disorders and violence in a total birth cohort: results from the Dunedin study. Archives of General Psychiatry 57: 979–986

Barnes, T.R. & Curson, D.A. (1994). Long-term depot antipsychotics: a risk-benefit assessment. Drug Safety 10: 464–479

Buckley, P.F., Bartell, J., Donenwirth, K., Lee, S., Torigoe, F., & Schulz, S. (1995). Violence and schizophrenia: clozapine as a specific anti-aggressive agent. Bulletin of the American Academy of Psychiatry and the Law 23: 607–611

Buckley, P.F., Hrouda, D.R., Friedman, L., Noffsinger, S.G., Resnick, P.J., & Camlin-Shingler, K. (2004). Insight and its relationship to violent behavior in patients with schizophrenia. American Journal of Psychiatry 161: 1712–1714

Buckley, P.F., Ibrahim, Z.Y., Singer, B., Orr, B., Donenwirth, K., & Brar, P.S. (1997). Aggression and schizophrenia: efficacy of risperidone. Journal of the American Academy of Psychiatry and Law 25: 173–181

Chue, P., Eerdekens, M., Augustyns, I., Lachaux, B., Molcan, P., Eriksson, L., Pretorius, H., & David, A.S. (2005). Comparative efficacy and safety of long-acting risperidone and risperidone oral tablets. European Neuropsychopharmacology 15: 111–117

Davis, J.M., Matalon, L., Watanabe, M.D., & Blake, L. (1994). Depot antipsychotic drugs. Place in therapy. Drugs 47: 741–773

Dencker, S.J. & Axelsson, R. (1996). Optimising the use of depot antipsychotics. CNS Drugs 6: 367–381

Fleischhacker, W.W., Eerdekens, M., Karcher, K., Remington, G., Llorca, P.-M., Chrzanowski, W., Martin, S., & Gefert, O. (2003). Treatment of schizophrenia with long-acting injectable risperidone: a 12-month open-label trial of the first long-acting second-generation antipsychotic. Journal of Clinical Psychiatry 64: 1250–1257

Gerlach, J. (1995). Depot neuroleptics in relapse prevention: advantages and disadvantages. International Clinical Psychopharmacology 9(Suppl. 5): 17–20

Glazer, W.M. & Kane, J.M. (1992). Depot neuroleptic therapy: an underutilized treatment option. Journal of Clinical Psychiatry 53: 426–433

Gray, R., Leese, M., Bindman, J., Becker, T., Burti, L., David, A., Gournay, K., Kikkert, M., Koeter, M., Puscher, B., Schene, A., Thornicroft, G., & Tansella, M. (2006). Adherence therapy for people with schizophrenia: European multicentre randomised controlled trial. British Journal of Psychiatry 189: 508–514

Haider, I. (1968). A controlled trial of fluphenazine enanthate in hospitalized chronic schizophrenics. British Journal of Psychiatry 114: 837–841

Healy, D. (2000). The birth of psychopharmacotherapy: explorations' in a new world 1952–1968. In: The Psychopharmacologists III. Interviews by Dr David Healy. Arnold, London, pp. 1–53

Heres, S., Hamann, J., Kissling, W., & Leucht, S. (2006). Attitudes of psychiatrists toward antipsychotic depot medication. Journal of Clinical Psychiatry 67: 1948–1953

Heres, S., Schmitz, F.S., Leucht, S., & Pajonk, F.G. (2007). The attitude of patients towards antipsychotic depot treatment. International Clinical Psychopharmacology 22: 275–282

Heysue, B.E., Levin, G.M., & Merrick, J.P. (1998). Compliance with depot antipsychotic medication by patients attending outpatient clinics. Psychiatric Services 49: 1232–1234

Hicks, R. & Ovenstone, I.M.K. (1996). Fluphenazine enanthate in the maintenance treatment of schizophrenia. British Medical Journal 29th Oct, 1071

Hirsch, S.R., Gaind, R., Rohde, P.D., Stevens, B.C., & Wing, J. (1973). Outpatient maintenance of chronic schizophrenic patients with long-acting fluphenazine: double-blind placebo controlled trial. British Medical Journal i: 633 –637

Hodgins, S. (1992). Mental disorder, intellectual deficiency and crime: evidence from a Danish birth cohort. Archives of General Psychiatry 49: 476–483

Hodgins, S., Hiscoke, U., & Freese, R., (2003). The antecedents of aggressive behavior among men with schizophrenia: a prospective investigation of patients in community treatment. Behavioral Sciences and the Law 21: 523

Hogarty, G.E, Schooler, N.R, Ulrich, R., Mussare, I., Ferro, P., & Herron, E. (1979). Fluphenazine and social therapy in the aftercare of schizophrenic patients. Archives of General Psychiatry 36: 1283–1294

Hosalli, P. & Davis, J.M. (2003). Depot risperidone for schizophrenia. Cochrane Database of Systematic Reviews, Issue 4. Art. No.: CD004161. DOI: 10.1002/14651858.CD004161

Ioannidis J.P.A., Haidich, A.B., & Lau, J. (2001). Any casualties in the clash of randomised and observational evidence? British Medical Journal 322: 879–880

Jones, P.B., Barnes, T.R.E., Davies, L., Dunn, G., Lloyd, H., Hayhurst, K.P., Murray, R.M., Markwick, A., & Lewis, S.W. (2006). Randomized controlled trial of the effect on quality of life of second- vs. first-generation antipsychotic drugs in schizophrenia: Cost Utility of the Latest Antipsychotic Drugs in Schizophrenia Study (CUtLASS 1). Archives of General Psychiatry 63: 1079–1087

Junginger, J., Parks-Levy, J., & Mcguire, L. (1998). Delusions and Symptom-Consistent Violence. Psychiatric Services 49: 218–220

Kane, J.M., Aguglia, E., Altamura, A.C., Ayuso Gutierrez, J.L., Brunello, N., Fleischhacker, W.W., Gaebel, W., Gerlach, J., Guelfi, J.D., Kissling, W., Lapierre, Y.D., Lindstrom, E., Mendlewicz, J., Racagni, G., Carulla, L.S., & Schooler, N.R. (1998). Guidelines for depot antipsychotic treatment in schizophrenia. European Neuropsychopharmacology 8: 55–66

Kane, J.M., Eerdekens, M., Lindenmayer, J.P., Keith, S.J., Lesem, M., & Karcher, K. (2003). Long-acting injectable risperidone: efficacy and safety of the first long-acting atypical antipsychotic. American Journal of Psychiatry 160: 1125–1132

Kinross-Wright, J., Vogt, A.H., & Charalampous, K.D. (2003). A new method of drug therapy. American Journal of Psychiatry 119: 779–780

Kemp, R., Hayward, P., Applewhaite, G., Everitt, B., & David, A. (1996). Compliance therapy in psychotic patients: randomised controlled trial. British Medical Journal 312: 345–349

Kemp, R., Kirov, G., Everitt, B., Hayward, P., & David, A. (1998). Randomised controlled trial of compliance therapy. 18-month follow-up. British Journal of Psychiatry 172: 413–419

Kissling, W. (1994). Compliance, quality assurance and standards for relapse prevention in schizophrenia. Acta Psychiatrica Scandinavica Supplement 382: 16–24

Kissling, W. (1997). Compliance, quality management and standards in the treatment of schizophrenia. Neuropsychobiology 35: 70–72

Lauriello, J., Lambert, T., Andersen, S., Lin, D., Taylor, C.C., & Mcdonnell, D. (2008). An 8-week, double-blind, randomized, placebo-controlled study of olanzapine long-acting injection in acutely ill patients with schizophrenia. Journal of Clinical Psychiatry 69: 790–799

Leff, J.P. & Wing, J.K. (1971). Trial of maintenance therapy in schizophrenia. British Medical Journal 11: 599–604

Lieberman, J.A., Stroup, T.S., Mcevoy, J.P., Swartz, M.S., Rosenheck, R.A., Perkins, D.O., Keefe, R.S.E., Davis, S.M., Davis, C.E., Lebowitz,B.D., Severe, J., & Hsiao, J.K. (2005). And the Clinical Antipsychotic Trials of Intervention Effectiveness (CATIE) Investigators, Effectiveness of antipsychotic drugs in patients with chronic schizophrenia. New England Journal of Medicine 353: 1209–1223

Link, B.G., Stueve, A., & Phelan, J. (1998). Psychotic symptoms and violent behavior: probing the components of "threat/control-override" symptoms. Social Psychiatry and Epidemiology 33: 55–60

Nose, M., Barbui, C., Gray, R., & Tansella, M. (2003). Clinical interventions for treatment non-adherence in psychosis: meta-analysis. British Journal of Psychiatry 183: 197–206

O'Donnell, C., Donohoe, G., & Sharkey, L. et al. (2003). Compliance therapy: a randomised controlled trial in schizophrenia. British Medical Journal 327: 834–838

Patel, M.X., Dezoysa, N., Bernadt, M., Bindman, J., & David, A.S. (2007). Voluntary out-patients and coercion: depot versus oral antipsychotics. Schizophrenia Bulletin 33: 452

Patel, M.X., & David, A.S. (2005). David AS. Why aren't depot antipsychotics prescribed more often and what can be done about it? Advances in Psychiatric Treatment 11: 203–211

Patel, M.X., Dezoysa, N., Baker, D., & David, A.S. (2005). Depot antipsychotic medication and attitudes of community psychiatric nurses. Journal of Psychiatric and Mental Health Nursing 12: 237–244

Patel, M.X., Dezoysa, N., Bernadt, M., & David, A.S. (2008). Patients' perspectives on adherence to antipsychotic medication: depots versus tablets. Journal of Clinical Psychiatry 69: 1548–1556

Patel, M.X., Dezoysa, N., Bernadt, M., & David, A.S. (2009) Depot and oral antipsychotics: patient preferences and attitudes are not the same thing. Journal of Psychopharmacology 23(7), 789–796. (published online ahead of print 26 June 2008, doi: 10.1177/0269881108092124)

Patel, M.X., Nikolaou, V., & David, A.S. (2003a). Psychiatrists' attitudes to maintenance medication for patients with schizophrenia. Psychological Medicine 33: 83–89

Patel, M.X., Nikolaou, V., & David, A.S. (2003b). Eliciting psychiatrists' beliefs about side effects of typical and atypical antipsychotic drugs. International Journal of Psychiatry in Clinical Practice 7: 117–120

Robinson, D., Woerner, M.G., Alvir, J.M. et al. (1999). Predictors of relapse following response from a first episode of schizophrenia or schizoaffective disorder. Archives of General Psychiatry 56: 241–7

Schanda, H., Knecht, G., Schreinzer, D., Stompe, T., Ortwein-Swoboda, G., & Waldhoer, T. (2004). Homicide and major mental disorders: a 25-year study. Acta Psychiatrica Scandinavica 110: 98–107

Shi, L., Ascher-Svanum, H., Zhu, B., Faries, D., Montgomery, W., & Marder, S.R. (2007). Characteristics and use patterns of patients taking first-generation depot antipsychotics or oral antipsychotics for schizophrenia. Psychiatric Services 58: 482–488

Simpson, G.M. (1974). A brief history of depot neuroleptics. Journal of Clinical Psychiatry 45: 3–4

Steinert, T., Sippach, T., & Gebhardt, R. (2000). How common is violence in schizophrenia despite neuroleptic treatment? Pharmacopsychiatry 33: 98–102

Swanson, J.W., Swartz, M.S., Van Dorn, R.A., Elbogen, E.B., Wagner, H.R., Rosenheck, R.A., Stroup, T.S., Mcevoy, J.P., & Lieberman, J.A. (2006). A national study of violent behavior in persons with schizophrenia. Archives of General Psychiatry 63: 490–499

Swanson, J.W., Swartz, M.S., Van Dorn, R.A., Volavka, J., Monahan, J., Stroup, T.S., Mcevoy, J.P., Wagner, H.R., Elbogen, E.B., & Lieberman, J.A. (2008). Comparison of antipsychotic medication effects on reducing violence in people with schizophrenia. British Journal of Psychiatry 193: 37–43

Swartz, M.S., Swanson, J.W., Hiday, V.A., Borum, R., Wagner, H.R., & Burns, B.J., (1998a). Taking the wrong drugs: the role of substance abuse and medication noncompliance in violence among severely mentally ill individuals. Social Psychiatry and Epidemiology 33: S75–S80

Swartz, M.S., Swanson, J.W., Hiday, V.A., Borum, R., Wagner, H.R., & Burns, B.J., (1998b).Violence and severe mental illness: the effects of substance abuse and nonadherence to medication. American Journal Psychiatry 155: 226–231

Swartz, M.S., Swanson, J.W., Wagner, H.R., Burns, B.J., & Hiday, V.A., (2001). Effects of involuntary outpatient commitment and depot antipsychotics on treatment adherence in persons with severe mental illness. Journal of Nervous and Mental Disease 189: 592

Tattan, T.M.G. & Creed, F.H. (2001). Negative symptoms of schizophrenia and compliance with medication. Schizophrenia Bulletin 27: 149–155

Taylor, D., Mir, S., Mace, S., & Hogman, G. (1999). Is Cost a Factor – II? A Survey of Psychiatrists and Health Authorities to Determine the Factors Influencing the Prescribing and Funding of Atypical Antipsychotics. London: National Schizophrenia Fellowship

Teasdale, B., Silver, E., & Monahan, J. (2006). Gender, threat/control-override delusions and violence. Law and Human Behavior 30: 649–658

Tiihonen, J., Walhbeck, K., Lonnqvist, J., Klaukka, T., Ioannidis, J.P.A., Volavka, J., & Haukka, J. (2006). Effectiveness of antipsychotic treatments in a nationwide cohort of patients in community care after first hospitalisation due to schizophrenia and schizoaffective disorder: observational follow-up study. British Medical Journal 333: 224

Valenstein, M., Copeland, L.A., Blow F.C., Mccarthy J.F., Zeber, J.E., Gillon, L., Bingham, C.R., & Stavanger, T. (2002). Pharmacy data identify poorly adherent patients with schizophrenia at increased risk for admission. Medical Care 40:630–639

Volavka, J. (1999). The effects of clozapine on aggression and substance abuse in schizophrenic patients. Journal of Clinical Psychiatry 60: 43–46

Walburn, J., Gray, R., Gournay, K., Quraishi, S., & David, A.S. (2001). A systematic review of patient and nurse attitudes to depot antipsychotic medication. British Journal of Psychiatry 179: 300–307

Walsh, E., Buchanan, A., & Fahy, T., (2002). Violence and schizophrenia: examining the evidence. British Journal of Psychiatry 180: 490–495

Weiden, P. & Glazer, W. (1997). Assessment and treatment selection for 'revolving door' inpatients with schizophrenia. The Psychiatric Quarterly 68: 377–392

Zygmunt, A., Olfson, M., Boyer, C.A., & Mechanic, D. (2002). Interventions to improve medication adherence in schizophrenia. American Journal of Psychiatry 159: 1653–1664

Modern Community Care Strategies for Schizophrenia Care: Impacts on Outcome

Tom Burns

Schizophrenia has been at the centre of psychiatry's development. The severity of schizophrenia's disabilities, in both its acute and more long-term phases, ensures its dominance in service planning. Self-neglect, apathy and disability derived from negative symptoms and cognitive dysfunction require social care and support as a central part of services. For practical purposes this means that the history and configuration of psychiatric services are broadly equivalent to the history and configuration of schizophrenia services.

It has recently been suggested that the dominance of the current comprehensive, integrated psychosocial approach has been to the detriment of the profession's image and potential (Goodwin et al. 2007). Goodwin and Geddes believe that the influence of schizophrenia has distracted psychiatry from a pragmatic and flexible medical model that accommodates better the full range of disorders we face. This perspective finds echo in some European systems such as traditional 'social psychiatry' in Germany where long-term psychosis community care was culturally separated from the medically dominated hospital settings and was often led by social workers.

It is customary to attribute the reduction in the mental hospital population to the introduction of chlorpromazine in the mid-1950s (Brill et al. 1962), but it is clear that far-reaching changes were afoot in psychiatry from the end of World War II. Some changes stemmed from greater attention to the course of schizophrenia and an increased understanding of the influences on the observed disabilities. The open-door movement gathered momentum in the late 1940s – Dingleton Hospital in Scotland started the process in 1945 and unlocked its last ward in 1948 (Ratcliffe 1962) until its final closure in 2004. It was soon followed by Mapperly Hospital in Nottingham and Warlingham Park Hospital in Croydon. Rehabilitation gained enormous impetus from Russell Barton's concept of 'institutional neurosis' to describe the

T. Burns (✉)
University of Oxford, Warneford Hospital, Oxford, OX3 7JX, UK
e-mail: tom.burns@psych.ox.ac.uk

W.F. Gattaz, G. Busatto (eds.), *Advances in Schizophrenia Research 2009*,
DOI 10.1007/978-1-4419-0913-8_24, © Springer Science+Business Media, LLC 2010

apathy and self-neglect of so many chronic schizophrenia patients (Barton 1959), supported by the Three Hospitals study demonstrating the impact of the social environment on schizophrenia outcomes (Wing and Brown 1970).

The running down and closure of mental hospitals has varied between different countries and cultures and is well documented (Leff et al. 2000). While essentially ubiquitous in developed countries there are some notable exceptions such as Belgium and Japan. In the United States, deinstitutionalisation and community services vary widely from state to state because state per capita costs for serious mental illness vary by 10-fold.

The main response to deinstitutionalisation has been the development of community services, but the picture is not straightforward. As mental hospitals have shrunk and closed, so the number of schizophrenia patients in prisons has risen (Draine et al. 2002; Fisher et al. 2006) together with an enormous growth in forensic facilities for mentally disordered offenders (Priebe et al. 2005).

Development of the Community Mental Health Team (CMHT)

The closure of mental hospitals soon demonstrated the need for effective care to be multi-faceted and to address both medical and social needs. It became rapidly apparent that no one individual or profession could adequately care for patients with schizophrenia and multidisciplinary team working soon evolved. Outpatient clinics took on new and expanded roles (e.g. depot clinics, day care, psychotherapy) and these were housed in Community Mental Health Centres (CMHCs). The earliest and most ambitious development of CMHCs was in the United States, introduced by President Kennedy (U.S. Congress 1963). These ran into early problems both with staffing and, more significantly, with a drift away from the care of individuals with severe mental illness, and schizophrenia particularly. A rejection of a medical role in the services made it impossible to recruit psychiatrists and consequently to treat psychotic patients.

Office-based care is increasingly rare for schizophrenia patients although not as rare as the research literature would suggest. It tends to be narrow in remit (usually either psychotherapy or pharmacotherapy) and is poorly equipped for managing such severe disorders. Similarly a focus on CMHTs should not blind us to the need for in-patient beds (which will not be dealt with here). It is fruitless to attempt to define the level of need for in-patient care as this is almost entirely driven by the extent of alternative services. Both acute and some long-term beds are an essential feature of all well-functioning services as is the need for a range of supported accommodation. The terminology for differing types of accommodation is confusing, but generally spans four basic forms:

1. *Group homes*: no regular staff, relatively independent patients, visits from community team staff.
2. *Day-staffed hostels*: one or two staff during the day, support and monitor patients (encouraging cooking and cleaning, etc.), usually no specific treatment but liaison with community team staff.
3. *Night-staffed hostels*: non-clinical staff sleep over, greater safety and availability.
4. *24-h-staffed/nursed hostels*: on-site clinical staff available overnight (sleeping in, sometimes, awake). These expensive hostels generally restricted to long-term severe illnesses (including compulsorily detained). Tend to be larger (10–20 residents as opposed to 4–8 in day-staffed hostels).

Case Management and CMHTs

Case management (Intagliata 1982) developed in the United States, initially as a non-clinician responsible for coordination of care ('brokerage case management'). This was rapidly superseded by 'clinical case management' where the case manager is a mental health clinician who both provides and coordinates care for the patient. The literature on case management is extensive. Several early studies compared 'stand-alone' case managers against multidisciplinary teams and found them wanting (e.g. the *Cochrane Reviews* contrasting ACT and case management (Marshall and Lockwood 1998; Marshall et al. 1997). Rapp and Goscha's (2004) review found a hierarchy of case management effectiveness in the United States.

Community Mental Health Teams (CMHTs)

Most case managers find themselves working in CMHTs (Burns 2004). The staffing of these teams vary, generally consisting of psychiatrists, nurses, social workers and often psychologists and occupational therapists. They hold regular meetings to assess and review individual patient care benefiting from their varied professional perspectives and tasks are distributed according to skills and needs. The basic CMHT originated in France and the United Kingdom, was refined in Italy and further developed in North America and Australia.

The generic or sector CMHT originated as mental hospital catchment areas were subdivided from whole cities into sectors of 50–100,000 inhabitants. Small sectors reduced travelling time and made it possible for all team members to know most of their complex and long-term patients. They could also establish personal relationships with local referrers and community resources. Sector size in Western Europe ranges from 20 to 100,000 population and varies according to resources (shrinking as investment increases) and parallel provision. As more specialised teams are established, the CMHT's remit may shrink and the sector size may increase, keeping its caseload the same. The clinical practice of these teams generally consists of assessment of new patients, providing their treatment, monitoring their progress, liaison with other important agents (social services, housing and rehabilitation) and varying degrees of social care (Burns 2004).

Specialised Teams for Schizophrenia Care

Generic CMHTs have functioned well for the care of schizophrenia patients in health-care systems where they have developed. In many respects this is because they have been formed around the needs of these patients (Goodwin et al. 2007). However, in high-income countries there has been a growth of specialised teams with segmentation of aspects of the care. There are numerous models of innovative teams and culturally specific teams but the main models that have gained ground are Assertive Community Treatment Teams, Rehabilitation Teams and Early Intervention Teams.

Assertive Community Treatment (ACT) Team

The ACT team is the most replicated and researched of any model of community care (Mueser et al. 1998). Stein and Test's original study showed improved clinical and social outcomes with substantially reduced hospitalisation at slightly lower cost (Test and Stein 1980; Weisbrod et al. 1980). Reduced hospital care is the common factor in all of these outcomes and meta-analyses of ACT and of case management (Marshall and Lockwood 1998; Marshall et al.2001) confirmed this hospital reduction (see Fig. 1).

This confirmation leads to their wholesale adoption throughout much of the Anglophone psychiatric community where they are central components of government policy in several countries (Department of Health 1999; US Department of Health and Human Services 1999). These bed reductions have, however, never been replicated in Europe (Burns et al. 1999; Thornicroft et al. 1998) and there is now convincing evidence that ACT has little to offer over well-functioning CMHTs in this respect (Wright et al. 2004; Burns et al. 2007). Combined health and social

Study	Treatment	Control	Peto Odds Ratio 95% CI	Weight %	Peto Odds Ratio 95% CI
Audini-London	9 / 33	9 / 33		6.5	1.00 [0.34, 2.93]
Bond-Chicago1	32 / 45	34 / 43		8.2	0.66 [0.25, 1.72]
Bond-Indiana1	12 / 50	33 / 53		12.6	0.21 [0.10, 0.47]
Chandler-California	49 / 252	57 / 264		41.5	0.88 [0.57, 1.34]
Lehman-Baltimore	42 / 77	46 / 75		18.4	0.80 [0.42, 1.52]
Test-Wisconsin	15 / 75	26 / 47		12.8	0.21 [0.10, 0.45]
Total (95% CI)	159 / 532	204 / 515		100.0	0.59 [0.45, 0.78]

Review: Assertive community treatment for people with severe mental disorders
Comparison: 01 ACT vs STANDARD CARE
Outcome: 03 Admitted to hospital during study

Test for heterogeneity chi-square= 18.78 df=5 p=0.0021
Test for overall effect Z=-3.74 p=0.00

0.1 0.2   1   5   10

Fig. 1 Cochrane meta-analysis of ACT vs. standard care against admissions

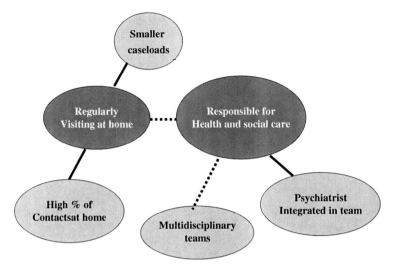

Fig. 2 Associations between service components and hospitalisation: regression analysis (Wright et al. 2004)

care and home visiting (Fig. 2) appear to be the core components of successful schizophrenia care and the bed reductions claimed for ACT appear to be essentially dependent on high local usage (with little gained over routine CMHT practice when beds are otherwise well controlled). High staffing levels with careful prescription of team structure seem to bring no clear benefit (Fig. 3).

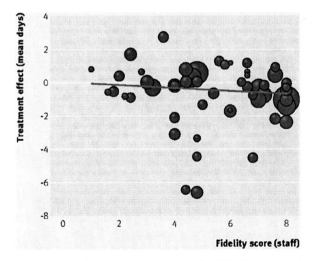

Fig. 3 Metaregression of intensive case management studies: IFACT team membership subscore vs. mean days per month in hospital. Negative treatment effect indicates reduction relative to control (Burns et al. 2007)

However, ACT does benefit from the precision of its description and the clarity of its focus (Boxes 1 and 2) and continues to be adopted as a model for services to care for schizophrenia patients. It is particularly valuable in helping change the focus of more diffuse services to the care of the severely ill and its 'evidence base' can overcome strong professional resistance.

Box 1 ACT Programme Principles

- Provision of material resources for patients
- Fostering patient coping skills
- Supporting patient motivation to persevere
- Freeing patient from pathological dependency relationships
- Support and education for those involved with the patient

Box 2 ACT Core components

- Assertive follow-up
- Small caseloads (1:10)
- Increased frequency of contact (weekly to daily)
- In vivo practice (care delivered at home or neighbourhood)
- Emphasis on medication
- Emphasis on engagement
- Support for family and carers
- Provision of services within the team whenever possible
- Liaison with other services when necessary
- Crisis stabilisation and availability 24/7

Rehabilitation and Recovery Teams

Rehabilitation teams evolved in response to the need to re-provide in the community comprehensive care, in particular support and social care for patients being discharged from downsizing and closing mental hospitals. However, the current focus is on the rise of a very different group of 'new long-stay' patients (Hirsch 1988). These are predominantly young schizophrenia patients (disproportionately men) who have poor treatment compliance, co-morbid drug and alcohol abuse and often behavioural disturbance. The two defining characteristics of separate rehabilitation services are predominantly their access to more long-term in-patient care for such individuals or a commitment to a defined patient group in long-term supported residential care.

Rehabilitation programmes are, of their nature, varied, but share common features to improve performance in the main adult social roles (Corrigan et al. 2007). Aspects of care that are more highly developed in rehabilitation teams include social skills training to help patients manage their survival (Liberman et al. 1998). Attempts to ameliorate cognitive impairments in schizophrenia have included Brenner's 'integrated psychological therapy' (Brenner et al. 1992) and more recently cognitive remediation (Pilling et al. 2002). However, these highly structured modularised approaches and highly structured social skills training approaches are currently losing influence and being replaced by supported housing, education, employment and socialisation plus self-help and consumer-run programmes in response to user preferences.

Early Intervention Services (EIS) First-Episode Psychosis Teams

Separate teams for first-episode care in schizophrenia are a relatively new development, championed in Australia and the United Kingdom (McGorry and Jackson 1999; Edwards et al. 2000; Birchwood et al. 1997), but now common internationally. EIS services vary considerably. The most basic ensure that all first-episode psychosis patients are treated in a dedicated team that is readily accessible and welcoming (these teams often have an expressly 'youth service' approach). They work hard to protect social and family supports and networks.

A strong case for the establishment of EIS services is that outcome is poorer if the duration of untreated psychosis is prolonged (Marshall et al. 2005). This basic EIS service is closely modelled on ACT (Department of Health 1999; Edwards et al. 2000), but with an explicit time limit (varying from 18 months to 5 years) for involvement before handing on to routine services.

Dual Diagnosis and Vocational Rehabilitation Services

In both the United States and Europe there is an emerging consensus that delivering substance abuse treatments separately from routine mental health care to schizophrenia patients is not successful. Research and service evolution over 20 years confirm that care needs to be integrated and the preferred location is the multidisciplinary CMHT (Drake et al. 2006, 2007, 2008). In such integrated services specified substance abuse workers can be responsible for this care or efforts can be made to skill-up most or all of the case managers.

Therapeutic aims in schizophrenia go beyond simple symptom control and embrace enhancing quality of life and promoting social inclusion (Morgan et al. 2007; Priebe 2007). Returning to work is probably one of the most effective means of radically improving quality of life and social inclusion. There is overwhelming evidence, however, that standardised supported employment, also called Individual Placement and Support (IPS), is more effective in helping patients with severe mental illnesses to achieve competitive employment (Bond et al. 2007, 2008; Burns et al. 2007).

Physical Health Care

Whether the physical health care in schizophrenia belongs in primary care or with mental health services depends on local and national policies. The strikingly increased standardised mortality in schizophrenia (particularly for cardiovascular and respiratory disorders; Kendrick 1996) means a reduced life expectancy of about 20 years. Many factors contribute to this reduced life expectancy – excess smoking, poor diet, inactivity and metabolic side effects of antipsychotic drugs. Almost invariably specialist mental health teams pick up much of this responsibility for the most severely ill patients (Saha et al. 2007).

Community Treatment Orders: Outpatient Commitment

With expanded community care, compulsion and coercion are now a pervasive feature of practice. (This can be either explicitly in the form of legal requirements or informally through professional or social pressure (Monahan et al. 2005).) Most developed common law countries have enacted forms of community treatment order ('mandated community treatment' and 'outpatient committal') (Dawson 2005). These are mainly applied in the care of established schizophrenia with high levels of self-neglect, poor treatment compliance and frequent relapse (Swartz et al. 1999; Gibbs et al. 2005). The introduction of these provisions has often been controversial (Kisely and Campbell 2007) and the evidence base for them is limited (Churchill et al. 2007). However, clinicians use and value them (Dawson 2005; Swartz et al. 2003) and families (Mullen et al. 2006) and, to some extent, patients (Gibbs et al. 2005) appreciate them. However, the only successful RCT was equivocal in its results (Swartz et al. 1999) although that subgroup of patients who received extended CTOs and regular care did appear to benefit (Swartz et al. 1999). Despite continuing concerns about the absence of a definitive RCT, the orders appear to be rapidly accepted by the clinical community as a key component in schizophrenia care although their frequency of use varies widely and inexplicably (Lawton-Smith 2005).

Informal Coercion

Community treatment orders have the advantage of legal scrutiny. Work by the MacArthur Group in the United States demonstrates that about half of all long-term psychiatric patients feel that they have been coerced in some form or other to comply with treatment (Monahan et al. 2005) and pilot work in the United Kingdom indicates very similar rates, although with somewhat different patterns. This is clearly an area of the care of schizophrenia patients that will need sustained scrutiny if sloppy or abusive practice is not to develop in community care as they did in some institutional care.

Conclusions

There is no single service structure that best suits schizophrenia care but there are some convincing basic principles. Care is inevitably multidisciplinary to reflect the complexity of patients' needs and their variation over time. The weight of evidence suggests these varied professionals need to work together in a multidisciplinary team. This team needs to draw on a range of perspectives and skills and address social as well as medical needs. This is particularly vital if patients are to be effectively engaged over the long periods that are required. Roles and responsibilities in these teams will remain in a dynamic equilibrium – each development in treatment (e.g. better, more complex, psychopharmacology, CBT for delusions, improved structured rehabilitation) will affect the balance of power and specialisation within the team. There needs to be clarity of purpose but good care is dependent on honest inter-professional relationships. These must permit acknowledgement and discussion of uncertainty and the team structures and practices must be flexible to accommodate advances in treatment.

Schizophrenia care is unrecognisable to that of 50 years ago when it was dominated by large asylums. After two decades of intense innovation and change, we are less naïve and have, belatedly, begun to improve the rigour of our mental health services research. Components of care are less the subject of heated polemic than of tailoring resources to needs. Schizophrenia care in 50 years time may be as different from that currently as it is now from the era before deinstitutionalisation.

References

Barton R. Institutional Neurosis. Bristol: John Wright; 1959.

Birchwood M, McGorry P, Jackson H. Early intervention in schizophrenia. Br J Psychiatry 1997 Jan; 170:2–5.

Bond GR, Drake RE, Becker DR. An update on randomized controlled trials of evidence-based supported employment. Psychiatric Rehabilitation J 2008; 31(4):280–290.

Bond GR, Xie H, Drake RE. Can SSDI and SSI beneficiaries with mental illness benefit from evidence-based supported employment? Psychiatr Serv 2007 Nov; 58(11):1412–1420.

Brenner HD, Hodel B, Roder V, Corrigan P. Treatment of cognitive dysfunctions and behavioral deficits in schizophrenia. Schizophr Bull 1992; 18(1):21–26.

Brill H, Patton RE. Clinical-statistical analysis of population changes in New York state mental hospitals since the introduction of psychotropic drugs. Am J Psychiatry 1962; 119:20.

Burns T, Catty J, Becker T, Drake RE, Fioritti A, Knapp M, et al. The effectiveness of supported employment for people with severe mental illness: a randomised controlled trial. Lancet 2007 Sep 29; 370(9593):1146–1152.

Burns T, Catty J, Dash M, Roberts C, Lockwood A, Marshall M. Use of intensive case management to reduce time in hospital in people with severe mental illness: systematic review and meta-regression. BMJ 2007 Aug 18; 335(7615):336.

Burns T, Creed F, Fahy T, Thompson S, Tyrer P, White I. Intensive versus standard case management for severe psychotic illness: a randomised trial. The Lancet 1999; 353:2185–2189.

Burns T. Community Mental Health Teams. Oxford: Oxford University Press; 2004.

Churchill R, Owen G, Singh S, Hotopf M. International experiences of using Community Treatment Orders. London: Institute of Psychiatry; 2007.

Corrigan PW, Mueser KT, Bond GR, Drake RE, Solomon P. The Principles and Practice of Psychiatric Rehabilitation. New York: Guildford Press; 2007.

Dawson J. Community Treatment Orders: International Comparisons. Dunedin: Otago University; 2005.

Department of Health. Modern Standards and Service Models: National Service Framework for Mental Health. London: Department of Health; 1999.

Draine J, Salzer MS, Culhane DP, Hadley TR. Role of social disadvantage in crime, joblessness and homelessness among persons with serious mental illness. Psychiatr Serv 2002 May; 53(5):565–573.

Drake RE, McHugo GJ, Xie H, Fox M, Packard J, Helmstetter B. Ten-year recovery outcomes for clients with co-occurring schizophrenia and substance use disorders. Schizophr Bull 2006 Jul; 32(3):464–473.

Drake RE, Mueser KT, Brunette MF. Management of persons with co-occurring severe mental illness and substance use disorder: programe implications. World Psychiatry 2007; 6:131–136.

Drake RE, O'Neal EL, Wallach MA. A systematic review of psychosocial interventions for people with co-occurring substance use and severe mental disorders. J Substance Abuse Treatment 2008; 34(1), 123–138.

Edwards J, McGorry PD, Pennell K. Models of early intervention in psychosis: an analysis of service approaches. In: Birchwood M, Fowler D, Jackson C (eds) Early Intervention in Psychosis: A Guide to Concepts, Evidence and Interventions. New York: John Wiley & Sons; 2000. pp. 281–314.

Fisher WH, Roy-Bujnowski KM, Grudzinskas AJ, Clayfield JC, Banks SM, Wolff N. Patterns and prevalence of arrest in a statewide cohort of mental health care consumers. Psychiatr Serv 2006 Nov; 57(11):1623–1628.

Gibbs A, Dawson J, Ansley C, Mullen R. How patients in New Zealand view community treatment orders. J Mental Health 2005; 14(4):357–368.

Gibbs A, Dawson J, Mullen R. Community treatment orders for people with serious mental illness: A New Zealand study. British Journal of Social Work 2006; 36(7): 1085–1100. Br J Social Work 2005.

Goodwin GM, Geddes JR. What is the heartland of psychiatry? Br J Psychiatry 2007 Sep; 191: 189–191.

Hirsch S. Psychiatric Beds and Resources: Factors Influencing Bed Use and Service Planning. London: Gaskell (Royal College of Psychiatrists); 1988.

Intagliata J. Improving the quality of community care for the chronically mentally disabled: the role of case management. Schizophr Bull 1982; 8(4):655–674.

Kendrick T. Cardiovascular and respiratory risk factors and symptoms among general practice patients with long-term mental illness. Br J Psychiatry 1996 Dec; 169(6):733–739.

Kisely S, Campbell LA. Does compulsory or supervised community treatment reduce 'revolving door' care? Br J Psychiatry 2007; 191:373–374.

Lawton-Smith S. A Question of Numbers. The Potential Impact of Community-Based Treatment Orders in England and Wales. London: King's Fund; 2005.

Leff J, Trieman N, Knapp M, Hallam A. The TAPS Project: A report on 13 years of research, 1985–1998. Psychiatric Bull 2000; 24:165–168.

Liberman RP, Wallace CJ, Blackwell G, Kopelowicz A, Vaccaro JV, Mintz J. Skills training versus psychosocial occupational therapy for persons with persistent schizophrenia. Am J Psychiatry 1998 Aug; 155(8):1087–1091.

Marshall M, Gray A, Lockwood A, Green R. Case management for severe mental disorders. The Cochrane Collaboration [2] 1997.

Marshall M, Gray A, Lockwood A, Green R. Case management for severe mental disorders (Cochrane Review). The Cochrane Library [1] 2001.

Marshall M, Lewis S, Lockwood A, Drake R, Jones P, Croudace T. Association between duration of untreated psychosis and outcome in cohorts of first-episode patients: a systematic review. Arch Gen Psychiatry 2005 Sep; 62(9):975–983.

Marshall M, Lockwood A. Assertive Community Treatment for people with severe mental disorders (Cochrane Review). The Cochrane Library [3]. 25-2-1998.

McGorry P, Jackson H. Recognition and Management of Early Psychosis. A Preventative Approach. Cambridge: Cambridge University Press; 1999.

Monahan J, Redlich AD, Swanson J, Robbins PC, Appelbaum PS, Petrila J, et al. Use of leverage to improve adherence to psychiatric treatment in the community. Psychiatr Serv 2005 Jan; 56(1):37–44.

Morgan C, Burns T, Fitzpatrick R, Pinfold V, Priebe S. Social exclusion and mental health. Conceptual and methodological review. Br J Psychiatry 2007; (191):477–483.

Mueser KT, Bond GR, Drake RE, Resnick SG. Models of community care for severe mental illness: A review of research on case management. Schizophr Bull 1998; 24(1):37–74.

Mullen R, Gibbs A, Dawson J. Family perspective on community treatment orders: A New Zealand study. Int J Soc Psychiatry 2006; 52:469–478.

Pilling S, Bebbington P, Kuipers E, Garety P, Geddes J, Martindale B, et al. Psychological treatments in schizophrenia: II. Meta-analyses of randomized controlled trials of social skills training and cognitive remediation. Psychol Med 2002 Jul; 32(5):783–791.

Priebe S, Badesconyi A, Fioritti A, Hansson L, Kilian R, Torres-Gonzales F, et al. Reinstitutionalisation in mental health care: comparison of data on service provision from six European countries. BMJ 2005; 330:123–126.

Priebe S. Social outcomes in schizophrenia. Br J Psychiatry 2007; 191(Suppl. 50):s15–s20.

Rapp CA, Goscha RJ. The principles of effective case management of mental health services. Psychiatric Rehabilitation J 2004; 27(4):319–333.

Ratcliffe R.A.W. The open door: Ten years' experience in Dingleton. Lancet 1962; ii:188–190.

Saha S, Chant D, McGrath J. A systematic review of mortality in schizophrenia: is the differential mortality gap worsening over time? Arch Gen Psychiatry 2007 Oct; 64(10):1123–1131.

Swartz MS, Swanson JW, Wagner HR, Burns BJ, Hiday VA, Borum R. Can involuntary outpatient commitment reduce hospital recidivism? Findings from a randomized trial with severely mentally ill individuals. Am J Psychiatry 1999 Dec; 156(12):1968–1975.

Swartz MS, Swanson JW, Wagner HR, Hannon MJ, Burns BJ, Shumway M. Assessment of four stakeholder groups' preferences concerning outpatient commitment for persons with schizophrenia. Am J Psychiatry 2003 Jun; 160(6):1139–1146.

Test MA, Stein LI. Alternative to mental hospital treatment. III. Social cost. Arch Gen Psychiatry 1980 Apr; 37(4):409–412.

Thornicroft G, Wykes T, Holloway F, Johnson S, Szmukler G. From efficacy to effectiveness in community mental health services. PRiSM Psychosis Study 10. Br J Psychiatry 1998;173: 423–427.

U.S. Congress. Public Law 88-164, 88th Congress, S-1576; 1963..

US Department of Health and Human Services. Mental Health: A Report of the Surgeon General. Rockville, MD; 1999.

Weisbrod BA, Test MA, Stein LI. Alternative to mental hospital treatment. II. Economic benefit-cost analysis. Arch Gen Psychiatry 1980 Apr; 37(4):400–405.

Wing JK, Brown GW. Institutionalism and Schizophrenia. Cambridge: Cambridge University Press; 1970.

Wright C, Catty J, Watt H, Burns T. A systematic review of home treatment services. Classification and sustainability. Soc Psychiatry Psychiatr Epidemiol 2004; 39:789–796.

Does Stigma Impair Treatment Response and Rehabilitation in Schizophrenia? The "Contribution" of Mental Health Professionals

Wulf Rössler

The fact that stigma and discrimination are the chief enemies of progress in providing adequate care and helping people to live a life of acceptable quality is becoming recognised in many countries. Patients and their families provide numerous examples of the effects that stigma can (and does) have on the chance of employment, marriage, renting an apartment, or receiving support from neighbours or the community (Sartorius 1998). For example, most European studies report employment rates among people with schizophrenia of around 10–20% (Marwaha and Johnson 2004). Thus persons, once diagnosed with a psychotic disorder, rarely have a chance to participate in the workforce relatively independent of their actual ability to work.

And on a societal level, the provision of health and social insurance systems for mental illness is less comprehensive than those for say physical illness of similar severity (Sartorius 1998). For example, Brazil only spends about 2.3% of its health budget on mental health, which is low by international standards (Andreoli et al. 2007, Mateus et al. 2008). In contrast, Switzerland spends about 16% of its health budget on mental health services (Jaeger et al. 2008). As a consequence of such a low resource allocation for mental health services in Brazil, patients are in the streets, jails and prisons, emergency services, or even locked up at home (Gentil 2007).

Basic social psychology research has shown that perceptions regarding specific health services – and about the people receiving those services – significantly influence allocation decisions (Corrigan and Watson 2003). Hence, the personal attitudes of political decision makers play a major role in the process of resource allocation as much as the assumed attitudes of the general population in whose name political decision makers "act". Negative attitudes towards the mentally ill by decision makers and the general population result in the above-mentioned form of structural stigmatisation.

W. Rössler (✉)
Department of General and Social Psychiatry, Psychiatric University Hospital Zurich, Switzerland
e-mail: roessler@dgsp.uzh.ch

W.F. Gattaz, G. Busatto (eds.), *Advances in Schizophrenia Research 2009*,
DOI 10.1007/978-1-4419-0913-8_25, © Springer Science+Business Media, LLC 2010

All these examples document the reduced chances of mentally ill persons for rehabilitation, i.e. to get (re-) integrated into societal life in general.

A Comprehensive Concept of Stigma

But discussing the stigma of mental illness and its impact on treatment and rehabilitation in more detail requires firstly a precise concept of the different components of stigma (Link and Phelan 2001, Corrigan 2000). For the conceptualisation of stigma it is most useful to separate stereotypes from prejudice and discrimination.

Actually we all use (and need) stereotypes in our daily lives. For accomplishing our daily work we often rely on preformed judgements in the form of categories or stereotypes about the functioning of the world, the reasons why people act as they act, etc. Stereotypes simplify our understanding of the world. We are generally not challenged to verify these stereotypes in our daily lives. We do not even have to agree on these stereotypes even if we know about them.

For instance we often use personality categories, which for example explain to us why men and women act differently. And we are aware of such stereotypes about groups, the white and the blacks, the Europeans and the Latin Americans, the Jews and the Muslims . . . and the mentally ill. The most prominent stereotypes regarding the mentally ill are the danger they pose, their unpredictability, and their unreliability. Among the mentally ill, persons with schizophrenia are the group most affected by these stereotypes (Link and Cullen 1986, Link et al. 1999).

This situation changes when we discuss the concept of prejudice. Prejudice is a consenting emotional reaction to a stereotype or a stereotyped person. Thus, the prejudice about the mentally ill comprises for instance the notion "I am afraid of schizophrenics, because they are dangerous and unpredictable". In this context we usually do not speak about a particular person who suffers from schizophrenia but predicate the group "schizophrenics", as if this illness could characterise the whole person.

Stereotypes and prejudice are necessary, but are not sufficient components of a comprehensive concept of stigma (Rüsch et al. 2005). In a comprehensive concept of stigma, stereotypes and prejudice lead in a subsequent step to discrimination, i.e. to behavioural consequences: "Mentally ill people should be locked away because of the danger they pose, and their unpredictability", or "we can't employ the mentally ill because they are unreliable". But according to Rüsch et al. (2005) discrimination can only be put into practice if the discriminating persons hold the social, economic, or political power to do so. For example mental health professionals are also affected by stigmatising attitudes. For instance there are expectations of the general public that mental health professionals can "contract" mental illness through their job. Others hold the view that mental health professionals have chosen their profession due to own "craziness". But such stereotypes and prejudices typically do not lead to consequences.

Conversely mental health professionals hold considerable power over the lives of mentally ill persons. Current laws in most countries around the world allow involuntary civil commitment to in-patient treatment, and often to outpatient treatment as well. Additionally, there is a remaining broad spectrum of informal coercive measures that are imposed on psychiatric patients outside judicial compulsory practices. Arguments for informal coercive interventions, which use threats of negative sanctions to compel the patient to accept treatment (Monahan et al. 2001), refer to the concept of paternalism in order to take the responsibility for patients' health (Veatch 1994). Or they refer to the concept of social control as a mandate by society to prevent or reduce undesired and disruptive behaviour (Lovell 1996). Hence the efficient use of treatment approaches heavily depends on mental health professionals' attitudes and their views regarding their patients.

Most of us health professionals consider ourselves in some way as partners of our patients with regard to decisions about treatment and rehabilitation. Concerning public representation, we intuitively follow the idea that we predominantly act as agents for our patients, who often are not capable of formulating their own needs. Thus, most research intended to reduce stigma and discrimination because of mental illness is in principle directed to the general public. We rarely ask what our "contribution" as mental health professionals could be in order to diminish stigma and discrimination that is engendered because of mental illness. Norman Sartorius (1998) gives a possible answer to it: "First, we should examine our own attitudes [. . .]".

The Impact of Stigmatisation on Social Networks of Mentally Ill

This is not only an academic question. Perceived stigmatisation of mentally ill people impairs their social relations and well-being. And mental health professionals are an important part of patients' social networks.

While perceived stigmatisation (both theoretically and empirically) has been accounted for as an independent and unalterable factor, we analysed data from a longitudinal study focusing on the reciprocal effects between stigmatisation and social relationships (Mueller et al. 2006). A sample of severely mentally ill persons ($n = 165$), mostly with a diagnosis of schizophrenia or a schizoaffective psychosis, took part in two psychiatric hospitals in Zurich in two structured interviews. One was conducted during their admission and the second 1 year later. Cross-lagged path models were designed to test the interrelations of (1) perceived stigmatisation, (2) a defensive stigma-coping orientation, (3) concrete stigmatising experiences, and either (4) social network or (5) perceived social support as dependent variables. Contrary to previous findings, neither of the three components of stigmatisation tested had any influence on social network or support. Social support, though, strongly predicted perceived stigmatisation 1 year later, but only in the group with a more recent onset of illness. This finding suggests that the perception of stigma is subject to modification in the course of new life circumstances and underlines the importance of activating social resources – including mental health professionals – especially in the first years of a severe mental illness.

Do Mental Health Professionals Stigmatise Their Patients?

Surprisingly there is little information about (stigmatising) attitudes of mental health professionals. Therefore we conducted several surveys among mental health professionals and compared these data with a previous own survey of the attitudes of the general population towards the mentally ill. Based on findings from our survey in the general population, we assumed that mental health professionals would have a more favourable attitude towards mentally ill persons, as contact with those mentally ill is associated with better attitudes towards the mentally ill (Lauber et al. 2004a).

We conducted one of our surveys among mental health professionals with psychiatrists in office practice. Out of all psychiatrists in office practice in the German-speaking part of Switzerland ($N = 855$), we drew a representative sample ($N = 100$) in terms of age and gender. After having received an informative letter, 90 psychiatrists, i.e. 90%, agreed to participate. The other survey among mental health professionals was conducted with professionals from psychiatric institutions, mainly psychiatric hospitals. We contacted in 29 hospitals a total of 3088 professionals, and they completed 1073 interviews (response rate: 34.7%). Following the above-proposed increments of stigma, some results concerning stereotypes, prejudice, and potentially discriminating behaviour among mental health professionals will be presented.

In one of our analyses (Lauber et al. 2006), we compared 12 stereotypes (abnormal, bedraggled, unreliable, weird, dangerous, unpredictable, healthy, self-controlled, reasonable, creative, stupid, and highly skilled) about the mentally ill rated by mental health professionals from psychiatric institutions, with the respective ratings of the general population. The mean value of the stereotypes scale of all professional groups and the general public is near the midpoint on a 5-point Likert scale, but in all cases, on the negative side. Considering the single stereotypes mental health professionals generally do not differ consistently in a negative or positive way from the public attitude. But there are significant differences between the professional groups: psychiatrists hold the most pronounced negative attitudes, whereas psychologists had the most positive ones. The result that stereotyping is evident in the mental health-care system is supported by findings from the United Kingdom where ethnic racism, another form of stereotyping, was found: involuntary admissions of young black men are more common than those of young white men, and schizophrenia is more commonly diagnosed in young black men although the prevalence in the community is not markedly different for black and white men (Minnis et al. 2001).

If mental health professionals (in particular psychiatrists) have negative attitudes towards the mentally ill, comparable to the negative attitudes of the general population, what does that mean about prejudices as a consenting emotional reaction to stereotypes held by psychiatrists? For that reason we asked psychiatrists in office practice some general questions about their attitudes towards community psychiatry according to Taylor and Dear's Inventory of Community Mental Health Ideology (Taylor and Dear 1981). The same inventory was applied in our survey with the general population. These questions measure the impact of mental health facilities on residential neighbourhoods, the danger to local residents posed by the mentally ill and the acceptance of the principle of psychiatric community care. The phrasing of the questions asked contains emotional reactions to the mentally ill. In detail the questions are as follows:

- Mental health facilities should be kept out of residential neighbourhoods.
- Locating mental health services in residential neighbourhoods endangers local residents.
- It is frightening to think of people with mental problems living in residential neighbourhoods.
- Local residents have good reasons to resist the location of mental health services in their neighbourhood.
- Local residents should accept the location of mental health facilities in their neighbourhood in order to serve the needs of the local community.
- Locating mental health facilities in a residential area downgrades the neighbourhood.

Psychiatrists and the general population have an overall positive (emotional) attitude to mental health facilities in the community. However, the psychiatrists' attitude was surprisingly significantly more positive than that of the general population (Lauber et al. 2004a). According to our above-introduced concept of stigma, we would have expected a consenting negative response to negative stereotypes as expressed by the psychiatrists and the general population. How can we interpret these results? A first cautious interpretation (because we are comparing two different samples on the side of the psychiatrists) is that psychiatrists have learnt their lesson. They know what they have to say, but it is not clear how much their statements are in this respect to be trusted.

This interpretation receives some support from other findings of our two studies with professionals addressing the question of discriminating behaviour as the third constituent of stigma. As a first measure of behavioural discrimination we assessed the social distance (Link et al. 1987). We assessed "social distance" in both samples of psychiatrists, i.e. in the sample of psychiatrists in office practice (Lauber et al. 2004a) and in the sample of psychiatrists in psychiatric institutions (Nordt et al. 2006). Social distance was assessed in both studies by the German version of the Social Distance Scale (Angermeyer and Matschinger 1997). This scale consists of seven questions assessing the willingness to interact with the person described in various social situations. Each question is rated on a 5-point Likert scale set by 1 "definitely willing" and 5 "definitely unwilling".

Beforehand the psychiatrists in office practice were presented with a vignette describing a person with schizophrenia. The psychiatrists of psychiatric institutions were presented with two vignettes, one describing a person with a depression and the other describing a person with schizophrenia. The psychiatrists from psychiatric institutions were asked to make their ratings for each of these vignettes.

The questions were as follows:
Would you...

- ...like to move next door to a person like Beat?
- ...make friends with a person like Beat?
- ...be willing to start work with a person like Beat?
- ...like your child to marry a person like Beat?
- ...recommend a person like Beat for a job?
- ...rent a room to a person like Beat?
- ...trust a person like Beat to take care of your child?

Overall, psychiatrists of both samples and the general population display no differences in their social distance to people with mental illness. Among psychiatrists and the general population, the level of social distance increases the more the situation described implies "social closeness". Most social distance was thus reported when the interviewee was asked whether the person depicted would look after the interviewee's child, rent a room from the respondent, or marry into the respondent's family. Having the depicted person as a co-worker or moving next door revealed the least social distance.

The reaction to the two vignettes did not differ between professionals of psychiatric institutions and the public. Both groups reacted with an increasing social distance towards the person in the schizophrenia vignette. Summarising our results concerning social distance, we must state that psychiatrists do not feel any closer to their patients than the general population. This is in spite of the fact that contact with mentally ill persons generally reduces the wish to be distant from the mentally ill (Lauber et al. 2004b).

As a second measure of behavioural discrimination, we assessed the willingness to restrict the individual rights of people who are mentally ill. We asked the mental health professionals from psychiatric institutions (Nordt et al. 2006) and the interviewees from our general survey (Lauber et al. 2000, 2002b), whether they approved or disapproved of the following four questions:

- What do you think: should a woman who had suffered severely from a mental illness have an abortion in the case of a pregnancy?
- Do you approve of the right to vote and to run for office for somebody who had suffered severely from a mental illness?
- What do you think: should somebody who is severely mentally ill have her/his driver's license revoked?
- What do you think: should somebody be admitted to a psychiatric hospital even against his/her will, and if necessary be restrained? Or, should a person under no circumstances whatever be compulsorily admitted to a psychiatric hospital?

The general public accepted restrictions as regards people with mental illness to a much higher degree, with the exception of compulsory admission. Compared with mental health professionals, the participants of the public survey endorsed these restrictions more strongly. Approximately three times as many people compared to professionals supported the withdrawal of the right to vote (19.6%) and recommended an abortion (29%) to women who had previously suffered from a severe mental illness. Almost all mental health professionals (> 98%) had a positive attitude towards compulsory admission, whereas every third person in the public was opposed to it (Nordt et al. 2006). At first sight we could easily form the impression that psychiatrists are on their patients' side, as they endorse much more liberal attitudes concerning restrictions imposed on the mentally ill compared to the general public. But actually they approve restrictions towards the mentally ill almost unanimously where their professional identity is affected. This attitude complies very much with a "coercion to undergo beneficial treatment" perspective (Torrey and Zdanowicz, 2001). The "coercion to detrimental stigma" perspective (Pollack 2004), however, claims that coercion increases stigmatisation and results in low self-esteem, a compromised quality of life and increased symptoms.

Self-Stigma

Persons with mental illness may internalise mental illness stigma and experience diminished self-esteem and self-efficacy. We refer to this process as self-stigma (Watson et al. 2007). Research suggests that perceived stigma results in a loss of self-esteem, self-efficacy, and presages limited prospects for recovery (Link 2001, Link et al. 1991, Markowitz 1998, Perlick et al. 2001, Rosenfield 1997, Sirey et al. 2001, Wright et al. 2000). These studies assume that prior to being labelled as "mentally ill", individuals have internalised cultural stereotypes about mental illness.

We could confirm this in our own study comparing chronically mentally ill patients' perception of devaluation and discrimination towards former mental patients, with the respective attitude of the general population (Graf et al. 2004). Subjective perception of stigma was measured by the German translation of Link's Perceived Devaluation and Discrimination Questionnaire (Link, 1987) that shows the respondent's assumption of how the general population ("the others") thinks about mentally ill people. The interviewees were asked to answer on a 5-point Likert scale ranging from "I fully disagree" (0) to "I fully agree" (4).

We asked the following questions:

- Most people would willingly accept a former patient as a close friend.
- Most people believe that a person who has been in a mental hospital is just as intelligent as the average person.
- Most young women would be reluctant to date a man who has been hospitalised for a serious mental disorder.
- Most people would not hire a former mental patient to take care of their children, even if he or she had been well for some time.

- Most people think less of a person who has been in a mental hospital.
- Most employers will pass over the application of a former mental patient in favour of another applicant.

The results showed that the chronically mentally ill and the general population share the belief that most people will reject former mental patients, although the degrees of agreement vary between the single statements. In a multiple regression analysis we further demonstrated that even when allowing for clinical factors and relevant demographic variables, the patients' perceived devaluation and discrimination has a significantly negative effect on their quality of life (the subjective Quality of Life was measured by the World Health Organization Quality of Life Instrument (WHOQOL)). Even the anticipation and fear of expected stigmatisation and discrimination leads to negative outcomes and reduces the life chances of mental patients.

Furthermore the perception of existent and nonexistent barriers is a major factor in help-seeking behaviour (Link et al. 1989). The fear of a mental illness label and the consequences of devaluation and discrimination may hamper many people in seeking help for mental or emotional problems (Hayward 1997; Link et al. 1999). These beliefs are directly relevant for people who enter psychiatric treatment, and in particular, in-patient treatment. At this point it matters to what extent one believes that most people will reject a mental patient. It often happens that a psychiatric hospitalisation labels a person as a mental patient with all negative consequences. This makes it clear why people sometimes strenuously oppose psychiatric hospitalisation.

Discussion

Stigma can affect mentally ill people through different ways and mechanisms. Structural discrimination refers to the fact that mental health care regularly does not receive an appropriate proportion of the total health budget. In many countries of the world, the mentally ill do not receive the treatment that could alleviate their symptoms and help them to become reintegrated in their previous lives. The reasons are mainly budgetary.

Because of direct discrimination throughout the general population, mentally ill persons are excluded from many activities of social life. This seriously impedes their rehabilitation. Therefore, several national and international psychiatric organisations have started campaigns against the stigmatisation of those mentally ill. The best-known anti-stigma programme comes from the World Psychiatric Association, which is directed towards the stigmatisation of persons with schizophrenia – the most stigmatised group among the mentally ill (http://www.openthedoors.com).

For many years, mental health professionals have not been considered an important source of discriminatory practices. But we could demonstrate in several studies that mental health professionals (in particular psychiatrists) do not hold less discriminatory attitudes towards the mentally ill than do the general population. It is not immoderate to expect more accepting attitudes and more understanding for the mentally ill among mental health professionals, when compared to the general population. We know from many studies with lay persons that contact with the mentally ill "normally" improves attitudes and social closeness with mentally ill. Why should this not work with mental health professionals? And finally, we health professionals have been trained for many years to better understand and deal with the disorders our patients suffer from. Nonetheless many professionals hold the pessimistic view that persons with severe mental illnesses are doomed to poor outcomes.

Holding negative attitudes towards the mentally ill can have serious implications for the lives of such people. Yet, mental health professionals hold the power to wield significant influence on the treatment and rehabilitation of severely mentally ill. Persons who endorse the stigma of mental illness are not going to support an individual's right to self-determination, the right to determine the kind of job they should pursue, the neighbourhood they want to live in, and the people with whom they want to have company.

We as psychiatrist often wonder why so many of our patients do not like us (particularly in-patients) – in contrast to almost all other medical disciplines. I personally find the answer not so difficult: Many patients simply do not think that they are treated with fairness, concern and respect. We use paternalistic approaches and do not believe in their ability to take responsibility for themselves. Thus we do not contribute to our patients' self-esteem and self-efficacy, which is a significant part of the recovery process.

PW Corrigan (2002) has proposed a heuristic model of how to improve treatment and community outcomes:

- Establishing a provider attitude of recovery, and developing collaborative treatment plans, will lead to a better use of medication and rehabilitation services.
- Replacing self-stigma with recovery expectations will lead to more self-efficacy, thereby making it more likely for our patients to pursue work and independent living opportunities.
- Challenging stigmatising attitudes and discriminatory behaviour will alleviate the chances of our patients to find reasonable accommodation, and to facilitate work and independent living opportunities.

These findings on the recovery process and the factors that impact on this process challenge our current policies and institutional practices developed to care for people with mental illnesses. All the progress we have made and will make in our field will be in vain if we do not find an alliance with those people affected.

References

Andreoli SB, Almeida-Filho N, Martin D, Mateus MD, Mari J. Is psychiatric reform a strategy for reducing the mental health budget? The case of Brazil. Rev Bras Psiquiat 2007; (29); 1: 43–46.

Angermeyer MC, Matschinger H. Social distance towards the mentally ill: results of representative survey in the Federal Republic of Germany. Psychol Med 1997; 27(1): 131–141.

Corrigan PW. Mental health stigma as social attribution: Implications for research methods and attitude change. Clin Psychol: Sci Pract 2000; 7(1): 48–67.

Corrigan PW. Empowerment and serious mental illness: Treatment partnerships and community opportunities. Psychiatric Quarter 2002; 73(3): 217–228.

Corrigan PW, Watson AC. Factors that explain how policy makers distribute resources to mental health services. Psychiatr Serv 2003 Apr; 54(4): 501–507.

Graf J, Lauber C, Nordt C, Ruesch P, Meyer PC, Rössler W. Perceived stigmatization of mentally ill people and its consequences for the quality of life in a Swiss population. J Nerv Ment Dis 2004; 192(8): 542–547.

Gentil V. More for the same? Rev Bras Psiquiat 2007; Jun; 29(2): 193–194.

Hayward P, Bright JA. Stigma and mental illness: A review and critique. J Ment Health 1997; 6: 345–354.

Jäger M, Sobocki P, Rössler W. Cost of disorders of the brain in Switzerland with a focus on mental disorders. Swiss Medical Weekly 2008; 138(1-2): 4–11.

Jäger M, Sobocki P, Rössler W. Cost of disorders of the brain in Switzerland. Swiss Medical Weekly 2008; 138: 4–11.

Lauber C, Nordt C, Sartorius N, Falcato L, Rössler W. Public acceptance of restrictions on mentally ill people. Acta Psychiatr Scand Suppl. 2000; 102: 26–32.

Lauber C, Nordt C, Falcato L, Rössler W. Determinants of attitude to volunteering in psychiatry: results of a public opinion survey in Switzerland. Int J Soc Psychiatry 2002a; 48: 209–219.

Lauber C, Nordt C, Falcato L, Rössler W. Public attitude to compulsory admission of mentally ill people. Acta Psychiatr Scand 2002b; 105: 385–389.

Lauber C, Anthony M, Ajdacic-Gross V, Rössler W. What about psychiatrists' attitude to mentally ill people? Eur Psychiatry 2004a; 19(7): 423–427.

Lauber C, Nordt C, Falcato L, Rössler W. Factors influencing social distance towards people with mental illness, Community Ment Health J 2004b; 40: 265–274.

Lauber C, Nordt C, Braunschweig C, Rössler W. Do mental health professionals stigmatize their patients? Acta Psychiatrica Scand 2006; 113(Suppl. 429): 51–59.

Link BG, Cullen FT. Contact with the mentally ill and perceptions of how dangerous they are. J Health Soc Behav 1986 Dec; 27(4): 289–302.

Link BG. Understanding labelling effects in the area of mental disorders: An empirical assessment of the effects of expectations of rejections. Am Sociol Rev 1987; 52: 96–112.

Link BG, Cullen FT, Frank J, Wozniak JF. The social rejection of former mental patients: understanding why labels matter. Am J Sociol 1987; 92: 146–150.

Link BG, Cullen FT, Struening E, Shrout PE, Dohrenwend BP. A modified labelling theory approach in the area of the mental disorders: An empirical assessment. Am Sociol Rev 1989; 54: 400–423.

Link BG, Mirotznik J, Cullen F. The effectiveness of stigma coping orientations: can negative consequences of mental illness labelling be avoided? J Health Soc Behav 1991; 32: 302–320.

Link BG, Phelan JC, Bresnahan M, Stueve A, Pescosolido BA. Public conceptions of mental illness: labels, causes, dangerousness, and social distance. Am J Public Health 1999; 89: 1328–1333.

Link BG. Stigma as a barrier to recovery: the consequences of stigma for the self-esteem of people with mental illness. Psychiatr Serv 2001; 52:1621–1626.

Link BG, Phelan JC. Conceptualizing stigma. Ann Rev Sociol 2001; 27: 363–385.

Lovell AM. Coercion and social control. A framework for research on aggressive strategies in community mental health. In Dennis DL & Monahan J (Eds). Coercion and Aggressive Community Treatment: A New Frontier in Mental Health Law. New York, Plenum Press, 1996.

Markowitz FE. The effects of stigma on the psychological well-being and life satisfaction of persons with mental illness. J Health Soc Behav 1998; 39: 335–347.

Marwaha S, Johnson S. Schizophrenia and employment. Soc Psychiatry Psychiatr Epidemiol 2004; 39: 337–349.

Mateus MD, Mari JJ, Delgado PG, Almeida-Filho N, Barrett T, Gerolin J, Goihman S, Razzouk D, Rodriguez J, Weber R, Andreoli SB, Saxena S. The mental health system in Brazil: Policies and future challenges. Int J Ment Health Syst 2008 Sep 5; 2–12.

Minnis H, McMillan A, Gillies M, Smith S. Racial stereotyping: survey of psychiatrists in United Kingdom. BMJ 2001; Oct; (20): 905–906.

Monahan J, Bonnie RJ, Appelbaum PS, Hyde PS, Steadman HJ, Swartz MS. Mandated community treatment: beyond outpatient commitment. Psychiatr Serv 2001 Sep; 52(9): 1198–1205.

Mueller B, Nordt C, Lauber C, Ruesch P, Meyer PC, Rössler W. Social support modifies perceived stigmatization in the first years of mental illness: a longitudinal approach. Soc Sci Med 2006; (62): 39–49.

Nordt C, Rössler W, Lauber C. Attitudes of mental health professionals toward people with schizophrenia and major depression. Schizophr Bull 2006 Oct; 32(4): 709-714.

Perlick D, Rosenheck R, Clarkin J, Sirey J, Salahi J, Struening E. Stigma as a barrier to recovery: adverse effects of perceived stigma on social adaption of persons diagnosed with bipolar affective disorder. Psychiatr Serv 2001; 52: 1627–1632.

Pollack, DA. Moving from Coercion to Collaboration in Mental Health Services DHHS (SMA) 04-3869. In Rockville, MD: Center for Mental Health Services, Substance Abuse and Mental Health Services Administration 2004.

Rosenfield S. Labelling mental illness: the effects of received services and perceived stigma on life satisfaction. Am Sociol Rev 1997; 62: 660–672.

Rüsch N, Angermeyer MC, Corrigan PW. The stigma of mental illness: concepts, forms, and consequences. Psychiatr Prax 2005; Jul; 32(5): 221–232.

Sartorius N. Stigma: what can psychiatrists do about it?. Lancet 1998; 352(9133): 1058–1059.

Sirey JA, Bruce ML, Alexopoulos GS, Perlick DA, Friedman SJ, Meyers BS. Stigma as a barrier to recovery: perceived stigma and patient-related severity of illness as predictors of antidepressant drug adherence. Psychiatr Serv 2001; 52: 1615–1620.

Taylor SM, Dear MJ. Scaling community attitudes toward the mentally ill. Schizophr Bull 1981; 7(2): 225–240.

Torrey EF, Zdanowicz M. Outpatient commitment: what, why, and for whom. Psychiatr Serv 2001; 52(3): 337–341.

Veatch R. Against paternalism in the patient-physician relationship. In Gilon R (Ed) Principles of Health Care Ethics. Chichester, John Wiley, 1994.

Watson AC, Corrigan P, Larson JE, Sells M. Self-Stigma in people with mental illness. Schizophr Bull 2007; 33(6): 1312–1318.

Wright ER, Gronfein WP, Owens TJ. Deinstitutionalization, social rejection, and the self-esteem of former mental patients. J Health Soc Behav 2000; 41: 68–90.

Treatment of Schizophrenia: Discussion

Shôn Lewis

New Drugs and Old

Rajiv Tandon reminds us that since chlorpromazine, no less than 60 antipsychotic drugs have been marketed. Clozapine proved a milestone in treatment effectiveness for patients with schizophrenia. The subsequently developed atypical antipsychotic drugs, now known as second-generation antipsychotics (SGAs), were heralded as the first major advance in the therapeutics of schizophrenia for 40 years. These drugs seemed to have important advantages over first-generation (FGA; typical or conventional) drugs, including better efficacy for positive, negative, and mood symptoms, with fewer adverse effects and the possibility of improving cognition. It was claimed that the increased cost of the newer drugs would be offset by savings resulting from decreased hospital stays and use of health-care services.

However, meta-analyses and systematic reviews yielded less clear results. Much of the evidence concerning the relative efficacy of FGA and SGA drugs came from relatively short-term, industry-funded trials where patients were highly selected, drop-out rates are high and outcomes are based predominantly on symptom ratings. As a result, health-care policy makers were undecided. Where was the independent evidence for saying that the SGA drugs were a major advance on the first-generation drugs in the population of patients receiving these drugs in routine mental health-care settings? Furthermore, how the SGA drugs compare? And is clozapine really superior to other drugs in practice? To address these questions, the National Institute of Mental Health in the United States and the NHS R&D Office in the United Kingdom each separately funded a "pragmatic," or practical, clinical trial in the late 1990s, with no sponsorship from industry. Pragmatic trials have characteristics of having broad inclusion criteria and long follow-up, aiming to mimic routine clinical practice as far as is consistent with a rigorous randomized design. Their purpose is to try better to clarify the real-life effectiveness, rather than the efficacy under ideal conditions, of an intervention.

S. Lewis (✉)
Professor of Adult Psychiatry and Head, Community-Based Medicine Research School University of Manchester
e-mail: shon.lewis@manchester.ac.uk

W.F. Gattaz, G. Busatto (eds.), *Advances in Schizophrenia Research 2009*,
DOI 10.1007/978-1-4419-0913-8_26, © Springer Science+Business Media, LLC 2010

In the United Kingdom, the CUtLASS trials (Jones et al., 2006; Lewis et al., 2006) were two medium-sized, open (that is, non-blind to patients and clinicians) randomized trials comparing classes of drug as grouped in most clinical guidelines: FGA versus non-clozapine SGA and non-clozapine SGA versus clozapine. The primary outcome was quality of life as measured on the Heinrichs scale at 1 year and symptoms were the main secondary outcome. Outcomes were assessed blind to treatment allocation. In the FGA versus SGA trial (CUtLASS 1), 227 people with schizophrenia, mostly outpatients, were randomized to either an FGA or a non-clozapine SGA drug (amisulpride, olanzapine, quetiapine, risperidone). The choice of individual drug within each class was made by the managing clinician in advance of randomization. The results showed that not only was there was no clinical advantage over 1 year to SGAs the data actually showed that those participants in the FGA arm did rather better. In addition, there were no significant differences in rates of objectively assessed EPS. Participants reported no preference for either class of drug. The similarly designed CUtLASS 2 trial of clozapine versus other SGAs, run at the same time in patients who had not responded well to two or more previous drugs, showed that there was a significant advantage to clozapine in symptom improvements over 1 year and patients significantly preferred it over other SGAs.

In the United States, the CATIE trial (Lieberman et al., 2005) was a double-blind trial in which 1,493 patients with chronic schizophrenia were randomized to one of the SGAs olanzapine, quetiapine, risperidone, ziprasidone (added to the design after the study had begun), or the medium-potency FGA, perphenazine. The objective of the trial was to compare the relative effectiveness of the FGA against several SGAs. The primary outcome for the trial, chosen to reflect real-world practice, was discontinuation of the drug and switching to another antipsychotic for any reason, be it lack of effectiveness, too many side effects, or patient choice. The trial was run over 57 sites between 2001 and 2004 and the sample size had 76% power to detect 12% differences in discontinuation rates. The results showed that no less than 74% of patients were discontinued from their randomized treatment over 18 months. Olanzapine proved to be the most effective in terms of having the lowest discontinuation rate (64%), but with the highest side effect burden overall. The remaining second-generation drugs differed neither from each other nor from the FGA perphenazine, in terms of effectiveness or (surprisingly) extrapyramidal side effects. There was no evidence that SGAs were better for negative symptoms. In terms of specific side effects, olanzapine caused most weight gain and dyslipidemia, quetiapine caused most anticholinergic effects, risperidone most hyperprolactinemia and sexual side effects, and perphenazine had highest rates of discontinuation for EPS, even though direct measures of EPS did not differ significantly between drugs.

In the subsequent trial for those participants who discontinued the first phase because of a lack of efficacy (CATIE phase 2: McEvoy et al., 2006), cases were re-randomized to a comparison of open-label clozapine versus other SGAs, with time to all-cause discontinuation again as the primary outcome. In the 99 participants entering CATIE phase 2, clozapine emerged as being significantly more effective than the other SGAs, with a median time to discontinuation of 10 months, twice the length of the next best, olanzapine.

The two trials have clearly different designs but also important similarities. The rationale for each trial was the lack of unbiased data to inform everyday clinical practice. The investigators in both trials predicted that SGAs would outperform FGAs and that clozapine would be the most effective. Both were government funded and both were designed to reflect routine clinical practice as much as possible, with broad inclusion criteria. Patient participants were similar clinically and demographically in the two trials. The core results were broadly the same in each trial and the primary hypotheses were not supported: SGAs were not found to be more effective than FGAs (with the exception of olanzapine in CATIE). Also, they did not produce measurably less EPS overall. In both trials, clozapine was the most effective.

Both trials have had criticisms leveled against them in terms of design detail. In particular, neither trial was powered to look at the issue of tardive dyskinesia. It is the convergence between the results of these two trials that is striking. The finding of clinical equivalence between SGAs and FGAs derives further support from two further trials with a similar pragmatic design. Rosenheck et al. (2003)found no advantage to olanzapine in comparison to haloperidol, given in lower doses than has been usual. The EUFEST trial (Kahn et al., 2008) showed no advantage to any SGA over haloperidol in symptom and functioning measures in first-episode patients in Europe.

Dr. Tandon concludes that there is no meaningful difference between first- and second-generation drugs and, as a result, the distinction can now be regarded as meaningless. But this is to overlook one key aspect, and one of the main reasons why CATIE and CUtLASS were undertaken. The chief distinction between the two classes in practice was the acquisition cost of the drugs, where FGAs were 20–30 times cheaper than SGAs (the C in CUtLASS stands for "Cost"). Was this extra cost really recouped through savings in other aspects of health care, such as inpatient stays?

In CUtLASS 1, the aim of the economic evaluation was to inform policy and treatment decision makers about the relative costs and utility (or value) of initiating treatment with FGAs or SGAs in people with schizophrenia. Specific research questions were: Are there differences in the direct costs of initiating treatment with FGAs and SGAs? Are there differences in the health states of people treated with FGAs and SGAs? Are SGAs more effective in a population with chronic schizophrenia?

Health status and service use data were collected from all patients enrolled in the trial to estimate resource use, costs, and utilities associated with FGAs and SGAs. The outcome measure for the economic evaluation was quality adjusted life years (QALYs). This was calculated from health states reported by patients, using a widely validated health status questionnaire (EQ-5D) at 12, 26, and 52 weeks from randomization. The EQ-5D is a validated generic health status measure covering five domains (mobility, self-care, usual activity, pain/distress, and anxiety/depression). The measure is used in national health surveys in the United Kingdom and in clinical trials in mental health. The utility values were used to estimate QALYs, based on the observed number of days patients were alive in the 12-month follow-up period of the trial.

Direct costs were measured as resource use multiplied by the unit cost or price of the resource item. Resource use data were collected for hospital in-patient and outpatient services, primary and community care services, and prescribed medications. Data on the use of psychiatric hospital care and medication were obtained by case note review in the relevant primary hospital or clinic for each patient. Patients also completed an economic questionnaire at each assessment to identify whether they had used any other hospital, primary, or community care services in the last 3 months. If additional services were used, patients were asked for details of type, name, and location of the services. The frequency and intensity of service use were then obtained from a detailed review of the relevant hospital, primary and community care records for each person. Descriptive analysis was used to compare utility values and QALYs and costs. The primary measure of interest for the economic analysis was the incremental cost effectiveness ratio (ICER). The QALY and cost data were inputs to estimate the ICER.

The primary and sensitivity analyses of the economic data indicate that FGAs were likely to be cost saving and associated with a gain in QALYs compared to SGAs. The cost-effectiveness acceptability analysis supported this conclusion. The analysis indicated that if the additional QALYs associated with FGAs were valued in monetary terms, using threshold cost per QALY values then FGAs were likely to be cost-effective. In other words, for people whose treatment needed to be changed, starting the new treatment with an FGA would be as effective as, or more effective than, initiating treatment with an SGA (Davies et al., 2007). The cost effectiveness data from the CATIE trial also indicated that perphenazine was significantly less costly and not less effective than the SGAs as a group (Rosenheck et al., 2006).

Depot Antipsychotic Drugs, Stigma, and Community Care

A thread might be detected to link the other three chapters. David and colleagues' excellent review of the history, development, and deployment of long-acting injectable medication points to large differences in rates of use between countries and makes the point that the development of community-based care in the United Kingdom, for instance, went hand in hand with the wider take-up of depots, one facilitating the other. It is important to note that the real value, effectiveness, and utility of depot medication have never properly been tested in comparison with oral medication in the population of patients in whom depots are most likely to be used: those with limited adherence. Trials are done in samples of participants who are generally adherent, thus minimizing real-life advantages and systematic reviews are therefore generally negative.

A chief objection to the use of depots is their inherently paternalistic and stigmatizing nature. Rossler reviews the impressive body of empirical work he and others have undertaken in the area of stigma, showing how stigma begins with us, the health professionals. Burns discusses how the general concept of coercion experienced by patients is alive even in community treatment settings. Using innovative meta-regression techniques in the context of meta-analysis, his own rigorous work has elucidated which are the key elements of an effective community service. He concludes that "Care must inevitably be multidisciplinary to reflect the complexity of patients' needs and their variation over time." The multidisciplinary team needs to draw on a range of perspectives and skills and address social as well as medical needs, particularly if patients are to be effectively engaged over the long periods that are required.

References

Davies LM, Lewis SW, Jones PB, Barnes TRE, Gaughran F, Hayhurst K, Markwick A, Lloyd H, on behalf of the CUtLASS team (2007). Cost effectiveness of first generation versus second generation antipsychotic drugs to treat psychosis: results from a randomised controlled trial in schizophrenia responding poorly to previous therapy. *Br J Psychiatry* 191: 14–22

Jones PB, Barnes TR, Davies L, Dunn G, Lloyd H, Hayhurst KP, Murray RM, Markwick A, Lewis SW (2006). Randomized controlled trial of effect on quality of life of second generation versus first generation antipsychotic drugs in schizophrenia – CUtLASS 1. *Arch Gen Psychiatry* 63: 1079–87

Kahn RS, Fleischhacker WW, Boter H, Davidson M, Vergouwe Y, Keet IP, Gheorghe MD, Rybakowski JK, Galderisi S, Libiger J, Hummer M, Dollfus S, López-Ibor JJ, Hranov LG, Gaebel W, Peuskens J, Lindefors N, Riecher-Rössler A, Grobbee DE (2008). EUFEST study group. Effectiveness of antipsychotic drugs in first-episode schizophrenia and schizophreniform disorder: an open randomised clinical trial. *Lancet* 371(9618): 1085–97

Lewis SW, Barnes TRE, Davies L, Murray RM, Dunn G, Kerwin R, Hayhurst K, Jones PJ (2006). Randomised controlled trial of effect on quality of life of prescription of clozapine versus other second generation antipsychotic drugs in resistant schizophrenia. *Schizophr Bull* 32: 715–23

Lieberman JA, Stroup TS, McEvoy JP, Swartz MS, Rosenheck RA, Perkins DO, Keefe RS, Davis SM, Davis CE, Lebowitz BD, Severe J, Hsiao JK (2005). Clinical Antipsychotic Trails of Intervention Effectiveness (CATIE) Investigators. Effectiveness of antipsychotic drugs in patients with chronic schizophrenia. *N Engl J Med* 353(12): 1209–23

McEvoy JP, Lieberman JA, Stroup TS, Davis SM, Meltzer HY, Rosenheck RA, Swartz MS, Perkins DO, Keefe RS, Davis CE, Severe J, Hsiao JK (2006). CATIE Investigators. Effectiveness of clozapine versus olanzapine, quetiapine, and risperidone in patients with chronic schizophrenia who did not respond to prior atypical antipsychotic treatment. *Am J Psychiatry* 163(4): 600–10

Rosenheck R, Perlick D, Bingham S, Liu-Mares W, Collins J, Warren S, Leslie D, Allan E, Campbell EC, Caroff S, Corwin J, Davis L, Douyon R, Dunn L, Evans D, Frecska E, Grabowski J, Graeber D, Herz L, Kwon K, Lawson W, Mena F, Sheikh J, Smelson D, Smith-Gamble V (2003). Department of Veterans Affairs Cooperative Study Group on the Cost-Effectiveness of Olanzapine. Effectiveness and cost of olanzapine and haloperidol in the treatment of schizophrenia: a randomized controlled trial. *JAMA* 290(20):2693-702

Rosenheck RA, Leslie D, Sindelar J, Miller EA, Lin H, Stroup S, McEvoy J, Davis S, Keefe RSE, Swartz M, Perkins D, Hsiao J, Lieberman JA (2006). Cost-effectiveness of second generation antipsychotics and perphenazine in a randomized trial of treatment for chronic schizophrenia. *Am J Psychiatry* 163(12): 2080–89

Index

A

Aalto, S., 104
Abercrombie, E. D., 182
Abi-Dargham, A., 100, 358
Abnormal stress responsivity in high-risk children, 183
Adams, B., 104
Adams, C. E., 406, 409, 411
Adams, E. K., 251
Adams, W., 151
Addington, J., 129, 253, 307, 311, 321
Adherence-related interventions, 411
Adhesio interthalamica (AI), 118–119
    absence of, 120
Adler, C. M., 100
α2A-Adrenoceptor (ADRA2A)-C1291G, 240
Adult-onset first-episode schizophrenia, longitudinal MRI studies on, 122–127
Aetiology and Ethnicity in Schizophrenia and Other Psychoses (ÆSOP) study, 5, 6, 7, 9, 81, 117
African-Caribbeans and Black-Africans schizophrenia and mania, rates for, 11
Agartz, I., 136
Age of onset distribution of schizophrenia, 359
Akbarian, S., 100, 103, 150, 156
Akil, M., 224
AKT1/GSK-3 signaling cascade, 225
Alexander, G. E., 225
Allardyce, J., 51–62, 70, 76, 83, 88–90
Allele-wise analysis, 238
Allen, D. N., 321
Allen, L. S., 120
Allen, N. C., 82
Alquicer, G., 361
Altar, C. A., 201
Altered hippocampal pyramidal cell alignment, 156–158

Alzheimer's disease pathology, 116
American Journal of Psychiatry, 273
Amminger, A., 303
Amminger, G. P., 5, 6, 7, 303
Amphetamine drug, 87, 180–182
    induced psychosis, 359–360
Andreasen, N. C., 99, 158
Andreoli, S. B., 429
Angermeyer, M. C., 433
Anglophone psychiatry, 309
Angrist, B., 175
Aniline, O., 104
Animal models, 153–154
Antagonism of dopamineric D_2 receptors, 105
Anterior cingulate cortex (ACC), 102–103
Antipsychotics, 236
    drugs, 99
    pharmacogenetics and, 237–240
        induced tardive dyskinesia, 240–241
    weight gain, 241–242
Anxiety-related processes, 289
Apelqvist, A., 195
Apolipoprotein E (APOE) ε4, 240
Appelbaum, P. S., 408
Apud, J. A., 224
Aradi, I, 100
Arango, C., 408, 409
Arion, D., 204, 207, 208, 209
Aripiprazole, 390
Arnsten, A., 100
Arnsten, A. F., 29, 100
Arolt, V., 235
Arranz, M. J., 41, 237, 239
Arseneault, L., 360, 369, 370
Asia
    Asian immigrants, schizophrenia study in, 75
    Asian women and schizophrenia incidence, 84

Ruaño, G., 242
Rubin, D. B., 348
Ruhrmann, G., 170, 301
Rüsch, N., 430
Ruscio, J, 334
Russell, V., 377–384
Rutten, B. P. F., 19–42
Rutter, M., 20, 21, 24, 29

S

Saha, S., 5, 70, 251, 252, 370, 371, 373, 424
Saijo, T., 135
Sallet, P. C., 130
Sampson, R. J., 83
Sams-Dodd, F., 153
São Paulo, psychoses study, 9–15
Sapolsky, R. M., 183
Sartorius, N., 3, 56, 429, 431
Schanda, H., 408
Schaufelberger, M. S., 113–138
Schizophrenia (SCZ), 3
    administrative rates, 77
    aetiological basis of, 70
    Afro-Caribbean patients, 31
    anatomical abnormalities in, 153
    cross-sectional architecture of, 319
    cytoarchitectural patterns in brains, 115
    developmental cascade toward, 362
    DTI studies of, 132
    genetic aspects of, 193
    genetic brain imaging in, 199–200
    incidence rates, 4
        cumulative distribution, 5
    incidence, variation in, 72
        age and sex, distribution by, 73, 359
        geographical, 77–78
        individual-level, 73–76
        temporal changes, 76–77
    intervention of, 300
    largest study of ToM in, 290
    lifetime prevalence, 70
    methodological difficulties associated with
        follow-up studies, 55–56
    migration and risk of, 11
        relative risk (RR) summary, 8–10
    neurogenesis-related genes and
        polymorphisms, 196–198
    neuropathological studies on, 114
    oligodendrocyte and myelin in pathogene-
        sis of, 157
    outcome of, 13
    postmortem SCZ brain tissue, gene and
        proteome expression, 204–206,
        208–209

SCZ-derived tags, 202
    undergraduate and school children,
        risk of, 348
    urbanization and neighbourhood, 11–12
Schley, C., 306
Schmidt-Kastner, R., 30
Schmitt, A., 149–158
Schooler, N. R., 339, 340
Schultz, L., 307
Schultz, W., 87, 178, 221
Schulze, K., 361
Scully, P. J., 78, 377–378, 381, 384
Secker, J. B., 307
Second-generation antipsychotics (SGA),
        389–390, 441–443
    in adverse effect, 394–395
    and FGAs efficacy, 392
    implications for clinical practice, 397–398
    in neuroleptic-refractory patients, 392–393
    treatment targets, 397–398
Seeman, P., 88, 100, 175, 210
Segal, D. S., 181, 207
Segal, P. N., 100
Segman, R. H., 241
Seidman, L. J., 154
Selection bias in immigrants, 74
Self-esteem, 289
Self-stigma, 435–436
Selten, J. P., 4, 5, 6, 7, 8, 28, 31, 33, 74, 82,
        88–90, 292, 361, 377
Semple, D. M., 255, 360
Serial analysis of gene expression (SAGE),
        201–202
Serotonin receptor 3B (HTR3B) promoter
        region, 238–239
Serotonin-transporter promoter region
        polymorphism (HTTLPR), 240
Serova, L. I., 182
Sertindole, 390
Shaikh, S., 239
Sham, P., 20, 31, 40, 41
Sham, P. C., 20, 31, 40, 41
Shanks, N., 182
Sharp, P. E., 177
Shenton, M. E., 117, 119, 150, 154, 176, 254
Shepherd, M., 56
Shevlin, M., 341
Shields, J., 31
Shi, L., 410
Shimizu, K., 195
Shively, C. A., 362
Shotgun peptide sequencing, 203
Signal transduction pathways, 101

Breinigsville, PA USA
19 February 2010
232802BV00004B/34/P